SHORT BOWEL SYNDROME

Practical Approach to Management

SHORT BOWEL SYNDROME

Practical Approach to Management

Edited by

John K. DiBaise
Mayo Clinic
Scottsdale, Arizona, USA

Carol Rees Parrish
University of Virginia Health System
Charlottesville, USA

Jon S. Thompson
University of Nebraska Medical Center
Omaha, USA

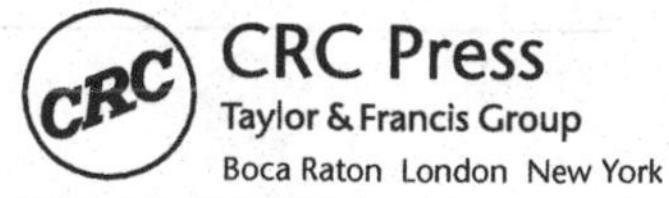

CRC Press
Taylor & Francis Group
Boca Raton London New York

CRC Press is an imprint of the
Taylor & Francis Group, an **informa** business

CRC Press
Taylor & Francis Group
6000 Broken Sound Parkway NW, Suite 300
Boca Raton, FL 33487-2742

First issued in paperback 2021

Version Date: 20160504

ISBN 13: 978-1-03-209785-5 (pbk)
ISBN 13: 978-1-4987-2078-6 (hbk)

Publisher's Note
The publisher has gone to great lengths to ensure the quality of this reprint but points out that some imperfections in the original copies may be apparent.

Library of Congress Cataloging-in-Publication Data

Names: DiBaise, John K., editor. | Parrish, Carol Rees., editor. | Thompson, Jon S., 1951- , editor.
Title: Short bowel syndrome : practical approach to management / [edited by] John K. DiBaise, Carol Rees Parrish, and Jon S. Thompson.
Description: Boca Raton : Taylor & Francis, 2016. | Includes bibliographical references and index.
Identifiers: LCCN 2015046178 | ISBN 9781498720786 (hardback : alk. paper)
Subjects: | MESH: Short Bowel Syndrome--therapy
Classification: LCC RC862.E52 | NLM WD 200.5.M2 | DDC 616.3/44--dc23
LC record available at http://lccn.loc.gov/2015046178

Visit the Taylor & Francis Web site at
http://www.taylorandfrancis.com

and the CRC Press Web site at
http://www.crcpress.com

Contents

Foreword

This is the first textbook that is exclusively about the issues experienced by patients with a short bowel. It covers all aspects of normal and abnormal physiology, the presenting features, and outcomes, including metabolic problems (acid-base and bone health), gallstones, and renal stones. It discusses both medical (diet and drugs) and surgical treatments, including intestinal transplantation. The use of growth factors, which is likely in the future to become increasingly important in promoting intestinal structural adaptation, is extensively discussed. Special emphasis is given to the psychosocial aspects of the quality of life of these patients, including support groups. Emphasis is rightly given to the importance of an experienced multidisciplinary team in caring for these patients.

Patients with a short bowel are regularly encountered in gastrointestinal medical and surgical practice. The length of small bowel remaining is not always known, so it may not be appreciated that a patient has problems associated with a shortened bowel. The presentation of patients with a short bowel depends upon the function of the remaining bowel (jejunum, ileum, and colon) and whether it is in continuity or not. Patients who have had several bowel resections, often for Crohn's disease, may present with diarrhea (steatorrhea) and weight loss. Patients with an ileostomy may present with dehydration and hypomagnesaemia due to high stomal losses and be labeled as having "ileostomy diarrhea." These two presentations may not be appreciated as problems of a short bowel, but, as this book describes, they are typical presenting features.

I have a long experience working and doing research in an intestinal failure unit and as a member of a hospital-based nutrition support team. In this book, I have found much new information and many original ideas about how to help these brave patients for whom I have much respect. This textbook is a must read not only by those with an interest in nutritional support but also by all those clinicians who see patients with gastroenterological problems.

Jeremy Nightingale, MD, FRCP
Co-chairman of the Intestinal Failure Unit
St Mark's Hospital
Harrow, UK

Preface

Short bowel syndrome is a rare and potentially overwhelming malabsorptive condition that threatens the quantity and quality of life of those affected. The management of patients with short bowel syndrome is complex and, despite its rarity, requires a wide range of healthcare providers to participate in the care of these patients. As such, there is a need to educate and inform healthcare providers about short bowel syndrome. Given recent advances in the management of short bowel syndrome, including the availability of pharmacologic agents to enhance intestinal absorption, refinements in parenteral nutrition, and surgical procedures designed to eliminate the need for parenteral nutrition support, we feel that now is a good time for such a book on the topic.

The goal of this international, multiauthor, interdisciplinary book is to bring the subject of short bowel syndrome to a wide audience. Physicians/surgeons, scientists, dietitians, nurses, pharmacists, patients, and their caregivers have all contributed to this book to provide a wide range of viewpoints on the state-of-the-art care of those with this condition. This book is not meant to be a comprehensive review of each chapter's topic; rather, an emphasis on a practical approach to diagnosis and treatment is provided. All issues related to the care of these patients, both in the hospital and community, are included. This book is intended not only for physicians and surgeons but also for nurses, ostomy/wound care nurses, nurse practitioners, physician assistants, dietitians, pharmacists, social workers, and other allied health professionals involved in the care of these complex patients.

We believe that this book will prove to be an invaluable resource to its readers and hope that it will improve the care of the patient with short bowel syndrome, advance knowledge in the field, and stimulate relevant research. We are grateful to the contributors of the book, all of whom have made significant contributions to the betterment of the lives of those affected by this condition.

John K. DiBaise, MD
Carol Rees Parrish, MS, RD
Jon S. Thompson, MD

Editors

John K. DiBaise, MD, is a professor of medicine and a consultant in the Division of Gastroenterology and Hepatology at the Mayo Clinic in Scottsdale, Arizona. Dr. DiBaise has published over 200 original articles, reviews, chapters, books, and editorials. In addition, he is an active clinical investigator and educator focusing on gastrointestinal motility and nutrition-related disorders. He is a Fellow of the American College of Gastroenterology and an active member of the American Gastroenterological Association, the American Society of Parenteral and Enteral Nutrition, and the American Society of Gastrointestinal Endoscopy. He is currently associate editor of the *American Journal of Gastroenterology* and recently completed serving as associate editor of *Nutrition in Clinical Practice*. He is on the editorial board of the *Journal of Parenteral and Enteral Nutrition*. He completed his gastroenterology and hepatology fellowship at the University of Nebraska Medical Center and his postgraduate training in internal medicine at the University of Iowa Hospitals and Clinics in Iowa City, Iowa. Dr. DiBaise received his medical degree from the University of Nebraska College of Medicine in Omaha, Nebraska, and his undergraduate degree from Northwestern University in Evanston, Illinois.

Carol Rees Parrish, MS, RD, has 35 years of clinical experience, the past 25 of which have been spent specializing in nutrition support and gastrointestinal disorders at the University of Virginia Health System, Digestive Health Center, Charlottesville, Virginia. Ms. Parrish founded the Medicine Nutrition Support Service in 1991, began the home nutrition support program at the University of Virginia Health System Home Health Company, developed the GI Nutrition Clinic, originated the University of Virginia Health System Celiac Support Group, and is the cofounder of the University of Virginia Health System Nutrition Support Traineeship, Weekend Warrior, and Webinar educational programs. She has been the nutrition series editor for the popular *Practical Gastroenterology Journal*'s Nutrition Series since 2003, having just published over 146 articles in the series.

She has also published 27 abstracts, 17 chapters, and 49 publications and given well over 200 presentations at local, state, regional, national, and international conferences.

Ms. Parrish's passion in gastrointestinal and nutrition support includes short gut/malabsorptive disorders, enteral and parenteral feeding modalities, small bowel bacterial overgrowth, pancreatitis, gastroparesis, refeeding syndrome, and many other gastrointestinal disorders.

Jon S. Thompson, MD, is Shackleford professor of surgery and chief of general surgery at the University of Nebraska Medical Center in Omaha, Nebraska. He received his medical degree and completed a residency in general surgery at the University of Colorado in Denver, Colorado. He received additional training in colorectal surgery at the Mayo Clinic. His clinical focus is on gastrointestinal surgery and especially surgical treatment of the short bowel syndrome. His research interests include short bowel syndrome and surgical nutrition. He is a founding member of the Intestinal Rehabilitation Program.

Contributors

Badr Al-Bawardy
Mayo Clinic
Rochester, Minnesota

James M. Badger
The Warren Albert Medical School of Brown University
and
Rhode Island Hospital
Providence, Rhode Island

Sue V. Beath
The Liver Unit including Small Bowel Transplantation
Birmingham Children's Hospital
W. Midlands, United Kingdom

Emilie Latour Beaudet
Beaujon Hospital
Assistance Publique—Hôpitaux de Paris
UFR de Médecine Paris Diderot
Clichy, France

Laura E. Beerman
Nebraska Medicine
Omaha, Nebraska

Christine T. Berke
Nebraska Medicine
Omaha, Nebraska

Lore Billiauws
Beaujon Hospital
Assistance Publique—Hôpitaux de Paris
UFR de Médecine Paris Diderot
Clichy, France

and

Centre de Recherche sur l'Inflammation Paris Montmartre
UFR de Médecine Paris Diderot
Paris, France

Joan Bishop
Oley Foundation
Albany Medical Center
New York, New York

Bethany E. Blalock
University of Virginia Health System
Digestive Health Center
Charlottesville, Virginia

Cathi Brown
Nebraska Medicine
Omaha, Nebraska

Sherilyn Gordon Burroughs
Sherrie and Alan Conover Center for Liver Disease and Transplantation
Houston Methodist Hospital
Houston, Texas

Lingtak-Neander Chan
University of Washington
Seattle, Washington

Matt Clark
University of Florida, Jacksonville
Jacksonville, Florida

Mandy L. Corrigan
Coram
St. Louis, Missouri

John K. DiBaise
Mayo Clinic
Scottsdale, Arizona

Douglas G. Farmer
Dumont-UCLA Transplant Center
David Geffen School of Medicine at UCLA
Los Angeles, California

Betsy Gallant
Cleveland Clinic
Cleveland, Ohio

Richard Gilroy
University of Kansas Medical Center
Kansas City, Kansas

Glenn Harvin
East Carolina University
Greenville, North Carolina

Ryan T. Hurt
Mayo Clinic
Rochester, Minnesota

Palle B. Jeppesen
Rigshospitalet
University Hospital of Copenhagen
Copenhagen, Denmark

Harlan Johnson
Oley Foundation
Albany Medical Center
New York, New York

Francisca Joly
Beaujon Hospital
Assistance Publique—Hôpitaux de Paris
UFR de Médecine Paris Diderot
Clichy, France

and

Centre de Recherche sur l'Inflammation Paris Montmartre
UFR de Médecine Paris Diderot
Paris, France

Darlene G. Kelly
Oley Foundation
Albany Medical Center
New York, New York

Deirdre A. Kelly
The Liver Unit including Small Bowel Transplantation
Birmingham Children's Hospital
W. Midlands, United Kingdom

Donald F. Kirby
Cleveland Clinic
Cleveland, Ohio

Denise Konrad
Cleveland Clinic
Cleveland, Ohio

Joe Krenitsky
University of Virginia Health System
Digestive Health Center
Charlottesville, Virginia

Berkeley N. Limketkai
Stanford University
Palo Alto, California

Lynn R. Mack
University of Nebraska Medical Center
Omaha, Nebraska

Laura Matarese
East Carolina University
Greenville, North Carolina

David F. Mercer
University of Nebraska Medical Center
Omaha, Nebraska

Jane Naberhuis
USDA/ARS Children's Nutrition Research Center
Baylor College of Medicine
Houston, Texas

Vandana Nehra
Mayo Clinic
Rochester, Minnesota

Jeremy Nightingale
St Mark's Hospital
Harrow, United Kingdom

Chaitanya Pant
Kansas University Medical Center
Kansas City, Kansas

Carol Rees Parrish
University of Virginia Health System
Digestive Health Center
Charlottesville, Virginia

Eamonn M.M. Quigley
Houston Methodist Hospital
Houston, Texas

John Rivas
Cleveland Clinic Florida
Weston, Florida

Fedja A. Rochling
University of Nebraska Medical Center
Omaha, Nebraska

Jim Ruse
Caregiver
Tustin, California

Lynn Ruse
SBS Patient
Tustin, California

James S. Scolapio
University of Florida, Jacksonville
Jacksonville, Florida

Kelly A. Tappenden
University of Illinois at Urbana-Champaign
Urbana, Illinois

Jon S. Thompson
University of Nebraska Medical Center
Omaha, Nebraska

Andrew Ukleja
Cleveland Clinic Florida
Weston, Florida

Jithinraj Edakkanambeth Varayil
Mayo Clinic
Rochester, Minnesota

Jordan Voss
University of Kansas School of Medicine
Kansas City, Kansas

Elizabeth A. Wall
The University of Chicago Medicine
Chicago, Illinois

Rebecca A. Weseman
University of Nebraska Medical Center
Omaha, Nebraska

Marion F. Winkler
The Warren Alpert Medical School of Brown University
and
Rhode Island Hospital
Providence, Rhode Island

1 Short Bowel Syndrome
Definition, Classification, Etiology, Epidemiology, Survival, and Costs

Palle B. Jeppesen

CONTENTS

KEY POINTS

- Patients with short bowel syndrome (SBS) and intestinal failure are heterogeneous regarding their postoperative convalescence, remnant bowel anatomy and function, and their need for parenteral support.
- The precise use of definitions and classifications for patients with SBS is a prerequisite for the optimal description, evaluation, and treatment of patients.
- The large differences in incidence and prevalence figures of SBS patients with intestinal failure among countries and regions illustrate that equity in its treatment may be restricted, even in areas where access to treatment for other organ failures is present.
- This discrimination by organ is not justifiable, since the costs and outcomes of treatment of SBS patients with intestinal failure with home parenteral nutrition resemble results seen in renal failure patients treated with dialysis.
- Due to the rarity and complexity of these heterogeneous patients, their management and care should ideally be provided by multidisciplinary centers of excellence within this field.

DEFINITION AND CLASSIFICATION

The primary function of the gastrointestinal (GI) tract is the adequate digestion and absorption of nutrients (macronutrients, fluid, electrolytes, trace elements, and vitamins) to meet the metabolic requirements of life, thereby preserving nutritional homeostasis, growth, body composition, function, and overall health. The intact, healthy GI tract possesses a large reserve capacity for nutrient assimilation (i.e., digestion and absorption). Indeed, in adults, the net absorption (i.e., dietary intake minus fecal excretion) of macronutrients exceeds 97%, and thc wet weight of fecal material remains below 300 g/day even after a substantial increase in oral intake.

Short bowel syndrome (SBS) refers to a condition characterized by malabsorption after intestinal resection [1–4]. In the event of malabsorption, SBS patients with mild so-called intestinal insufficiency easily compensate for this by increasing oral intake (hyperphagia) [5–7]. In SBS patients with more extensive intestinal resections and moderate malabsorption, the need for hyperphagia may be more substantial, and dietary advice, pharmacological interventions, and medical treatments may be needed to maintain nutritional homeostasis. In patients with severe intestinal insufficiency, supplemental enteral nutrition may be necessary [8–11]. In those patients where nutritional homeostasis is challenged by a small negative balance, homeorhetic regulatory mechanisms may allow the body to change from one homeostatic, stable condition to another without the loss of vital body functions, thereby preserving normal physiologic functions, growth, and health. It is believed that the resting energy expenditure may decrease in SBS patients who are unable to compensate orally for their energy malabsorption, similar to individuals exposed to semistarvation conditions [12]. Under conditions of fluid restriction, physiological compensatory mechanisms will ensue in an attempt to decrease body fluid and electrolyte losses. For instance, aldosterone will stimulate renal sodium reabsorption, sustaining blood volume and pressure in the face of fluid and sodium depletion [13].

In SBS patients, who experience even more severe disturbances in nutritional homeostasis, deficiencies are associated with an accommodation characterized by detrimental pathophysiological and, potentially, pathological changes in body function, clinical symptoms, and eventually disease. Depending on the presence of body stores, a subclinical deficiency state may exist for a prolonged period of time, before the body stores are depleted and biochemical deficiencies and clinical symptoms become overt. A subclinical deficiency state may also become overt in a situation where the metabolic requirements suddenly increase due to changes either in the environment or in the physical activity of the patient or as a result of a disease process. Thus, in these SBS patients with so-called intestinal failure, the absolute intestinal absorption is so limited that, in spite of optimal management and metabolic adaptation, parenteral support (PS) of fluids or nutrition (i.e., parenteral nutrition [PN]) is required to maintain nutritional homeostasis, body function, and health [1,2,10,14,15]. Thus, SBS is a spectrum ranging from relatively preserved intestinal function through various degrees of intestinal insufficiency (i.e., mild, moderate, and severe) to intestinal failure, as illustrated in Figure 1.1.

Absolute intestinal absorption may be impaired by intestinal resection, but a variety of other pathophysiological conditions may contribute to the development of intestinal failure. Examples include extensive mucosal disease caused by inflammatory bowel disease, radiation enteritis, celiac disease, or microvillus atrophy. Furthermore, absorptive surface area may be bypassed by the presence of intestinal fistula. In addition, intestinal obstruction or pseudo-obstruction could diminish the oral intake of the patient, thereby limiting his or her capacity for compensatory hyperphagia. Nutrient assimilation could also be diminished by impairment of digestion caused by disturbances in the production of bile acids [16] and digestive enzymes [17]. Likewise, small intestinal bacterial overgrowth could contribute to the malabsorptive disorder [18,19]. Thus, all of these potential

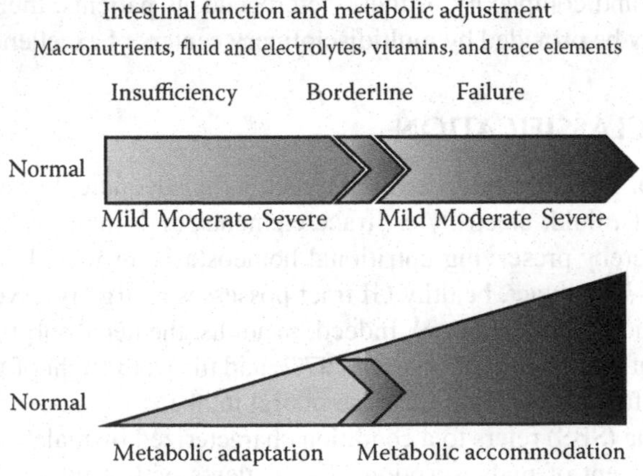

FIGURE 1.1 The SBS clinical spectrum ranging from normal through various degrees of intestinal insufficiency to various degrees of intestinal failure.

contributors to the clinical condition should be considered and addressed when evaluating and treating SBS patients with intestinal failure.

In an attempt to objectively demonstrate the spectrum of malassimilation, Jeppesen and Mortensen [10] measured the absolute intestinal absorption by performing metabolic balance studies in adult patients with intestinal insufficiency and failure. Duplicate portions of oral intakes and fecal excretions were quantified and absolute energy and wet weight absorption were determined. The results of these balance studies allowed the spectrum of intestinal insufficiency or failure to be determined, and objective discrimination between the two conditions was made possible (Figure 1.2a) [10]. These balance studies, however, also illustrated the heterogeneity of the patients within the spectrum. Functional intestinal failure was present in most patients when absolute wet weight absorption (diet wet weight minus fecal wet weight) was below 1.4 kg/day or when absolute energy absorption was below 5 MJ/day (~1200 kcal/day) (~84% of calculated basal metabolic rate). These wet weight and energy absorption values are minimally required for normal perspiration, renal function, and protein-energy metabolism in most SBS patients. Based on results from these and other balance studies, a urine volume above 800 mL/day with a sodium concentration above 20 mmol/L and a body mass index above 20 kg/m^2 is desired in adults with SBS [10,20,21].

The ability to compensate for malabsorption by hyperphagia varies considerably among SBS patients. In fact, some SBS patients with intestinal insufficiency are able to compensate by hyperphagia for a malabsorption of more than 75% by increasing their oral wet weight and energy intake to more than 7 kg/day and 22 MJ/day (5250 kcal/day), respectively. Others fail to compensate orally for their more moderate malabsorption and thus depend on PS (Figure 1.2b and c) [10].

Metabolic balance studies are more difficult to perform in infants and children than in adults. In a small study employing the same set-up for metabolic balance studies as described by Jeppesen and Mortensen [10], children who required PS absorbed less than 150% of their calculated basal metabolic rate and less than 50% of their calculated basal fluid requirements [22].

Only a few centers around the world routinely perform these metabolic balance studies as part of their clinical practices. As a result, other more subjective descriptive classifications of SBS have been suggested to harmonize the shared knowledge and understanding of this condition, an important objective to set a uniform template for comparing clinical data between centers with an interest in patients with intestinal failure [15]. This is a primary requisite for comparing outcome results. These SBS classifications are based on the postoperative convalescence condition of the patient, the remaining bowel anatomy, or the need of the patient for PS.

Regarding the postoperative convalescence of SBS patients, three types are described according to the recovery duration, the need for postsurgical handling (i.e., sepsis management, nutrition, anatomy mapping, and planning), and reversibility [23–25]. Type 1 SBS-intestinal failure patients are those who experience a short-term, self-limiting, perioperative, acute disturbance in intestinal function often related to motility disturbances such as paralytic ileus. These patients require PS for a limited period of time before making a full recovery without complications. Type 2 SBS-intestinal failure patients are those who experience a more severe postoperative condition where a prolonged, complex, multidisciplinary intervention and in-hospital specialized PS are required. Type 2 is often seen in the setting of an abdominal catastrophe such as mesenteric ischemia, volvulus, or trauma. Type 2 patients have considerable associated morbidity (e.g., wounds, bowel obstruction, anastomotic leak, and fistula) and a high mortality due to systemic sepsis and metabolic and/or nutritional complications. Once the perioperative complications have resolved, weaning from PS is eventually achieved in relation to the multidisciplinary efforts of intestinal rehabilitation. The spontaneous adaptation after surgery may be accelerated, and even a state of hyperadaptation may be achieved by the use of a modified diet, oral rehydration solution, conventional pharmacological therapy such as antimotility and antisecretory agents, and hormonal trophic factor therapy [26]. Type 3 SBS-intestinal failure is defined as a chronic, stable situation where home PN (HPN) is required for months/years or even lifelong in spite of intestinal rehabilitation efforts. Efforts should be made, even years after surgery, since a reduction in the daily PN volume and days off PN may improve the

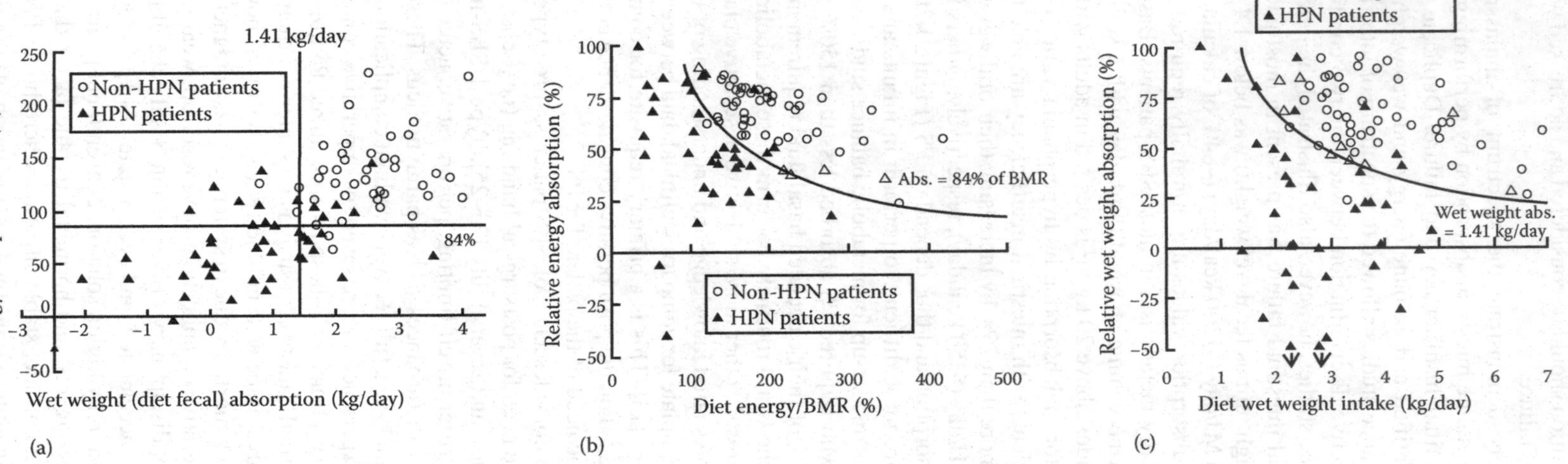

FIGURE 1.2 Differentiation between non-HPN (intestinal insufficiency) and HPN (intestinal failure patients) based on objective measurements of intestinal energy and wet weight absorption. (a) Presents the borderlines given by an energy absorption of 84% of calculated basic metabolic rate (BMR). (b and c) Demonstrate the large heterogeneity between patients regarding their ability to orally compensate for malabsorption. (From Jeppesen, P.B. et al., *Gut*, 46, 701–706, 2000. With permission.)

quality of life in intestinal failure patients [27]. Attempts at surgical rehabilitation [28] or intestinal transplantation [2,29,30] may be considered in such patients when continuing PN is deemed hazardous or impossible.

According to a technical review from the American Gastroenterological Association, SBS in adults can be defined as a condition where there is less than 200 cm of functional small intestine remaining [2]. As such, SBS patients may be classified according to their remnant bowel anatomy. Group 1 consists of patients with an end-jejunostomy, group 2 consists of those patients who have a jejuno-colonic anastomosis, and group 3 consists of those with a jejuno-ileo-colonic anastomosis. Employing conventional dietary and pharmacological therapies, the adult SBS patients at greatest risk for permanent dependence on PS/PN are those with an end-jejunostomy and less than 115 cm of small bowel, those with a jejuno-colonic anastomosis and less than 60 cm, and those with a jejuno-ileo-colonic anastomosis and less than 35 cm of residual small intestine [31,32]. In infants, consideration of the gestational age is imperative when reporting residual bowel length. To account for gestational age, it has been suggested that residual bowel should be presented as a percentage of original total bowel length or of that expected for a particular age [33]. The likelihood of gradually regaining intestinal autonomy by gaining adaptive effects on top on those achieved by the conventional dietary and pharmacological therapies seems to be best in patients with a preserved segment of the ileum and colon-in-continuity, whereas improvements in intestinal absorption over time are less likely in patients with end-jejunostomies [34,35]. This may relate to the findings that mucosal nerve ends and endocrine cells within the GI tract pass information via the enteric nervous system in response to the passing of luminal contents, thereby regulating the highly coordinated processes of nutrient assimilation. The neuroendocrine feedback mechanisms, often referred to as the "gastric, ileal, and colonic brakes," may be disrupted by distal intestinal resections or mucosal disease [36,37]. The attenuation of the meal-stimulated secretion of hormones in SBS patients with jejunostomies may result in some of the pathophysiological features of SBS: accelerated GI motility, gastric and intestinal hypersecretion, diminished intestinal blood flow, disturbed immunological and barrier functions, impaired mucosal replacement, repair, and adaptation [38]. Therefore, once patients are discharged from the hospital on HPN, the likelihood of regaining intestinal autonomy after 2 years of HPN is less than 10% in adults [32]. More recent data, however, suggest that HPN weaning may be as high as 26% 1 year after bowel resection and, rarely, can be reversed even 5 years after surgery [39]. In children, the ability to wean was highest in patients with preservation of >10% of their expected small bowel (83%) compared with those patients who had less (11%) [40]. Patient selection and differences in the number of SBS patients with a preserved colon may explain differences between study outcomes. The likelihood of weaning SBS patients from HPN probably relates to the location and proximity of the patients to the borderline between intestinal insufficiency and failure. Thus, SBS patients with the longest remnants of small intestine, the presence of a colon, and the lowest PS/PN volumes perhaps should be candidates for the most diligent intestinal rehabilitation efforts in an attempt to restore enteral autonomy.

Based on these considerations, characterization of adult intestinal failure patients according to their need for PS/PN has been suggested [4]. In postadaptive SBS patients in a steady-state condition, the degree of intestinal failure could be indirectly or reciprocally evaluated by calculation of the need for PS. A more simple and modified classification based on the requirements for PS of energy and volume was subsequently proposed by the European Society for Clinical Nutrition and Metabolism chronic intestinal failure working group [15]. In this classification, intestinal failure patients are grouped according to 16 subtypes in a simple 4 × 4 table categorized by the requirement for PS based on energy (0, 1–10, 11–20, and >20 kcal/kg/day; category A, B, C, and D, respectively) and volume (≤1000, 1001–2000, 2001–3000, and >3000 mL/day; category 1, 2, 3, and 4, respectively) needs. A summary of all these classification systems is given in Figure 1.3.

Having summarized these contemporary ideas regarding the terminologies that should be used in the field, it is obvious that a clear understanding and the precise use of these definitions and classifications within the spectrum of intestinal insufficiency and failure are prerequisites for the

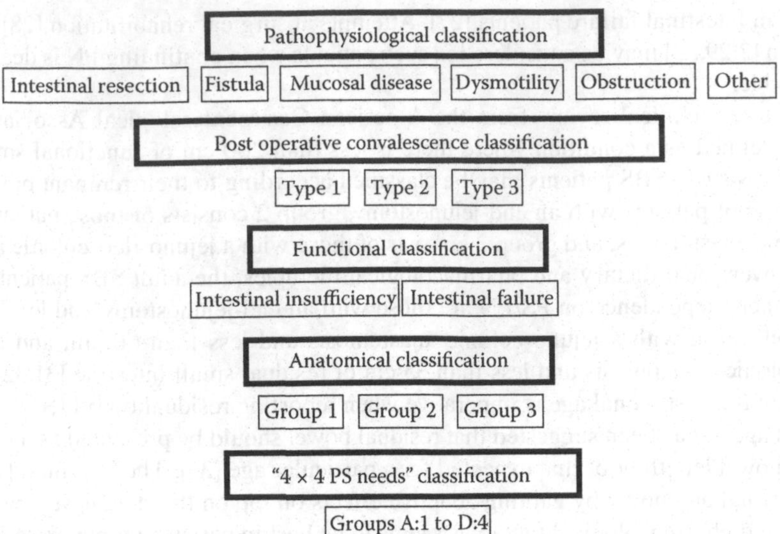

FIGURE 1.3 Suggested classification systems of SBS.

optimal description and evaluation of the SBS patient. This, in turn, is important for the optimal individualized and differentiated management of these highly complex, heterogeneous patients.

ETIOLOGY

The relative distribution among the etiologies of SBS patients in a cohort may depend on economic, cultural, historical, political, geographical, religious, medical, and educational factors within a country or region as well as individual interests and efforts of healthcare providers. In infants, SBS may result from congenital diseases (gastroschisis, intestinal atresia, intestinal malformation, and omphalocele) and midgut volvulus, but necrotizing enterocolitis is still considered the most common indication for surgery that leads to SBS and intestinal failure [41]. Approximately 80% of patients in the pediatric population develop SBS within the neonatal period [40]. Trauma, surgical complications, volvulus, intussusception, and mesenteric thrombosis are more common in older children [42].

In adults, SBS most frequently occurs as a consequence of intestinal resections in the setting of acute mesenteric vascular disease (arterial or venous thrombosis), Crohn's disease, trauma, and complications of other intraabdominal surgery (e.g., bariatric surgery). Less frequently, intestinal volvulus and intussusception are responsible for SBS in adults. With a more aggressive approach to the treatment of cancer in many countries, complications of cancer surgery or surgery due to radiation enteritis seem to be contributing to the increasing incidence and prevalence of SBS seen [15].

EPIDEMIOLOGY

Since the introduction of HPN for the treatment of SBS and intestinal failure in the early 1970s [43–45], the management of these patients has evolved dramatically in many parts of the world, especially in the United States [46], Canada [47], European countries [48,49], Australia [50], New Zealand [51], and Japan [52], whereas developments in lower-income countries such as several African countries, India, and China [53] have been more gradual. It has recently been estimated that the number of adult SBS patients who require chronic PS is approximately 10,000 to 15,000 in the United States. With an estimated population of approximately 320 million inhabitants, the point prevalence would be around 45 adult SBS patients/million [54]. The very low incidence and prevalence of SBS in some countries and regions [48] may be due to underreporting or to regional differences in the underlying causes, but it may also suggest that healthcare professionals in these areas lack the knowledge that a life without a bowel is indeed possible if PS is provided. Unfortunately, it may also indicate that many patients, when faced with SBS and intestinal failure, are not yet considered for PS or PN as long-term, life-saving therapy. Other reasons to decline or rationalize PS or PN may include inability to manage the care for these patients in the acute post-surgical setting; financial or logistical barriers may also be limiting factors.

The ability to safely provide PN in the homes of patients has improved their rehabilitation, thus providing better long-term survival and quality of life at a lower cost [55]. Initially, HPN was limited to the younger adults with benign causes of SBS, but the indication was soon expanded to include all age groups within a wider range of conditions (e.g., congenital disorders, dysmotility disorders, intestinal fistulas, mechanical obstruction, and extensive mucosal diseases) and even to elderly patients with malignant diseases. The reported incidence and prevalence seem to be higher in areas where the long-term management of SBS historically has been in multidisciplinary referral organizations with the knowledge, strategy, and facilities to alleviate the distress of these patients [56]. In some countries and regions, it is worrying to see low incidence and prevalence of SBS and poor access to home PS and PN, since the access is given for treatment of other organ failures such as the kidney, heart, liver, and lungs. When comparing SBS-intestinal failure patients with patients receiving renal replacement therapy (RRT; hemodialysis and peritoneal dialysis) due to chronic end-stage renal disease, this discrimination by organ cannot be justified based on financial or outcome data. SBS-intestinal failure patients do equally well or even better in these respects [57,58].

In Denmark (population: 5.6 million inhabitants), where treatments for organ failures are funded by a tax-financed healthcare system and a centralized referral system exist, 400 adult patients currently receive HPN due to chronic intestinal failure, and 250 of these patients have SBS. Thus, the point prevalence of intestinal failure in adults is around 70 patients/million inhabitants and 45 SBS-intestinal failure patients/million inhabitants. In comparison, as of December 31, 2012, the prevalence of adult patients on RRT in Denmark was approximately 800/million inhabitants (70% hemodialysis and 30% peritoneal dialysis) [59]. Thus, in an environment with free equity to organ failure treatment and a long tradition of RRT and intestinal failure treatment in a well-defined population, the ratio of patients receiving HPN to patients receiving RRT is approximately 10%. Since Denmark has one of the highest prevalences of intestinal failure patients in the world, it is likely that the ratio between intestinal failure and RRT may be somewhat lower in other countries; however, since the number of RRT patients is known in most countries, this ratio still may provide an estimate of the number of intestinal failure patients that would be anticipated to be present in the same country. The relative rarity of chronic type 3 intestinal failure patients compared with patients with chronic end-stage renal disease in the general population suggests that regional and national strategies should ideally facilitate the referral and centralization of these patients to dedicated "Centers of Excellence." In many countries, the treatment of intestinal failure patients is dispersed and decentralized, and as such, the patient volume at any one center is often insufficient to obtain and maintain the expertise of the organization that is required to be able to provide the optimal, individualized care required in this heterogeneous, complex patient population [60,61]. A sufficient patient volume and adequate resources should allow multidisciplinary centers to adapt the organization and requirements needed to provide proper quality of care and the best possible mental and physical rehabilitation of these unfortunate patients [62,63]. Three tertiary referral intestinal failure treatment centers exist in Denmark.

With the global increase in incidence and prevalence of intestinal failure patients due to the increased awareness of the life-saving option of HPN and the gradual expansion of the indications for PS/PN, an increasing comorbidity of the patients is anticipated. The increase in heterogeneity and complexity of this patient population will further add to the requirements of knowledge, education, and support for the successful, long-term, multidisciplinary management of these patients.

SURVIVAL

A comparison between survival rates in different case series and cohorts is significantly influenced by the relative differences in patient groups treated and reported on [64].

In general, intestinal failure in the pediatric population is associated with considerable morbidity and mortality, and in contrast to adults, much of this is attributable to the adverse effects of HPN, mainly central venous catheter-related sepsis and intestinal failure-associated liver disease. In a Canadian study including neonates with SBS, a mortality rate of 37% was found among 175 patients referred to a surgical regional referral center [65]. Mortality in these patients seemed to be bimodally distributed. The neonates who died shortly after surgery were typically those who had a small bowel resection of more than 75%. A second period for increased mortality was observed 8–12 months after the resection and was attributed to HPN-related sepsis and liver failure, before the survival plateaued at 63%. In 389 pediatric patients with intestinal failure referred to a highly specialized center in Pittsburgh, the survival rate at 5 years was 95% in the patients who were weaned from PN by 2.5 years after referral compared with 52% in those patients who were not weaned [66]. Improved care for infants on PN over the last years, however, seems to have led to a dramatic decrease in the number of patients referred for combined liver and intestinal transplantation [67].

In a cohort of 124 adult patients with nonmalignant SBS enrolled within a 13-year period from 1980 to 1992 in a referral center in Paris, the survival rates were 86% and 75% at 2 and 5 years, respectively [32]. The causes of death were related to PN in 7 of 40 cases; two patients died of septicemia and two died of liver failure. In a multivariate analysis, the presence of an end-enterostomy, a small bowel length <50 cm, and a diagnosis of arterial mesenteric infarction as the cause for SBS were negatively associated with survival. Almost identical findings were demonstrated in a more mixed cohort of 188 adult intestinal failure patients from a UK referral center. In these patients, survival rates of 86%, 77%, 73%, and 71% at 1, 3, 5, and 10 years, respectively, were found [68]. An increased probability of death with increasing age was observed; however, there was no association with the presence of a stoma. Much of the mortality in patients receiving adult HPN patients again resulted from the underlying disease; only two deaths were of HPN-related causes (9%). In patients with benign diseases such as Crohn's disease, the 10-year survival was above 85%.

In another French study of a mixed cohort of 268 adult SBS patients followed up over a 25-year period, the survival probability rates were 94%, 70%, and 52% at 1, 5, and 10 years, respectively [39]. Factors contributing to decreased survival rates were age >60 years, diagnosis of arterial mesenteric infarction, a history of cancer, and the presence of an end-ostomy; HPN-related complications accounted for only 13% of deaths. Similar finding have been reported in surveys from Denmark and the United States [49,56,69,70].

COSTS

HPN is the adaptation to the home setting of the in-hospital PN technique. Although life-saving and providing improved quality of life and a better social rehabilitation, the provision of HPN also incurs significant healthcare utilization and substantial cost [47,71]. The costs of HPN are, however, much lower compared with providing the service in the hospital [55,72]. Over a 12-year time frame, Detsky et al. [73] estimated that HPN resulted in a net savings in healthcare costs of $19,232 per patient and an increase in survival, adjusted for quality of life, of 3.3 years compared with the alternative of treating these patients in the hospital with intermittent nutritional support when needed. HPN resulted in incremental costs of $48,180 over 12 years, $14,600 per quality-adjusted life-year gained. The authors concluded that the cost-utility of HPN compared favorably with that of other healthcare programs when HPN was used to treat patients with intestinal failure secondary to conditions such as Crohn's disease or acute volvulus [73].

Huge differences exist regarding the organization, payment structure, and quality of healthcare service provided to SBS HPN patients between nations and even regions [74–78]. In some countries, a centralized referral system to centers of excellence exists, whereas in others, the care of SBS patients on HPN is decentralized. Combining this with the large heterogeneity of SBS patients regarding background diagnosis, remnant intestinal anatomy and function, the personalized nature for PS requirements, and a high variance in the likelihood of complications, an estimation of the mean cost of HPN is highly challenging [69].

Direct costs may be attributed to the establishment and implementation of an "intestinal failure unit" with its multidisciplinary involvement. As illustrated in Figure 1.4, a wide range of ancillary support staff is necessary in the ideal organization. Surgical and medical services as well as radiologists, microbiologists, anesthesiologists, pharmacists, dietitians, and nurses may be required for resolution of postoperative complications. The inclusion of a pain management team and wound and stoma care nurses is ideal. A bowel anatomy mapping team is essential to provide the best knowledge before considering reconstructive surgery. A service for the placing of long-term indwelling, central venous catheters is needed. A protocolized training program with standardized procedures for patients, family members, and/or external home care nurses to administer PN at home is required. Staffing for general care and rehabilitation, physiotherapy, and supportive mental care is ideal for these patients who suffer from a chronic, often lifelong, condition. A discharge liaison nurse may be required to ease the successful transition from the hospital to the home environment of the patient. A link to the outpatient clinic as well as to the general practitioner of the patient is important and needs to be established. In addition, this ideal organization would have the hospital network of complication specialists to interact with in case of readmissions due to intestinal failure- or PN-related complications. The quality of the provision of the healthcare should be ensured by the continuous review of well-defined, relevant outcome parameters, and research within the organization should focus on the development and implementation of better treatment strategies.

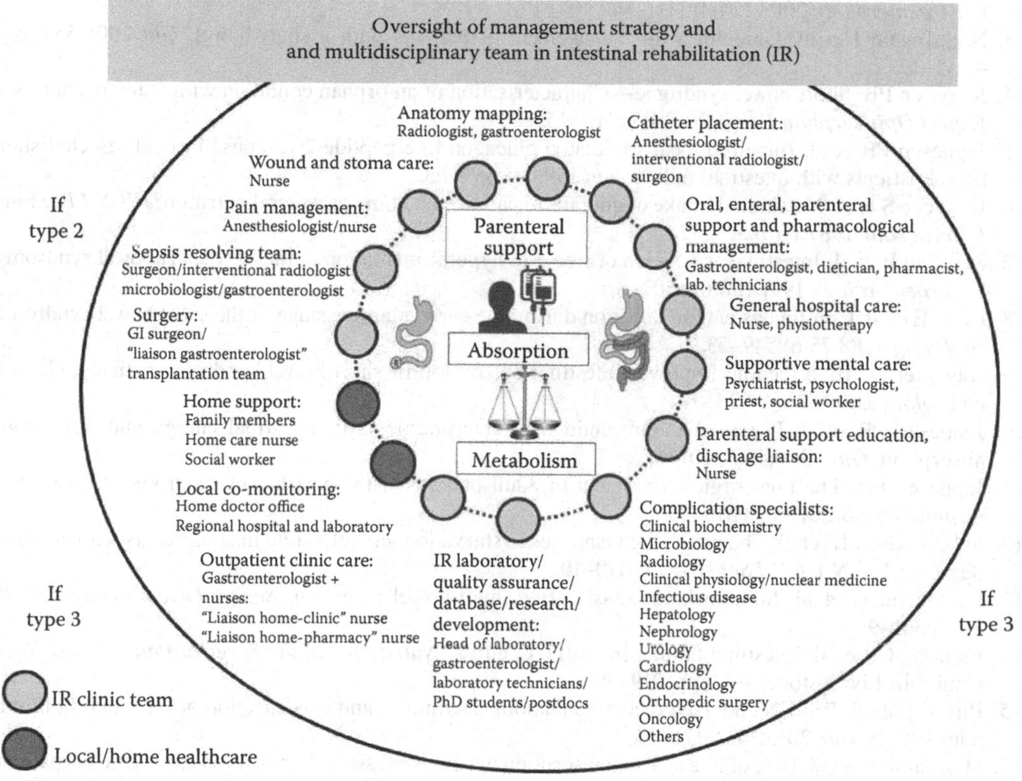

FIGURE 1.4 "Center of Excellence" management strategy and multidisciplinary involvement.

The running costs and profits of solutions and equipment vary, as do the home healthcare service, the outpatient follow-up (laboratory tests, etc.), and readmissions due to complications [73]. In some countries, the cost of PN solutions and infusion equipment has been estimated to be from US$75,000 to US$150,000 per year [79]. In other countries, these estimates are 5 to 10 times less. In some countries, the average costs for the in-hospital management of complications have been estimated to be US$10,000 to US$50,000 per patient per year, and in others, from US$0 to US$140,000 per year [71,80,81]. In comparison, in the United States, the total Medicare expenditures for patients with end-stage renal disease receiving hemodialysis have been estimated at approximately US$60,000 per year [82].

CONCLUSIONS

In conclusion, the treatment of SBS patients with HPN has proved not only its clinical value but also its cost superiority in comparison with in-hospital treatment. Furthermore, compared with hemodialysis, the cost-effectiveness is comparable; however, since SBS patients with intestinal failure and need for HPN are rare compared with patients receiving hemodialysis, the impact on the overall economic healthcare burden is at least 10 times less. Healthcare providers taking care of SBS patients with intestinal failure should ensure that their patients receive care that is comparable with the standards of treatments of other organ failure treatments within their respective regions and countries.

REFERENCES

1. O'Keefe SJ et al. Short bowel syndrome and intestinal failure: Consensus definitions and overview. *Clin Gastroenterol Hepatol* 2006;4(1):6–10.
2. Buchman AL et al. AGA technical review on short bowel syndrome and intestinal transplantation. *Gastroenterology* 2003;124(4):1111–34.
3. Nightingale J et al. Guidelines for management of patients with a short bowel. *Gut* 2006;55(Suppl 4):iv1–12.
4. Jeppesen PB. Short bowel syndrome—Characterisation of an orphan condition with many phenotypes. *Expert Opin Orphan Drugs* 2013;1(7):515–25.
5. Jeppesen PB et al. Impaired meal stimulated glucagon-like peptide 2 response in ileal resected short bowel patients with intestinal failure. *Gut* 1999;45:559–63.
6. DiCecco S et al. Nutritional intake of gut failure patients on home parenteral nutrition. *JPEN J Parenter Enteral Nutr* 1987;11(6):529–32.
7. Messing B et al. Intestinal absorption of free oral hyperalimentation in the very short bowel syndrome. *Gastroenterology* 1991;100(6):1502–8.
8. Levy E et al. Continuous enteral nutrition during the early adaptive stage of the short bowel syndrome. *Br J Surg* 1988;75(6):549–53.
9. Joly F et al. Tube feeding improves intestinal absorption in short bowel syndrome patients. *Gastroenterology* 2009;136(3):824–31.
10. Jeppesen PB et al. Intestinal failure defined by measurements of intestinal energy and wet weight absorption. *Gut* 2000;46(5):701–6.
11. Jeppesen PB. The non-surgical treatment of adult patients with short bowel syndrome. *Expert Opin Orphan Drugs* 2013;1(7):515–25.
12. Schebendach JE et al. The metabolic responses to starvation and refeeding in adolescents with anorexia nervosa. *Ann N Y Acad Sci* 1997;817:110–19.
13. Ladefoged K et al. Sodium homeostasis after small-bowel resection. *Scand J Gastroenterol* 1985; 20(3):361–9.
14. Fleming CR et al. Intestinal failure. In: Hill GL, editor. *Nutrition and the Surgical Patient.* New York: Churchill Livingstone; 1981, pp. 219–35.
15. Pironi L et al. ESPEN endorsed recommendations. Definition and classification of intestinal failure in adults. *Clin Nutr* 2015;34(2):171–80.
16. Hofmann AF et al. Role of bile acid malabsorption in pathogenesis of diarrhea and steatorrhea in patients with ileal resection. I. Response to cholestyramine or replacement of dietary long chain triglyceride by medium chain triglyceride. *Gastroenterology* 1972;62(5):918–34.

17. Malagelada JR et al. Regulation of pancreatic and gallbladder functions by intraluminal fatty acids and bile acids in man. *J Clin Invest* 1976;58(2):493–9.
18. Cole CR et al. Small bowel bacterial overgrowth: A negative factor in gut adaptation in pediatric SBS. *Curr Gastroenterol Rep* 2007;9(6):456–62.
19. Ziegler TR et al. Small bowel bacterial overgrowth in adults: A potential contributor to intestinal failure. *Curr Gastroenterol Rep* 2007;9(6):463–7.
20. Hill GL et al. Long term changes in total body water, total exchangeable sodium and total body potassium before and after ileostomy. *Br J Surg* 1975;62(7):524–7.
21. Ng DH et al. The 'not so short-bowel syndrome': Potential health problems in patients with an ileostomy. *Colorectal Dis* 2013;15(9):1154–61.
22. Aunsholt L et al. Bovine colostrum to children with short bowel syndrome: A randomized, double-blind, crossover pilot study. *JPEN J Parenter Enteral Nutr* 2014;38(1):99–106.
23. Shaffer J. Definition and service development. *Clin Nutr* 2002;21(Suppl 1):144–5.
24. Lal S et al. Review article: Intestinal failure. *Aliment Pharmacol Ther* 2006;24(1):19–31.
25. Gardiner KR. Management of acute intestinal failure. *Proc Nutr Soc* 2011;70(3):321–8.
26. Jeppesen PB. Growth factors in short-bowel syndrome patients. *Gastroenterol Clin North Am* 2007;36(1):109–21.
27. Jeppesen PB et al. Quality of life in patients with short bowel syndrome treated with the new glucagon-like peptide-2 analogue teduglutide—Analyses from a randomised, placebo-controlled study. *Clin Nutr* 2013;32(5):713–21.
28. Rege AS et al. Autologous gastrointestinal reconstruction: Review of the optimal nontransplant surgical options for adults and children with short bowel syndrome. *Nutr Clin Pract* 2013;28(1):65–74.
29. Kaufman SS et al. Indications for pediatric intestinal transplantation: A position paper of the American Society of Transplantation. *Pediatr Transplant* 2001;5(2):80–7.
30. Sudan D. The current state of intestine transplantation: Indications, techniques, outcomes and challenges. *Am J Transplant* 2014;14(9):1976–84.
31. Carbonnel F et al. The role of anatomic factors in nutritional autonomy after extensive small bowel resection. *JPEN J Parenter Enteral Nutr* 1996;20(4):275–80.
32. Messing B et al. Long-term survival and parenteral nutrition dependence in adult patients with the short bowel syndrome. *Gastroenterology* 1999;117(5):1043–50.
33. Wales PW et al. Short bowel syndrome: Epidemiology and etiology. *Semin Pediatr Surg* 2010;19(1):3–9.
34. Nightingale JM et al. The short bowel syndrome: What's new and old? *Dig Dis* 1993;11(1):12–31.
35. Hill GL et al. Impairment of 'ileostomy adaptation' in patients after ileal resection. *Gut* 1974;15(12):982–7.
36. Spiller RC et al. The ileal brake—Inhibition of jejunal motility after ileal fat perfusion in man. *Gut* 1984;25(4):365–74.
37. Nightingale JM et al. Disturbed gastric emptying in the short bowel syndrome. Evidence for a 'colonic brake'. *Gut* 1993;34(9):1171–6.
38. Jeppesen PB et al. Impaired meal stimulated glucagon-like peptide 2 response in ileal resected short bowel patients with intestinal failure. *Gut* 1999;45(4):559–63.
39. Amiot A et al. Determinants of home parenteral nutrition dependence and survival of 268 patients with non-malignant short bowel syndrome. *Clin Nutr* 2013;32(3):368–74.
40. Spencer AU et al. Pediatric short bowel syndrome: Redefining predictors of success. *Ann Surg* 2005;242(3):403–9.
41. Squires RH et al. Natural history of pediatric intestinal failure: Initial report from the Pediatric Intestinal Failure Consortium. *J Pediatr* 2012;161(4):723–8.
42. Sigalet DL. Short bowel syndrome in infants and children: An overview. *Semin Pediatr Surg* 2001;10(2):49–55.
43. Shils ME et al. Long-term parenteral nutrition through an external arteriovenous shunt. *N Engl J Med* 1970;283(7):341–4.
44. Jeejeebhoy KN et al. Home parenteral nutrition. *Can Med Assoc J* 1980;122(2):143–4.
45. Jarnum S et al. Long-term parenteral nutrition. I. Clinical experience in 70 patients from 1967 to 1980. *Scand J Gastroenterol* 1981;16(7):903–11.
46. Howard L. A global perspective of home parenteral and enteral nutrition. *Nutrition* 2000;16(7–8):625–8.
47. Raman M et al. Canadian home total parenteral nutrition registry: Preliminary data on the patient population. *Can J Gastroenterol* 2007;21(10):643–8.
48. Van Gossum A et al. Home parenteral nutrition in adults: A multicentre survey in Europe in 1993. *Clin Nutr* 1996;15(2):53–9.

49. Ugur A et al. Home parenteral nutrition in Denmark in the period from 1996 to 2001. *Scand J Gastroenterol* 2006;41(4):401–7.
50. Gillanders L et al. AuSPEN clinical practice guideline for home parenteral nutrition patients in Australia and New Zealand. *Nutrition* 2008;24(10):998–1012.
51. Gillanders L et al. Benchmarking home parenteral nutrition in Scotland and New Zealand: Disparities revealed. *N Z Med J* 2008;121(1284):28–33.
52. Takagi Y et al. Report on the first annual survey of home parenteral nutrition in Japan. *Surg Today* 1995;25(3):193–201.
53. Zhu W et al. Rehabilitation therapy for short bowel syndrome. *Chin Med J (Engl)* 2002;115(5):776–8.
54. NPS Pharmaceuticals. http://www.fda.gov/downloads/AdvisoryCommittees/CommitteesMeetingMaterials /Drugs/GastrointestinalDrugsAdvisoryCommittee/UCM323506.pdf.
55. Richards DM et al. Cost-utility analysis of home parenteral nutrition. *Br J Surg* 1996;83(9):1226–9.
56. Jeppesen PB et al. Adult patients receiving home parenteral nutrition in Denmark from 1991 to 1996: Who will benefit from intestinal transplantation? *Scand J Gastroenterol* 1998;33(8):839–46.
57. Jeppesen PB et al. Quality of life in patients receiving home parenteral nutrition. *Gut* 1999;44(6):844–52.
58. Laupacis A et al. A study of the quality of life and cost-utility of renal transplantation. *Kidney Int* 1996;50(1):235–42.
59. Noordzij M et al. Renal replacement therapy in Europe: A summary of the 2011 ERA-EDTA Registry Annual Report. *Clin Kidney J* 2014;7(2):227–38.
60. Messing B et al. Prognosis of patients with nonmalignant chronic intestinal failure receiving long-term home parenteral nutrition [see comments]. *Gastroenterology* 1995;108(4):1005–10.
61. Pironi L et al. Candidates for intestinal transplantation: A multicenter survey in Europe. *Am J Gastroenterol* 2006;101(7):1633–43.
62. Matarese LE et al. Short bowel syndrome in adults: The need for an interdisciplinary approach and coordinated care. *JPEN J Parenter Enteral Nutr* 2014;38(1 Suppl):60S–4S.
63. Smith CE et al. Home parenteral nutrition: Does affiliation with a national support and educational organization improve patient outcomes? *JPEN J Parenter Enteral Nutr* 2002;26(3):159–63.
64. Pironi L et al. Outcome on home parenteral nutrition for benign intestinal failure: A review of the literature and benchmarking with the European prospective survey of ESPEN. *Clin Nutr* 2012;31(6):831–45.
65. Wales PW et al. Neonatal short bowel syndrome: Population-based estimates of incidence and mortality rates. *J Pediatr Surg* 2004;39(5):690–5.
66. Nucci A et al. Interdisciplinary management of pediatric intestinal failure: A 10-year review of rehabilitation and transplantation. *J Gastrointest Surg* 2008;12(3):429–35.
67. Khan KM et al. Developing trends in the intestinal transplant waitlist. *Am J Transplant* 2014;14(12):2830–7.
68. Lloyd DA et al. Survival and dependence on home parenteral nutrition: Experience over a 25-year period in a UK referral centre. *Aliment Pharmacol Ther* 2006;24(8):1231–40.
69. Howard L. Home parenteral nutrition: Survival, cost, and quality of life. *Gastroenterology* 2006;130(2 Suppl 1):S52–9.
70. Scolapio JS et al. Survival of home parenteral nutrition-treated patients: 20 years of experience at the Mayo Clinic. *Mayo Clin Proc* 1999;74(3):217–22.
71. Reddy P et al. Cost and outcome analysis of home parenteral and enteral nutrition. *JPEN J Parenter Enteral Nutr* 1998;22(5):302–10.
72. Marshall JK et al. Economic analysis of home vs hospital-based parenteral nutrition in Ontario, Canada. *JPEN J Parenter Enteral Nutr* 2005;29(4):266–9.
73. Detsky AS et al. A cost-utility analysis of the home parenteral nutrition program at Toronto General Hospital: 1970–1982. *JPEN J Parenter Enteral Nutr* 1986;10(1):49–57.
74. Schalamon J et al. Mortality and economics in short bowel syndrome. *Best Pract Res Clin Gastroenterol* 2003;17(6):931–42.
75. Tu Duy Khiem-El Aatmani A et al. Home parenteral nutrition: A direct costs study in the approved centres of Montpellier and Strasbourg. *Gastroenterol Clin Biol* 2006;30(4):574–9.
76. Piamjariyakul U et al. Complex home care: Part I—Utilization and costs to families for health care services each year. *Nurs Econ* 2010;28(4):255–63.
77. Smith CE et al. Complex home care: Part III—Economic impact on family caregiver quality of life and patients' clinical outcomes. *Nurs Econ* 2010;28(6):393–414.
78. Piamjariyakul U et al. Complex home care: Part 2—Family annual income, insurance premium, and out-of-pocket expenses. *Nurs Econ* 2010;28(5):323–9.
79. Sudan D. Cost and quality of life after intestinal transplantation. *Gastroenterology* 2006;130(2 Suppl 1):S158–62.

80. Wateska LP et al. Cost of a home parenteral nutrition program. *JAMA* 1980;244(20):2303–4.
81. Brakebill JI et al. Pharmacy department costs and patient charges associated with a home parenteral nutrition program. *Am J Hosp Pharm* 1983;40(2):260–3.
82. Just PM et al. Reimbursement and economic factors influencing dialysis modality choice around the world. *Nephrol Dial Transplant* 2008;23(7):2365–73.

2 Psychological, Social, and Quality of Life Considerations in Short Bowel Syndrome

James M. Badger and Marion F. Winkler

CONTENTS

KEY POINTS

- Short bowel syndrome (SBS) is a complex disorder that often has associated psychological and social factors that may contribute to a patient's experience of symptoms.
- SBS impacts these patients' independence, performance status, socialization, and interpersonal relationships, including sexuality; poses an economic burden; and requires adapting to the need for medical equipment and healthcare personnel for assistance.
- SBS patients are generally very knowledgeable about their condition and should be included in any discussion regarding treatment changes.
- Psychiatric management is most effective when there is a collaborative relationship between mental health clinicians and the clinicians primarily responsible for the patient's medical care.
- The goals of treatment are directed toward mitigating symptoms, reducing medical hospitalizations and unnecessary diagnostic tests, and fostering self-management. Therapeutic options should be individualized and based in the context of providing comprehensive care.
- Assessing quality of life is important to identify the range of problems that affect those who are receiving home parenteral nutrition (PN).

- Peer support and empathy can be an important strategy to foster coping skills and increase knowledge and confidence for individuals with SBS and home PN dependency.
- Understanding the need to maintain normalcy in life can help healthcare professionals facilitate an SBS patient's adaptation to home PN by offering strategies and interventions to address problems as they occur while promoting hope and optimism for the future.

INTRODUCTION

Short bowel syndrome (SBS) is a complex disorder that often has associated psychological and social factors that may contribute to a patient's experience of symptoms. There is a paucity of information available about how to best address the psychological distress that most individuals with SBS experience. Although a variety of psychological treatments are often recommended, their effectiveness is unclear and untested in SBS. Research in this area that can be extrapolated to the SBS population has focused predominantly on chronic gastrointestinal (GI) conditions associated with SBS (e.g., inflammatory bowel disease), individuals with ostomies, and patients requiring home parenteral nutrition (HPN). In this chapter, we explore the physical, emotional, technological, and financial burdens affecting patients with SBS; review coping and treatment strategies; and discuss peer support to assist clinicians caring for these complex patients.

Medical illness and psychiatric comorbidities often coexist in SBS. Some patients may have underlying psychiatric conditions, substance abuse/dependence, or a history of childhood abuse and later develop an acute or chronic medical condition that leads to SBS. For others, the result of an acute or chronic medical event resulting in SBS and the subsequent treatments may lead to the development of substance abuse/dependence and/or psychiatric disorders. Patients with SBS commonly struggle with a myriad of symptoms, including recurrent diarrhea, steatorrhea, malabsorption, malnutrition, chronic pain, or alterations in fluid and electrolyte balance. They also experience a need for more frequent visits to healthcare providers and recurrent hospitalizations, and some must adapt to life with an ostomy and central venous (and sometimes enteral) catheter for administration of nutrition support and the need to alter their lifestyle to accommodate technology dependence. SBS impacts these patients' independence, performance status, socialization, and interpersonal relationships, including sexuality; poses an economic burden; and requires adapting to the need for medical equipment and healthcare personnel for assistance.

BRAIN–GUT AXIS

Wilhelmsen [1] suggests that psychosocial factors play a role in how GI disorders are experienced and interpreted. The idea that there is a connection between the brain and the GI system has existed for over a century [2]. Early researchers investigated the impact of stress and emotions on GI function. More recently, emphasis has focused on exploring signaling from visceral afferent neurons to the brain. Emerging data suggest that bidirectional signaling occurs between the brain and the GI system [3,4].

An individual's response to stress or emotional reaction can impact GI function. How patients attribute the cause of their symptoms may influence both self-management and seeking of medical care. Intentional self-monitoring of symptoms combined with heightened awareness of bodily sensations (somatic awareness) creates a feedback loop that can self-perpetuate anxiety. Lackner et al. [5] report that many patients with functional GI symptoms experience a unique type of anxiety related to fear that these symptoms may signal imminent threat of adverse consequences. Somatic vigilance may heighten the intensity or frequency of symptoms and potentially create avoidance of activities or situations where GI symptoms could occur. Additionally, altered gut motility and enteric nervous system (ENS) response may also play a role in SBS. Efferent and afferent nerves connect the enteric and central nervous systems. The brain has the capacity via neural connections to affect GI sensation, motility, secretion, and inflammation. Conversely, viscerotropic effects via visceral afferent signaling reciprocally can affect central pain perception, mood, and behavior [4]. The current thinking is that the gut is affected by an interaction between serotonin and cholinergic neurotransmitters via the ENS [6,7]. Grundmann et al. [8] support the notion that serotonin and cholinergic neurotransmitters affect both intestinal motility and mood regulation.

PHYSICAL BURDEN

The physical burden of living with SBS revolves around maintaining homeostasis through adequate fluid, electrolyte, and nutritional balance. Many patients develop metabolic bone disease resulting in chronic weakness and bone and muscle pain. Malabsorption of other micronutrients may result in a variety of systemic symptoms, including gait disturbances, muscle weakness, and visual and mental status changes. Severe fatigue related to malnutrition, chronic anemia, or changes in fluid balance may impact functional ability. Ostomy patients struggle often with peristomal skin irritation, pouch leakage, offensive odor, and embarrassment from appliance noise [9].

EMOTIONAL BURDEN

The multiple symptoms present in the patient with SBS and the need for HPN present multiple emotional challenges. Most HPN patients have altered oral intake of both food and liquids. Stern et al. [10] point out that a large portion of human socialization revolves around the process of eating or drinking and that not participating in such routine activities can result in social isolation. Although HPN satisfies a person's fluid and nutrient requirements, this therapy does not replace the taste, sensation, enjoyment, or socialization that one experiences from food and mealtimes. Family members also report mixed emotions and feelings of guilt at mealtimes when they are in the presence of a person who requires HPN [11,12].

Similar to losing a limb, the loss of intestine may require a period of mourning or grief before acceptance [10]. Clinicians should explain that relearning to eat in the setting of altered bowel function might be difficult, requiring patience and determination. It is important to empower individuals to take responsibility for seeking, finding, and trying foods they can tolerate. Additionally, SBS patients may also need to develop a new way of eating. Pharmacologic and dietary strategies to help manage disabling diarrhea or high stoma output are necessary to improve quality of life (QOL) along with the ability to participate in daily activities.

TECHNOLOGY BURDEN

Patients requiring HPN pose many challenges related to the need for strict hygiene, alteration of eating patterns, and functional limitations associated with being tethered to an infusion pump [10]. Carlsson et al. [13] reported that not only did SBS patients have poor QOL, but also those patients having SBS and HPN dependence fared worse, with the lowest ratings on QOL scales. Most patients experience sleep disturbance due to alarm noise from pumps or equipment, frequent urination, and concern about accidental catheter dislodgement [14]. Silver [11] reports that the combination of recurrent diarrhea, food intolerance, and HPN dependence commonly restricts travel and participation in leisure-time activities. Although the availability of portable infusion pumps that can be carried in a backpack has allowed increased freedom of movement, the weight of the backpacks, combined with the effects of metabolic bone disease when present, may result in back pain or injury.

Both patients and families must adapt to the time-consuming nature of HPN. Infusions typically last 12 to 24 hours and often occur overnight. Individuals frequently plan their daily activities around their infusion schedule, home care nursing visits, and medical appointments, leaving little time for enjoyable activities or socialization. Any strategy to shorten the parenteral nutrition (PN) administration time is considered important for good QOL [15].

FINANCIAL BURDEN

Individuals who require HPN experience substantial economic burden. Part of this economic distress relates to the cost of medical expenses, fear of losing insurance coverage, and shrinking capitation for catastrophic health care. Gaskamp [16] specifically reported increased depression and decreased QOL related to declining HPN insurance benefits. Lower family QOL also correlates with financial distress as measured by inability to pay monthly bills [17]. Additional psychosocial stress may result from the paradox of being able to work due to improved physical function and nutritional recovery because of the PN, yet being unable to work because of the need for disability insurance to cover PN-related expenses.

COPING STRATEGIES

Individuals with chronic GI disorders use a variety of coping techniques to assuage the signs and symptoms of their disease, to increase daily functioning and to improve QOL [18]. Patients often become experts in coping with their condition and figuring out how to best manage their symptoms. They are generally very knowledgeable about their condition and should be included in any discussion regarding treatment changes. Most patients acquire knowledge and skills about medical management through living with their condition. Psychological adaptation generally occurs gradually.

Stern et al. [10] caution that not all patients are "psychologically robust," and some may demonstrate maladaptive coping behavior. In the setting of SBS requiring HPN, they warn that central venous catheters meant to keep patients alive and provide nourishment could also become the focus of neglect, self-harm, or abuse. For instance, some patients may use catheter access as a portal for injecting substances with or without the intent to cause self-harm. Patients with known or suspected illicit drug abuse history will require careful monitoring.

Some patients have difficulty differentiating between their emotions and physical symptoms. Thus, they tend to describe all difficulties in terms of somatic language, which involves a preoccupation on physical symptoms. These individuals are extremely sensitive to bodily cues and have a low threshold to seek out medical attention for symptoms. Healthcare professionals often struggle to sort out acute from chronic symptoms, symptoms that do not make physiological sense, and those that are in excess of what would be expected based on physical exam. Making the situation even more difficult, somatizing patients commonly deny any emotional component to their physical problems.

The traditional medical approach to symptom investigation only serves to exacerbate the problem when no clear organic etiology for symptoms is identified and no specific treatment can be recommended. The patient often feels misunderstood and the healthcare provider feels helpless to make the situation better. Family members may express their own frustration about the healthcare provider's inability to figure out what is wrong with their loved one.

TREATMENT STRATEGIES

There are several different psychotherapies and medication treatments that may be helpful for patients with SBS. Rollman et al. [19] found that patients with both a chronic medical condition and a mood or other psychiatric disorder report more symptoms and experience poorer treatment outcomes than do those without psychiatric conditions. Somatizing patients are best viewed as representing a mixture of physical, emotional, and interactional processes [20]. Psychosocial distress is often expressed in terms of physical complaints. Healthcare providers struggle to be vigilant to the possibility of a symptom signaling a new medical diagnosis and balancing that concern with avoiding unnecessary medical testing for an emotionally based problem. Therefore, psychiatric management is most effective when there is a collaborative relationship between mental health clinicians and the clinicians primarily responsible for the patient's medical care. The goals of treatment are directed toward mitigating symptoms, reducing medical hospitalizations and unnecessary diagnostic tests, and fostering self-management. Therapeutic options should be individualized and based in the context of providing comprehensive care.

Education

Patients may experience the need for ongoing education about their clinical status due to alterations in mental status, medication effects, anxiety, or secondary to selective hearing. Perhaps one way to approach patients during follow-up appointments would be to review what has been done surgically, where they are clinically in their course of recovery, and expectations of what they may experience in the future. Efforts should be made to not focus solely on bowel function during these discussions. Instead, expand queries to include current social environment, available support, general functioning, and mood and ask specifically about any other concerns.

Provide honest responses to questions regarding recovery, prognosis, and potential treatment complications. Reinforce that the goal for patients with HPN-dependent SBS when possible is to eventually resume enteral autonomy and reduce or discontinue PN. Highlight the fact that intestinal adaptation occurs in the first one or more years after massive bowel resections and may increase GI absorptive capacity and, therefore, may help some individuals with the process of transitioning off of PN and onto oral feeding. Acknowledge that for many SBS patients with differing bowel lengths and bowel anatomies, the road to recovery and freedom from PN is less predictable, requiring adherence to treatment recommendations and close medical monitoring and communication. Offering reassurance, scheduling regular medical follow-up opportunities, and discussing symptom parameters that would warrant contact provides patients with a framework for dealing with future medical uncertainties.

Self-Management

Self-management is defined as a process in which individuals actively manage a chronic illness [21]. This includes management of both physical and emotional challenges. Physical care often involves maintaining hydration and nutrition status as well as intravenous access and ostomy care when present. Emotional self-management involves how one psychologically adapts to expected and unexpected life events. It is generally accepted that individuals who are problem focused, as compared with those who are more emotionally focused, tend to cope better with adversity.

Four personal characteristics associated with improved coping ability include hardiness, locus of control, learned resourcefulness, and optimism [22]. Resilient or hardy people take action, believe that life experiences are controllable, and view problems as a challenge to be solved. Locus of control refers to an individual's perception about control of life events. Internal locus of control means that an individual believes that he or she can control external events through his or her behavior or action. Conversely, individuals with external locus of control believe that outcomes of life events are determined by factors outside their control. Learned resourcefulness refers to an individual's degree of self-confidence and ability to problem solve, reach out to others, and self-regulate emotional responses when dealing with highly stressful situations. Lastly, optimism plays a role in how an individual will respond to life's uncertainty or adversity. Those individuals demonstrating high optimism view the cup as half full. They tend to have a general expectation that good will happen. When confronted with adversity, they view the situation as a temporary "bump in the road" or setback, resulting in renewed efforts to overcome the problem. Success enhances self-confidence and reinforces that good things will indeed happen. Alternately, pessimists view any deviation toward their goal as representing defeat, and this reinforces the notion that more bad things are likely to happen. These events in turn become self-fulfilling prophecies.

Winkler et al. [15] proposed that living with HPN dependency is a continually shifting process in which individuals seek to achieve normalcy in life by creating a balance between self-identity and the identity shaped by the need for PN, the underlying disease, and life events. On the basis of an adaptation of the Shifting Perspectives Model of Chronic Illness [23], individuals who view their illness, underlying medical condition, or PN dependency as a dominant focus in life and as a significant burden shift more toward the "illness in the foreground" perspective and more frequently describe HPN as burdensome, their infusion schedule as confining, lack of energy and physical weakness, self-pity, and social isolation (Figure 2.1). Conversely, HPN-dependent adults who praise the beneficial aspects of HPN and downplay the inconvenience, alter their infusion schedules, describe feeling strong and good stamina, have a positive attitude, and report more enjoyable social interactions shift the focus of HPN more toward the "wellness in the foreground" perspective. These individuals are able to go about their lives in a "normal" way and place HPN in the background.

Thus, patients need to be encouraged to do their best in controlling symptoms and learning ways to maintain their independence. Setting small achievable goals provides confidence and self-mastery. This will also serve to counter restrictive activity and hopefully improve social functioning. Distraction is another way to dampen preoccupation with physical symptoms and worry. Distraction provides the opportunity to focus on something outside of one's health. For those unable to physically leave their environment, there are ways to mentally free themselves from illness burden such as meditating, using guided imagery, writing journals, reading books, listening to music, or pursuing hobbies.

Psychotherapy

Chronic GI illness, such as SBS, with associated treatment requirements, creates a burden for both patient and family members. Patients may also experience grief related to surgical interventions, change in normal eating patterns, and body image changes related to having a stoma and/or central venous catheter. Psychotherapy can provide an opportunity for catharsis, learning new ways to cope with life stressors and provide social support. Therapy interventions can focus on the individual, a couple, and/or the entire family. Therapy referrals should ideally be made directly through the clinician providing the patient's primary care. The patient benefits most when there are open lines of communication between the therapist and this healthcare provider. Types of therapy offered will vary depending on the goals of treatment and patient needs (Table 2.1).

Psychopharmacological Therapy

Patients with SBS often experience anxiety or depression symptoms. Although treatment may seem straightforward, there are several issues that should be considered. First, it would be best to have the patient evaluated by a mental health professional so that an accurate diagnosis can be made. Second, the patient may benefit from psychotherapy alone without the addition of any new medications.

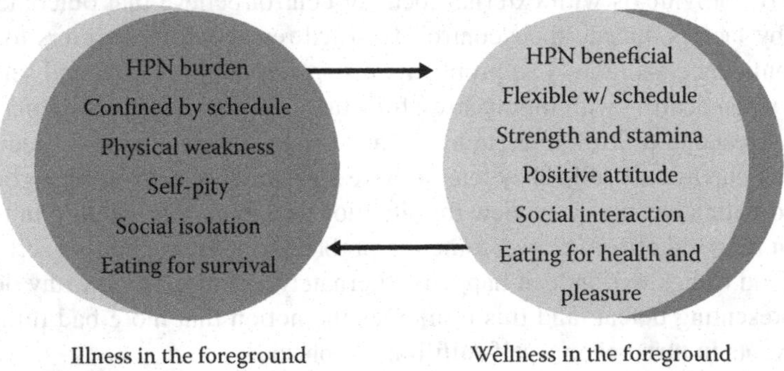

FIGURE 2.1 Shifting perspectives model of chronic illness applied to home parenteral nutrition (HPN) dependency. (Reprinted with permission of Wolters Kluwer Health from Winkler MF et al., *J Infus Nurs.* 2015; 38:290–300, page 296.)

TABLE 2.1
Types of Psychotherapy

Therapy Type	Description
Cognitive therapy	Therapy based on the belief that thoughts influence behavior and feelings. Changing unhelpful thoughts or faulty thinking can result in changes to both behavior and feelings.
Behavioral therapy	Therapy based on the notion that behavior is learned and can be changed. Behavioral therapies focus on addressing faulty learning and subsequent behavior. Change in behavior leads to changes in feelings and thoughts.
Cognitive behavioral therapy	This is a problem-focused therapy that uses a blended approach of therapeutic interventions.

Lastly, patients with SBS are at risk for impaired absorption of oral medications. Although most drugs are normally absorbed in the stomach and proximal small bowel, enteric-coated and delayed-release medications may not be absorbed properly and should be avoided if alternatives are available [24]. Alternatively, medications that can have serum drug levels monitored could be considered. Any medication prescribed will need to be closely monitored and titrated to achieve optimal benefit.

Table 2.2 illustrates commonly prescribed psychotropic medications, dosage range, drug classification, mechanism of action, indications, and most common side effects. The choice of which antidepressant to use is based largely on personal preference from clinical experience; however, side effect profiles of each medication should be considered when making a decision.

Selective serotonin reuptake inhibitors (SSRIs) and selective serotonin-noradrenergic reuptake inhibitors (SNRIs) are generally well tolerated. To minimize GI side effects, it is best to start at lower-than-usual dosage range. Sertraline is the only SSRI whose absorption is increased with food; however, food may help reduce GI side effects related to all SSRIs [25]. Nausea and vomiting may occur during the first few weeks of treatment but generally resolve when receptor rebalancing takes place. Therapeutic effects will usually take 3–6 weeks. SSRIs and SNRIs should be gradually tapered over the course of a few weeks prior to stopping to avoid withdrawal symptoms. Mirtazapine is an atypical antidepressant with an added benefit of being an appetite stimulant and is also available as an orally disintegrating tablet [26]. It has been shown in rodent models to ameliorate visceral hypersensitivity and improve delayed gastric emptying at high doses [27]. Further research is required to see if these findings apply to humans. Tricyclic antidepressants (TCAs) are known to slow movement of contents through the GI tract and may be most helpful in people who have diarrhea. It is believed that these drugs also reduce pain perception, although the exact mechanism is unknown. Olden [28] reports that another key action may be the reduction of somatization and a reduced tendency to regard gut sensations as indicating illness. Iskandar et al. [29] found that low-dose TCAs might be helpful for residual bowel symptoms in irritable bowel–disordered patients without structural abnormalities irrespective of their mood effects [29]. Nortriptyline and desipramine have fewer side effects than other TCAs do. Desipramine is the TCA of choice in functional diarrhea [30]. All TCAs can lower the seizure threshold, which is dose related. Unfortunately, TCAs are associated with many cholinergic side effects. Therefore, they should be started at a low dose and gradually increased to the desired effect. Their full effect may not be seen for 4–6 weeks. They should be used in caution with patients who have major depressive disorders due to overdose toxicity risk. Because some antidepressants in this class can cause cardiac conduction problems, it would be wise to screen patients for cardiac issues prior to initiating these drugs.

QUALITY OF LIFE

QOL is a multidimensional construct that generally includes an assessment of physical health status, psychological well-being, illness perception, social functioning, and cognitive function. As shown

TABLE 2.2
Psychopharmacological Therapy

Drug Classification	Medication, Dosage, and Frequency	Mechanism of Action	Indications	Side Effects
Benzodiazepines	Lorazepam 0.5–1 mg daily, four times per day Diazepam 2.5–10 mg daily, three times per day Clonazepam 0.5–1 mg daily, three times per day	Effect: benzodiazepine receptors that modulate gamma-aminobutyric acid activity	Short-term relief of anxiety symptoms	• Increased sedation • Amnestic effects • Tolerance • Withdrawal symptoms if abruptly stopped • Use with caution in patients with known substance abuse history or regular opiate use
Selective serotonin reuptake inhibitors (SSRIs)	Fluoxetine 10–40 mg daily Sertraline 25–200 mg daily Paroxetine[a] 10–40 mg daily Citalopram 10–40 mg daily Escitalopram 5–20 mg daily	5-HT reuptake inhibition	Anxiety or depressive symptoms Prokinetic effects	• Sexual dysfunction • Sweating • Hyponatremia • Avoid abrupt discontinuation • Can effect platelet aggregation • Risk of bleeding especially post-operatively and with use of non-steroidal anti-inflammatory drugs
Selective serotonin-noradrenergic reuptake inhibitors (SNRIs)	Venlafaxine[b] 37.5–225 mg daily, two times per day Duloxetine 20–30 mg, two times per day	Inhibits serotonin and norepinephrine uptake	Depression May help mitigate pain	• Insomnia/anxiety/activation • Nausea or decreased appetite • Avoid abrupt discontinuation • Hyponatremia • Sweating • Headache/dizziness • Hypertension (higher dose)

(Continued)

TABLE 2.2 (CONTINUED)
Psychopharmacological Therapy

Drug Classification	Medication, Dosage, and Frequency	Mechanism of Action	Indications	Side Effects
Atypical antidepressant	Mirtazapine[c] 7.5–45 mg at hour of sleep	Increases release of norepinephrine and serotonin by blocking presynaptic α2-adrenergic receptors	Anxiety or depressive symptoms Appetite stimulant Sleep improvement	• Somnolence at lower doses • Dizziness • Potentiate sedation of alcohol or benzodiazepine
Norepinephrine dopamine reuptake inhibitor (NDRI)	Buproprion 75–100 mg, two times per day	Norepinephrine and dopamine inhibition	Depression	• Weight loss • Loss of appetite • Dry mouth • Nausea • Constipation • Insomnia • Dizziness • Sweating • Hypertension
Tricyclic antidepressants (TCAs)	Amitriptyline[d] 10–150 mg at hour of sleep Imipramine 10–150 mg at hour of sleep Desipramine 10–200 mg at hour of sleep Nortriptyline 10–150 mg at hour of sleep (has therapeutic window)	Blocks the transporter site for norepinephrine and serotonin increasing synaptic levels	Anxiety and depressive symptoms Slow movement of contents through GI tract and may help diarrhea Reduce pain perception Antiemetic Improve sleep	• Increased appetite • Weight gain • Constipation • Orthostatic hypotension • Dry mouth • Seizure • Tremor • Conduction abnormalities • Avoid abrupt discontinuation

[a] Paroxetine may cause weight gain.
[b] Venlafaxine may cause constipation.
[c] Mirtazapine may cause constipation.
[d] Amitriptyline may cause excessive sedation.

in the list below, many factors impact QOL. An individual's expectations regarding health status and how one copes with physical limitations and disability influence life satisfaction and perceived QOL. In a recent study of HPN-dependent adults with SBS, factors commonly mentioned affecting their QOL included enjoyment, happiness, satisfaction with life, and whether or not they were able to participate in daily activities [14].

Factors that impact quality of life

Age
Coping skills
Dependency on others
Depression
Diarrhea
Disease
Drug dependency (opiates/narcotics)
Family and peer support systems
Fatigue
Feelings toward technology dependency
Financial insecurity and insurance status
Frequent infections
Gender
Goals and expectations
Health
Inability to eat normally
Inability to work or keep a job
Length of home PN dependency
Pain
Performance and functional status
Polyuria
Presence of a stoma
Rehospitalization
Regular healthcare and professional visits
Quality relationships
Satisfaction with life
Self esteem
Sleep disruption
Social isolation

QOL among HPN-dependent individuals is most frequently measured as part of a research study or as an outcome in response to pharmacological or surgical treatment. Until recently, no validated SBS or HPN-specific QOL instruments were available for this purpose [31]. Instead, most studies used generic measures of health status, such as the Short-Form 36 Questionnaire, Quality of Life Index, or Sickness Impact Profile [32]. More recently, Baxter et al. developed a new patient and treatment-specific questionnaire called the HPN-QOL instrument that incorporates functional scales (general health, physical function, ability to eat and drink, employment, travel, emotional function, and sexual function), symptom scales (body image, weight, immobility, fatigue, sleep pattern, GI symptoms, pain, presence of stoma, and financial issues), and HPN administration items with the goal of differentiating between QOL affected by HPN therapy and that of the underlying illness or disease [33,34].

Poor physical function, disabling diarrhea, alterations in eating and/or appetite, and depression are generally associated with chronic illness and disease factors. Sleep disturbance, nocturia, fear of catheter malposition, and infection are usually attributed to HPN administration. Catheter-related complications necessitating hospital admission are strongly associated with impaired QOL and the presence of depression, fatigue, and social impairment [35]. Dreesen et al. [36] studied a cohort of 300 chronic intestinal failure patients requiring HPN and identified incidence of catheter-related infection, survival, and QOL as the most important indicators for their care. These patients also associated improved QOL with a reduction in disease-related symptoms such as diarrhea, fistula output and fatigue, as well as a reduction in HPN-related problems.

Assessing QOL is important to identify the range of problems that affect those who are receiving HPN. This process does not always require a validated instrument; rather, it can be initiated with a general discussion of how the patient defines QOL and his or her expectations about his or her illness or medical therapy and is integrated into a routine medical appointment. Patients tend to enjoy communication about their emotional state, psychosocial concerns, and the nonmedical aspects of living with HPN [37]. Patients often view their medical appointments as being nothing more than a "TPN tune-up" that focuses primarily on the medical or disease aspects of their care. Yet, they desire a more holistic approach to HPN management incorporating physical, spiritual, and emotional support [15,38].

Use of a visual analog scale is a good technique for patients to illustrate their level of psychosocial distress or problems associated with SBS and HPN. Roskott et al. [38] validated an HPN version of an oncology distress thermometer and problem list. Emotional and physical problems were most strongly associated with psychological distress, while not being able to work was related to elevated distress. Regular use of these visual analog instruments was helpful to gain insight into distress and to identify patients who were interested in referral. Improved QOL was associated with facilitating support to patients who most need and want it.

PEER SUPPORT

There are many organizations that provide important outreach services, educational materials, and emotional support to patients, families, and caregivers with HPN dependency. These support systems provide a sense of normalcy by enabling PN-dependent individuals to be part of a home nutrition community [39]. When in-person group support is not available, online social support offers an opportunity to connect with others who are facing similar challenges. People who participate in online social support feel empowered and find value in communicating with others, locating resources, navigating the healthcare system, learning how to resolve conflict, and developing self-knowledge [40]. Peer support and empathy can be an important strategy to foster coping skills and increase knowledge and confidence for individuals with SBS and HPN dependency, thereby improving QOL. Further details on support groups and other useful resources for SBS patients and their providers can be found in Chapter 28.

CONCLUSION

SBS patients experience many physical, emotional, and economic burdens related to their underlying disease and treatment. There are important coping and treatment strategies that may help these patients better deal with the GI symptoms and lifestyle changes associated with this complex disorder and need for PN. Psychological support is most effective when there is a collaborative relationship between mental health clinicians and medical providers. Clinicians need to continually review treatment goals, lifestyle adjustments, and the patient's personal expectations during each patient encounter. Inquiring about concerns unrelated to routine medical issues can be very therapeutic for both patients and family members. Understanding the need to maintain normalcy in life can help healthcare professionals facilitate an SBS patient's adaptation to HPN by offering strategies and interventions to address problems as they occur while promoting hope and optimism for the future.

REFERENCES

1. Wilhelmsen I. The role of psychosocial factors in gastrointestinal disorders. *Gut* 2000;47(Suppl IV):73–75.
2. DaCosta JM. Mucous enteritis. *Am J Med Sci* 1871;89:321–325.
3. Mayer EA. Gut feelings: The emerging biology of the gut–brain communication. *Nat Rev Neurosci.* 2011;12:453–466.
4. Drossman DA. The functional gastrointestinal disorders and the ROME III process. *Gastroenterology* 2006;130:1377–1390.
5. Lackner JM et al. Fear of GI symptoms has an important impact on quality of life in patients with moderate-to-severe IBS. *Am J Gastroenterol* 2014;109:1815–1823.
6. Gershon MD. Nerves, reflexes, and the enteric nervous system: Pathogenesis of the irritable bowel syndrome. *J Clin Gastroenterol* 2005;39(5 Suppl III):S184–S193.
7. Kern MK et al. Cerebral cortical registration of subliminal visceral stimulation. *Gastroenterology* 2002;122:290–298.
8. Grundmann O et al. Complementary and alternative medicines in irritable bowel syndrome: An integrated view. *World J Gastroenterol* 2014;20:346–362.
9. Richbourg L et al. Difficulties experienced by the ostomate after hospital discharge. *J Wound Ostomy Continence Nurs* 2007;34:70–79.
10. Stern JM et al. Psychological aspects of home parenteral nutrition, abnormal illness behavior, and risk of self-harm in patients with central venous catheters. *Aliment Pharmacol Ther* 2007;27:910–918.
11. Silver HJ. The lived experience of home total parenteral nutrition: An online qualitative inquiry with adults, children, and mothers. *Nutr Clin Pract* 2004;19:297–304.
12. Winkler MF et al. The meaning of food and eating among home parenteral nutrition dependent adults with intestinal failure: A qualitative inquiry. *J Am Diet Assoc* 2010;110:1676–1683.
13. Carlsson E et al. Quality of life and concerns in patients with short bowel syndrome. *Clin Nutr* 2003;22:445–452.
14. Winkler MF et al. An exploration of quality of life and the experiences of living with home parenteral nutrition. *JPEN J Parenter Enteral Nutr* 2010;34:395–407.
15. Winkler MF et al. The impact of long term home parenteral nutrition on the patient and the family: Achieving normalcy in life. *J Infus Nurs* 2015;38:290–300.
16. Gaskamp CD. Quality of life and changes in health insurance in long-term home care. *Nurs Econ* 2004;22:135–139, 146.
17. Smith CE et al. Complex home care, part III: Economic impact on family caregiver quality of life and patients' clinical outcomes. *Nurs Econ* 2010;28:393–399, 414.
18. Fletcher PC et al. I am doing the best that I can: Living with inflammatory bowel disease and/or irritable bowel syndrome (part II). *Clin Nurse Spec* 2008;22:278–285.
19. Rollman BL et al. Treating anxiety in the presence of medical comorbidity: Calmly moving forward. *Psychosom Med* 2013;75:710–712.
20. McDaniel SH et al. Somatizing patients and their families. In: *Medical Family Therapy: A Biopsychosocial Approach to Families with Health Problems.* Eds., McDaniel SH, Hepworth J, Doherty WJ. New York: Basic Books, 1992, Chapter 6, pp. 122–151.
21. Schulman-Green D et al. Processes of self-management in chronic illness. *J Nurs Scholarsh* 2012;44:136–144.
22. Auerbach SM, Gramling SE, Eds. *Stress Management: Psychological Foundations.* Upper Saddle River, NJ: Prentice-Hall, 1998.
23. Paterson BL. The shifting perspectives model of chronic illness. *J Nurs Scholarsh* 2001;33:21–26.
24. Crone CC et al. Gastrointestinal disorders. In: *Clinical Manual of Psychopharmacology in the Medically Ill.* Eds., Ferrando SJ, Levenson JL, Owen JA. Washington, DC: American Psychiatric Publishing, 2010, Chapter 4, pp. 103–148.
25. Stahl SM, Ed. *Stahl's Essential Psychopharmacology—The Prescribers Guide.* Third Edition. New York: Cambridge University Press, 2009.
26. Sadock BJ, Sadock VA, Sussman N, Eds. *Kaplan & Sadock's Pocket Handbook of Psychiatric Drug Treatment.* Fourth Edition. Philadelphia, PA: Lippincott Williams & Wilkins, 2006, pp. 72–81, 82–86, 157–159, 187–192, 193–207, 235–237, 238–249.
27. Yin J et al. Ameliorating effects of mirtazapine on visceral hypersensitivity in rats with neonatal colon sensitivity. *Neurogastroenterol Motil* 2014;22:1022–1068.

28. Olden KW. The use of antidepressants in functional gastrointestinal disorders: New uses for old drugs. *CNS Spectr* 2005;10:891–896.
29. Iskandar HN et al. Tricyclic antidepressants for management of residual symptoms in inflammatory bowel disease. *J Clin Gastroenterol* 2014;48:423–429.
30. Dellon ES et al. Treatment of functional diarrhea. *Curr Treat Options Gastroenterol* 2006;9:331–342.
31. Baxter JP et al. A review of the instruments used to assess the quality of life of adult patients with chronic intestinal failure receiving parenteral nutrition at home. *Br J Nutr* 2005;94:633e8.
32. Winkler MF. Quality of life in adult home parenteral nutrition patients. *JPEN J Parenter Enteral Nutr* 2005;29:162–170.
33. Baxter JP et al. The development and translation of a treatment-specific quality of life questionnaire for adult patients on home parenteral nutrition. *e-SPEN Eur E J Clin Nutr Metab* 2008;3:e22–e28.
34. Baxter JP et al. The clinical and psychometric validation of a questionnaire to assess the quality of life of adult patients treated with long-term parenteral nutrition. *JPEN J Parenter Enteral Nutr* 2010;34:131–142.
35. Huisman-de Waal G et al. Psychosocial complaints are associated with venous access-device related complications in patients on home parenteral nutrition. *JPEN J Parenter Enteral Nutr* 2011;35: 588–595.
36. Dreesen M et al. Outcome indicators for home parenteral nutrition (HPN) care: Point of view from adult patients with benign disease. *JPEN J Parenter Enteral Nutr* 2015;39:828–836.
37. Huisman-de Waal G et al. Predicting fatigue in patients using home parenteral nutrition: A longitudinal study. *Int J Behav Med* 2011;18:268–276.
38. Roskott AMC et al. Screening for psychosocial distress in patients with long-term home parenteral nutrition. *Clin Nutr* 2013;32:396–403.
39. Chopy K et al. A qualitative study of the perceived value of membership in the Oley Foundation by home parenteral and enteral nutrition consumers. *JPEN J Parenter Enteral Nutr* 2015;39:426–433.
40. Paterson BL et al. Engagement of parents in on-line social support interventions. *J Pediatr Nurs* 2013;21:2419–2428.

3 Short Bowel Syndrome
Anatomical and Physiological Considerations

Jeremy Nightingale

CONTENTS

KEY POINTS

- In the patient undergoing small bowel resection, knowing the length and segment of small bowel remaining is more important than the length resected given the highly variable small intestinal length.
- There are two common types of patient with a short bowel, those with an end-jejunostomy, whose major problem is of high stomal losses of water and sodium causing dehydration,

and patients with a jejunum in continuity with the colon, who have problems with steatorrhea and malnutrition.

- Twenty-four-hour upper gut secretions (saliva, gastric, and pancreatobiliary) total about 4 L when consuming a normal diet.
- The colon absorbs sodium, water, and magnesium within its lumen and also participates in the synthesis and absorption of short-chain fatty acids and amino acids produced by colonic bacterial fermentation.
- Nutrients stimulate small intestinal growth (via glucagon-like peptide-2); within the colon, they act to slow gastric emptying and small bowel transit (via the ileal and colonic brakes mediated by peptide YY).
- Patients with a colon show improvement in gut absorption over time (1–3 years), while those with an end-jejunostomy do not.

INTRODUCTION

The gastrointestinal (GI) tract of humans aims primarily to digest and absorb food and water. To do this, it has complex and interrelated neurological, endocrine, and immunological systems [1]. The entire gut acts as one integrated unit and may be referred to as an "intestinal orchestra" [2]. If any part fails, then reduced intestinal absorption may result in a reduction in macronutrient, micronutrient, and water absorption, so that malnutrition and/or dehydration result (i.e., intestinal failure).

In this chapter, the anatomical and physiological components relevant to patients with a short bowel will be considered. In general, patients with short bowel syndrome (SBS) fall into one of two groups, those with an end-jejunostomy (less than 200 cm jejunum) or those with jejunum anastomosed to the colon (Figure 3.1). Sometimes, the ileocecal valve and a short length of ileum remain (i.e., jejunoileocolic anastomosis), as occurs in some patients after a mesenteric infarction or small bowel volvulus; their outcome is similar, or better, in terms of absorption to those with a jejunocolic anastomosis.

NORMAL BOWEL STRUCTURE AND LENGTH

The proximal two-fifths of small bowel is named jejunum; the distal three-fifths is the ileum. The normal nonobstructed jejunal and ileal diameters are 4 and 3.5 cm, respectively. The small intestinal absorptive area is increased by the villi, of which there are 20–40 per mm of small bowel.

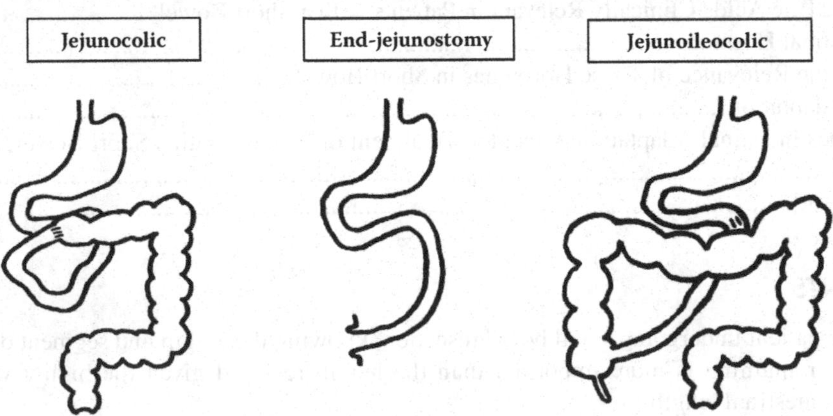

FIGURE 3.1 Types of remnant bowel anatomy in patients with a short bowel.

The human small intestinal length has been measured at autopsy, by small bowel enema, and at surgery from the duodenojejunal flexure (i.e., ligament of Treitz) to the ileocecal valve and varies from 275 to 1049 cm (Table 3.1). In most studies, the small bowel length correlates with height and thus tends to be shorter in women. Postmortem measurements of small bowel length are generally about a meter longer as the bowel is easily stretched. Radiological measurements of small bowel length give shorter results than obtained at autopsy or surgery, partly because radiographs are only in two dimensions and because a small bowel enema [3] causes bowel distension, thus shortening the bowel. Measurements of remaining small bowel length can be made with an opisometer on a contrast (e.g., barium) follow-through examination and are relatively accurate when <200 cm small bowel remains [4]. While the use of magnetic resonance imaging or computed tomography scans here not been carefully evaluated for this purpose, they are likely to be equally as accurate.

Functioning bowel length can be assessed by measuring a fasting plasma citrulline level [5]. Citrulline is a nonessential amino acid that is synthesized in the enterocyte from glutamine, and thus, all the citrulline in the systemic circulation is derived from the enterocytes. Serial plasma citrulline levels have been suggested for use to monitor progress in patients after a small bowel transplant but otherwise are not measured routinely in patients with a short bowel.

What Bowel Length Is Considered Short?

An appreciation of the large range of normal small intestinal length emphasizes the need after a bowel resection to refer to the *remaining* length of small intestine rather than to the amount resected. With knowledge of the remaining small intestinal length, predictions about the long-term need for fluid/nutritional support can be made (Table 3.2, [6,7]). In general, a patient with <100 cm to an end-jejunostomy is likely to need long-term parenteral fluid and/or nutrition, with those with

TABLE 3.1
Measured Lengths of Small Intestine from Duodenojejunal Flexure in Men and Women

Author	Date	Number	Small Intestinal Length, Mean (Range) (cm)
		Autopsy[a]	
Bryant [8]	1924	160	620 (300–850)
Underhill [9]	1955	100	620 (340–790)
		Surgery	
Backman and Hallberg [10]	1974	42	660 (400–850)
Slater and Aufses[b] [11]	1991	38	500 (300–780)
Teitelbaum [12]	2013	24	506 (285–845)[c]
Tacchino [13]	2015	443	690 (350–1049)[c]
		Radiological	
Intubation			
Hirsch et al. [14]	1956	10	260 (210–320)
Small Bowel Enema			
Fanucci et al. [3]	1988	158	290 (160–430)

[a] Autopsy measurements from the pylorus; all others from the duodenojejunal flexure (duodenum = 25 cm).
[b] 21 of these patients had small bowel and 4 others colonic Crohn's disease, but their small intestinal lengths were not different from that of 13 patients without Crohn's disease.
[c] Length correlated with height. Tacchino [13] also showed stretching the bowel increased length by 137 cm.

TABLE 3.2
Guide to Small Bowel Length and the Long-Term Fluid/Nutritional Support Needed by Patients with a Short Bowel

Jejunal Length (cm)	Jejunum–Colon	Jejunostomy
0–50	PN	PN + PS
51–100	ON	PN + PS[a]
101–150	None	ON + OGS
151–200	None	OGS

Source: Nightingale, J.M.D. et al., *Gut*, 55, 1–12, 2006; Nightingale, J.M.D. et al., *Gut*, 33, 1493–1497, 1992; Gouttebel, M.C. et al., *Dig. Dis. Sci.*, 31, 718–723, 1986; Messing, B. et al. *Gastroenterology*, 117, 1043–1050, 1999.

Note: OGS, oral (or enteral) glucose/saline solution; ON, oral (or enteral) nutrition; PN, parenteral nutrition; PS, parenteral saline (±magnesium).

[a] At 85–100 cm may need PS only.

100–200 cm likely to need oral therapy to reduce sodium and water loss from their stoma. This contrasts to patients with jejunum in continuity with a colon who may need parenteral nutrition (PN) if <50 cm jejunum remains, but with >50 cm (providing normal function), parenteral support is rarely needed.

ILEOCECAL VALVE

The ileocecal valve consists of two semilunar flaps projecting into the lumen of the large bowel at the junction of the caecum and colon. Two main functions are attributed to the ileocecal valve: to control the passage of ileal contents into the caecum, allowing adequate time for digestion and absorption, and to prevent the reflux of caecal contents into the small bowel [15]. Studies in patients who have had a right hemicolectomy for colon cancer, however, call this concept into question as transit of a scrambled egg meal from the small to the large bowel was qualitatively and quantitatively the same as in healthy subjects and there was no significant coloileal reflux [16]. Ileal peristalsis, rather than the ileocecal valve, is likely the main factor that keeps the number of bacteria in the small bowel much lower than that in the colon.

COLON

The average length of the colon at autopsy is about 1.6 m (range, 1.0–3.3 m) [8,9]. The unstretched colon at colonoscopy is much shorter at about 0.9 m. In addition to its role as a storage chamber for stool until defecation occurs, the colon serves the functions of absorbing water (up to 6 L/day) [17] and minerals (sodium, magnesium, and calcium), the manufacture of vitamin K by bacteria in residence, fermenting unabsorbed complex carbohydrates to short-chain fatty acids (acetate, propionate, and butyrate), and absorbing amino acids and medium-chain triglycerides. The colon avidly absorbs sodium and chloride against a high-concentration gradient; hence, normal stool contains very little sodium and chloride. The left colon (descending) absorbs more water/sodium than the right colon (ascending) does [18]. Twenty-five percent of body urea is salvaged within the colonic lumen, more if a patient is consuming a low oral protein intake. Urea is converted to ammonia in the colonic epithelium and secreted into the colonic lumen, where bacteria synthesize it into amino acids, which are then reabsorbed [19]. The function of the colon in absorbing macronutrients has been recognized for many years, and the first enteral nutrition (including by the ancient Egyptians) was given rectally (milk, egg, beef broth, wine, or brandy) [20].

What Is the Clinical Importance of the Colon Being in Circuit in Patients with a Short Bowel?

As the colon absorbs water and sodium avidly, the SBS patient with some colon remaining in continuity with the small intestine typically requires less water and sodium supplementation. The principal clinical problem related to having a short bowel and colon in circuit is steatorrhea with an increased absorption of dietary oxalate, which can give rise to calcium oxalate renal stones. As such, patients with a jejunum in continuity with a colon may benefit from a diet rich in complex carbohydrates, moderate in fat [21], and low in oxalate. Rarely, colonic bacteria manufacture the D-isomer of lactic acid, causing a neurologic syndrome characterized by confusion, ataxia, and acidosis with high anion gap [22]. Patients with a colon are less likely to develop cholestasis when receiving PN [23], while those who have their intestinal continuity restored after a mesenteric infarction (i.e., colon brought back into continuity) require less, or even no, parenteral support [24].

VOLUME OF GASTROINTESTINAL SECRETIONS

An estimate of the daily volume of intestinal secretions produced when a normal diet is consumed comes from the seminal work of Borgström et al. [25] and Fordtran and Locklear [26]. Using nonabsorbed markers in healthy subjects, they demonstrated that about 4 L of endogenous secretions pass the duodenojejunal flexure daily, including about 0.5 L saliva, 1–2 L gastric juice [27], and 1.5 L of pancreaticobiliary secretions (0.6 L of which is pancreatic juice) [28]. Although there is experimental evidence in animals that a denervated gastric pouch will hypersecrete acid after a massive resection of small intestine, the evidence for this occurring in humans is poor [29]. Each day, about 6 L of chyme will pass the duodenojejunal flexure, and most of this is absorbed in the first 100 cm of the jejunum [25]. About 1–2 L enters the colon, and in individuals with normal functioning colon, <200–250 mL (g)/day is excreted in the stool (Table 3.3).

TABLE 3.3
Approximate Daily Volume and Composition of Intestinal Secretions Produced in Response to Food Ingestion

	Volume (L)	pH	Na (mmol/L)	K (mmol/L)	Cl (mmol/L)	HCO_3 (mmol/L)	Mg (mmol/L)	Ca (mmol/L)
Saliva	0.5	7	45	20	44	60	0.7	1.3
Gastric juice	2.0	2	10	10	130	0	0.5	2.0
Pancreatic juice	0.6	8	140	10	30	110	0.2	0.3
Hepatic bile	0.9	7	145	5	100	28	0.6	2.5
Small bowel secretion	1.8[a]	7	138	6	141	<5	<0.1	2.5
Serum		7.4	140	4	100	24	1.0	2.4

Source: Borgström, B. et al., *J. Clin. Invest.*, 36, 1521–1536, 1957; Fordtran, J.S. et al., *Am. J. Dig. Dis.*, 11, 503–521, 1966; Carlson, A.J., *The Control of Hunger in Health and Disease*, The University of Chicago Press, Chicago, 1916; McCaughan, J.M. et al., *Arch. Int. Med.*, 61, 739–754, 1938.

[a] This fluid is released and absorbed on the mucosa and rarely needs to be taken into account in calculating fluid losses; estimates of its electrolyte composition are unreliable.

Why Are Gastrointestinal Secretions Important in Patients with a Short Bowel?

Patients with <100 cm of small intestine remaining may not be able to absorb the volume of secretions produced after food ingestion. Less drink/food will result in less secretions and lower stomal/fecal losses. This fluid reduction is the most important step in managing a patient with a high output stoma, followed by giving a glucose-electrolyte (i.e., oral rehydration) solution to sip. While a reduction in oral fluid intake can be very helpful in controlling stool output, it may not always be possible unless the patient is receiving PN, because of the concomitant reduction in oral energy intake. Antisecretory drugs, particularly proton pump inhibitors, can reduce gastric acid secretion and are an integral part of the regimen to reduce the stomal output of patients with a high-volume end-jejunostomy whose stomal output exceeds their oral intake.

Secretions produced by the small intestine are not usually clinically important as they are reabsorbed completely by the functioning intestine; however, if the small bowel is obstructed, it secretes fluid, which will be lost when the obstruction resolves. These secretions may take time (hours/days) to return to their normal volume. Therefore, many patients with a high-output stoma and intermittent obstruction will have the problem of salt and water depletion after the obstructive symptoms have resolved. A low-fiber diet reduces the chance of obstructive episodes occurring.

GASTROINTESTINAL MOTILITY

The gut is innervated by the vagus nerve (parasympathetic), which contains 90% sensory (afferent) and 10% motor (efferent) neurons. Additional innervation to the gut is from the spinal (sympathetic) nerves. Villus cells whose microvilli extend into the gut lumen respond to a range of stimuli, including bacterial toxins, pH, osmolality, and nutrients. There is an interchange of information between the submucosal and myenteric plexi comprising the enteric nervous system and the brain. The pattern of gastrointestinal motility (i.e., migrating myoelectrical complex [MMC]) is affected by the interactions between the enteric and autonomic nervous systems and depends upon whether an individual is in a fasted or a fed state.

Stomach and Small Intestine Motility

The stomach divides into two functionally different parts: the fundus, where solid food is held while it is being broken down by gastric secretions, and the antrum, which acts as a grinding unit that allows only food particles of <2 mm to pass through the pylorus. During fasting, the interdigestive MMC occurs about every 90–120 minutes (range, 50–140) and lasts for 5–10 minutes in any one area and takes about 90 minutes to travel from the stomach to the ileum. The MMC is strongly propulsive and is responsible for clearing the last part of a meal and indigestible materials from the stomach and small intestine, thus serving a "housekeeper" function [30]. Loss of the MMC may occur in some gut dysmotility disorders and is associated with small intestinal bacterial overgrowth. After an extensive distal ileal resection, the MMC cycle was found to be shorter, but jejunal contraction frequency and amplitude were not changed [31].

After a meal, liquid from a mixed liquid–solid meal starts to empty immediately. If the liquid is taken alone, the rate of gastric emptying is much faster. Solid emptying usually occurs in a linear fashion after an initial lag phase of 20–30 minutes, during which the meal remains in the fundus undergoing trituration and dilution by gastric secretions as previously described.

The frequency of the electrical slow wave regulating gut motility varies from 3/min in the stomach to 12/min in the jejunum to 8/min in the ileum. Small bowel contractions can be segmental or peristaltic (rate, 2–25 cm/sec); peristalsis predominates in the duodenum, while segmental contractions predominate further distally. Peristalsis can cause very rapid transit if there is no inhibitory feedback from nutrients; thus, water can reach the caecum in 15 minutes. Even with nutrients, the first part of a liquid meal can travel very rapidly, reaching the caecum in just 14 minutes for the liquid and 24 minutes for the solid components [32]. This first contact with nutrients in the distal small bowel then initiates an inhibitory humorally mediated (glucagon-like peptides [GLP-1 and GLP-2] and peptide YY; see "Gastrointestinal

Hormones" below) feedback response, which slows gastric emptying to allow more time for digestion and absorption. After the bulk of a meal has been emptied from the stomach, the "fasting" activity resumes until another meal is ingested.

Colonic Motility

Most of the time, there is segmental contracting nonpropulsive activity within the colon, which allows mixing of the colonic contents and time for absorption. Several times a day, a high-pressure propulsive peristaltic wave propels some of the colonic contents to the rectum ("mass movement") in anticipation of defecation. Isotopic studies have shown that the first part of a meal remains in the colon for a median of 31 hours (range, 24–48). In normal subjects, most of a meal will have left the bowel within 3 days of being eaten. Colonic transit is slower in women than in men [33].

Why Is Gut Motility Important in Patients with a Short Bowel?

Patients with a jejunostomy have rapid transit of liquid from the stomach to the stoma. Drugs are frequently given to slow small bowel transit, allowing more time for absorption. Loperamide (often in very high doses), codeine phosphate, and clonidine have this function. Restoring bowel continuity to bring the colon into circuit can result in slower gastric emptying and small bowel transit. This effect may be due to the distal bowel-produced hormones, GLP-1, GLP-2 and peptide YY [34].

GASTROINTESTINAL DIGESTION AND ABSORPTION

Water, Sodium, and Magnesium

Most meals have a low sodium content (10–40 mmol/L), generating a steep concentration gradient between the lumen and plasma. Sodium-rich salivary and pancreaticobiliary secretions raise the luminal level, as do intestinal secretions, so that the sodium concentration at the duodenojejunal flexure reaches about 90 mmol/L and increases further toward 140 mmol/L in the terminal ileum [26]. Although some water and sodium may be absorbed before chyme reaches the jejunum, in most individuals with a normal bowel anatomy, a meal continues to be diluted by secretions until a distance of 100 cm distal to the duodenojejunal flexure [25,26]. This distance is clinically important in the short bowel setting because if a patient has a stoma situated in the upper 100 cm of the jejunum, the volume of stomal output is likely to be greater than the volume taken by mouth. Such a patient, sometimes referred to as a "net secretor," will be in negative fluid and sodium balance after any food or drink [35].

Jejunal mucosa is more permeable to water, sodium, and chloride than is ileal mucosa. It allows back-diffusion through leaky intercellular junctions so the jejunal contents become iso-osmolar. Thus, water movement in response to an osmotic gradient in the jejunum is 9 times [36] and sodium fluxes 2 times [37] as great as in the ileum. As such, sodium absorption in the jejunum can occur only against a small concentration gradient, depends upon water movement, and is coupled to the absorption of glucose and some amino acids [38]. When the small bowel is intubated and perfused with solutions containing different amounts of sodium, absorption of sodium from the perfusate occurs mainly when the sodium concentration is 90 mmol/L or more, while secretion of sodium into the lumen occurs when the concentration is less. Several studies have shown that maximal jejunal absorption of sodium from a perfused solution occurs at a concentration around 120 mmol/L [39–41]. These studies formed the basis for the development of oral rehydration solutions (ORS). In contrast, the ileum can absorb sodium against a concentration gradient and movement of sodium is not coupled with glucose or other nutrients. The ileum is important in conserving sodium and water when the body becomes depleted since, unlike the jejunum, the ileal mucosa can increase its sodium absorption in response to aldosterone [42].

Magnesium is an intracellular cation that is a cofactor for many enzymatic reactions; 50% resides in bone. Each day, about 10–20 mmol of magnesium is consumed, of which about a third is absorbed mainly by a gradient-driven saturable process occurring primarily in the distal small intestine and colon [43]. The proportion absorbed is variable according to the amount of magnesium in the diet. When the total dietary magnesium is increased to 24 mmol in a healthy person, only 24% is absorbed. If the dietary intake is reduced to 1 mmol, 76% is absorbed [44]. The jejunal absorption of magnesium, like that of calcium, is increased by 1,25-dihydroxycholecalciferol [45]. The kidney, under conditions of magnesium deprivation, can reduce magnesium excretion to <0.5 mmol/day [46]. Aldosterone increases [47] and parathormone reduces renal magnesium excretion [48]. Very little magnesium is found in intestinal secretions (Table 3.3). Magnesium present within the circulation is 30% bound to albumin. As such, serum levels of magnesium may not reliably indicate body magnesium status; measuring red blood cell magnesium may be helpful in this situation.

How Does Water, Sodium, and Magnesium Physiology Affect the Clinical Care of Patients with a Short Bowel?

Patients with an end-jejunostomy are advised to restrict oral hypotonic fluids (0.5–1.0 L/24 hours) to prevent net efflux of sodium into the bowel lumen (Figure 3.2). Instead, an ORS is recommended to be sipped throughout the day (often cold and flavored to improve palatability) so that sodium and water absorption is enhanced. The concentration of sodium in the solution aims to be 90–120 mmol/L to optimize net absorption. Hypertonic fluids must also be restricted, as they have the effect of drawing water into the bowel lumen to dilute the tonicity, thereby adding to the sheer volume of stool/ostomy output.

Magnesium deficiency occurs commonly in patients with an end-jejunostomy [49], although, surprisingly, even those with very low serum levels can be asymptomatic. The low magnesium is due to a combination of factors that include hyperaldosteronism (from sodium depletion), loss of magnesium absorbing bowel, too much dietary fat, low vitamin D, and proton pump inhibitor therapy. Treatments, other than parenteral infusion, include reducing sodium depletion, using oral magnesium and alpha-cholecalciferol supplements, reducing oral fat intake, and considering the discontinuation of proton pump inhibitors if possible.

Carbohydrate, Protein, and Lipids

Saliva, gastric, and pancreaticobiliary secretions break down carbohydrates and proteins to oligosaccharides and oligopeptides within the gut lumen. They are not designed to create small molecules (e.g., amino acids, monosaccharides), as these would be hyperosmolar and result in water secretion and osmotic diarrhea. Instead, the final breakdown into small molecules occurs at the

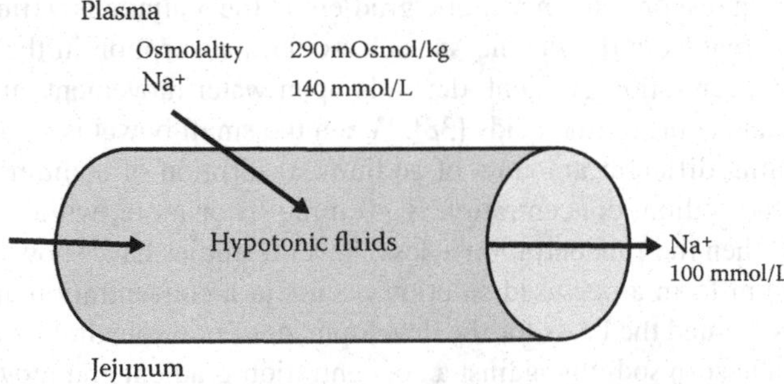

FIGURE 3.2 Diagram to show how drinking hypotonic fluid (tea, coffee, water, etc.) leads to sodium secretion/diffusion into the jejunum; this sodium is then lost through the stoma. Thus, the more hypotonic the fluid drunk is, the more sodium is lost through the stoma and the patient becomes yet more thirsty.

mucosal brush border (e.g., by disaccharidases for carbohydrates) immediately before absorption. In the jejunum, glucose and galactose absorption is partly coupled with that of sodium; that of fructose is by an independent mechanism. Protein digestion is mediated by endopeptidases that cleave protein at specific points in the middle of proteins (e.g., pepsin, trypsin, chymotrypsin, and elastase), and exopeptidases that work systematically from the ends.

Intubation studies in healthy subjects have shown that most polysaccharides and proteins are digested and absorbed within the proximal 100 cm of the small intestine [25]. Fats, however, are less completely absorbed and require a longer length of bowel depending upon how much is ingested. Long-chain fatty acids (C14–C20) form micelles with bile salts; these are absorbed and formed into chylomicrons within the enterocyte, which then pass via the thoracic duct to the systemic circulation. Medium-chain fatty acids (C6–12) are absorbed by both the small and large bowels and pass directly into the portal venous system; they are readily oxidized in the liver via a carnitine-independent pathway.

The colonic bacteria can ferment unabsorbed, complex carbohydrates to produce short-chain fatty acids, which can then be absorbed and utilized as energy (up to 1000 kcal/day in some cases) by the host.

What Is the Dietary Advice for Patients with a Short Bowel?

Patients with a jejunum and colon are encouraged to consume a diet high in complex carbohydrates (which, as previously mentioned, can be fermented and used for energy) but not too high in fat, as fatty acids cause salt and water secretion into the colon [21]. A low oxalate diet to reduce the chance of developing calcium oxalate renal stones is also advised. Patients with a jejunostomy do not require these dietary restrictions but should follow a low osmolality diet (large molecules) that is high in sodium to prevent salt and water losses [22].

Vitamins, Calcium, and Iron Absorption

Most water-soluble vitamins are actively absorbed from the upper intestine, except food-bound vitamin B_{12}, which is bound by an intrinsic factor (a mucoprotein produced by parietal cells in the stomach) and is predominantly selectively absorbed from the distal 60 cm of the ileum [50]. The fat-soluble vitamins, A, D, E, and K; essential fatty acids; and cholesterol do not have specific active uptake mechanisms but dissolve in the lipophilic center of the micelles. This allows the hydrophobic molecules to diffuse through the aqueous chyme to reach the lipid outer membrane of the brush border into which these lipophilic substances readily diffuse [1].

Thirty to eighty percent of ingested calcium is absorbed mainly by active transport in the upper small intestine. The transport is facilitated by 1,25 dihydroxycholecalciferol, lactose, and protein. Phosphates, phytates, and oxalate form insoluble complexes with calcium and thus inhibit calcium absorption.

Only 3–6% of the iron ingested is usually absorbed; this keeps up with losses of 0.6 mg/day in men and double this in women. Gastric acid dissolves insoluble iron salts and facilitates the reduction of ferric iron (Fe^{3+}) present in most food to ferrous iron (Fe^{2+}), which can be actively absorbed in the proximal small bowel. This reduction depends on ascorbic acid, which is actively secreted in gastric juice, and other reducing agents in the diet. The amount of iron entering the circulation is carefully controlled; much is bound to apoferritin to form ferritin within the mucosal cells. This poorly absorbable complex is shed into the gut lumen when the mucosal cells are sloughed and is lost from the body.

What Are the Clinical Implications for Vitamin B_{12}, Calcium, and Iron Treatment in Patients with a Short Bowel?

Most patients with a short bowel will have had their terminal ileum resected and, if not receiving PN, will need regular B_{12} supplementation, usually 3 monthly (or once every 3 months in the United

Kingdom) injection although daily high dose oral supplementation may also be successful. Calcium problems are rare, but a good dietary intake is necessary to ensure bone health and to bind oxalate if a residual colon segment is present. Iron deficiency is common, even in patients requiring PN as it does not routinely provide iron, and may necessitate regular iron infusions.

BILE ACIDS

Bile acids are natural soaps that put lipids into an aqueous solution so that they can be absorbed. The liver synthesizes two primary bile acids, cholic and chenodeoxycholic acid. These are conjugated with glycine or taurine in a ratio of 3:1; the taurine conjugates are more soluble. Each day, one-quarter to one-third of the primary bile acids undergo anaerobic bacterial dehydroxygenation within the terminal ileum and colon, resulting in the formation of the secondary bile acids, deoxycholic and a small percentage of insoluble lithocholic acid. Normal human bile consists of 50% cholic acid, 39% chenodeoxycholic acid, 15% deoxycholic acid, and 5% lithocholic acid. There is 3–5 g of bile acids in an individual, 95% of which circulates through the enterohepatic circulation 5–14 times daily.

How Are Bile Acids Clinically Relevant in Patients with a Short Bowel?

The enterohepatic circulation is important for the action of some drugs such as loperamide, which enter this circulation, and, if disrupted by ileal resection, bypass, or disease, higher than normal doses of loperamide are needed to achieve the same effect. Unabsorbed bile acids within the colon (e.g., after an ileal resection) stimulate salt and water secretion and motility, thereby worsening diarrhea. A bile acid sequestrant may occasionally be beneficial; however, in the setting of short bowel, there is often bile acid deficiency, and use of a bile acid sequestrant will only worsen fat malabsorption and steatorrhea. Conjugated bile acid replacement therapy (e.g., cholylsarcosine) has been used to improve fat absorption in patients with a short bowel but is not widely available [51–53].

GASTROINTESTINAL HORMONES

Many hormones are produced by cells within in the GI tract. These hormones participate in many physiological roles, including the control of secretomotor activity, and are closely linked with the nervous system. Most of the gut hormones fall into one of two families according to their molecular structure: the gastrin family (e.g., gastrin and cholecystokinin) or the secretin family (e.g., gastric inhibitory peptide [GIP], GLP, secretin, and vasoactive intestinal peptide). The hormones are produced in response to luminal stimuli (primarily nutrient contact) and have five main areas of function, including the control of gastric emptying/secretion (gastrin, somatostatin), regulating the rate of digestion (cholecystokinin, secretin, GIP, and motilin), slowing the rate of GI transit (GLP-1, neurotensin, and peptide YY), promoting intestinal growth (GLP-2 and neurotensin), and control of blood glucose (insulin, GLP-1, GIP).

Motilin promotes gastrointestinal activity and may induce the MMC [54]. Motilin analogs such as macrolide antibiotics (e.g., erythromycin) cause premature phase III-like intense contractions of the gastric antrum and small bowel and have been used to treat gastroparesis and constipation.

Somatostatin has been referred to as "endocrine cyanide" as it reduces the circulating levels of all known GI peptide hormones, most anterior pituitary hormones, and many others (e.g., calcitonin and renin). By endocrine, paracrine, and neurotransmitter actions, it inhibits most GI functions, including the reduction of gastric, pancreatic, and biliary secretions [55], as well as pentagastrin-stimulated salivary flow [56]. Somatostatin also slows small bowel transit, may delay gastric emptying, and reduces GI blood flow and the absorption of carbohydrate, lipid, and amino acids. As somatostatin and its analogs suppress trophic (i.e., growth) hormones, it can be postulated that they may reduce intestinal adaptation after a small bowel resection; however, there is no evidence for this in humans, and rat studies show no such effect [57].

Peptide YY has structural similarities to pancreatic polypeptide and consists of 36 amino acids with a tyrosine at each end, hence the name peptide YY [58]. It is distributed throughout the small and large intestines (duodenum to rectum) and increases in concentration from the ileum to the rectum [59]. It coexists in the L cells with GLP-2 [60,61]. High levels of peptide YY are observed in situations when unabsorbed nutrients reach the colon, such as tropical sprue or chronic pancreatitis [62], dumping syndrome [63], and after an ileal resection leaving the colon in situ [34,64]. Low levels are seen in jejunostomy and ileostomy patients due to the absence of their colon [34,64]. Peptide YY may be the major hormone responsible for the ileal and colonic brakes [24,39], which slow gastric and small bowel transit when unabsorbed nutrients reach the ileum or colon.

GLP-2 is an enterocyte-specific growth hormone that causes small and large bowel villus and crypt growth, increases small and large bowel length and weight, and reduces gastric antral motility [65,66]. GLP-2 levels have been shown to be low in patients with a jejunostomy and high in patients with a colon-in-continuity [67,68].

What Is the Relevance of These Hormones in Short Bowel?

The somatostatin analog octreotide has been used to reduce GI secretions and slow motility in patients with a jejunostomy; however, its effect does not appear to be superior to that of a proton pump inhibitor and it is more expensive and requires what some describe as painful subcutaneous administration [35].

Both peptide YY and GLP-2 levels are very low in patients with a jejunostomy and high in patients with a jejunocolic anastomosis. If either or both were administered to patients with a jejunostomy, they would be expected to reduce output by slowing transit and stimulating upper gut growth. A longer-acting analog of GLP-2, teduglutide, is currently available for use in clinical practice for selected patients to facilitate weaning of parenteral support [69]. At present, there is no published research to show if peptide YY or an analog reduces jejunostomy output or facilitates the weaning from PN.

INTESTINAL ADAPTATION

Intestinal adaptation is the process that attempts to restore the total gut absorption of nutrients, electrolytes, and water to that prior to an intestinal resection [70]. This takes place over the first few years after resection and occurs by several mechanisms, including the patient eating more food than normal (hyperphagia), an increase in the absorptive area of the remaining bowel (structural adaptation), and by slower GI transit (functional adaptation). There is no evidence that any adaptation occurs in patients with a jejunostomy; however, in patients with a retained colon, functional adaptation occurs with slowing of gastric emptying and small bowel transit [49], probably due to high circulating peptide YY, GLP-1, and GLP-2 levels [34,68]. There is increased jejunal absorption of macronutrients (e.g., carbohydrates), water, sodium, and calcium with time and an increased chance of the patient being able to discontinue PN [22]. Thus, patients with a colon-in-continuity may show a gradual reduction in nutritional requirements over the 1–3 years after continuity is established.

How Does Intestinal Adaptation Affect the Treatment of Patients with a Short Bowel?

Patients with a jejunostomy can be expected to need the same nutrient/fluid management indefinitely after surgery. Patients with a colon show improved absorption and may be able to stop or reduce parenteral support with time. Care must be made to monitor these patients closely during the adaptation period to make appropriate changes in their PN, so they do not become overweight or fluid overloaded.

CONCLUSION

An understanding of normal anatomy and physiology and the way in which it is disrupted in patients with a short bowel is helpful in the understanding of how to optimize the treatment of these patients.

REFERENCES

1. Nightingale JMD et al. Normal intestinal anatomy and physiology. In: Nightingale JMD, ed. *Intestinal Failure*. London: Greenwich Medical Media., 2001, pp. 15–36.
2. Jeejeebhoy KN. What is intestinal failure? Lecture at Royal College of Physicians, London, in conference: Acute intestinal failure and short term nutrition support. September 2009.
3. Fanucci A et al. Normal small-bowel measurements by enteroclysis. *Scand J Gastroenterol* 1988;23: 574–576.
4. Nightingale JMD et al. Length of residual small bowel after partial resection: Correlation between radiographic and surgical measurements. *Gastrointest Radiol* 1991;16:305–306.
5. Crenn P et al. Postabsorptive plasma citrulline concentration is a marker of absorptive enterocyte mass and intestinal failure in humans. *Gastroenterology* 2000;119:1496–1505.
6. Gouttebel MC et al. Total parenteral nutrition needs in different types of short bowel syndrome. *Dig Dis Sci* 1986;31:718–723.
7. Messing B et al. Long-term survival and parenteral nutrition dependence in adult patients with the short bowel syndrome. *Gastroenterology* 1999;117:1043–1050.
8. Bryant J. Observations upon the growth and length of the human intestine. *Am J Med Sci* 1924;167: 499–520.
9. Underhill BML. Intestinal length in man. *Br Med J* 1955;2:1243–1246.
10. Backman L et al. Small intestinal length. An intraoperative study in obesity. *Acta Chir Scand* 1974;140: 57–63.
11. Slater G et al. Small bowel length in Crohn's disease. *Am J Gastroenterol* 1991;8:1037–1040.
12. Teitelbaum EN et al. Intraoperative small bowel length measurements and analysis of demographic predictors of increased length. *Clin Anat* 2013;26:827–32.
13. Tacchino RM. Bowel length: Measurement, predictors, and impact on bariatric and metabolic surgery. *Surg Obes Relat Dis* 2015;11:328–334.
14. Hirsch J et al. Measurement of the human intestinal length in vivo and some causes of variation. *Gastroenterology* 1956;31:274–284.
15. Phillips SF et al. Motility of the ileocolonic junction. *Gut* 1988;29:390–406.
16. Fich A et al. Ileocolonic transit does not change after right hemicolectomy. *Gastroenterology* 1992;103: 794–799.
17. Debongnie JC et al. Capacity of the colon to absorb fluid. *Gastroenterology* 1978;74:698–703.
18. Bowling TE et al. Reversal by short-chain fatty acids of colonic fluid secretion induced by enteral feeding. *Lancet* 1993;342:1266–1268.
19. Jackson AA. Salvage of urea–nitrogen and protein requirements. *Proc Nutr Soc* 1995;54:535–547.
20. Randall HT. Enteral nutrition: Tube feeding in acute and chronic illness. *JPEN J Parenter Enteral Nutr* 1984;8:113–136.
21. Nordgaard I et al. Colon as a digestive organ in patients with short bowel. *Lancet* 1994;343:373–376.
22. Nightingale JMD et al. Guidelines for the management of patients with a short bowel. *Gut* 2006;55(suppl IV):1–12.
23. Adaba F et al. Chronic cholestasis in patients on parenteral nutrition: The influence of restoring bowel continuity after mesenteric infarction. *Euro J Clin Nutr* 2016;70:189–193.
24. Adaba F et al. Mesenteric infarction: Clinical outcomes after restoration of bowel continuity. *Ann Surg* 2015;262:1059–1064.
25. Borgström B et al. Studies of intestinal digestion and absorption in the human. *J Clin Invest* 1957;36: 1521–1536.
26. Fordtran JS et al. Ionic constituents and osmolality of gastric and small intestinal fluids after eating. *Am J Dig Dis* 1966;11:503–521.
27. Carlson AJ. *The Control of Hunger in Health and Disease*. Chicago: University of Chicago Press, 1916:232–247.
28. McCaughan JM et al. The external secretory function of the human pancreas. Physiologic observations. *Arch Int Med* 1938;61:739–754.

29. Windsor CWO et al. Gastric secretion after massive small bowel resection. *Gut* 1969;10:779–786.
30. Itoh Z et al. The interdigestive migrating complex and its significance in man. *Clin Gastroenterol* 1982;11:497–521.
31. Schmidt T et al. Effect of intestinal resection on human small bowel motility. *Gut* 1996;38:859–863.
32. Nightingale JMD et al. Disturbed gastric emptying in the short bowel syndrome. Evidence for a "colonic brake." *Gut* 1993;34:1171–1176.
33. Kamm MA. The small intestine and colon: Scintigraphic quantitation of motility in health and disease. *Eur J Nucl Med* 1992;19:902–912.
34. Nightingale JMD et al. Gastrointestinal hormones in the short bowel syndrome. PYY may be the "colonic brake" to gastric emptying. *Gut* 1996;39:267–272.
35. Nightingale JMD et al. Jejunal efflux in short bowel syndrome. *Lancet* 1990;336:765–768.
36. Fordtran JS et al. Permeability characteristics of the human small intestine. *J Clin Invest* 1965;44: 1935–1944.
37. Davis GR et al. Permeability characteristics of human jejunum, ileum, proximal colon and distal colon: Results of potential difference measurements and unidirectional fluxes. *Gastroenterology* 1982;83: 844–850.
38. Fordtran JS et al. The mechanisms of sodium absorption in the human small intestine. *J Clin Invest* 1968;47:884–900.
39. Spiller RC et al. Jejunal water and electrolyte absorption from two proprietary enteral feeds in man: Importance of sodium content. *Gut* 1987;28:681–687.
40. Sladen GE et al. Interrelationships between the absorptions of glucose, sodium and water by the normal human jejunum. *Clin Sci* 1969;36:119–132.
41. Rodrigues CA et al. What is the ideal sodium concentration of oral rehydration solutions for short bowel patients? *Clin Sci* 1988;74(suppl 18):69.
42. Levitan R et al. Water and electrolyte content of human fluid after D-aldosterone administration. *Gastroenterology* 1967;52:510–512.
43. Kayne LH et al. Intestinal magnesium absorption. *Miner Electrolyte Metab* 1993;19:210–217.
44. Graham LA et al. Gastrointestinal absorption and excretion of magnesium in man. *Metabolism* 1960;9:646–659.
45. Krejs GJ et al. Effect of 1,25-dihydroxyvitamin D3 on calcium and magnesium absorption in the healthy human jejunum and ileum. *Am J Med* 1983;75:973–976.
46. Shils ME. Experimental human magnesium depletion. I. Clinical observations and blood chemistry alterations. *Am J Clin Nutr* 1964;15:133–143.
47. Horton R et al. Effect of aldosterone on the metabolism of magnesium. *J Clin Endocrinol Metab* 1962;22:1187–1192.
48. Zofková I et al. The relationship between magnesium and calciotropic hormones. *Magnes Res* 1995; 8:77–84.
49. Nightingale JMD et al. Colonic preservation reduces the need for parenteral therapy, increases the incidence of renal stones but does not change the high prevalence of gallstones in patients with a short bowel. *Gut* 1992;33:1493–1497.
50. Thompson WG et al. The relation between ileal resection and vitamin B12 absorption. *Can J Surg* 1977;20:461–464.
51. Gruy-Kapral C et al. Conjugated bile acid replacement therapy for short-bowel syndrome. *Gastroenterology* 1999;116:15–21.
52. Heydorn S et al. Bile acid replacement therapy with cholylsarcosine for short-bowel syndrome. *Scand J Gastroenterol* 1999;34:818–23.
53. Kapral C et al. Conjugated bile acid replacement therapy in short bowel syndrome patients with a residual colon. *Z Gastroenterol* 2004;42:583–589.
54. Vantrappen G et al. Motilin and the interdigestive migrating motor complex in man. *Dig Dis Sci* 1979;24:497–500.
55. Reichlin S. Somatostatin. *N Engl J Med* 1983;309:1495–1501, 1556–1563.
56. Loguercio C et al. Effect of somatostatin on salivary secretion in man. *Digestion* 1987;36:91–95.
57. Vanderhoof JA et al. Lack of inhibitory effect of octreotide on intestinal adaptation in short bowel syndrome in the rat. *J Pediatr Gastroenterol Nutr* 1998;26:241–244.
58. Tatemoto K. Isolation and characterization of peptide YY (PYY), a candidate gut hormone that inhibits pancreatic exocrine secretion. *Proc Natl Acad Sci USA* 1982;79:2514–2518.
59. Adrian TE et al. Human distribution and release of a putative new gut hormone, peptide YY. *Gastroenterology* 1985;89:1070–1077.

60. Ali-Rachedi A et al. Peptide YY (PYY) immunoreactivity is co-stored with glucagon-related immunoreactants in endocrine cells of the gut and pancreas. *Histochemistry* 1984;80:487–491.
61. Bottcher G et al. Co-existance of peptide YY and glicentin immunoreactivity in endocrine cells of the gut. *Regul Pept* 1984;8:261–266.
62. Adrian TE et al. Peptide YY abnormalities in gastrointestinal diseases. *Gastroenterology* 1986;90:379–384.
63. Adrian TE et al. Plasma peptide YY (PYY) in dumping syndrome. *Dig Dis Sci* 1985;30:1145–1148.
64. Adrian TE et al. Release of peptide YY (PYY) after resection of small bowel, colon or pancreas in man. *Surgery* 1987;101:715–719.
65. Baldassano S et al. GLP-2: What do we know? What are we going to discover? *Regul Pept* 2014;194–195:6–10.
66. Wøjdemann M et al. Glucagon-like peptide-2 inhibits centrally induced antral motility in pigs. *Scand J Gastroenterol.* 1998;33:828–832.
67. Jeppesen PB et al. Impaired stimulated glucagon-like peptide 2 response in ileal resected short bowel patients with intestinal failure. *Gut* 1999;45:559–563.
68. Jeppesen PB et al. Elevated plasma glucagon-like peptide 1 and 2 concentrations in ileum resected short bowel patients with a preserved colon. *Gut* 2000;47:370–376.
69. Jeppesen PB et al. Teduglutide reduces need for parenteral support among patients with short bowel syndrome with intestinal failure. *Gastroenterology* 2012;143:1473–1481.
70. Goodlad RA et al. Intestinal adaptation. In: Nightingale JMD, ed. *Intestinal Failure*. London: Greenwich Medical Media, 2001:243–260.

4 Intestinal Adaptation
The Contemporary Treatment Goal for Short Bowel Syndrome

Jane Naberhuis and Kelly A. Tappenden

CONTENTS

KEY POINTS

- Intestinal adaptation is a natural process stimulated by massive small bowel resection wherein structural and functional changes allow for enhanced nutrient and fluid digestion and absorption in the remaining intestine.
- Maximizing the degree of intestinal adaptation achieved is critically important for reducing a patient's long-term dependence on parenteral nutrition.
- Many factors influence the degree of intestinal adaptation achieved, including the magnitude and site of the resection, and postsurgical nutrition and medical therapy.
- Intestinal adaptation occurs most notably in the first 1–2 years after resection; however, exogenous stimuli may be used to facilitate adaptation several years later.

INTRODUCTION

Intestinal adaptation is a natural process that occurs after massive small bowel resection, where structural and functional changes allow for enhanced nutrient and fluid digestion and absorption in the residual intestine [1,2]. Many factors influence the degree of intestinal adaptation achieved, including the magnitude and site of the resection, and postsurgical nutrition and medical therapy. Maximizing the intestinal adaptation achieved is critically important for reducing a patient's long-term dependence on parenteral nutrition (PN). As such, clinicians must gain a strong understanding of the multifaceted process of intestinal adaptation (Figure 4.1) and its importance in the successful management of patients with short bowel syndrome (SBS).

INTESTINAL ADAPTATION AFTER RESECTION

Structural Adaptations

While comprehensive study of intestinal adaptation has occurred mainly in animal models, postresection adaptation in humans is demonstrated by the majority of patients who progress from PN dependence postsurgery to enteral autonomy within months/years [3]. Indeed, available evidence indicates that gross changes in intestinal morphology, including small bowel lengthening and dilation, occur after resection in humans [4]. To quantify the extent of these changes, McDuffie and associates [5] evaluated intestinal morphology in 33 infants with necrotizing enterocolitis at the time of resection and again at ostomy reversal. In these patients, villus height and crypt depth increased by 32% and 22%, respectively, at ostomy reversal compared with baseline. Structural adaptation of the intestinal mucosa also occurs in adults. Doldi [6] reported enterocyte hyperplasia and a 75% increase in villus height in the small intestine of 13 patients 2 years after jejunoileal bypass surgery. Joly and associates [7] documented a 35% increase in crypt depth and a 22% increase in cell number/crypt in the colon of 12 patients with jejuno-colonic anastomosis, compared with healthy controls, 10 years after resection.

In-depth study in preclinical models of SBS indicate that the mechanisms of structural adaptation after massive resection include

- Faster rate of proliferation in the epithelial crypt [8–10];
- Expanded crypt depth and villus height [11,12];
- Increased residual intestinal mucosal mass, diameter, and length [11,13,14];
- Amplified intestinal DNA, RNA, and protein concentrations [14,15]; and
- Angiogenesis with subsequent increase in blood flow [16–18].

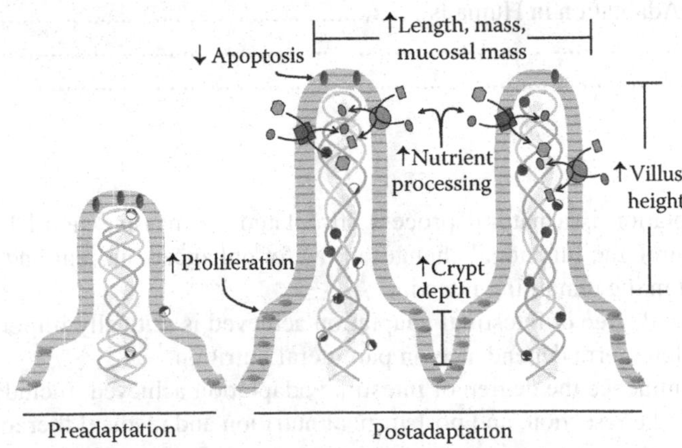

FIGURE 4.1 Structural and functional intestinal adaptations after massive intestinal resection.

Functional Adaptations

Increased Cellular Capacity

After resection, the human intestine is capable of increased absorptive capacity through mucosal surface area expansion and enhancement of absorptive efficiency of each cell [19–22]. It is important to note that while structural adaptations alone allow for increased nutrient processing capacity of the intestinal epithelium due to increased surface area (i.e., more enterocytes), functional adaptations have a multiplier effect by allowing for increased nutrient processing action per unit surface area (i.e., by each enterocyte).

Animal studies indicate that intestinal resection is associated with increased expression of transporter proteins and exchangers involved in nutrient, electrolyte, and water absorption, including the sodium glucose cotransporter, Na^+/H^+ exchangers, and Na^+/K^+ adenosine triphosphatases, which is not solely a result of increased enterocyte mass [23–26]. Furthermore, epithelial cell maturation may be accelerated with adaptation, as developing enterocytes express digestive enzymes and amino acid transporters more rapidly after small bowel resection than in an intact bowel [27,28]. The net result of these changes in protein expression and activity is to increase the digestive and absorptive capacity of the remnant bowel.

Recruitment of Nutrient Processing by the Colon

The enhanced nutrient processing capacity of the residual colon after resection represents another mechanism of functional adaptation after massive intestinal resection. For example, the colon has been described as a salvage organ for harvesting malabsorbed carbohydrates via fermentation to short-chain fatty acids (SCFAs) when patients with SBS consume a diet high in complex carbohydrates [29]. In another striking example of colonic adaptation, Ziegler and associates [30] report a 5-fold increased expression of PepT1, a transporter of dipeptides and tripeptides, in the colon of patients with SBS compared with controls.

Motility Shifts Facilitate Nutrient Processing

A slowing in small bowel transit represents yet another mechanism of functional adaptation allowing for increased contact time between luminal nutrients and the absorptive mucosa. In dogs, small intestinal transit time increased by 35% between weeks 4 and 12 after a 50% resection [31]. Plasma concentration of peptide YY (responsible for the phenomenon known as the "ileal brake"), a hormone released by the distal small intestine and proximal colon that delays gastric emptying and intestinal transit, is elevated in patients with an ileal resection and colon-in-continuity [32]. After intestinal resection, patients typically experience less diarrhea over time [33]; slowed gastrointestinal transit, in addition to the other structural and functional changes described, likely contributes to this reduction.

DETERMINANTS OF INTESTINAL ADAPTATION

Several factors influence the magnitude of intestinal adaptation that occurs postresection, including residual anatomy, route and composition of nutrition therapy, and various trophic factors (Table 4.1).

TABLE 4.1
Determinants of Intestinal Adaptation

Residual Anatomy	Enteral Nutrients	Intestinotrophic Factors
Segmental plasticity	Route of nutrient administration	Growth hormone
Extent of resection	Nutrient complexity	Glucagon-like peptide-2
	Dietary fat	
	Short-chain fatty acids	
	Glutamine	

Residual Anatomy

Segmental Plasticity

The segment of intestine resected influences the adaptation of the residual tissue, with the ileum displaying greater adaptive potential than the jejunum [11,34,35]. Clinically, this fact results in proximal intestinal resections being associated with less diarrhea and steatorrhea compared with distal resections [36] despite the jejunum typically processing far more nutrients than the ileum in the intact healthy intestine. The increased adaptive capacity of the ileum may be because the distal intestine is typically exposed to fewer luminal nutrients, which act as potent stimuli for intestinal growth, under normal conditions. Indeed, in the intact intestine, villus length gradually decreases along the proximal–distal axis. In support of this fact, surgical transposition of an ileal segment to a proximal location results in structural and function adaptation of that segment, even without loss of tissue and overall intestinal length [37]. In contrast, villus length decreases in jejunal segments that are transposed distally [1,37].

Extent of Resection

The extent of resection also impacts adaptation of the residual intestine. As a rule, the magnitude of resection positively correlates with adaptation after surgery [5,38,39]. McDuffie and colleagues [5] report that the magnitude of the change in villus height correlated with the length of the small bowel removed in infants after resection necessitated by necrotizing enterocolitis. However, the ability of the intestine to fully compensate for tissue loss is nonetheless limited. In a retrospective study of 268 patients with intestinal failure (IF), remnant small bowel length of less than 75 cm was associated with greater probability of permanent dependence on PN, whereas the presence of a colon-in-continuity was associated with PN independence [40]. As such, the clinical prognosis for PN independence is highly individual, depending upon both the length of the remaining intestine and the presence of a functional colon.

Enteral Nutrients

Route of Nutrient Administration

The stimulation provided by nutrients in the intestinal lumen is required to maintain the structure of the intestinal mucosa. The absence of enteral nutrients induces mucosal atrophy and decreases digestive enzyme and nutrient transporter activity in animals and humans, even when adequate energy is provided via PN [41–43]. PN-induced mucosal atrophy reverses upon reintroduction of enteral nutrition [41,42], whereas luminal nutrients stimulate adaptation postresection [44,45]. In combination with PN, enteral trophic nutrients can be used to stimulate intestinal adaptation and promote enteral autonomy. In adult patients with SBS, continuous tube feeding (exclusively or in conjunction with oral feeding) has been shown to increase the net absorption of lipids, proteins, and energy compared with oral feeding alone [46]. In the pediatric population, hypocaloric trophic tube feeding can be used in conjunction with PN to stimulate intestinal adaptation and promote enteral autonomy. Despite agreement that earlier initiation of feeds promotes intestinal adaptation and minimizes PN-associated complications [47,48], the timing of initial feeding in SBS remains a point of contention. In general, enteral feeding should be started when the postoperative ileus resolves [49,50]. Initially, continuous, rather than bolus, feeds are preferred due to the lower risk of osmotic diarrhea [51] and increased absorption and tolerance [46]; however, bolus feeds, when tolerated, may eventually be preferred due to their promotion of hormonal stimulation [52].

Nutrient Complexity

Complex nutrients stimulate adaptation to a greater extent than monomeric nutrients do, likely because of the additional digestive activity required prior to nutrient absorption [53]. For example, rats and pigs fed a chow diet after intestinal resection showed greater structural adaptation and digestive enzyme activity than did similar animals that received an elemental diet [45,54]. Similarly, Weser and colleagues [53] demonstrated that disaccharides are more trophic to the rat small bowel than monosaccharides. Such data indicate that nutrients requiring digestive processing prior to absorption serve as important stimuli for intestinal adaptation.

Dietary Fat

Dietary lipids appear to be the most intestinotrophic macronutrient [55,56]. However, long-chain triglycerides require micelle formation for absorption and are not well absorbed in the small intestine of SBS patients due to bile acid deficiency related to extensive distal ileal resection and loss of enterohepatic circulation. A high-fat diet was associated with increased bowel weight and villus height at 14 days postresection in rats [56]. In contrast, a low-fat diet reduced markers of intestinal adaptation compared with a higher-fat isocaloric diet [57].

Certain fats may stimulate adaptation more than others. Long-chain fatty acids are superior to medium-chain fatty acids in inducing epithelial hyperplasia after intestinal resection [58,59]. Among long-chain fatty acids, the relative stimulation provided by saturated versus polyunsaturated fatty acids is not clear. Vanderhoof and associates [60] reported that a diet high in menhaden oil, a polyunsaturated fatty acid, induces greater structural adaptations when compared with safflower oil, a less highly unsaturated fatty acid, or beef tallow, a saturated fatty acid. Similarly, diets high in the polyunsaturated fatty acids docosahexaenoic acid and arachidonic acid stimulated greater increases in mucosal mass than did diets high in safflower oil or hydrogenated coconut oil [55]. In contrast, Keelan and colleagues [61] report that resected rats receiving diets high in saturated fatty acids had increased jejunal glucose transport compared with animals receiving diets high in polyunsaturated fatty acids. Similarly, Sukhotnik et al. [62] showed that villus height and crypt depth increased in resected rats receiving a diet high in palmitic acid, a saturated fatty acid, compared with those receiving a diet with low palmitic acid content. Clinically, patients with SBS and a colon-in-continuity are generally unable to tolerate high-fat diets because of steatorrhea and reduced nutrient absorption. As such, medium-chain triglycerides are sometimes used, despite the fact that they do little to stimulate intestinal adapatation. However, MCTs do not require micelle formation for absorption and may therefore enhance lipid absorption, particularly in the event of cholestasis or bile salt malabsorption. Consequently, a ratio of 30:70 of medium- to long-chain triglyceride has been recommended for SBS patients [63].

Short-Chain Fatty Acids

SCFAs are an important colonic energy source [64] and decrease fluid loss by stimulating sodium and water absorption in the colon [65]. Most SCFAs in the human diet are derived from nonabsorbed carbohydrates that undergo bacterial fermentation in the colon [66]. In unresected rats maintained on PN, supplementation with SCFAs mitigated PN-induced declines in mucosal weight and DNA and RNA content [67]. Furthermore, SCFA supplementation of PN increases nutrient transporter expression and nutrient absorption [68,69]. After experimental resection, PN supplemented with SCFAs enhances intestinal adaptation in mature rats and neonatal piglets [70,71]. The volatile nature of butyrate precludes its direct inclusion in nutritional formulations. Providing carbohydrates that are rapidly fermentable, such as certain prebiotics or fermentable fibers [72], has been shown to be a clinically feasible means to supply SCFAs via fermentation in the lumen of the distal intestine. In a neonatal piglet model of SBS in which animals received 20% of nutrient needs enterally and the reminder parenterally [73], supplementation with short-chain fructooligosaccharides at a level (10 g/L enteral formula) known to produce physiologically relevant butyrate concentrations within the distal intestine [74,75] augmented both structural and functional indices of intestinal adaptation. Humans with SBS and colon-in-continuity also appear to benefit from SCFAs. In a study of six patients with SBS, dietary supplementation for 20 days with pectin, a starch that acts as a substrate for bacterial SCFA production, increased colonic levels of SCFAs and tended to increase fluid absorption [76].

Glutamine

The amino acid glutamine is the primary energy source for enterocytes and appears to have a role in intestinal growth [77]. In animal studies, the impact of glutamine depends on the route of administration. When administered with PN, glutamine counteracts PN-induced intestinal atrophy and improves parameters of postresection adaptation [78–81]. However, enteral glutamine has not been shown to induce intestinal adaptation [82–85], likely because any modest effects of glutamine are masked by the greater trophic stimulation provided by luminal nutrition. Scolapio et al. [86] studied eight SBS patients who received 8 weeks of treatment with oral glutamine (0.45 g/kg/day) and a high-carbohydrate, low-fat diet and found that it did not improve intestinal morphology, gastrointestinal transit, D-xylose absorption, and stool losses.

Intestinotrophic Factors

A variety of putative intestinotrophic factors have been studied for their role in intestinal adaptation. Those studied for clinical use in patients with SBS are the focus of the discussion here. Others are discussed in a recent review by McMellen and colleagues [87].

Preclinical Results

Recombinant Human Growth Hormone

In 2003, the U.S. Food and Drug Administration (FDA) approved recombinant human growth hormone (rhGH; somatropin; Zorbtive, EMD Serono, Rockland, Massachusetts) as a short-term (4-week) treatment for adult SBS patients to facilitate weaning from PN. Preclinical animal studies demonstrate enhanced bowel growth and ion transport with rhGH treatment [88,89], and excised human intestinal tissue displays enhanced amino acid transport and intestinal protein content after growth hormone treatment [90]. The FDA approval of rhGH was based on reductions in PN energy content and frequency of PN administration with rhGH (with or without concomitant glutamine use) compared with placebo [91]. When used in conjunction with rhGH, glutamine (Nutrestore, Emmaus Medical, Inc., Torrance, California) is also approved for treatment of SBS. Despite the impressive reductions in PN use with this combination treatment [91,92], the widespread clinical use of these two therapies has been limited. This seems to be due to concerns regarding the frequency of treatment-emergent adverse events and the attenuation of therapeutic gains after treatment discontinuation [93]. The clinical effects and use of rhGH and glutamine in SBS are discussed in detail in Chapter 20.

Glucagon-Like Peptide-2

First reported to stimulate enterocyte proliferation in 1996 [94], GLP-2 is an intestinotrophic mediator capable of increasing absorptive surface area, preventing mucosal atrophy, and increasing DNA, RNA, and protein concentrations in the intestinal cells of animals sustained on PN [95–97]. In other preclinical models, GLP-2 enhanced nutrient and fluid absorption [98], opposed inflammatory insults [99,100], increased intestinal barrier function [101], and inhibited gastric emptying and stimulated intestinal blood flow [102–104]. In adult SBS subjects, GLP-2 increases intestinal absorption and decreases diarrhea and reduces fecal wet weight, energy, nitrogen, sodium, and potassium losses [105,106]. Additionally, both intravenous and subcutaneous GLP-2 administration increases mesenteric blood flow in healthy adult subjects [103]. Despite these promising effects in adults, only limited data are available regarding GLP-2 use in infants. In piglet models of SBS receiving 40 μg/kg/day split into two daily doses over a 42-day study period, GLP-2 administration had no effect on weight gain, feed intake, or behavior [107], indicating that administration of exogenous GLP-2 may be safe for growing infants. Villus height, crypt depth, and crypt cell proliferation throughout the small intestine and colon were increased, while the rate of apoptosis was decreased throughout both the small and large intestine in GLP-2- versus vehicle control-treated animals. Overall, pharmacological levels of GLP-2 were well tolerated in these piglets, and its trophic effects appear to be confined, as desirable, to the gastrointestinal tract. Additional details, including the clinical use of teduglutide, a longer-acting GLP-2 analog, in humans are discussed in Chapter 19.

EVALUATING INTESTINAL ADAPTATION IN HUMANS

Compared with the wealth of animal studies investigating intestinal adaptation, there are far fewer human studies due to the small population with SBS and the invasive nature of direct assessments. For assessing functional adaptation in patients with SBS, 72-hour nutrient balance studies, with fecal and urinary analyses at baseline and after an intervention, are the gold standard to assess digestion and absorption. This method is, however, complex, costly, and neither patient- nor clinician-friendly. Other parameters that have also been used as indirect surrogate markers of postresection adaptation include PN weaning, enhanced urine output and stool weight after oral intake, and absorption of inert sugars. Inexpensive, valid, and reliable indicators of intestinal adaptation and subsequent long-term dependence on PN are needed.

Citrulline is a nonessential amino acid produced primarily by enterocytes. Therefore, plasma concentration is considered to be a surrogate biomarker for enterocyte mass. In several studies, plasma citrulline concentration was strongly correlated with remnant small bowel length [108–111]. In patients with SBS, a postabsorptive plasma citrulline concentration of <20 μmol/L was predictive of permanent PN dependence when measured more than 2 years after surgery [108]. The clinical value of this test is, however, limited given that several subsequent studies have refuted the utility of plasma citrulline concentration as an accurate assessment of postresection functional adaptation [110–112].

TIMING OF INTESTINAL ADAPTATION IN HUMANS

Intestinal adaptation in adults is thought to occur within 2 years after resection and, perhaps, longer in infants [19]. Messing and associates [3] reported that 95% of patients (n = 64) with SBS on PN achieved enteral autonomy within 2 years postresection. However, some evidence indicates that significant adaptation can occur beyond the 2-year mark. Gouttebel and associates [113] report progressive increases in calcium absorption repeatedly assessed from 1.5 through 120 months in 30 patients after intestinal resection. Similarly, in a cohort of 268 patients with SBS, 26% were weaned from PN more than 2 years after the restoration of digestive continuity [40]. In another report of 72 patients with SBS who achieved enteral autonomy, 47% had been PN dependent for 2 to 5 years and 18% had been PN dependent for >5 years [114]. Finally, trophic factor use may enhance this latent adaptive response. In an open-label, long-term study of teduglutide in patients with SBS treated for up to 30 months, 13/65 (20%) achieved complete independence from PN. As such, although marked intestinal adaptation occurs early in the postoperative course, continued improvements in intestinal absorptive capacity are possible and can occur with trophic factor stimulation many years after resection.

CONCLUSION

A wealth of preclinical data has highlighted many of the mechanisms responsible for adaptation in nonhuman animals, including accelerated enterocyte differentiation, increased expression and activity of nutrient transporters, angiogenesis, and slowed intestinal transit. However, the precise molecular factors contributing to intestinal adaptation in humans remain incompletely understood. Newer, less invasive techniques for assessing intestinal microarchitecture and improved methods of evaluating intestinal absorptive function may provide additional insights into the attributes, timing, and stimuli of postresection adaptation in humans with SBS.

REFERENCES

1. Dowling RH, Booth CC. Functional compensation after small-bowel resection in man. Demonstration by direct measurement. *Lancet.* 1966;2:146–147.
2. Weinstein LD et al. Enhanced intestinal absorption after small bowel resection in man. *Arch Surg.* 1969;99:560–562.
3. Messing B et al. Long-term survival and parenteral nutrition dependence in adult patients with the short bowel syndrome. *Gastroenterology.* 1999;117:1043–1050.
4. Thompson JS et al. Surgical approach to short-bowel syndrome. Experience in a population of 160 patients. *Ann Surg.* 1995;222:600–605.
5. McDuffie LA et al. Intestinal adaptation after small bowel resection in human infants. *J Pediatr Surg.* 2011;46:1045–1051.
6. Doldi SB. Intestinal adaptation following jejuno-ileal bypass. *Clin Nutr.* 1991;10:138–145.
7. Joly F et al. Morphological adaptation with preserved proliferation/transporter content in the colon of patients with short bowel syndrome. *Am J Physiol Gastrointest Liver Physiol.* 2009;297:G116–G123.
8. Loran M, Crocker T. Population dynamics of intestinal epithelia in the rat two months after partial resection of the ileum. *J Cell Biol.* 1963;19:285–291.
9. Pereira-Fantini P et al. Short- and long-term effects of small bowel resection: A unique histological study in a piglet model of short bowel syndrome. *Histochem Cell Biol.* 2011;135(2):195–202.
10. Sacks A et al. Early proliferative events following intestinal resection in the rat. *J Pediatr Gastroenterol Nutr.* 1995;21:158–164.
11. Dowling RH, Booth CC. Structural and functional changes following small intestinal resection in the rat. *Clin Sci.* 1967;32:139–149.
12. Lauronen J et al. Intestinal adaptation after massive proximal small-bowel resection in the pig. *Scand J Gastroenterol.* 1988;33:152–158.
13. O'Connor T et al. Magnitude of functional adaptation after intestinal resection. *Am J Physiol.* 1999;276:R1265–R1275.
14. Vanderhoof J et al. Potential for mucosal adaptation following massive small bowel resection in 3-week-old versus 8-week-old rats. *J Pediatr Gastroenterol Nutr.* 1983;2:672–676.
15. Yang Q, Kock N. Intestinal adaptation following massive ileocecal resection in 20-day-old weanling rats. *J Pediatr Gastroenterol Nutr.* 2010;50:16–21.
16. Martin C et al. Intestinal resection induces angiogenesis within adapting intestinal villi. *J Pediatr Surg.* 2009;44:1077–1083.
17. Rowland K et al. Immediate alterations in intestinal oxygen saturation and blood flow after massive small bowel resection as measured by photoacoustic microscopy. *J Pediatr Surg.* 2012;47:1143–1149.
18. Ulrich-Baker M et al. Blood flow responses to small bowel resection. *Am J Physiol.* 1986;251:G815–G822.
19. Buchman AL et al. AGA technical review on short bowel syndrome and intestinal transplantation. *Gastroenterology.* 2003;124:1111–1134.
20. Buchman A. The medical and surgical management of short bowel syndrome. *Med Gen Med.* 2004;6:12–20.
21. Drucker D et al. Intestinal response to growth factors administered alone or in combination with human [Gly2] glucagon-like peptide 2. *Am J Physiol* 1997;273:G1252–G1262.
22. Yazbeck R et al. Growth factor based therapies and intestinal disease: Is glucagon-like peptide-2 the new way forward? *Cytokine Growth Factor Rev.* 2009;20:175–184.
23. Sigalet DL, Martin GR. Mechanisms underlying intestinal adaptation after massive intestinal resection in the rat. *J Pediatr Surg.* 1998;33:889–892.
24. Hines OJ et al. Adaptation of the Na+/glucose cotransporter following intestinal resection. *J Surg Res.* 1994;57:22–27.
25. Hines OJ et al. Up-regulation of Na+,K+ adenosine triphosphatase after massive intestinal resection. *Surgery.* 1994;116:401–407.
26. Musch MW et al. Region-specific adaptation of apical Na/H exchangers after extensive proximal small bowel resection. *Am J Physiol Gastrointest Liver Physiol.* 2002;283:G975–985.
27. Chaves M et al. Increased activity of digestive enzymes in ileal enterocytes adapting to proximal small bowel resection. *Gut.* 1987;28:981–987.
28. Menge H et al. Cellular adaptation of amino acid transport following intestinal resection in the rat. *J Physiol.* 1983;334:213–223.
29. Nordgaard I et al. Colon as a digestive organ in patients with short bowel. *Lancet.* 1994;343:373–376.
30. Ziegler TR et al. Distribution of the H+/peptide transporter PepT1 in human intestine: Up-regulated expression in the colonic mucosa of patients with short-bowel syndrome. *Am J Clin Nutr.* 2002;75:922–930.

31. Quigley EM, Thompson JS. The motor response to intestinal resection: Motor activity in the canine small intestine following distal resection. *Gastroenterology.* 1993;105:791–798.
32. Nightingale JM et al. Gastrointestinal hormones in short bowel syndrome. Peptide YY may be the "colonic brake" to gastric emptying. *Gut.* 1996;39:267–272.
33. Cosnes J et al. Functional adaptation after extensive small bowel resection in humans. *Eur J Gastroenterol Hepatol.* 1994;6:197–202.
34. Thompson JS et al. Factors affecting outcome following proximal and distal intestinal resection in the dog: An examination of the relative roles of mucosal adaptation, motility, luminal factors, and enteric peptides. *Dig Dis Sci.* 1999;44:63–74.
35. Appleton GV et al. Proximal enterectomy provides a stronger systemic stimulus to intestinal adaptation than distal enterectomy. *Gut.* 1987;28(Suppl):165–168.
36. Cosnes J et al. Role of the ileocecal valve and site of intestinal resection in malabsorption after extensive small bowel resection. *Digestion.* 1978;18:329–336.
37. Altmann GG, Leblond CP. Factors influencing villus size in the small intestine of adult rats as revealed by transposition of intestinal segments. *Am J Anat.* 1970;127:15–36.
38. Porus RL. Epithelial hyperplasia following massive small bowel resection in man. *Gastroenterology.* 1965;48:753–757.
39. Juno RJ et al. A serum factor(s) after small bowel resection induces intestinal epithelial cell proliferation: Effects of timing, site, and extent of resection. *J Pediatr Surg.* 2003;38:868–874.
40. Amiot A et al. Determinants of home parenteral nutrition dependence and survival of 268 patients with non-malignant short bowel syndrome. *Clin Nutr.* 2013;32:368–374.
41. Buchman AL et al. Parenteral nutrition is associated with intestinal morphologic and functional changes in humans. *JPEN J Parenter Enteral Nutr.* 1995;19:453–460.
42. Guedon C et al. Decreased brush border hydrolase activities without gross morphologic changes in human intestinal mucosa after prolonged total parenteral nutrition of adults. *Gastroenterology.* 1986;90:373–378.
43. Levine GM et al. Role of oral intake in maintenance of gut mass and disaccharide activity. *Gastroenterology.* 1974;67:975–982.
44. Feldman EJ, Dowling RH, McNaughton J, Peters TJ. Effects of oral versus intravenous nutrition on intestinal adaptation after small bowel resection in the dog. *Gastroenterology.* 1976;70:712–719.
45. Ford WD et al. Total parenteral nutrition inhibits intestinal adaptive hyperplasia in young rats: Reversal by feeding. *Surgery.* 1984;96:527–534.
46. Joly F et al. Tube feeding improves intestinal absorption in short bowel syndrome patients. *Gastroenterology.* 2009;136:824–831.
47. Gutierrez I et al. Neonatal short bowel syndrome. *Semin Fetal Neonatal Med.* 2011;16:157–163.
48. Kocoshis S. Medical management of pediatric intestinal failure. *Semin Pediatr Surg.* 2010;19:20–26.
49. Andorsky D et al. Nutritional and other postoperative management of neonates with short bowel syndrome correlates with clinical outcomes. *J Pediatr.* 2001;139:27–33.
50. Quiros-Tejeira R et al. Long-term parenteral nutritional support and intestinal adaptation in children with short bowel syndrome: A 25-year experience. *J Pediatr.* 2004;145:157–163.
51. Vanderhoof J, Matya S. Enteral and parenteral nutrition in patients with short-bowel syndrome. *Eur J Pediatr Surg.* 1999;9:214–219.
52. Rudolph J, Squires R. Current concepts in the medical management of pediatric intestinal failure. *Curr Opin Organ Transplant.* 2010;15:324–329.
53. Weser E et al. Intestinal adaptation. Different growth responses to disaccharides compared with monosaccharides in rat small bowel. *Gastroenterology.* 1986;91:1521–1527.
54. Bines JE et al. Influence of diet complexity on intestinal adaptation following massive small bowel resection in a preclinical model. *J Gastroenterol Hepatol.* 2002;17:1170–1179.
55. Kollman K et al. Dietary lipids influence intestinal adaptation after massive bowel resection. *J Pediatr Gastroenterol Nutr.* 1999;28:41–45.
56. Sukhotnik I et al. Effect of dietary fat on early morphological intestinal adaptation in a rat with short bowel syndrome. *Pediatr Surg Int.* 2004;20:419–424.
57. Sukhotnik I et al. Low-fat diet impairs postresection intestinal adaptation in a rat model of short bowel syndrome. *J Pediatr Surg.* 2003;38:1182–1187.
58. Vanderhoof JA et al. Effect of high percentage medium-chain triglyceride diet on mucosal adaptation following massive bowel resection in rats. *JPEN J Parenter Enteral Nutr.* 1984;8:685–689.
59. Chen WJ et al. Effects of lipids on intestinal adaptation following 60% resection in rats. *J Surg Res.* 1995;58:253–259.

60. Vanderhoof JA et al. Effects of dietary menhaden oil on mucosal adaptation after small bowel resection in rats. *Gastroenterology.* 1994;106:94–99.
61. Keelan M et al. Intestinal morphology and transport after ileal resection in rat is modified by dietary fatty acids. *Clin Invest Med.* 1996;19:63–70.
62. Sukhotnik I et al. Dietary palmitic acid modulates intestinal re-growth after massive small bowel resection in a rat. *Pediatr Surg Int.* 2008;24:1313–1321.
63. Jeppesen P, Mortensen P. The influence of a preserved colon on the absorption of medium chain fat in patients with small bowel resection. *Gut.* 1998;43:478–483.
64. Nordgaard I et al. Importance of colonic support for energy absorption as small-bowel failure proceeds. *Am J Clin Nutr.* 1996;64:222–231.
65. Byrne T et al. Bowel rehabilitation: An alternative to long-term parenteral nutrition and intestinal transplantation for some patients with short bowel syndrome. *Transplant Proc.* 2002;34:887–890.
66. Macfarlane S, Macfarlane GT. Regulation of short-chain fatty acid production. *Proc Nutr Soc.* 2003; 62:67–72.
67. Koruda MJ et al. Parenteral nutrition supplemented with short-chain fatty acids: Effect on the small-bowel mucosa in normal rats. *Am J Clin Nutr.* 1990;51:685–689.
68. Tappenden KA, McBurney MI. Systemic short-chain fatty acids rapidly alter gastrointestinal structure, function, and expression of early response genes. *Dig Dis Sci.* 1998;43:1526–1536.
69. Tappenden KA et al. Short-chain fatty acid-supplemented total parenteral nutrition alters intestinal structure, glucose transporter 2 (GLUT2) mRNA and protein, and proglucagon mRNA abundance in normal rats. *Am J Clin Nutr.* 1998;68:118–125.
70. Bartholome AL et al. Supplementation of total parenteral nutrition with butyrate acutely increases structural aspects of intestinal adaptation after an 80% jejunoileal resection in neonatal piglets. *JPEN J Parenter Enteral Nutr.* 2004;28:210–223.
71. Tappenden KA et al. Short-chain fatty acid-supplemented total parenteral nutrition enhances functional adaptation to intestinal resection in rats. *Gastroenterology.* 1997;112:792–802.
72. Stewart M et al. Fructooligosaccharides exhibit more rapid fermentation than long-chain inulin in an in vitro fermentation system. *Nutr Res.* 2008;28:329–334.
73. Barnes J et al. Intestinal adaptation is stimulated by partial enteral nutrition supplemented with the prebiotic short-chain fructooligosaccharide in a neonatal IF piglet model. *JPEN J Parenter Enteral Nutr.* 2012;36:524–537.
74. Flickinger EA et al. Glucose-based oligosaccharides exhibit different in vitro fermentation patterns and affect in vivo apparent nutrient digestibility and microbial populations in dogs. *J Nutr.* 2000;130:1267–1273.
75. Correa-Matos NJ et al. Fermentable fiber reduces recovery time and improves intestinal function in piglets following *Salmonella typhimurium* infection. *J Nutr.* 2003;133:1845–1852.
76. Atia A et al. Macronutrient absorption characteristics in humans with short bowel syndrome and jejunocolonic anastomosis: Starch is the most important carbohydrate substrate, although pectin supplementation may modestly enhance short chain fatty acid production and fluid absorption. *JPEN J Parenter Enteral Nutr.* 2011;35:229–240.
77. Windmueller HG, Spaeth AE. Identification of ketone bodies and glutamine as the major respiratory fuels in vivo for postabsorptive rat small intestine. *J Biol Chem.* 1978;253:69–76.
78. O'Dwyer ST et al. Maintenance of small bowel mucosa with glutamine-enriched parenteral nutrition. *JPEN J Parenter Enteral Nutr.* 1989;13:579–585.
79. Tamada H et al. The dipeptide alanyl-glutamine prevents intestinal mucosal atrophy in parenterally fed rats. *JPEN J Parenter Enteral Nutr.* 1992;16:110–116.
80. Tamada H et al. Alanyl glutamine-enriched total parenteral nutrition restores intestinal adaptation after either proximal or distal massive resection in rats. *JPEN J Parenter Enteral Nutr.* 1993;17:236–242.
81. Gu Y et al. Effects of growth hormone (rhGH) and glutamine supplemented parenteral nutrition on intestinal adaptation in short bowel rats. *Clin Nutr.* 2001;20:159–166.
82. de Souza Neves J et al. Glutamine alone or combined with short-chain fatty acids fails to enhance gut adaptation after massive enterectomy in rats. *Acta Cir Bras.* 2006;21(Suppl 4):2–7.
83. Michail S et al. Effect of glutamine-supplemented elemental diet on mucosal adaptation following bowel resection in rats. *J Pediatr Gastroenterol Nutr.* 1995;21:394–398.
84. Vanderhoof JA et al. Effects of oral supplementation of glutamine on small intestinal mucosal mass following resection. *J Am Coll Nutr.* 1992;11:223–227.

85. Yang H et al. No effect of bolus glutamine supplementation on the postresectional adaptation of small bowel mucosa in rats receiving chow ad libitum. *Dig Surg*. 2000;17:256–260.
86. Scolapio JS et al. Effect of glutamine in short-bowel syndrome. *Clin Nutr*. 2001;20:319–323.
87. McMellen ME et al. Growth factors: Possible roles for clinical management of the short bowel syndrome. *Semin Pediatr Surg*. 2010;19:35–43.
88. Benhamou P et al. Human recombinant growth hormone increases small bowel lengthening after massive small bowel resection in piglets. *J Pediatr Surg*. 1997;32:1332–1336.
89. Guarino A et al. In vivo and in vitro effects of human growth hormone on rat intestine ion transport. *Pediatr Res*. 1995;37:576–580.
90. Inoue Y et al. Growth hormone enhances amino acid uptake by the human small intestine. *Ann Surg*. 1994;219:715–724.
91. Byrne TA et al. Growth hormone, glutamine, and an optimal diet reduces parenteral nutrition in patients with short bowel syndrome: A prospective, randomized, placebo-controlled, double-blind clinical trial. *Ann Surg*. 2005;242:655–661.
92. Byrne T et al. A new treatment for patients with short-bowel syndrome. *Ann Surg*. 1995;222:243–255.
93. Wales PW et al. Human growth hormone and glutamine for patients with short bowel syndrome. *Cochrane Database Syst Rev*. 2010;(6):CD006321.
94. Drucker D et al. Induction of intestinal epithelial proliferation by glucagon-like peptide-2. *Proc Natl Acad Sci USA*. 1996;93:7911–7916.
95. Burrin D et al. Glucagon-like peptide-2 dose-dependently activates intestinal cell survival and proliferation in neonatal piglets. *Endocrinology*. 2005;146:22–32.
96. Litvak D et al. Glucagon-like peptide-2 is a potent growth factor for small intestine and colon. *J Gastrointest Surg*. 1998;2:146–150.
97. Tsai C et al. Intestinal growth-promoting properties of glucagon-like peptide-2 in mice. *Am J Physiol*. 1997;273:E77–E84.
98. Brubaker P et al. Intestinal function in mice with small bowel growth induced by glucagon-like peptide-2. *Am J Physiol*. 1997;272:E1050–E1058.
99. Ivory C et al. Interleukin-10-independent anti-inflammatory actions of glucagon-like peptide 2. *Am J Physiol Gastrointest Liver Physiol*. 2008;295:G1202–G1210.
100. Sigalet D et al. Enteric neural pathways mediate the anti-inflammatory actions of glucagon-like peptide 2. *Am J Physiol Gastrointest Liver Physiol*. 2007;293:G211–G221.
101. Moran G et al. GLP-2 enhances barrier formation and attenuates TNFα-induced changes in a Caco-2 cell model of the intestinal barrier. *Regul Peptides*. 2012;178:95–101.
102. Bremholm L et al. The effect of glucagon-like peptide-2 on mesenteric blood flow and cardiac parameters in end-jejunostomy short bowel patients. *Regul Pept*. 2011;168:32–38.
103. Bremholm L et al. Glucagon-like peptide-2 increases mesenteric blood flow in humans. *Scand J Gastroenterol*. 2009;44:314–319.
104. Hoyerup P et al. Glucagon-like peptide-2 stimulates mucosal microcirculation measured by laser Doppler flow-metry in end-jejunostomy short bowel syndrome patients. *Regul Peptides*. 2013;180:12–16.
105. Jeppesen P et al. Glucagon-like peptide 2 improves nutrient absorption and nutritional status in short-bowel patients with no colon. *Gastroenterology*. 2001;120:806–815.
106. Naimi R et al. A dose-equivalent comparison of the effects of continuous subcutaneous glucagon-like peptide 2 (GLP-2) infusions versus meal related GLP-2 injections in the treatment of short bowel syndrome (SBS) patients. *Regul Peptides*. 2013;184:47–53.
107. Sigalet D et al. Effects of chronic glucagon-like peptide-2 therapy during weaning in neonatal pigs. *Regul Peptides*. 2014;88:70–80.
108. Crenn P et al. Postabsorptive plasma citrulline concentration is a marker of absorptive enterocyte mass and intestinal failure in humans. *Gastroenterology*. 2000;119:1496–1505.
109. Santarpia L et al. Citrulline blood levels as indicators of residual intestinal absorption in patients with short bowel syndrome. *Ann Nutr Metab*. 2008;53:137–142.
110. Jianfeng G et al. Serum citrulline is a simple quantitative marker for small intestinal enterocytes mass and absorption function in short bowel patients. *J Surg Res*. 2005;127:177–182.
111. Papadia C et al. Plasma citrulline concentration: A reliable marker of small bowel absorptive capacity independent of intestinal inflammation. *Am J Gastroenterol*. 2007;102:1474–1482.
112. Peters JH et al. Poor diagnostic accuracy of a single fasting plasma citrulline concentration to assess intestinal energy absorption capacity. *Am J Gastroenterol*. 2007;102:2814–2819.

113. Gouttebel MC et al. Intestinal adaptation in patients with short bowel syndrome. Measurement by calcium absorption. *Dig Dis Sci.* 1989;34:709–715.
114. Pironi L et al. Survival of patients identified as candidates for intestinal transplantation: A 3-year prospective follow-up. *Gastroenterology.* 2008;135:61–71.
115. Schwartz L et al. Long-term teduglutide for the treatment of patients with intestinal failure associated with short bowel syndrome. *Clin Transl Gastroenterol.* 2016;7:e142. doi: 10.1038/ctg.2015.69.

5 Diarrhea in Short Bowel Syndrome

Badr Al-Bawardy and Vandana Nehra

CONTENTS

KEY POINTS

- Diarrhea is the predominant symptom in short bowel syndrome (SBS).
- Diarrhea in SBS may result in volume depletion, nutritional deficiencies, and/or metabolic complications and negatively impacts patient quality of life.
- Understanding the multiple underlying mechanisms contributing to diarrhea in SBS is essential to allow tailoring of management.
- Management of diarrhea in SBS involves excluding readily treatable causes and addressing the associated complications of diarrhea followed by symptomatic treatment.

INTRODUCTION

Diarrhea is the predominant symptom in patients with short bowel syndrome (SBS). There are multiple underlying pathophysiologic mechanisms that interact to cause diarrhea in these patients. Diarrhea is an important problem in SBS as it may result in electrolyte disturbances, volume depletion, weight loss, and numerous nutritional deficiencies and represents an important source of frustration negatively affecting these patients' quality of life. Indeed, when severe, diarrhea may require frequent intravenous (IV) fluid supplementation or parenteral nutrition (PN). Even in the absence of long-term PN, patients with SBS have a significantly lower quality of life in terms of social functioning and mental health in comparison with matched controls [1]. This is mainly due to the diarrhea and the resulting need for hospitalization for dehydration and management of nutritional deficiencies. In addition, SBS patients with large-volume diarrhea often decrease their oral intake to prevent high stool output or ingest increased oral fluids that result in a worsening of the diarrhea, further contributing to the detriment in their quality of life [2]. Therefore, identifying and treating the underlying cause(s) of diarrhea in these patients is essential to implement a successful management strategy. Fortunately, the majority of patients with SBS are able to control the diarrhea, at least to a degree, and maintain social functioning in the form of employment and activities of daily living [3].

MECHANISMS OF DIARRHEA IN SBS

There are multiple mechanisms contributing to the diarrhea that occurs in SBS. These factors often interact so that the diarrhea in SBS patients is typically multifactorial (see list below). These are discussed in more detail in the following section.

Major causes of diarrhea in short bowel syndrome

- Loss of intestinal absorptive area
- Small intestinal bacterial overgrowth
- Gastric hypersecretion (up to 6 months postresection)
- Rapid gastrointestinal transit (modulating hormones: PYY and GLP-1/2)
- Bile acid deficiency
- Pancreatic enzyme/nutrient mismatch
- Miscellaneous causes
    - Infection (e.g., *Clostridium difficile*)
    - Medications (e.g., sorbitol containing)
    - Active underlying bowel disease (e.g., Crohn's disease, radiation enteritis)
    - Partial small bowel obstruction (ostomy)

Loss of Absorptive Area

One of the most important mechanisms of diarrhea in SBS is loss of intestinal absorptive area. The small bowel is responsible for absorption of the majority of the nutrients and the 7–9 L of water and electrolytes it receives daily from both endogenous and exogenous sources. The normal length of the small bowel is highly variable but is estimated to be between 3 and 8 m [4]. To maintain a positive water balance, at least 100 cm of intact jejunum is required [5]. In addition, the colon has inherent absorptive capacity, and patients with an intact colon are less likely to require fluid supplementation [6]. Presence of the colon-in-continuity after small bowel resection has an important role in energy salvage as unabsorbed carbohydrates are converted by bacterial fermentation to short-chain fatty acids, which not only provide an energy source but also promote colonic absorption of water and electrolytes [7]. Individuals generally tolerate more extensive resections of small intestine if the colon is maintained in continuity. Studies have shown that patients can live independent of PN with about 70 cm of small intestine in colonic continuity; however, in the absence of colonic continuity, about 110 cm of healthy small intestine is required for patients to survive independent of PN [8].

The site of small bowel resection (i.e., jejunal vs. ileal) plays an important pathophysiologic role. As described in detail in Chapter 4, after major resection, the small intestine undergoes adaptive changes to enhance the absorptive surface. Most of the adaptation, however, occurs in the ileum, with only minimal (if any) changes observed in the jejunum [9]. Absorption of many electrolytes and micronutrients including iron, calcium, magnesium, phosphorus, and folic acid takes place in the duodenum and jejunum. The proximal 100–200 cm of the jejunum is also the main site for absorption of carbohydrates, protein, and water-soluble vitamins [10].

The distal 60 cm of the ileum is a specialized site for absorption of intrinsic factor-bound vitamin B_{12}. The terminal ileum is also responsible for bile acid absorption and maintenance of the enterohepatic circulation. Approximately 95% of the bile acids are reabsorbed and transported back to the liver. Resection of <100 cm of terminal ileum may result in bile acid malabsorption and choleric diarrhea because of impairment of the enterohepatic circulation and entry of unabsorbed bile acids into the colon [11]. The α hydroxyl groups of the unabsorbed bile acids, deoxycholic acid and chenodeoxycholic acid, are responsible for enhanced fluid and electrolyte secretion into the colon and increased colonic contractility [12]. The mechanisms that promote this secretory effect in the colon resulting in diarrhea include activation of adenylate cyclase and increased colonic mucosal permeability [13]. The bile acid pool is maintained by supplementation of the enterohepatic circulation by accelerated hepatic bile acid synthesis. Use of bile acid binders in this setting may control the diarrhea; however, patient acceptance can be problematic. In contrast, resection of >100 cm of ileum results in interruption of the enterohepatic circulation of bile acids and eventual depletion of bile acids, resulting in fat malabsorption and steatorrhea. Use of bile acid binders in this setting, which is far more common in SBS, may worsen the diarrhea by binding already depleted bile acids, further increasing fat malabsorption. In this situation, dietary fat restriction and supplementation with medium chain triglycerides should be considered to reduce the diarrhea and steatorrhea. Importantly, in patients with SBS and absence of colon, there is no role for use of bile acid binders, and dietary restriction of fat is also unnecessary as it will only decrease calories available for absorption.

Loss of Ileocecal Valve (or Terminal Ileum)

The ileocecal valve has been suggested to function to allow more nutrient and water absorption by slowing intestinal transit. Although this property is often attributed to the ileocecal valve, it may actually be mediated by the secretion of hormones that are produced in the terminal ileum and proximal colon, including glucagon-like peptides 1 and 2 (GLP-1 and GLP-2) and peptide YY (PYY). Loss of the distal ileum and proximal colon (and ileocecal valve by necessity), a common situation in SBS, causes more rapid intestinal transit leading to diarrhea.

Small Intestinal Bacterial Overgrowth

The ileocecal valve does serve to prevent reflux of colonic content into the small bowel, and resection of the ileocecal valve with colonic anastomosis increases the risk of small intestinal bacterial overgrowth (SIBO)-related diarrhea [4]. Other factors that contribute to the increased risk of SIBO in SBS patients include decreased effective peristalsis in the remaining bowel as it dilates in an effort to adapt to loss of absorptive area and use of antidiarrheal and antisecretory agents [14]. These complex surgical patients are also at risk for intestinal strictures (e.g., anastomotic) and blind loops, which may also facilitate SIBO.

SIBO is common in patients with SBS, although data regarding the exact prevalence are lacking. There are multiple factors that contribute to the development of diarrhea secondary to SIBO in patients with SBS. Deconjugation of bile acids in the intestinal lumen will result in fat malabsorption and diarrhea. Deconjugation of bile acids can result in the production of substances that exert deleterious effects on the intestinal epithelium, causing protein and carbohydrate malabsorption [14]. In addition, gut bacteria can have direct inflammatory effects on the intestinal epithelium, resulting in villous atrophy and malabsorption [14].

The diagnosis of SIBO can be made by culturing small bowel aspirates or hydrogen breath testing. Both tests have their limitation. For example, false-positive cultures can occur due to contamination during sample collection, while false-negative results can also occur due to sampling error or from difficulty culturing anaerobic microorganisms. In the setting of rapid intestinal transit, an expected situation in SBS, false-positive hydrogen breath test can occur due to metabolism of glucose by normal colonic flora and essentially precludes its usefulness in this setting [14].

Patients with SBS are at risk for development of a rare neurological disorder caused by an accumulation in D-lactic acid after ingestion of a large carbohydrate load. While not necessary related to SIBO, D-lactic acidosis occurs when the unabsorbed carbohydrates are metabolized by colonic bacteria to D-lactic acid, which is then absorbed and results in an unexplained anion gap metabolic acidosis [15]. These patients present with neurologic symptoms, including altered mental status, slurred speech, ataxia, and memory loss. The diagnosis is confirmed by a special assay for detection of D-lactate since the conventional lactate assay only measures the L-isomer. As such, a high index of suspicion for this condition should be present in SBS patients presenting with neurologic symptoms, anion-gap metabolic acidosis, and normal L-lactate level. Similar to SIBO, management often includes treatment with oral antimicrobial agents. A low-carbohydrate diet and correction of dehydration, if present, are also commonly advised, as is administration of sodium bicarbonate in cases of severely symptomatic D-lactic acidosis. Anecdotal reports have also suggested a benefit from use of probiotics, synbiotics, and autologous gastrointestinal reconstruction [16]. D-Lactate toxicity has been reported in patients with SBS after the administration of probiotics consisting of D-lactate-producing species and with the use of antibiotics that select for *Lactobacillus* [17].

Gastric Hypersecretion

Gastric secretion is increased in the immediate postoperative period in SBS and can last up to 6 months. An increase in the basal acid output and pentagastrin-stimulated acid output has been reported after resection of >60 cm of the terminal ileum in males with Crohn's disease [18]. Basal acid hypersecretion has also been demonstrated in a pediatric SBS population [19].

The primary mechanism for increased acid secretion after intestinal resection is the loss of negative feedback; cholecystokinin and secretin signaling to gastrin-producing cells in the gastric antrum is lost and gastrin secretion is unopposed, leading to an increase in gastric acid production. This hypersecretory state contributes to diarrhea and steatorrhea primarily by increasing the sheer volume delivered to the upper gut; however, it also stimulates intestinal peristalsis, deactivates pancreatic enzymes secondary to the low pH, and precipitates bile salts, thereby disrupting micelle formation.

Loss of Intestinal Motility-Modulating Hormones

Dysmotility and rapid intestinal transit play a central role in promoting diarrhea in SBS. Intestinal motility is influenced by multiple gut hormones that are affected in the setting of massive intestinal resections. GLP-1, GLP-2, and PYY are examples of such motility-modulating gut hormones. These hormones are produced by L cells in the distal ileum and proximal colon, both common sites of resection in SBS, as previously mentioned, and are released in response to intraluminal nutrients including fat. One of the roles of these hormones is to slow gastric and intestinal transit. These hormones are responsible for what is referred to as the jejunal and ileal brakes. Therefore, rapid gastrointestinal transit is an expected consequence contributing to diarrhea in SBS patients with ileal and colonic resection.

A study of jejunostomy patients has demonstrated slower gastric emptying of liquids in jejunostomy patients with a preserved colon compared with those with colonic resection [20]. In addition, a subsequent study has correlated a decrease in PYY concentration in SBS patients with rapid gastric emptying and an absent colon [21]. It has also been demonstrated that SBS patients with colonic preservation have higher GLP-1 and GLP-2 concentrations and slower gastric emptying than do SBS patients without a colon [22].

Other Causes

Diarrhea in SBS can also occur as a consequence of infections, medications, and underlying bowel disease. SBS patients have multiple risk factors that increase their chances for developing *Clostridium difficile* infection, including [23]

- A high rate of hospitalization and institutionalization for management of fluid and electrolyte derangements as well as nutritional deficiencies; and
- Frequent exposure to antibiotics to treat infectious complications, such as catheter-related bloodstream infections and SIBO.

There is also a common misconception that patients with an end-jejunostomy or ileostomy cannot acquire *C. difficile*; however, numerous reports refute this notion [24].

Underlying bowel disease such as Crohn's disease or radiation enteritis can also contribute to diarrhea present in SBS. As a result of multiple resections, Crohn's disease remains one of the most common causes of SBS, accounting for up to 21% of all causes of intestinal failure [25]. The recurrence rate of Crohn's disease after surgical resection is highly variable and has ranged between 11% and 32% at 5 years [26]. Therefore, in Crohn's patients with SBS, investigating for disease recurrence or activity as a contributor to diarrhea with radiographic imaging and/or endoscopy is imperative as the disease, and thus the diarrhea, can often be improved with medical therapy.

A detailed review of the medication profile is valuable in SBS patients with diarrhea as many different medications may contribute. Antibiotic-induced diarrhea unrelated to *C. difficile* infection is common. Other medications frequently implicated include elixirs containing sorbitol (or other sugar alcohols), selective serotonin reuptake inhibitors, nonsteroidal anti-inflammatory drugs, and proton pump inhibitors [27].

CONSEQUENCES OF DIARRHEA IN SBS

Diarrhea in SBS may result in significant fluid, electrolyte, and acid-base derangements; metabolic disorders; and multiple micronutrient and macronutrient deficiencies (see list below). This section will discuss these consequences briefly as they will be covered thoroughly in other chapters in this book.

Major consequences of diarrhea in short bowel syndrome

- Fluid, electrolyte and acid-base imbalances
  - Hypokalemia, hypocalcemia, hypomagnesemia and metabolic acidosis
- Macronutrient deficiencies
- Micronutrient deficiencies
- Metabolic complications
  - Cholelithiasis, liver disease, nephrolithiasis, metabolic bone disease

Fluid, Electrolyte, and Acid-Base Imbalances

Fluid losses leading to dehydration and hypovolemia can result in many complications, including chronic kidney disease. The major contributor to fluid loss in SBS is the loss of absorptive area; the capability to maintain a positive net fluid balance is related to the length of healthy bowel remaining and degree of intestinal adaptation that has occurred. The presence of remaining colon-in-continuity is particularly important. A negative water balance does not typically occur in the setting of an intact colon due to its inherent absorptive capacity. Sodium losses in patients with a proximal jejunostomy can approach 100 mEq/L of small bowel effluent [28]. This will lead to net water losses as water absorption through the intestinal lumen is coupled to sodium. Therefore, use of oral rehydration solutions (ORSs), described further in Chapter 11, plays a central role in fluid and electrolyte replacement in SBS patients with high stool output, especially in those without colon remaining.

The main electrolyte abnormalities encountered in patients with SBS include hypokalemia, hypocalcemia, hypomagnesemia, and hypophosphatemia. Hypokalemia generally results from large-volume diarrhea, which can also be associated with loss of bicarbonate and development of hyperchloremic metabolic acidosis. Hypocalcemia is occasionally seen due to low vitamin D levels that result from malabsorption of fat-soluble vitamins and binding of calcium to the unabsorbed fatty acids and being excreted in the stool. Hypomagnesemia also results from high gastrointestinal fluid losses, most commonly in SBS patients with an ostomy, and can be challenging to correct via oral supplementation given its diarrheagenic effect. Magnesium is chelated in the lumen of the bowel by fatty acids, resulting in malabsorption [3]. Secondary hyperaldosteronism develops in SBS due to chronic dehydration from significant losses of water and sodium. This contributes to magnesium deficiency by increasing urinary losses. In addition, long-term use of proton pump inhibitors has also been associated with development of hypomagnesemia [29]. Lastly, hypophosphatemia may occur as a result of malabsorption or refeeding syndrome and can precipitate critical cardiovascular and neuromuscular compromise. Phosphorus levels must be monitored closely, particularly in the period immediately after initiating nutrition support, and deficiency recognized and replaced promptly. Electrolyte and acid-base disorders in SBS are discussed in more detail in Chapter 6.

Macronutrient and Micronutrient Deficiencies

Both macronutrient and micronutrient deficiencies frequently complicate the clinical course in patients with SBS as a result of chronic diarrhea and/or malabsorption. SBS patients mainly manifest with deficiencies of the fat-soluble vitamins A, D, E, and K in the setting of fat malabsorption and steatorrhea [30]. Water-soluble vitamin deficiencies are less common, as they are absorbed in the proximal small bowel, except for vitamin B_{12}. Because vitamin B_{12} is predominantly absorbed by active transport by receptors in the distal ileum, most SBS patients will require vitamin B_{12} supplementation or deficiency will inevitably follow. Diarrhea in SBS can also result in a variety of trace element deficiencies, including zinc, copper, and selenium. Vitamin and trace element deficiencies in SBS are described in detail in Chapters 12 and 13.

Metabolic Consequences

Metabolic consequences associated with the diarrhea and malabsorption occurring in SBS include, but are not limited to, cholelithiasis, nephrolithiasis, metabolic bone disease, and liver disease. These disorders are discussed further in Chapters 7, 8, and 26, respectively.

MANAGEMENT OF DIARRHEA IN SBS

The management of diarrhea in SBS involves not only the reduction in stool output but also the correction of existing fluid and electrolyte imbalances and macronutrient and micronutrient deficiencies while monitoring and, whenever possible, preventing metabolic complications. As the details of the individual treatments will be covered in other chapters, we focus here on summarizing the overall approach to management of the diarrhea that often occurs in patients with SBS.

The approach to diarrhea in SBS starts with an evaluation of the potential etiology excluding readily correctable causes not directly related to the altered bowel anatomy. This includes a careful review of the medication list and discontinuing possible offending medications. In addition, underlying gastrointestinal infection, particularly *C. difficile*, should be evaluated. The presence of active underlying bowel disease such as Crohn's disease, radiation enteritis, celiac disease, or microscopic colitis should be investigated and treated when present. Partial or intermittent small bowel obstruction, especially in ostomy patients, can result in diarrhea and should be investigated with radiographic and/or endoscopic imaging. Once this initial evaluation is completed, when diarrhea persists, the management should focus on the altered bowel anatomy and the variety of mechanisms potentially contributing to the diarrhea as described previously. This includes incorporating dietary and fluid modifications based on the remaining bowel anatomy, treating gastric acid hypersecretion, judicious use of antimotility agents, treating SIBO when identified, and, occasionally, considering a trial of pancreatic enzymes if there is concern of mismatch of nutrient and enzyme mixing (Figure 5.1).

Diet Considerations

After a resection of the small bowel, most patients who develop SBS experience significant malabsorption. A low simple sugar diet decreases luminal fluid shifts, which contribute to osmotic diarrhea. Hypertonic substances promote influx of water into the intestinal lumen, particularly the jejunum, which results in fluid losses as diarrhea. In absence of colon-in-continuity, fat restriction only limits ingested calories; hence, in patients with an end-jejunostomy, there is no benefit from restriction of dietary fat or oxalate. However, when the colon is present in continuity, the increased concentration of unabsorbed fatty acids entering the colon would predispose to worsening diarrhea and hyperoxaluria. Therefore, this group will benefit from a low-fat, oxalate-restricted diet.

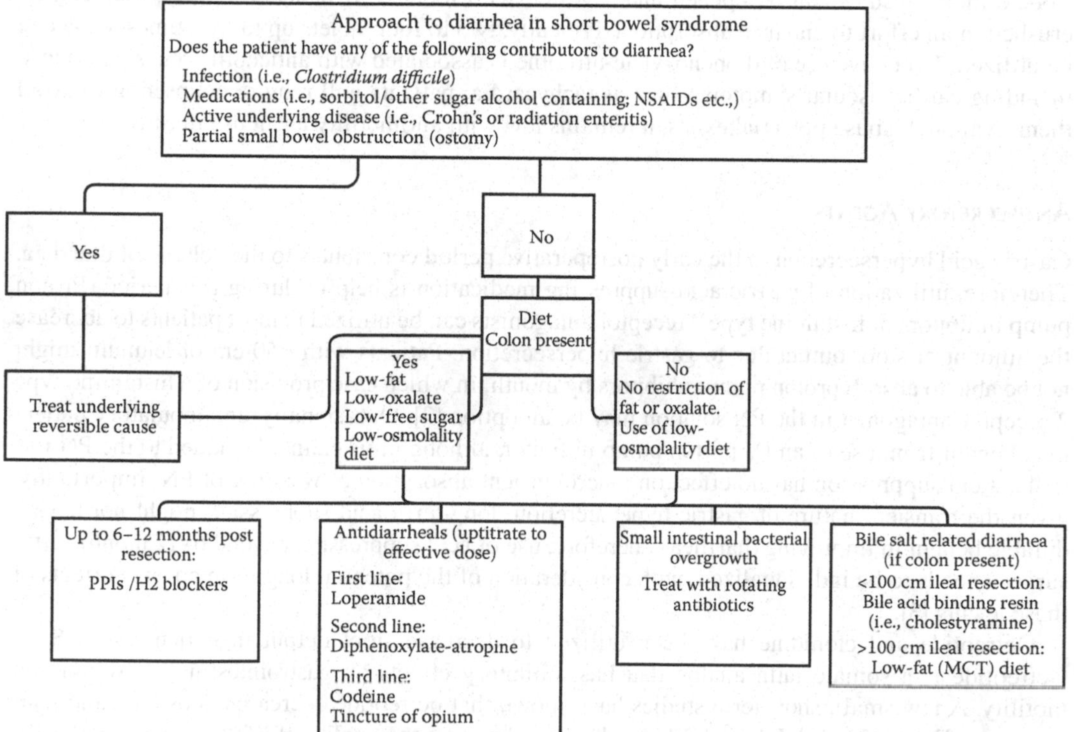

FIGURE 5.1 Suggested algorithmic approach to diarrhea in short bowel syndrome. MCT, medium chain triglyceride; NSAIDs, non-steroidal anti-inflammatory drugs; PPIs, proton pump inhibitors.

Oral Rehydration Solutions

In addition to dietary modifications, utilization of ORSs should be pursued in patients with significant volume depletion secondary to diarrhea. ORSs are often helpful in decreasing the need for IV fluids in SBS patients, particularly those with an end-jejunostomy. ORSs promote absorption of fluid and electrolytes via glucose-mediated active and passive sodium absorption in the jejunum via the sodium glucose cotransporter (SGLT1) and other mechanisms such as solvent drag and active sodium absorption [31]. Although a sodium concentration of 120 mmol/L is optimal for jejunal absorption, its use is limited by palatability. Concentrations of 70–90 mmol/L are generally acceptable from both effectiveness and adherence perspectives [32]. ORS is recommended to be used as a sipping solution throughout the day to promote absorption. Several tips are available to enhance palatability and, thus, adherence with its use (e.g., mix with sugar-free flavoring, refrigerate).

Antimotility Agents

Antimotility agents play an important role in slowing intestinal transit time and promoting absorption of nutrients by prolonging mucosal contact time, thus decreasing stool output. These agents include loperamide, diphenoxylate-atropine, codeine phosphate, and tincture of opium. These medications should generally be administered 30–60 minutes prior to meals for maximal benefit. Titration of the dosage is recommended until the desired effect or maximal amount is achieved. Adjustments can be made every 3–5 days. Patients occasionally benefit from using a combination of these medications. Loperamide and diphenoxylate-atropine are typically the first-line option due to their efficacy and benign side effect profile. Multiple formulations are available. While liquid formulations are available, most are sorbitol-based elixirs that may actually aggravate the diarrhea. Loperamide capsules can be opened and ingested with food or, if tablets are used, they can be crushed in an effort to enhance absorption. Typically, two to four tablets up to four times a day can be utilized. Excessive use of diphenoxylate-atropine is associated with anticholinergic side effects, including cardiovascular symptoms such as tachycardia; patients will require counseling to avoid them. Although abuse potential exists, it remains low with antimotility agent use in SBS.

Antisecretory Agents

Gastric acid hypersecretion in the early postoperative period contributes to the volume of diarrhea. Therefore, utilization of gastric acid-suppressing medication is helpful during this period. Proton pump inhibitors or histamine type 2 receptor antagonists can be utilized in most patients to decrease the amount of stool output due to gastric hypersecretion. Patients with <50 cm of jejunum might not be able to absorb proton pump inhibitors by mouth, in which case provision of a histamine type 2 receptor antagonist in the PN solution may be an option [3]. Occasionally, an ambulatory patient may benefit from use of an IV proton pump inhibitor, although this cannot be added to the PN formula. Acid suppression has no effect on macronutrient absorption or weaning of PN. Importantly, given the transient nature of gastric hypersecretion, long-term acid suppression might not have a durable benefit in improving diarrhea. Therefore, use of acid suppression beyond 6–12 months after surgery needs to be individualized, with consideration of the potential long-term adverse effects of these agents [3].

Octreotide and clonidine have been utilized to decrease stool output in patients with SBS. Octreotide is a somatostatin analog that has inhibitory effects on gastrointestinal secretion and motility. A few small, short-term studies have shown that octreotide decreases ileostomy and jejunostomy effluent [33–35]. It has also been shown to improve the quality of life in patients with SBS [36]. Although octreotide reduces stool volume, it does not improve nutrient and fat absorption and it has not been shown to aid in the weaning of PN [37]. There are drawbacks to the use of octreotide, including possible interference with intestinal adaptation after resection by decreasing splanchnic blood flow, an increased risk of cholelithiasis, and its expense, discomfort at the injection site, and inconvenience [38–40]. Octreotide is available in short- and long-acting formulations. The short-acting formulation is generally administered subcutaneously three times per day at a dose range of 50–250 μg each. The long-acting formulation is typically dosed as 20 mg once monthly given intramuscularly.

Clonidine is an α2-adrenergic agonist used primarily to treat hypertension that also has demonstrated antimotility effects that slow intestinal transit. Two small trials have shown that clonidine decreases fecal fluid and electrolyte loss and stool volume in patients with SBS [41,42]. Anecdotal reports suggest a clinical benefit of clonidine in reducing diarrhea. Clonidine can be given orally at doses between 0.1 and 0.3 mg up to three times a day. An advantage of clonidine is that it is also available in a transdermal delivery system, which may be preferred if medication absorption is in question.

Antimicrobials to Treat SIBO

The exact prevalence of SIBO in patients with SBS remains unclear. As alluded to previously, diagnosis can be made by culturing a small bowel aspirate or by glucose or lactulose hydrogen breath testing; however, both have substantial limitations. In particular, those with SBS and remaining colon generally have rapid intestinal transit; thus, hydrogen detected by breath testing typically reflects production by colon bacteria and erroneous results. As such, empiric treatment in the setting of typical symptoms such as worsening flatulence, bloating, and diarrhea is commonly employed. Treatment most commonly consists of the use of antibiotics. Patients with SBS will typically require recurrent treatment for SIBO as the underlying mechanism responsible for the condition remains unaltered. Therefore, one strategy is to treat with a 7- to 10-day course of three or four alternating broad-spectrum (given the polymicrobial nature of SIBO) antibiotics once monthly. The antibiotics can be rotated to decrease the risk of developing antibiotic resistance. There are insufficient data to recommend one antibiotic regimen over another. The risk of antibiotic use (e.g., *C. difficile* infection) should be weighed against the benefits. The options for patients who fail to respond to antibiotics are unclear particularly after an empiric trial since it has not been confirmed whether the patient's symptoms are actually due to SIBO. Nevertheless, considerations include a trial of a different antibiotic or the collection of a small bowel aspirate with speciation and identification of the sensitivity pattern of the causative microorganism(s) to ensure the absence of resistance to the antibiotic.

Bile Acids and Sequestrants

The management of bile acid-related diarrhea depends on the length of ileal resection and whether an intact colon remains in place. Resection of <100 cm of terminal ileum in patients with an intact colon, an uncommon situation in SBS, may result in secretory bile acid-induced diarrhea. In this setting, a bile acid binder such as cholestyramine, colestipol, or colesevelam should be considered. Caution should be exercised with the use of cholestyramine and colestipol, as they can interfere with the absorption of certain medications and fat-soluble vitamins [43]. Importantly, the use of cholestyramine should be reserved for those with colon present. When the ileal resection is >100 cm, a far more common situation in SBS, bile acid deficiency develops and use of a bile acid binder may worsen the diarrhea and exacerbate steatorrhea and loss of fat-soluble vitamins. Unfortunately, there are no readily available, effective bile acids that can be used to supplement the deficiency and improve fat absorption. Instead, management in this setting involves dietary restriction of fat with or without the use of medium-chain triglycerides if colonic continuity is maintained.

Pancreatic Enzyme Replacement

Pancreatic enzyme replacement is rarely needed in patients with SBS unless the patient has a history of concomitant pancreatic insufficiency. The provision of pancreatic enzymes when a nutrient–enzyme mismatch is suspected, such as may occur in the setting of a Roux-en-Y gastroenterostomy or Billroth II anastomosis, might be warranted. Prior to enzyme supplementation, use of acid suppression should be provided to prevent denaturation of the enzymes [44]. Alternatively, an enteric-coated formulation can be used.

Trophic Factors

Trophic factors, including recombinant human growth hormone and recombinant GLP-2, have been shown to promote intestinal adaptation and enhance fluid and nutrient absorption in patients with SBS and are commercially available as aids to facilitate the weaning of PN [45,46]. These agents are discussed in depth in Chapters 19 and 20.

CONCLUSION

In conclusion, diarrhea in patients with SBS is the predominant symptom and is a source of considerable consternation for both the patient and the treating clinician. It is quite often the source of volume depletion, nutrient deficiencies, and metabolic complications. Management of diarrhea in SBS involves first excluding other readily treatable causes of diarrhea and then correcting the consequences such as water and electrolyte imbalances and nutrient deficiencies. An understanding of the underlying mechanisms contributing to the diarrhea in SBS is critical to allow tailored management. In addition, close follow-up and frequent reassessment of the efficacy of therapy is needed.

REFERENCES

1. Carlsson E et al. Quality of life and concerns in patients with short bowel syndrome. *Clin Nutr* 2003; **22**(5):445–52.
2. Winkler MF et al. The meaning of food and eating among home parenteral nutrition-dependent adults with intestinal failure: a qualitative inquiry. *J Am Diet Assoc* 2010;**110**(11):1676–83.
3. Nightingale J et al. Guidelines for management of patients with a short bowel. *Gut* 2006;**55**(Suppl 4): 1–12.
4. Buchman AL et al. AGA technical review on short bowel syndrome and intestinal transplantation. *Gastroenterology* 2003;**124**(4):1111–34.
5. Sleisenger MH et al. *Sleisenger and Fordtran's Gastrointestinal and Liver Disease: Pathophysiology, Diagnosis, Management.* 9th ed. Philadelphia, PA: Saunders/Elsevier, 2010.
6. Nightingale JM et al. Colonic preservation reduces need for parenteral therapy, increases incidence of renal stones, but does not change high prevalence of gall stones in patients with a short bowel. *Gut* 1992;**33**(11):1493–7.
7. Jorgensen JR et al. In vivo absorption of medium-chain fatty acids by the rat colon exceeds that of short-chain fatty acids. *Gastroenterology* 2001;**120**(5):1152–61.
8. Dudrick SJ et al. Management of the short-bowel syndrome. *Surg Clin N Am* 1991;**71**(3):625–43.
9. Thompson JS et al. Factors affecting outcome following proximal and distal intestinal resection in the dog: an examination of the relative roles of mucosal adaptation, motility, luminal factors, and enteric peptides. *Dig Dis Sci* 1999;**44**(1):63–74.
10. Borgstrom B et al. Studies of intestinal digestion and absorption in the human. *J Clin Invest* 1957;**36**(10):1521–36.
11. Poley JR et al. Role of fat maldigestion in pathogenesis of steatorrhea in ileal resection. Fat digestion after two sequential test meals with and without cholestyramine. *Gastroenterology* 1976;**71**(1):38–44.
12. Chadwick VS et al. Effect of molecular structure on bile acid-induced alterations in absorptive function, permeability, and morphology in the perfused rabbit colon. *J Lab Clin Med* 1979;**94**(5):661–74.
13. Fromm H et al. Bile acid-induced diarrhoea. *Clin Gastroenterol* 1986;**15**(3):567–82.

14. DiBaise JK et al. Enteric microbial flora, bacterial overgrowth, and short-bowel syndrome. *Clin Gastroenterol Hepatol* 2006;**4**(1):11–20.
15. Halperin ML et al. D-Lactic acidosis: Turning sugar into acids in the gastrointestinal tract. *Kidney Int* 1996;**49**(1):1–8.
16. Takahashi K et al. A stand-alone synbiotic treatment for the prevention of D-lactic acidosis in short bowel syndrome. *Int Surg* 2013;**98**(2):110–3.
17. White L. D-lactic acidosis: More prevalent than we think? *Pract Gastroenterol* 2015;**39**(9):26–45.
18. Fielding JF et al. Gastric acid secretion in Crohn's disease in relation to disease activity and bowel resection. *Lancet* 1971;**1**(7709):1106–7.
19. Hyman PE et al. Gastric acid hypersecretion in short bowel syndrome in infants: Association with extent of resection and enteral feeding. *J Pediatr Gastroenterol Nutr* 1986;**5**(2):191–7.
20. Nightingale JM et al. Disturbed gastric emptying in the short bowel syndrome. Evidence for a "colonic brake." *Gut* 1993;**34**(9):1171–6.
21. Nightingale JM et al. Gastrointestinal hormones in short bowel syndrome. Peptide YY may be the "colonic brake" to gastric emptying. *Gut* 1996;**39**(2):267–72.
22. Jeppesen PB et al. Elevated plasma glucagon-like peptide 1 and 2 concentrations in ileum resected short bowel patients with a preserved colon. *Gut* 2000;**47**(3):370–6.
23. Freiler JF et al. *Clostridium difficile* small bowel enteritis occurring after total colectomy. *Clin Infect Dis* 2001;**33**(8):1429–31; discussion 1432.
24. Williams RN et al. Enteral *Clostridium difficile*, an emerging cause for high-output ileostomy. *J Clin Pathol* 2009;**62**(10):951–3.
25. Lal S et al. Review article: Intestinal failure. *Aliment Pharmacol Ther* 2006;**24**(1):19–31.
26. Elriz K et al. Crohn's disease patients with chronic intestinal failure receiving long-term parenteral nutrition: A cross-national adult study. *Aliment Pharmacol Ther* 2011;**34**(8):931–40.
27. Sweetser S. Evaluating the patient with diarrhea: A case-based approach. *Mayo Clin Proc* 2012;**87**(6):596–602.
28. Ladefoged K et al. Fluid and electrolyte absorption and renin–angiotensin–aldosterone axis in patients with severe short-bowel syndrome. *Scand J Gastroenterol* 1979;**14**(6):729–35.
29. Hess MW et al. Systematic review: Hypomagnesaemia induced by proton pump inhibition. *Aliment Pharmacol Ther* 2012;**36**(5):405–13.
30. Edes TE et al. Essential fatty acid sufficiency does not preclude fat-soluble-vitamin deficiency in short-bowel syndrome. *Am J Clin Nutr* 1991;**53**(2):499–502.
31. Atia AN et al. Oral rehydration solutions in non-cholera diarrhea: A review. *Am J Gastroenterol* 2009;**104**(10):2596–604; quiz 2605.
32. Rodrigues CA et al. What is the ideal sodium concentration of oral rehydration solutions for short bowel patients. *Clin Sci* 1988;**74**(s18):69.
33. Cooper JC et al. Effects of a long-acting somatostatin analogue in patients with severe ileostomy diarrhoea. *Brit J Surg* 1986;**73**(2):128–31.
34. Kusuhara K et al. Reduction of the effluent volume in high-output ileostomy patients by a somatostatin analogue, SMS 201–995. *Int J Colorect Dis* 1992;**7**(4):202–5.
35. Ladefoged K et al. Effect of a long acting somatostatin analogue SMS 201–995 on jejunostomy effluents in patients with severe short bowel syndrome. *Gut* 1989;**30**(7):943–9.
36. Nightingale JM et al. Octreotide (a somatostatin analogue) improves the quality of life in some patients with a short intestine. *Aliment Pharmacol Ther* 1989;**3**(4):367–73.
37. O'Keefe SJ et al. Octreotide as an adjunct to home parenteral nutrition in the management of permanent end-jejunostomy syndrome. *JPEN J Parenter Enteral Nutr* 1994;**18**(1):26–34.
38. Sukhotnik I et al. Sandostatin impairs postresection intestinal adaptation in a rat model of short bowel syndrome. *Dig Dis Sci* 2002;**47**(9):2095–102.
39. Bass BL et al. Somatostatin analogue treatment inhibits post-resectional adaptation of the small bowel in rats. *Am J Surg* 1991;**161**(1):107–11; discussion 111–12.
40. Redfern JS et al. Octreotide-associated biliary tract dysfunction and gallstone formation: pathophysiology and management. *Am J Gastroenterol* 1995;**90**(7):1042–52.
41. Buchman AL et al. Clonidine reduces diarrhea and sodium loss in patients with proximal jejunostomy: A controlled study. *JPEN J Parenter Enteral Nutr* 2006;**30**(6):487–91.
42. McDoniel K et al. Use of clonidine to decrease intestinal fluid losses in patients with high-output short-bowel syndrome. *JPEN J Parenter Enteral Nutr* 2004;**28**(4):265–8.
43. Kumpf VJ. Pharmacologic management of diarrhea in patients with short bowel syndrome. *JPEN J Parenter Enteral Nutr* 2014;**38**(1 Suppl):38S–44S.

44. Parrish CR. The Clinician's guide to short bowel syndrome. *Pract Gastroenterol* 2005;**31**:67–107.
45. Byrne TA et al. Growth hormone, glutamine, and an optimal diet reduces parenteral nutrition in patients with short bowel syndrome: A prospective, randomized, placebo-controlled, double-blind clinical trial. *Ann Surg* 2005;**242**:655–61.
46. Jeppesen PB et al. Teduglutide reduces need for parenteral support among patients with short bowel syndrome with intestinal failure. *Gastroenterology* 2012;**143**(6):1473–81.

6 Electrolyte and Acid-Base Disturbances

Lingtak-Neander Chan and Berkeley N. Limketkai

CONTENTS

KEY POINTS

- In patients with short bowel syndrome, the intestine typically has a reduced capacity to absorb adequate amount of fluids and electrolytes. Together with increased gastrointestinal fluid loss, this greatly increases the risk of developing fluid, electrolyte, and acid-base disorders.
- Conditions that lead to large volume loss of gastrointestinal fluid and electrolytes can overwhelm the kidney's ability to regulate serum pH, thus potentially contributing to metabolic acidosis or alkalosis.
- Clinical manifestations of these electrolyte and acid-base disorders tend to be mild and nonspecific; however, when severe, significant neuromuscular, respiratory, and cardiac complications may occur, sometimes resulting in death.
- The goals of therapy include replacing volume or electrolyte deficits and treating the underlying causes leading to these disorders.

INTRODUCTION

The intestine plays an important role in regulating the homeostasis of fluid, electrolytes, and acid-base balance. The intestinal mucosa contains polarized epithelial cells with ion transporters designed to regulate the flow of fluid and electrolytes and maximize their net absorption, while maintaining an electrochemical gradient across the epithelial barrier. The junction between epithelial cells is highly regulated with variable permeability along the length of the gastrointestinal (GI) tract to optimize nutrient and fluid absorption. These physiologic features account for the impressive ability of the GI tract to reduce up to 10 L of food and fluid volume that passes through it daily to just 100 to 200 mL of stool output [1]. GI tract surgery, such as bowel resection or ostomy creation, can decrease the intestinal absorption of fluid and electrolytes and increase their losses, resulting in dehydration, electrolyte disturbances, and acid-base disorders. Fluid and electrolyte disorders are common complications in patients with short bowel syndrome (SBS), and their management is an important aspect of care for these patients, particularly in preventing hospitalization. This chapter begins with an overview on the homeostasis of fluid; key electrolytes, namely, sodium (Na^+), potassium (K^+), chloride (Cl^-), and magnesium (Mg^{2+}); and acid-base disturbances. This is followed by a discussion on treatment that will emphasize the management of dehydration, common electrolyte deficiencies (e.g., hyponatremia, hypokalemia, and hypomagnesemia), and acidemia/alkalemia that occur in SBS patients.

FLUID AND ELECTROLYTE HOMEOSTASIS

Under normal physiological conditions, approximately 8 to 10 L of isotonic fluid enters the proximal small bowel daily. The sources of fluid include food and drinks, along with secretions from the GI tract in response to this oral intake [2]. About 90% of this fluid is absorbed along the length of the gut and reincorporated into the extracellular fluid through the enterosystemic fluid cycle to prevent dehydration (Figure 6.1). Interruptions to this fluid cycle, such as the presence of a fistula or ostomy or rapid intestinal transit, may affect fluid and electrolyte balance. SBS patients with <100 cm of residual jejunum without a colon are particularly at risk for developing dehydration if oral fluid intake is limited as more sodium and fluid are being secreted than absorbed (i.e., net secretors). In general, patients with a significant amount of ileum and/or colon removed are at risk for developing dehydration and electrolyte disorders [3].

In the GI tract, water is primarily absorbed through a passive process accompanied by the active transport of electrolytes and nutrients across the intestinal epithelial tissues. Mechanistically, water absorption is mediated through the (i) intercellular route, which occurs through the tight junctions between the enterocytes, and (ii) transcellular route, which is regulated by the aquaporins and carrier-mediated transporter system (e.g., sodium-dependent glucose transporter) [4]. The efficiency of water absorption depends on the tight junction of the GI epithelial cells, the regulation of transluminal solute transporters—especially the sodium transporter—and GI transit time. The duodenum and proximal jejunum have high bidirectional permeability to water and solutes, resulting in very low efficiency for water absorption [5]. The distal jejunum and the ileum have tighter epithelial cell junctions and a highly regulated sodium transport system, resulting in a more efficient fluid absorption process than the proximal small intestine. Compared with the small intestine, the colon has the slowest transit and tightest epithelial cell junctions. Therefore, the efficiency of water and sodium reabsorption is also the highest. In healthy individuals, approximately 1 to 2 L of fluid is reabsorbed in the colon daily. In patients with SBS, the colon may reabsorb up to 6 L of fluid daily [6].

The transluminal transport of electrolytes and trace elements in the GI tract is highly regulated by carrier-mediated transport proteins. Although there appears to be a regional specificity for the absorption efficiency of some micronutrients (e.g., duodenum and proximal jejunum for zinc, duodenum for non-heme iron), the most abundant electrolytes, such as sodium, chloride, and potassium, can be absorbed along the entire length of the intestine. Under normal physiological conditions,

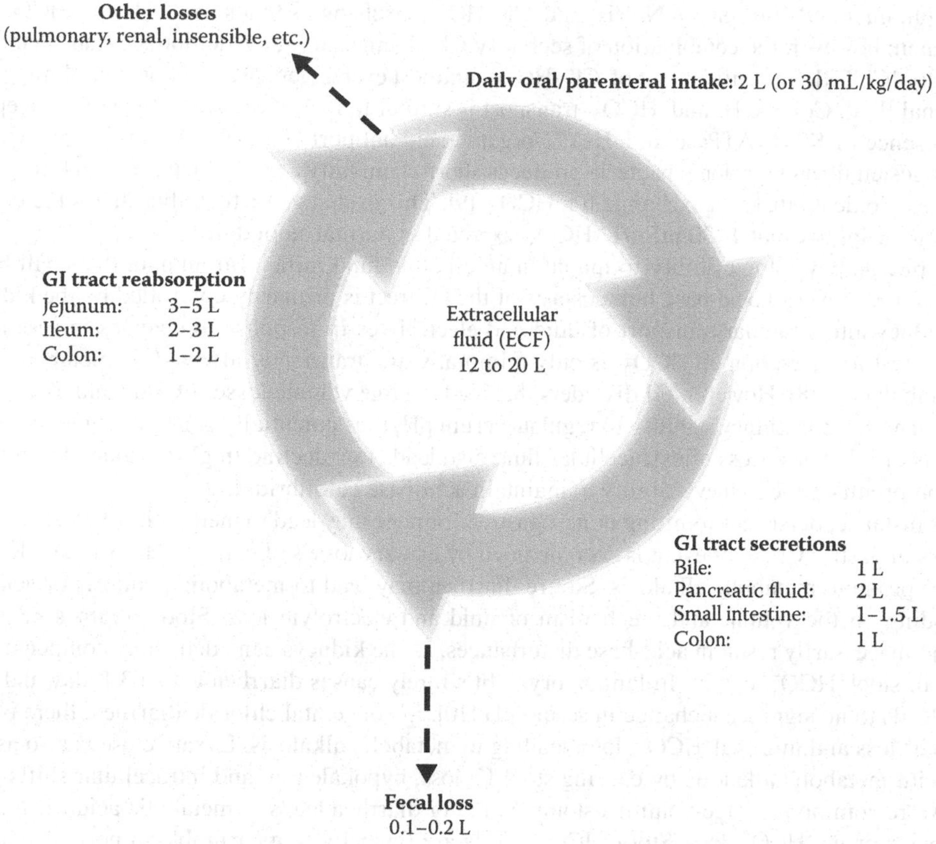

FIGURE 6.1 The human enterosystemic fluid cycle.

total sodium loss is determined by the combined effect on intestinal sodium secretion and renal sodium handling through the regulation of the renin–angiotensin–aldosterone system and natriuretic peptides. Additionally, antidiuretic hormone (vasopressin), secreted by the posterior pituitary gland, also affects plasma sodium concentration by regulating renal water handling. Daily potassium loss is primarily determined by renal function, although intestinal fluid may also contribute to its loss. With respect to magnesium, urinary loss accounts for approximately one-third of the total output, whereas intestinal secretion accounts for about 60% of total daily loss. Approximately 90% of the eliminated phosphate is excreted renally, with about 10% secreted into the gut [7]. Thus, in SBS patients with severe GI fluid loss, sodium and magnesium are at greater risk of depletion than potassium and phosphorus.

ACID-BASE REGULATION

The pH of the GI tract fluid varies according to location along the digestive tract. Large volumes of hydrogen (H^+) and bicarbonate $\left(HCO_3^-\right)$ ions bidirectionally traverse the intestinal epithelium continuously to produce a net alkaline stool [8]. Gastric parietal cells produce acid via the apical H^+/K^+-ATPase. Food intake stimulates gastrin release, which results in the secretion of up to 1.5 L of gastric acid daily, and reduces gastric pH to 1.0 [8]. Unlike the acidic gastric milieu, fluid in the small intestine and colon is either neutral or alkaline. The duodenum contains Brunner's glands that secrete HCO_3^- into the lumen to alkalinize the gastric effluent. In addition, the pancreas secretes 1 to 2 L of a highly alkaline fluid (70 to 120 mEq/L HCO_3^-) into the duodenum daily, bringing the luminal pH up to 7 or higher, an important factor for maximal function of pancreaticobiliary secretions.

The jejunum and ileum contain Na^+/H^+ and Cl^-/HCO_3^- exchangers that secrete H^+ and HCO_3^- into the lumen; however, the combination of secretory Cl^- channels (e.g., cystic fibrosis transmembrane regulator [CFTR]) and enrichment of Cl^-/HCO_3^- antiport exchangers promotes net alkalinity of the intestinal fluid. Colonic H^+ and HCO_3^- transport is similar to that of the small intestine, except for the presence of K^+/H^+-ATPase and HCO_3^-/organic acid antiport channels. Anaerobic metabolism of undigested fibers by colonic bacteria produces short-chain fatty acids, which are then transported into the colonic epithelia in exchange for HCO_3^- [9]. This exchange further alkalinizes the colonic lumen with approximately 30 mEq/L HCO_3^- excreted in normal stool daily.

Despite its physiologic ability to maintain an alkaline fluid milieu throughout the small bowel and colon, the overall acid-base homeostasis of the GI tract is primarily controlled by the kidneys. The kidney alters tubular transport of fluid and electrolytes in response to changes in serum pH, while intestinal secretion of HCO_3^- is only minimally and transiently affected by metabolic acid-base imbalances [8]. However, GI disorders that lead to large volume losses of fluid and electrolytes can overwhelm the kidney's ability to regulate serum pH, thus potentially contributing to metabolic acidosis or alkalosis. Loss of extracellular fluid also leads to a decline in glomerular filtration rate and compromises the kidney's ability to maintain acid-base equilibrium.

For instance, persistent vomiting or nasogastric drainage may lead to metabolic alkalosis through the loss of gastric Cl^-. This event is accompanied by urinary losses of cations (H^+, Na^+, and K^+) that further promote metabolic alkalosis. Severe diarrhea may lead to metabolic alkalosis or acidosis, depending on the volume and mechanism of fluid and electrolyte loss. Stool volumes <3 L/day may not necessarily result in acid-base disturbances, as the kidneys can adequately compensate for shifts in stool HCO_3^- output. Inflammatory colitis rarely causes diarrhea above 3 L/day and typically leads to no significant change in serum pH [10]. In congenital chloride diarrhea, there is high stool Cl^- loss and minimal HCO_3^- loss, leading to metabolic alkalosis. Laxative use is also associated with metabolic alkalosis by causing stool K^+ loss, hypokalemia, and intracellular shifts of H^+ [11]. More commonly, large-volume ostomy output or diarrhea leads to metabolic acidosis through disproportionate HCO_3^- loss. Stool HCO_3^- levels are typically immeasurable in normal stool but can rise to 30 mEq/L in patients with recently constructed ileostomies and upward to 75 mEq/L in those with secretory diarrhea (Table 6.1). In cholera, for instance, constitutive activation of the CFTR channel leads to increased luminal Cl^-, Cl^-, and HCO_3^- exchange and subsequent HCO_3^- secretion into stool.

TABLE 6.1
Volume and Electrolyte Composition in Diarrheal and Ostomy Fluid

	Volume (L/day)	[Na+] (mEq/L)	[K+] (mEq/L)	[Cl−] (mEq/L)	$[HCO_3^-]$ (mEq/L)
Normal stool	<0.15	20–30	55–75	15–25	0
Diarrhea					
Colitis	1–3	50–100	15–20	50–100	10
Osmotic	1–5	5–20	20–30	5–20	10
Secretory	1–20	40–140	15–40	25–105	20–75
Congenital Cl−	1–5	30–80	15–60	120–150	<5
Ileostomy Output					
New	1	115–140	5–15	95–125	30
Adapted	0.5	40–90	5	20	15–30

Source: Charney, A.N. et al., in: Gennari, F.J., Adrogue, H.J., Galla, J.H., Madias, N.E., eds., *Acid-Base Disorders and Their Treatment*, Taylor & Francis, Boca Raton, FL, 2005, 209–240.

Acid-base disturbances in SBS depend largely on stool output. In the setting of significant malabsorption and large-volume diarrhea, metabolic acidosis can occur through similar mechanisms of HCO_3^- loss as described with other severe diarrheal diseases. In addition, relative carbohydrate malabsorption in SBS patients leads to fermentation by colonic bacteria into L- and D-isomers of lactic acid [9,12]. While humans can rapidly metabolize L-lactic acid, metabolism for D-lactic acid occurs more slowly and is then allowed to accumulate in the bloodstream, thus further contributing to metabolic acidosis. Lactic acidosis can also arise from vascular hypoperfusion in severe volume depletion. A fourth mechanism for potential acid-base imbalance in SBS is iatrogenic metabolic acidosis or alkalosis through the provision of excessive amount of chloride or acetate in parenteral nutrition.

Individuals with a new ileostomy secrete, on average, 95 to 125 mEq/L Cl^- and 30 mEq/L HCO_3^- daily. Metabolic acidosis can arise when there is a net HCO_3^- loss. In contrast, a mature ileostomy will, on average, have a reduced anionic loss of 20 mEq/L Cl^- and 15 to 30 mEq/L HCO_3^-. The process of intestinal adaptation that occurs over time after intestinal resection confers a reduced risk for acid-base disturbance.

LABORATORY INTERPRETATION

Fluid Disorders

In patients with dehydration, one of the most commonly identified laboratory changes is an increased ratio of serum blood urea nitrogen (BUN) to creatinine (SCr) at >20:1 (normal, ~10:1 to 15:1). However, SCr concentration can be reduced in patients with chronic liver disease, malnutrition, or low muscle mass, which may be present in some SBS patients. Elderly individuals also have lower SCr. Therefore, a patient's fluid status should not be evaluated solely based on BUN:SCr ratio [7]. Other nonspecific laboratory changes suggesting the presence of dehydration may include a sudden increase in hematocrit with no other explanations, hypernatremia (serum sodium >150 mEq/L—albeit rare in SBS), and elevated urine-specific gravity. In contrast, laboratory tests are rarely used as an effective surrogate indicator of fluid overload, unless congestive heart failure is also suspected. Overall, fluid overload is rare in SBS patients. Therefore, the discussion on treatment of fluid disorders later in this chapter will focus on dehydration. In SBS, adequate hydration is considered to be present when urine output is >1 L/day and urinary sodium concentration is >20 mEq/L.

Electrolyte Disorders

Electrolyte disorders involving potassium, chloride, magnesium, and phosphorus can generally be determined based on their serum concentrations. Low serum concentrations strongly suggest clinical deficiencies. Serum potassium concentration can also be affected by acid-base status. Acidemia causes transient hyperkalemia due to shifting of intracellular potassium into the extracellular compartment. Serum potassium concentration will generally decrease once the acidemia is corrected [7]. Untreated acidemia can lead to chronic efflux of intracellular potassium, which may increase renal potassium wasting, leading to intracellular potassium depletion over time. Conversely, alkalemia can cause hypokalemia. In SBS patients with chronic diarrhea, severe hypokalemia may be present not only from increased GI potassium loss but also from intracellular shifting due to metabolic alkalosis associated with concomitant GI bicarbonate loss. Serum sodium concentration should be interpreted with caution. While severe dehydration or fluid overload can cause mild hypernatremia or hyponatremia, respectively, more severe cases of sodium disorders are likely the result of defects in free water regulation, such as in the case of syndrome of inappropriate antidiuretic hormone or diabetes insipidus. In these patients, sodium disorders should be managed with concurrent interventions in correcting water handling. In patients with abnormal serum sodium concentration, a thorough assessment of fluid status including physical examination for the presence/absence of edema should be undertaken, and diseases involving abnormal water handling should be excluded. In SBS, hyponatremia can be a significant and underrecognized problem.

Acid-Base Disorders

While acid-base status is most thoroughly evaluated by arterial blood gas analysis, the serum HCO_3^- concentration, typically provided together with electrolytes, BUN, and SCr, in a basic metabolic panel, also gives an estimation of acid-base balance. Serum HCO_3^- concentration <24 mEq/L or arterial pH <7.35 represents acidemia and suggests metabolic acidosis. Additionally, serum chloride concentration and the ratio between Cl^- and HCO_3^- may also be used to guide clinical assessment. An elevated serum Cl^- concentration is often associated with a decrease in serum HCO_3^- and vice versa. This is a physiological compensatory mechanism to prevent excess anion accumulation. Therefore, hyperchloremia may suggest the presence of metabolic acidosis without an increased anion gap (see below). For example, excessive use of an intravenous (IV) saline solution or chloride salts in parenteral nutrition may lead to hyperchloremic metabolic acidosis.

The serum anion gap, most commonly calculated as ($[Na^+] - [Cl^-] - [HCO_3^-]$), is useful to assess the etiology of metabolic acidosis and to guide treatment approaches. An alternative formula that includes K^+ ($[Na^+] + [K^+] - [Cl^-] - [HCO_3^-]$) is sometimes used, particularly by nephrologists. When not including K^+ in the equation, the average normal anion gap is 12 mEq/L and ranges from 8 to 16 mEq/L depending upon a few variables, including the laboratory technique used. An elevated anion gap suggests the presence of unmeasured anions, such as lactate or strong organic acids. Important for the patient with SBS, D-lactic acidosis, which cannot be detected by the standard serum lactate test used in the clinical setting, may cause an elevated anion gap but normal L-lactate level [12]. Metabolic acidosis from diarrhea usually has a normal anion gap.

CLINICAL MANIFESTATIONS

Fluid Disorders

Patients with dehydration may present with altered mental status, ranging from lethargy in moderate dehydration to obtunded in severe cases. Abnormal physical findings may include dry mucous membrane, absence of tears, and reduced skin turgor. The patient's eyes may be sunken and the magnitude parallels the severity of dehydration. From a cardiovascular standpoint, the patient may present with cool limbs, hypotension, and tachycardia. Other findings may include sudden weight loss (usually over a few days) and decreased urination. In contrast, the most common signs and symptoms of hypervolemia include peripheral edema and sudden weight gain. In more severe cases, pulmonary edema may develop, which manifests as dyspnea and orthopnea.

Electrolyte Disorders

Sodium

Clinical manifestations of disorders of sodium homeostasis (both hypernatremia and hyponatremia), while often asymptomatic, may include neurocognitive changes ranging from malaise, agitation, and apathy to disorientation, seizure, or coma. The severity of the symptoms correlates with the magnitude of sodium deficit or excess. In patients with SBS, because of low intake and increased loss from the GI tract, the typical presentation is hypovolemic hyponatremia. Patients with an end-jejunostomy are especially at risk for developing hyponatremia. Most patients with hyponatremia present with no or very mild and nonspecific symptoms, until serum sodium concentration approaches 120 mEq/L [7]. Hypernatremia occurs less commonly in patients with SBS. As such, when present, an evaluation of other causes of hypernatremia should be undertaken.

Potassium

Most patients with disorders of potassium homeostasis present with mild, nonspecific symptoms such as muscle cramps, dizziness, or fatigue. Palpitations may present intermittently in some patients. The most serious clinical problems related to potassium disorders are cardiac conduction problems (detectable by electrocardiogram) that, when severe, can result in death. Therefore, a comprehensive assessment of recent nutrient intake and duration of diarrhea is an important process in triaging ambulatory patients who are at risk for developing potassium disorders. Patients with continued diarrhea, uncontrolled ostomy output, vomiting, or poor oral/enteral intake for 3 days or more, especially those with clinical signs of dehydration, should be evaluated for hypokalemia.

Magnesium

Similar to the clinical manifestations of hypocalcemia, patients with hypomagnesemia may present with neuromuscular symptoms such as weakness, tremor, tetany, or hyperreflexia. In some cases, magnesium depletion can present with disorientation, psychosis, stupor, or coma. Hypomagnesemia may also precipitate hypocalcemia as the release of parathyroid hormone is partially regulated and affected by serum magnesium. Since the GI tract accounts for up to two-thirds of the daily magnesium loss, patients with SBS are at increased risk for developing hypomagnesemia. Specifically, a significant amount of magnesium is lost in the jejunal and ileal effluent in patients with severe GI fluid loss. SBS patients without a colon are at the highest risk for developing chronic hypomagnesemia [13]. Hypermagnesemia is uncommon in patients with SBS unless an excessive amount of magnesium is inadvertently administered in IV fluid or parenteral nutrition solutions.

Acid-Base Disorders

Tight regulation of plasma hydrogen ion concentration is necessary to optimize the physiological functions of the human body. Serum pH needs to be maintained within the range of 7.35 to 7.40 in order to allow enzymes, transport proteins, and ion channels to function at maximal capacity. Change in pH outside this range will generally cause serious disruptions to critical metabolic pathways and impair cellular processes [14].

Metabolic acidosis generally causes nonspecific symptoms; however, it can also lead to diverse multiorgan effects, such as disturbances in endocrinologic, cardiovascular, musculoskeletal, and neurologic function. Metabolic acidosis is associated with hypercatabolism and inhibition of protein synthesis, thus leading to protein–calorie malnutrition [11]. Endocrinological derangements include insulin resistance, impaired glucose tolerance, and alterations in thyroid and parathyroid hormone secretion (see list below) [10]. Cardiovascular effects of metabolic acidosis include increased catecholamine release and resistance, which could present with perturbations in cardiac contractility, arrhythmias, arterial vasodilation, and hypotension [15]. Tachypnea occurs as the body strives to exhale CO_2. Finally, chronic metabolic acidosis leads to progressive bone degradation and metabolic bone disease, manifested as osteopenia or osteoporosis.

Consequences of metabolic acidosis

1. Altered nutrient dynamics
   a. Catabolic effects, especially on protein synthesis
   b. Insulin resistance
   c. Impaired intracellular uptake of certain nutrients
   d. Decreased adenosine triphosphate (ATP) synthesis and oxidative phosphorylation
2. Metabolic bone disease (chronic)
   a. Physiochemical dissolution of bone
   b. Decreased osteoblast function
   c. Increased osteoclast function

   d. Increased level and effect of parathyroid hormone
   e. Possible decreased activity of 1-α-hydroxylase and production of active vitamin D
3. Altered homeostasis of neuroendocrine functions
   a. Decreased growth hormone secretion and insulin-like growth factor-1 (IGF-1) response
   b. Suppressed insulin action on glucose metabolism
   c. Increased glucocorticoid production and release
   d. Suppressed plasma T3 and T4 concentrations

TREATMENT APPROACHES

FLUID DISORDERS

The goal of fluid therapy for dehydration is to restore euvolemia without inducing or worsening electrolyte disorders. The treatment includes controlling precipitating factors, replacing the fluid deficit, and providing sufficient maintenance fluid to prevent a recurrence of dehydration. Depending upon the primary cause, pharmacotherapy with antidiarrheal agents, antisecretory drugs, or antiemetics may be indicated. Fluid deficit generally can be replenished using oral rehydration therapy; however, IV fluid is preferred in patients with significant cardiovascular signs/symptoms (e.g., severe hypotension), altered mental status, inability to tolerate oral/enteral fluid due to refractory nausea and vomiting, or uncontrolled diarrhea. Importantly, oral rehydration therapy is more effective in preventing and delaying dehydration rather than treating dehydration associated with severe diarrhea [16].

Oral rehydration solutions (ORSs) are glucose-electrolyte solutions that utilize a principle called solvent drag; the presence of glucose (or its polymer) allows passive absorption of electrolytes and water in the jejunum through the sodium–glucose cotransport system when the luminal electrolyte concentrations are higher than those in the plasma [13,17] (Table 6.2) [18]. Hypertonic fluids (e.g., fruit juices) with unbalanced electrolyte content should be avoided in SBS patients because the hypertonicity results in an influx of sodium and water across the jejunum epithelium and worsens fluid and electrolyte imbalance. Since the jejunum is highly permeable, as discussed previously, fluid absorption is negligible with hypotonic fluids. Therefore, both hypotonic and hypertonic fluids should generally be avoided in SBS patients with an end-jejunostomy. For SBS patients with residual ileum and colon (i.e., jejunoileocolonic anatomy), ORS may not be necessary; however, even these SBS patients should avoid hypertonic solutions. Tolerability and palatability are important factors in determining the successful adherence to ORS use. They should be consumed slowly and continuously throughout the day to minimize GI discomfort. Commercially available, flavored ORS may still not be palatable to some

TABLE 6.2
Electrolyte Composition of Various Bodily Fluids

	$[Na^+]^a$	$[K^+]^a$	$[Cl^-]^a$	$[HCO_3^-]^a$	pH
Plasma	135–145	3.5–5	95–110	22–26	7.35–7.45
Bile	135–155	5–10	85–110	40	5.0–6.5
Pancreatic juice	120–160	5–10	30–75	70–120	8.0–8.3
Distal jejunum/ileum	75–120	5–10	70–125	30	6.8–7.8
Colon	50–115	10–30	35–70	15–25	5.7–6.7

Source: Wesson, D.E. et al., in: Gennari, F.J., Adrogue, H.J., Galla, J.H., Madias, N.E., eds., *Acid-Base Disorders and Their Treatment*, Taylor & Francis, Boca Raton, FL, 2005, 489–490.

[a] mEq/L.

patients, especially children. Recipes for homemade ORS are available through a number of well-respected sources. These alternative ORS options may provide more flexibility to increase adherence [19,20]. Chapter 11 provides further details on the management of fluid disturbances in SBS, including the use of ORS.

Use of IV fluids should be the preferred approach when treating severe dehydration, especially in the presence of cardiovascular or neurological deficits. Sodium-based IV fluids, such as sodium chloride 0.9% (i.e., physiologic saline solution), are preferred. Ringers' lactate solution contains a lower chloride concentration than do physiologic saline solution and lactate, which is a precursor of bicarbonate ion. This may be beneficial in patients with underlying metabolic acidosis; however, its potassium content (4 mEq/L) may limit its role in patients with hyperkalemia or renal dysfunction (Table 6.3). The use of sodium chloride 0.45% (i.e., "half normal saline"), however, may be justified in the absence hyponatremia in some cases, especially in children. Plain dextrose solution without sodium (e.g., dextrose 5%) should be avoided as these solutions are functionally an IV version of free water and will further reduce serum sodium concentration.

For acute resuscitation, up to 1 L of saline solution (20 mL/kg for children) can be administered intravenously over 20 to 30 minutes [21]; however, when used chronically, 1 L of IV fluid is usually administered more slowly (e.g., over 3–4 hours). Vital signs and clinical symptoms should be reassessed to determine the follow-up actions. The patient's maintenance fluid requirement can be estimated by using the Holliday-Segar equation or a weight-based method (25–30 mL/kg/day). Combined dextrose–saline solutions (e.g., D5W-NaCl 0.9%) may be used as a maintenance fluid to prevent ketosis.

Electrolyte Disorders

Hyponatremia

For most patients with hyponatremia, depending upon the severity, the initial goal of therapy is to raise the serum sodium concentration to 130 mEq/L over a few days. Patients with mild hyponatremia (>125 mEq/L) who are asymptomatic can usually be managed with a sodium-containing ORS or an increase in oral sodium intake, provided that the oral/enteral route is viable (i.e., vomiting and diarrhea are controlled, evidence of functional intestine). Oral sodium chloride tablets may also be useful for patients with hypovolemic hyponatremia who are treated as outpatients with concurrent therapy to reverse the fluid disorder. The principles in determining the amount of IV sodium can be applied to the dose calculation for oral salt tablets. Every 9 g (~1.5 teaspoons) of oral sodium chloride (table salt) provides a similar quantity of sodium as 1 L of sodium chloride

TABLE 6.3
Summary of Characteristics of Commonly Used IV Fluids

IV Fluid	Ingredients	Peripheral IV Access Ok	Bolus Ok	Comment
Dextrose 5%	Dextrose 50 g/L	Yes	No	Can cause hyponatremia
Sodium chloride 0.9%	Sodium 154 mEq/L, chloride 154 mEq/L	Yes	Yes	Preferred IV fluid
Sodium chloride 0.45%	Sodium 77 mEq/L, chloride 77 mEq/L	Yes	No	Can cause hyponatremia
Ringer's lactate solution	Sodium 130 mEq/L, potassium 4 mEq/L, calcium 2.7 mEq/L, chloride 109 mEq/L, lactate 28 mEq/L	Yes	Not recommended because of K^+ and Ca^{2+}	Not preferred in renal failure or hyperkalemia

0.9% solution (i.e., 154 mEq of sodium). For comparison purposes, salt tablets have ~1 g of NaCl per tablet. Commercially available salt tablets often contain 1 g of sodium chloride (15.4 g) per tablet, which provide 17.1 mEq of sodium. Sodium chloride tablets readily dissolve in water to form an oral saline solution; however, some patients may not find salt tablets or salt solution palatable.

IV sodium therapy is preferred in more severe cases of hyponatremia. In most cases, sodium chloride 0.9% is used. Hypertonic saline solutions (e.g., NaCl 3% or 5%) are usually not necessary unless serum sodium is <120 mEq/L, severe altered mental status is present, or fluid restriction is necessary—rarely the case in patients with SBS. Because of the high osmolarity, a hypertonic saline solution must be infused via a central venous catheter.

In patients requiring urgent treatment for hyponatremia, (e.g., seizure, loss of consciousness, and severe disorientation with serum sodium <120 mEq/L), the initial goal is to increase serum sodium by 4 to 6 mEq/L within 24 hours of baseline [22]. In most cases, neurological deficits improve with this target. Although total sodium deficit can be estimated using established equations, the rate of change in serum sodium concentration is the most important factor in determining the appropriateness of the therapeutic regimen. The average rate of increase in serum sodium should not exceed 1–2 mEq/L/hour and 9 mEq/L in any given 24-hour period. There is no evidence that correction of serum sodium by >10 mEq/L in 24 hours or 18 mEq/L in 48 hours improves the outcomes in patients with acute or chronic hyponatremia [23]. Importantly, if hyponatremia is corrected too rapidly, it outpaces the brain's ability to adapt to the changes in serum osmolality and may lead to a potentially irreversible, sometimes lethal, complication called central pontine myelinolysis, also referred to as osmotic demyelination syndrome (ODS). The clinical manifestations of ODS are typically delayed for 2 to 6 days after overly rapid elevation of the serum sodium concentration. The symptoms of ODS vary but may include dysarthria, dysphagia, paraparesis or quadriparesis, behavioral disturbances, lethargy, confusion, disorientation, obtundation, and coma; seizures may also be seen but are less common. Severely affected patients may become "locked in"; they are awake but are unable to move or communicate.

It is also important to remember that concurrent with sodium replacement therapy, other medications that induce sodium wasting, such as loop diuretics, should be withheld. A thorough evaluation should be conducted to determine the exact cause(s) of hyponatremia and whether additional therapeutic modalities are warranted.

Hypokalemia

The goals of therapy in hypokalemia are to prevent or treat life-threatening complications and replace potassium deficit. The severity of hypokalemia positively correlates with the magnitude of potassium deficit. It is generally accepted that for every 100 mEq of potassium salt given, the corresponding increase in serum potassium concentration is approximately 0.27 mEq/L. In chronic hypokalemia, 200 to 400 mEq of elemental potassium is required to increase the serum potassium concentration by 1 mEq/L [24]. Mild hypokalemia can be treated with oral potassium supplementation. Potassium chloride is the preferred salt form, whereas potassium phosphate may be considered in patients with concurrent hypophosphatemia. Potassium chloride is available as an oral liquid or in a slow-release tablet or capsule. Liquid forms of potassium chloride are inexpensive and preferred in patients with an enteral feeding tube but are often poorly palatable. Although slow-release potassium tablets are generally well tolerated by patients without any major GI tract surgeries, their use in SBS patients is not recommended, as the generally rapid intestinal transit may lead to incomplete absorption. Interventions utilizing potassium-rich foods (e.g., bananas) are not as reliable or effective as potassium salt replacement, in part, because dietary potassium is predominantly in the form of potassium phosphate or potassium citrate, which contains a lower amount of elemental potassium on a per gram basis. Potassium content in banana is about 2.2 mEq/inch; approximately two to three bananas provide 40 mEq of potassium [25].

IV potassium supplementation is highly effective, although it carries risks. The most serious risk associated with IV potassium is arrhythmia, which is closely associated with the rate of infusion. As a general rule, the rate of potassium infusion should *never* exceed 10 mEq/hour in the absence of continuous electrocardiographic monitoring. Infusion rates >10 mEq/hour should be given only in settings with continuous cardiac monitoring, such as the intensive care unit. Rates above 20 mEq/hour are highly irritating to peripheral veins. An infusion rate >40 mEq/hour is not recommended. The preferred vehicle in delivering potassium is saline solution, as infusing large amount of dextrose may stimulate insulin release, which would drive plasma potassium intracellularly. Potassium acetate should be considered in patients with hypokalemia who also have metabolic acidosis or a bicarbonate deficit. Similarly, potassium phosphate can be used in hypokalemic patients with concomitant hypophosphatemia. To maximize potassium retention, serum magnesium concentration should be monitored and deficiency corrected.

Hypomagnesemia

Although a number of magnesium salts are available for oral administration, their bioavailability is relatively limited. The typical oral magnesium dose in a patient with normal renal function is 20 to 80 mEq/day (approximately 240 to 1000 mg of elemental magnesium). Diarrhea is a common dose-related side effect of oral magnesium supplements. Typically, daily doses of elemental magnesium of 100 mEq/day or higher cause diarrhea. For reference purposes, every 400 mg magnesium oxide provides about 20 mEq of elemental magnesium.

IV magnesium replacement is a more effective approach and better tolerated in the treatment of hypomagnesemia. Unfortunately, the rate of intracellular magnesium uptake is slow and an abrupt elevation in the plasma magnesium concentration can block the magnesium reabsorption in the renal loop of Henle. Thus, the commonly used IV bolus of magnesium (e.g., 8 mEq of magnesium sulfate over 15 to 20 minutes) is inefficient in raising serum magnesium concentration, with up to 50% of the infused magnesium dose lost in the urine. Therefore, the most effective approach to treat hypomagnesemia is to give IV magnesium as continuous infusion. Providing 4 to 8 g of magnesium sulfate (32 to 64 mEq) slowly over 12 to 24 hours is a highly effective regimen and is associated with much higher magnesium retention than using the bolus approach. This dose can be repeated as necessary to maintain the plasma magnesium concentration above 1 mg/dL [26]. Other treatment considerations for hypomagnesemia are summarized in the list below [27].

Summary of treatment considerations for hypomagnesemia

1. Correct metabolic acidosis—chronic acidosis reduces the synthesis of a protein needed for the kidney to reabsorb magnesium in the distal convoluted tubules, thereby causing urinary wasting.
2. Replete vitamin D deficiency—hypovitaminosis D may worsen hypomagnesemia and decrease magnesium retention in the body.
3. Rule out hyperthyroidism—hyperthyroidism can increase magnesium depletion.
4. Control diarrhea—oral magnesium supplements can increase in diarrhea/stool output. Steatorrhea may also cause an increase of magnesium loss through binding of magnesium to fatty acids in stool—consume less fat in diet.
5. Review medication list—proton pump inhibitors may cause hypomagnesemia.
6. Rule out secondary hyperaldosteronism as this may lead to increased urinary magnesium losses—check for sodium depletion by obtaining a 24-hour urinary sodium. A urinary sodium value <20 mEq/L suggests sodium depletion.
7. Control blood glucose—hyperglycemia can result in an increase in magnesium loss.
8. If previous interventions cannot improve magnesium absorption, this may suggest a renal component to magnesium loss and consultation with a nephrologist may be warranted.
9. Determine total magnesium loss if necessary—consider checking 24-hour urinary magnesium.

Acid-Base Disorders

Correction of metabolic acidosis in SBS hinges on improved control of diarrheal output and repletion of lost fluids and electrolytes. Dietary strategies may include modification of eating patterns to smaller and more frequent meals (see Chapter 10). A reduction in carbohydrate intake helps reduce the osmotic load into the lumen while concurrently reducing the substrates for bacterial fermentation into lactic acid. Pharmacologic strategies may include the use of antidiarrheal agents to reduce motility, improve absorption, and decrease volume and electrolyte loss. Oral or IV supplementation with sodium bicarbonate or a base equivalent (e.g., citrate) can be used to help correct metabolic acidosis, although the optimal threshold for initiating therapy is currently unclear [14]. The dose of bicarbonate supplementation can be estimated by calculating the base deficit: (0.6 × body weight) × (desired bicarbonate − actual bicarbonate). Serum $\left[HCO_3^-\right]$ levels will require several hours to equilibrate. For patients on parenteral nutrition, acetate anions (e.g., potassium acetate, sodium acetate), which serve as the precursor of bicarbonate *in vivo*, can be used in place of chloride anions to help alkalinize the serum (Table 6.4). Because the conversion of acetate to bicarbonate takes place primarily in the liver, patients with end-stage liver disease may have a reduced capacity in preventing metabolic acidosis with acetate salt alone. Importantly, bicarbonate salt should never be used in compounding parenteral nutrition solutions as the bicarbonate salt dramatically increases the pH of the solution and disrupts the solubility of the other salts.

TABLE 6.4
Bicarbonate and Equivalent Replacement Suggestions

Bicarbonate Source	Dose for 1 mEq Bicarbonate	Dose for 20 mEq Bicarbonate
Sodium bicarbonate tablets	• Approximately 100 mg • Each 650-mg tablet contains 7.74 mEq of bicarbonate	Approximately 3 × 650 mg tablets
Citrate, Bicitra, Cytra-2, Shohl's solution, Oracit, Polycitra-K	• All contain 1–2 mEq/mL of bicarbonate equivalent (citrate is a precursor of bicarbonate)	Approximately 20 mL Note: It is important to note whether the solution contains potassium or not to avoid inadvertent potassium excretion.
Acetate added to PN or IV fluids Sodium bicarbonate added to IV fluids (but not PN)	• Each mEq of acetate theoretically generates 1 mEq of bicarbonate (depending on hepatic function and serum pH; acetate is a precursor of bicarbonate)—the dose depends on the specific dilution in the fluid given • Acetate may be preferred over bicarbonate if the IV fluid also contains calcium or other drugs as there are no concerns about precipitation or compatibility • Bicarbonate can be added to D_5W. Adding 150 mEq (one ampule of 7.5% sodium bicarbonate = 44.6 mEq HCO_3^-) of $NaHCO_3$ to 1 L of D_5W would make it equivalent to D_5W-NS except that it contains HCO_3^- instead of Cl^- ions • Bicarbonate can also be added to sodium containing IV fluid. Adding 75 mEq of $NaHCO_3$ to 1 L of NaCl 0.45% would make an isotonic saline solution • Never add bicarbonate salt to PN solutions as it would cause precipitation due to its high pH	

Source: Rosner, M., *Pract. Gastroenterol.*, 33, 42, 2009.

CONCLUSION

SBS patients are at risk for developing fluid, electrolyte, and acid-base disorders. The most common conditions include dehydration, hyponatremia, and hypomagnesemia. Excessive loss of GI fluid may also lead to metabolic acidosis. The risk in developing these disorders is related to the ability to tolerate oral intake and the residual GI tract anatomy, particularly the presence/absence of the colon. Fluid and electrolyte disorders can generally be managed by oral replacement therapy, although IV therapy is preferred in patients with severe clinical manifestations or who are unable to tolerate oral therapy. When combined with correcting the underlying causes leading to these disorders, an improvement in fluid balance, electrolyte deficits, and acid-base derangements is usually successful.

REFERENCES

1. Rao MC et al. Intestinal electrolyte absorption and secretion. In: Feldman M, Friedman LS, Brandt LJ, eds. *Sleisenger and Fordtran's Gastrointestinal and Liver Disease.* 10th ed. Philadelphia, PA: WB Saunders; 2015:1713–1735.
2. Matarese LE. Nutrition and fluid optimization for patients with short bowel syndrome. *JPEN J Parenter Enteral Nutr* 2013;37:161–170.
3. Nightingale JM et al. Jejunal efflux in short bowel syndrome. *Lancet* 1990;336:765–768.
4. Phillips SF et al. Water and electrolyte transport during maintenance of isotonicity in human jejunum and ileum. *J Lab Clin Med* 1967;70:686–698.
5. Leiper JB. Fate of ingested fluids: factors affecting gastric emptying and intestinal absorption of beverages in humans. *Nutr Rev* 2015;73(Suppl 2):57–72.
6. Debongnie JC et al. Capacity of the colon to absorb fluid. *Gastroenterology* 1978;74:698–703.
7. Chan L-N et al. Interpretation of electrolytes, mineral and trace elements in the body. In: Lee M.W-L. ed. *Basic Skills in Interpreting Laboratory Data.* 5th ed. Bethesda, MD: American Society of Health-System Pharmacists 2013;125–159.
8. Charney AN et al. Gastrointestinal influences on hydrogen ion balance. In: Gennari FJ, Adrogue HJ, Galla JH, Madias NE, eds. *Acid-Base Disorders and Their Treatment.* Boca Raton, FL: Taylor & Francis; 2005:209–240.
9. Charney AN et al. Acid-base effects on colonic electrolyte transport revisited. *Gastroenterology* 1996;111:1358–1368.
10. Caprilli R et al. Consequence of colonic involvement on electrolyte and acid-base homeostasis in Crohn's disease. *Am J Gastroenterol* 1985;80:509–512.
11. Galla JH. Metabolic alkalosis. *J Am Soc Nephrol* 2000;11:369–375.
12. White L. D-Lactic acidosis: more prevalent than we think? *Pract. Gastroenterol* 2015;39(9):14.
13. Buchman AL et al. Dietary management in short bowel syndrome (Chapter 30). In: Buchman AL, ed. *Clinical Nutrition in Gastrointestinal Disease.* Thorofare, NJ: SLACK Incorporated; 2006:357–365.
14. Rosner M. Metabolic acidosis in patients with gastrointestinal disorders: metabolic and clinical consequences. *Pract Gastroenterol* 2009;33(4):42.
15. Kraut JA, Madias NE. Metabolic acidosis: Pathophysiology, diagnosis and management. *Nat Rev Nephrol.* 2010;6:274–285.
16. World Health Organization. WHO position paper or oral rehydration salts to reduce mortality from cholera. http://www.who.int/cholera/technical/en/ (accessed September 9, 2015).
17. Fortran JS. Stimulation of active and passive sodium absorption by sugars in human jejunum. *J Clin Invest* 1975;55:728–737.
18. Wesson DE et al. Hyperchloremic metabolic acidosis due to intestinal loss and other nonrenal causes (Chapter 15). In: Gennari FJ, Adrogue HJ, Galla JH, Madias NE, eds. *Acid-Base Disorders and Their Treatment.* Boca Raton, FL: Taylor & Francis; 2005:489–490.
19. Oley Foundation. Oral rehydration solution (ORS) recipes. http://www.oley.org/lifeline/ORS.html (accessed September 9, 2015).
20. University of Virginia Health System, Digestive Health Center. Homemade oral rehydration solution. http://www.medicine.virginia.edu/clinical/departments/medicine/divisions/digestive-health/nutrition-support-team/patient-education/Homemade%20Oral%20Rehydration%20Solutions%2012-8-14.pdf (accessed September 9, 2015).
21. National Institute for Health and Care Excellence. Intravenous fluid therapy in over 16s in hospital. https://www.nice.org.uk/guidance/cg174/chapter/recommendations (accessed September 15, 2015).

22. Sterns RH et al. The treatment of hyponatremia. *Semin Nephrol* 2009;29:282–299.
23. Verbalis JG et al. Hyponatremia treatment guidelines 2007: Expert panel recommendations. *Am J Med* 2007;120(11 Suppl 1):S1–S21.
24. Sterns RH et al. Internal potassium balance and the control of the plasma potassium concentration. *Medicine (Baltimore)* 1981;60:339–354.
25. Kopyt N et al. Renal retention of potassium in fruit. *N Engl J Med* 1985;313:582–583.
26. Kraft MD et al. Treatment of electrolyte disorders in adult patients in the intensive care unit. *Am J Health Syst Pharm* 2005;62:1663–1682.
27. Parrish, CR. *A Patient's Guide to Managing a Short Bowel.* 3rd ed. Westwood, MA: Universal Wilde; 2015:1–66.

7 Cholelithiasis and Nephrolithiasis

Andrew Ukleja and John Rivas

CONTENTS

KEY POINTS

- Gallstones and renal stones occur commonly in patients with short bowel syndrome (SBS).
- Interruption of enterohepatic circulation of bile acids, parenteral nutrition use, and bowel rest/fasting are major contributors to gallstone formation in SBS.
- Preventive measures for gallstone formation include oral and enteral intake, ursodeoxycholic acid, cholecystokinin, and treatment of small intestinal bacterial overgrowth when present.
- SBS patients with remnant bowel anatomy including colon-in-continuity, but not end-jejunostomy, are at risk of oxalate renal stones as a result of hyperoxaluria.
- Increased fluid intake and optimizing parenteral nutrition volume for all forms of renal stones is of utmost importance.
- A diet low in oxalate and fat is the primary strategy for prevention of oxalate stones.

CHOLELITHIASIS

Gallstone disease is common in short bowel syndrome (SBS), occurring in 25–45% of patients [1–3]. The main factors responsible for the development of gallstones in SBS include reduced gallbladder contractility, cholesterol supersaturation of bile, and enhanced cholesterol nucleation and crystallization. Patients at highest risk within this population tend to be those without a terminal ileum (with or without a colon) and those receiving long-term parenteral nutrition (PN). Furthermore, because some of these patients may have abnormal liver enzymes prior to the development of SBS due to critical illness or polypharmacy, significant gallbladder/biliary disease in this patient population may be overlooked and not diagnosed until more complicated disease develops. This delay can increase morbidity and mortality in patients with SBS and gallstone disease [4,5]. The purpose of this part of the chapter is to review the etiopathogenesis, risk factors, clinical presentation, diagnosis, and management of gallstone disease occurring in patients with SBS.

Etiopathogenesis and Risk Factors

The liver produces approximately 1.5 L of bile, a complex mixture of organic and inorganic material, daily. This mixture contains electrolytes, water, bile acids, calcium bilirubinate, phospholipids, cholesterol monohydrate crystals, and proteins. Cholesterol excretion into bile and bile acid synthesis are the two main pathways by which the body eliminates cholesterol. At normal body pH, the liver synthesizes bile acids and bile salts from cholesterol [6]. The liver is also responsible for the production of cholesterol. A fine line exists between production of cholesterol and production of bile acids, the mechanism of which is beyond the scope of this chapter.

Bile acids are water soluble (hydrophilic); cholesterol is water insoluble (hydrophobic). Therefore, for cholesterol to be eliminated from the body, it has to be solubilized in the form of mixed micelles, which are made up of hydrophilic lecithin and bile acids surrounding the hydrophobic cholesterol. For this to occur, the cholesterol, bile acids, and lecithin have to exist in a specific molar ratio. It would be reasonable then to expect that any disproportion of this molar ratio among said factors would lead to micellar insolubility; however, that is not the case. Biliary cholesterol supersaturation by itself is not a sufficient factor for gallstone development. In general, at least three factors are necessary for the formation of gallstones: (1) bile supersaturated with cholesterol, (2) stasis of bile within the gallbladder, and (3) nucleation (self-assembly) of cholesterol molecules. Bile within the gallbladder that is supersaturated with cholesterol stimulates the gallbladder to secrete mucin, which, in excess, provides the perfect environment for cholesterol nucleation. Crystals subsequently form that will, in turn, aggregate to form biliary sludge and, ultimately, stones [7].

Since approximately 95% of bile is absorbed in the terminal ileum as part of the enterohepatic circulation, any interruption in this pathway will cause a reduction in the bile acid pool [6]. This, in turn, will initially result in a relative and temporary increase in bile acid synthesis, a reduction in cholesterol synthesis, and fat malabsorption. Over time, the rate-limiting enzyme for cholesterol biosynthesis, 3-hydroxy-3-methyl-glutaryl-CoA (HMG-CoA) reductase, is upregulated, leading to a disproportion of the molar ratios described previously with subsequent development of gallstones.

Other important factors leading to the development of gallstones in patients with SBS are PN and bowel rest [8]. These two factors are independent of each other, as patients with either factor are prone to develop gallstones. The incidence of biliary sludge in patients on PN is dependent upon the duration of PN and has been reported to occur from 6% at 3 weeks to 100% at 6–13 weeks [9]. Other reports have quoted an overall 23% incidence of gallstone while on PN [10]. The proposed mechanism is due mainly to a reduction in cholecystokinin (CCK) production, leading to reduced gallbladder motility and bile stasis within the gallbladder [1]. Similarly, lack of oral/enteral intake may also cause a reduction in the circulating gastrointestinal hormones such as CCK, affecting gallbladder function, leading to bile stasis. Small intestinal bacterial overgrowth (SIBO) also appears to contribute to intrahepatic cholestasis and gallstone development by enhancing bile acid production and reducing bile flow [11].

SBS patients who are not PN dependent tend to produce cholesterol stones, while those receiving long-term PN typically develop pigmented calcium bilirubinate gallstones [12]. The difference in gallstone composition has to do with the underlying mechanism leading to stone formation. In patients with SBS who do not require PN, cholesterol stones form because of a relative decrease in bile acid synthesis, with subsequent cholesterol supersaturation. An exception would be in patients with SBS secondary to ileal resection and who are not on PN. These patients may develop pigmented gallstones instead of cholesterol stones because the increased bile acids reaching the colon cause solubilization of unconjugated bilirubin, which will then be absorbed and contribute to calcium bilirubinate stone formation. In general, calcium bilirubinate stones are more common in PN-dependent patients because long-term PN (continuous or cyclic) leads to a decrease in gallbladder contraction and failure of sphincter of Oddi relaxation, leading to preferential bile flow into the gallbladder and bile stasis within the gallbladder [13]. These factors, along with altered bowel anatomy and degree of enteral nutritional intake, may result in gallstone formation within 3 to 4 months of initiating PN [14]. Interestingly, while pigment stones are more commonly found in men with SBS, cholesterol stones occur more often in women, possibly due to the higher estrogen concentration [15].

The risk of cholelithiasis is higher in SBS patients receiving octreotide, a long-acting somatostatin analog, independent of bowel anatomy [16]. Octreotide reduces postprandial contractility of the gallbladder and increases small bowel transit time, causing more lithogenic bile production [17]. Other drugs commonly used by SBS patients such as opiates and anticholinergics may also increase the risk of gallstones secondary to reduced gallbladder contractility.

Clinical Presentation and Diagnosis

Diagnosing cholelithiasis, whether symptomatic or complicated (e.g., acute cholecystitis), in patients with SBS can be challenging, as many of these patients are likely to have abnormal liver enzymes at baseline and will often experience chronic dyspeptic complaints. As a consequence, a delay in the diagnosis is not uncommon and translates to an increase in morbidity and mortality in this patient population. There is also a negative correlation between the length of the remnant small bowel and abnormal liver enzymes, since abnormal enzymes and elevated bilirubin levels are most common in those with a small bowel length less than 100 cm, given that most of these patients are also receiving PN [18–24]. For this reason, a high degree of clinical suspicion is necessary for prompt diagnosis and appropriate treatment.

Although many patients with SBS and gallstones are asymptomatic, approximately 10% will eventually develop episodic biliary pain and/or gallstone-related complications [3,25]. Biliary colic is the main complaint in approximately 75% of symptomatic patients; most do not have concomitant abnormal laboratory or physical exam findings. As such, a high index of clinical suspicion and early referral for diagnostic testing are needed. Right upper quadrant abdominal ultrasound is often the initial test of choice; however, magnetic resonance cholangio-pancreatography should be considered if there is an inconclusive ultrasound, a high index of suspicion, or high pretest probability of choledocholethiasis in the face of a negative ultrasound.

Management and Prevention

As previously described, there are three basic underlying mechanisms that lead to gallstone formation: (1) production of cholesterol supersaturated bile, (2) stasis of bile within the gallbladder, and (3) nucleation of cholesterol molecules. Targeting these factors may help reduce the likelihood of gallstone formation. Gallbladder stasis may be prevented chemically, hormonally, or mechanically by oral/enteral feeding, use of CCK infusion, or prophylactic cholecystectomy (see list below).

- Chemical
  - Small intestinal bacterial overgrowth treatment
  - Amino acid infusion
  - Ursodeoxycholic acid
  - Oral and enteral feeding
- Hormonal
  - Cholecystokinin
- Mechanical
  - Prophylactic cholecystectomy

Oral and Enteral Feeding

Providing even minimal intake, either orally or enterally via a feeding tube, of nutrients that include protein or long-chain triglycerides will stimulate sufficient release of CCK and potentially prevent gallstones. In a study by Messing et al. [26], resuming oral diet 4 weeks after bowel rest and stopping PN resulted in disappearance of PN-induced biliary sludge.

Ursodeoxycholic Acid

Production of lithogenic bile can be decreased by administration of the secondary bile acid ursodeoxycholic acid (UDCA), 600 mg daily. This results from a reduction in cholesterol crystallization by decreasing levels of promoting factors, including haptoglobin and aminopeptidase N [27,28]. Some evidence suggests that oral UDCA may be an effective preventive therapy and treatment for gallstones, possibly by reducing PN-associated cholestasis [29,30].

Small Intestinal Bacterial Overgrowth

The presence of small bowel dilatation, dysmotility, loss of ileocecal valve, and anatomical changes, combined with acid suppression and antimotility drugs, all increase the risk of SIBO in SBS patients. SIBO may contribute to formation of lithogenic bile acids (lithocholic acid). Drugs enhancing intestinal transit and antibiotics may be beneficial in the setting of SIBO in patients with SBS [31,32].

Prophylactic Cholecystectomy

An invasive method of decreasing the potential for gallstone-related complications in the SBS patient who either has asymptomatic gallstones or no gallstones would be to perform prophylactic cholecystectomy [29,33]. Prophylactic cholecystectomy should mainly be considered only when another abdominal surgery is being considered [3,25]. Such prophylactic measures may be reasonable given that SBS patients, particularly those on PN, appear to be at higher risk of gallstone-related morbidity. Prophylactic sphincterotomy, another option to facilitate the passage of gallstones that migrate into the common bile duct, is generally considered only in those patients thought to be too high risk for surgery.

Cholecystokinin

The proposed mechanism for gallbladder stasis in patients with SBS on long-term PN is a reduction of CCK production, since CCK is the main hormone responsible for gallbladder contraction. Therefore, one obvious strategy to prevent gallstones would be to increase CCK levels. CCK octapeptide (CCK-8) administered twice daily has been shown to be efficacious and cost-effective [34]. An elevation in CCK levels could also be accomplished either by feeding patients small amounts of foods high in long-chain triglycerides or by amino acid infusion (see below), both of which would lead to gallbladder contraction and subsequent decrease in bile stasis and ultimate sludge or stone formation [35,36].

Amino Acid Infusion

Pulsed rapid intravenous amino acid infusions stimulate human gallbladder contraction in a dose-related manner and prevent biliary stasis and sludge formation [37–39]. The mechanism of stimulation is related to the release of CCK. The magnitude of response may be similar to that seen after meal stimulation [40]. In a study of healthy volunteers, intravenous administration of amino acids and enteral administration of long-chain triacylglycerols both increased gallbladder contraction by 17% and 37%, respectively [41]. These findings suggest that an intravenous infusion of amino acids may be useful for the prophylaxis of gallstones and sludge formation in PN-dependent patients.

Summary

Gallstone disease is common in patients with SBS. The primary factors leading to the production of "lithogenic bile" and gallstones include reduced gallbladder contractility, supersaturation of bile, and enhanced nucleation and crystallization of cholesterol. SBS patients at highest risk tend to be those without a terminal ileum and those receiving long-term PN. Importantly, patients with SBS are at increased risk for gallstone-related complications because of delayed or missed diagnosis. Therefore, the approach for patients with SBS presenting with a clinical picture suggestive of biliary disease should prompt the clinician to order appropriate testing to rule out gallstones and associated biliary complications such as pancreatitis, cholangitis, or cholecystitis when indicated. Understanding the principle mechanisms responsible for the development of gallstone formation in this patient population helps target specific risk factors and may reduce the likelihood of their formation and associated morbidity and mortality.

NEPHROLITHIASIS

Like gallstones, renal stones also occur commonly in patients with SBS [1,42]. In a study of SBS patients with a jejunocolonic anastomosis, the prevalence of symptomatic oxalate kidney stones was as high as 24% [1]. In patients with SBS and a colon-in-continuity, calcium oxalate stones are the most prevalent, while patients with an end-jejunostomy or ileostomy are prone to both oxalate and uric acid stones. In comparison, the prevalence of renal stones in the general population is approximately 8.4%; nearly 80% of the stones are composed primarily of calcium oxalate or, less often, calcium phosphate [43,44].

Etiology and Risk Factors

There are multiple factors associated with an increased risk of nephrolithiasis present in SBS. Sodium and water reabsorption capacity varies from patient to patient after major small bowel resection. Dehydration leading to reduced urine volumes is associated with kidney stone formation. [45,46]. Particularly at risk are patients with an end-jejunostomy as they often have significant fluid losses resulting in chronic salt and water depletion. In the setting of high stomal output, volume depletion and stool losses of bicarbonate result in metabolic acidosis, reduced citrate excretion, and acidic urine [47,48]. A persistently low urine pH promotes uric acid precipitation and leads to the formation of uric acid stones [49].

Both uric acid and calcium oxalate stones are seen in patients with ileostomy mainly due to chronic dehydration. In contrast, SBS patients with colon-in-continuity form mainly calcium oxalate kidney stones [42,50–52]. Approximately 25% of SBS patients with oxalate stones become symptomatic [1]. Hyperoxaluria, with or without nephrolithiasis, is often observed after small bowel resection. Hyperoxaluria can lead to nephrocalcinosis and renal parenchymal disease characterized by deposition of calcium oxalate crystals in the renal parenchyma, profound tubular damage, interstitial inflammation, and fibrosis, leading to chronic renal failure and end-stage renal disease [53]. Patients may present with pain related to renal colic as a result of obstructive uropathy, symptomatic urinary tract infection leading to pyelonephritis, or chronic renal failure.

The risk of nephrolithiasis increases as a result of enhanced absorption of enteric oxalate in those with colon remaining. Oxalate absorption in the colon is increased by high oxalate intake in the diet. Up to 40% of the daily excretion of oxalate in the urine is from a dietary source; however, oxalate absorption in the intestine depends linearly on the concomitant dietary intake of calcium and is influenced by the bacterial degradation by several bacterial species of intestinal microbiota. The gut-dwelling obligate anaerobe *Oxalobacter formigenes* has been an area of research interest because of its oxalate-degrading property [54]. A reduction in bacterial breakdown of oxalate due to decreased *O. formigenes* in the colon of SBS patients has been described [55]. By altering the intestinal bacterial population, probiotics may have the potential to lower oxalate absorption and urinary excretion and may be beneficial in the treatment or prevention of oxalate stones as shown in healthy subjects [56].

The combination of distal ileal resection (>100 cm), colon-in-continuity, and fat malabsorption leads to increased absorption of dietary oxalate by the colon [57,58]. This is due to reduced bile acid secretion from a marked reduction of bile acid pool size because of interruption in the enterohepatic circulation of bile acids. This process decreases the micellar solubilization of dietary fatty acids. The malabsorbed free fatty acids bind to calcium rather than oxalate, forming insoluble calcium soaps, and lower free intraluminal calcium, leaving oxalate in soluble form. High concentrations of soluble oxalate in the colon promote its absorption by passive diffusion or by oxalate transporters and lead to hyperoxaluria [59]. Increased luminal concentration of long-chain fatty acids in the colon enhances the absorption of oxalate by increasing the permeability of the colon mucosa to oxalate [60]. A positive correlation between fecal fat and hyperoxaluria has been found [61]. Mechanisms of oxalate renal stones formation and potential targets for therapy are shown in Figure 7.1.

Most oxalate in urine is derived from amino acid catabolism and ascorbic acid metabolism. Hypercalciuria, oxaluria, hypocitraturia, alkaline urine, and chronic dehydration all seem to increase the risk of calcium oxalate stone formation [62–64]. A critical regulator of calcium absorption is luminal calcium since only free ionized calcium can be absorbed. Therefore, increased luminal load of calcium is accompanied by an increase in calcium absorption [65,66]. Calcium flux across the intestine is regulated by acute luminal load and by an adaptation to chronic changes in dietary calcium intake. Dietary calcium also affects oxalate absorption. The intestinal calcium–oxalate interactions are complex. Supersaturation of urine with calcium and oxalate is a critical step in kidney stone formation. Renal excretion of calcium, oxalate, phosphate, water, and urine pH are primary determinants of stone formation. The need to conserve water in SBS patients often results in excretion of ions, including calcium, oxalate, and phosphate, in relatively small volumes of urine, leading to a substantial supersaturation with calcium oxalate and phosphate. Inhibitors of crystallization, including multivalent metallic cations (e.g., magnesium), small organic acids (e.g., citrate),

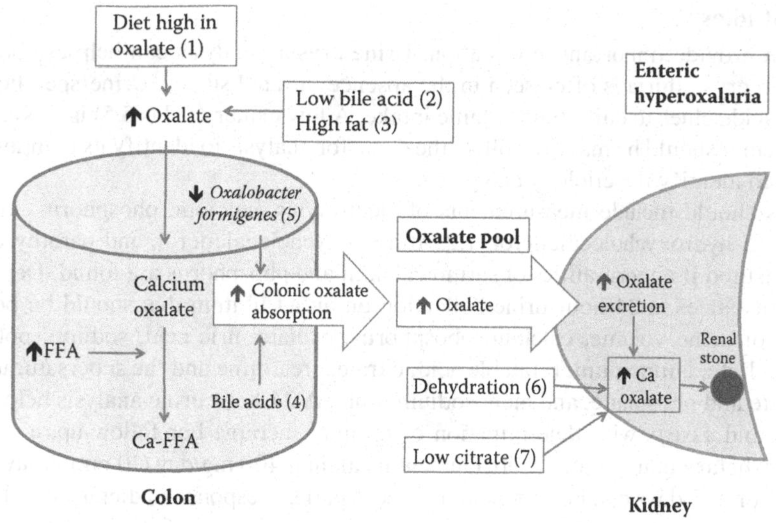

FIGURE 7.1 Mechanisms of oxalate renal stone formation and potential targets for therapy.

and inorganic anions (e.g., pyrophosphate) and macromolecules (e.g., osteopontin), may prevent stone formation [49,54,67].

Clinical Manifestations

In the majority of cases, nephrolithiasis is asymptomatic. The most characteristic symptom of nephrolithiasis is pain, which is often associated with hematuria, nausea, and vomiting. The classic ureteral colic is characterized by a mild and barely noticeable ache initially followed by an intense pain that typically waxes and wanes in severity and occurs in waves. Severe pain usually lasts 20–60 minutes. The site of obstruction determines the location of pain. The abrupt severe flank pain resolves after passage or removal of the stone. Gross or microscopic hematuria occurs in the majority of patients presenting with symptomatic nephrolithiasis but can also be present in asymptomatic patients. This finding is the single most discriminating predictor of a kidney stone in patients presenting with unilateral flank pain. Other manifestations include urinary tract infection and acute renal failure due to outflow obstruction. In SBS patients, the recurrence rate of stones is unknown but is most likely higher than in the general population (5-year recurrence rate, 40%) [68].

Diagnosis

A thorough history often provides the clues necessary for the accurate diagnosis of nephrolithiasis. Volume contraction and oliguria from low fluid intake and excessive stool output need to be recognized. A diet history, including estimated dietary intake of calcium, oxalate, sodium, protein, purine, and potassium-rich citrus fruits, should be determined. Recurrent urinary tract infection with urease-positive organisms (e.g., *Proteus*, *Haemophilus*, *Corynebacterium*, *Ureaplasma*) should be identified. Attention should be paid to the drugs associated with hypercalcuria (e.g., corticosteroids, vitamin D, calcium supplements, and antacids) or hyperoxaluria (e.g., vitamins C and B_6) [49]. Additional evaluation consists of tests to identify both kidney stones and the predisposing factors to stone formation in the individual.

Laboratory Studies

Urinalysis can provide important information. Urine crystal analysis can help establish the diagnosis; however, crystalluria is often seen in the absence of renal stones. Urine-specific gravity and osmolality provide clues to daily fluid volume intake. A low urinary pH (<5.5) is linked to uric acid stones. An attempt should be made to collect the stone for analysis to identify its composition, which can then help to identify the etiology and prognosis.

Blood tests should include measurements of electrolytes, calcium, phosphorus, and uric acid. The levels of 25-hydroxycholecalciferol, 1,25-dihydroxycholecalciferol, and parathyroid hormone should be measured if abnormalities of serum calcium and phosphorus are found. Depending upon clinical circumstances, a 24-hour urine collection on an ad libitum diet should be performed for measurement of urine volume, calcium, phosphorus, oxalate, uric acid, sodium, potassium, pH, bicarbonate, sulfate, ammonium, titratable acid, citrate, creatinine and the supersaturation ratios of calcium oxalate and phosphate, and monosodium urate. A 24-hour urine analysis helps to establish the diagnosis and assists with determination of optimal therapy. For follow-up, a 24-hour urine analysis under dietary manipulation with elemental calcium 400 mg/day (10 mmol/day) and sodium 100 mEq/day for 4–7 days can be beneficial to assess patient response to dietary modification.

Radiological Studies

Plain radiography of the abdomen can detect renal stones and their certain characteristics but has poor sensitivity. Intravenous pyelography (IVP) has been the standard diagnostic procedure for decades and served well. Another noninvasive imaging modality used for stone detection is renal ultrasonography [69]. At present, noncontrast helical computed tomography is the preferred diagnostic test since it is more sensitive than ultrasonography for stone detection and can identify other important anatomical details such as ureteral dilatation, hydronephrosis, and location of the stone(s) but is less cumbersome than IVP [70].

Treatment and Prevention of Renal Stones

Acute Therapy

Most patients with renal colic can be managed conservatively with pain medication and hydration until the stone passes. Forced intravenous hydration has not been associated with reduced pain medication use or increase in stone passage [71]. The likelihood of ureteral stone passage will depend on the size and location of the stone. Smaller stones are more likely to pass without intervention [72]. The probability of spontaneous passage is 97% for stones smaller than 2 mm in size [73]. For stones larger than 6 mm, spontaneous passage is rare (only 1%), and urologic intervention is often required [74]. In patients with urosepsis, acute renal failure, anuria, and nausea or vomiting, urgent urologic consultation is warranted. Therapeutic options for stones that have not passed include extracorporeal shock wave lithotripsy, ureteroscopic lithotripsy, percutaneous nephrolithotomy, and laparoscopic stone removal [75].

Chronic Therapy and Renal Stone Prevention

The therapy to minimize stone recurrence is based on measurements of urinary supersaturation and determination of stone type (oxalate versus uric acid). General advice on fluid and dietary modification is directed at lowering urinary supersaturation with the goal of preventing future stone formation. The principal strategies used to reduce oxalate absorption in SBS patients with colon-in-continuity include avoidance of dehydration and oxalate-rich foods. Therefore, nonpharmacologic measures include an increase in fluid intake (concomitant increase in urine volume), restriction of dietary oxalate (reduction in urinary oxalate excretion), restriction of dietary sodium (reduction of urine calcium excretion), restriction of animal protein (reduction of urine calcium excretion), and an increase in excretion of the citrate (a calcification inhibitor). Other preventive strategies include a low-fat diet and oral calcium supplementation with meals. Pharmacologic therapy is aimed to reduce both oxalate and uric acid stone formation and includes cholestyramine, bile acids, and xanthine oxidase inhibitors. These strategies are discussed in more detail later in the chapter.

Increased Fluid Intake

Controlled trials have demonstrated the benefit of increased fluid intake for all forms of renal stone disease. Urine volume should be increased as much as possible to reduce the concentrations of calcium and oxalate in the urine. Most SBS patients require increased oral fluid intake or proper PN volume adjustments. An increase in fluid intake that results in a urine volume of more than 2 L/day has been linked to reduction in the incidence of stone formation [76,77]. In SBS patients, however, such a high urine volume is often difficult to achieve. In healthy individuals, the urine volume is lowest at night, when there is minimal or no fluid intake, leading to maximal urine supersaturation and stone formation. Urine volumes may be the opposite in SBS patients on cyclic PN, in whom urine volume is higher at night. SBS patients with a history of renal stones should be encouraged to drink fluids throughout the day with a target volume of ≥2 L/day. For those without a history of renal stones, adequate volume is necessary to keep the urine volume above 1 L/day. Urine volumes should be monitored regularly on a periodic basis in SBS patients. Episodes of dehydration should be corrected early by the addition of intravenous fluid infusions when needed.

Oxalate and Purine Restriction

A reduction in dietary oxalate in SBS patients with colon-in-continuity is of foremost importance (Table 7.1). It should be recognized that adherence to a low-oxalate diet is a challenge because of abundance of oxalate-rich foods. In the setting of uric acid stones, avoidance of foods high in purines is also occasionally recommended since high purine intake is a cause of hyperuricosuria.

TABLE 7.1
Foods and Beverages High in Oxalates

Food Type	Examples
Fruits	• Apricots, figs, rhubarb, kiwi fruit
Vegetables	• Artichoke, green and wax beans, beets, raw red cabbage, celery, chives, eggplant, endive, leeks, okra, green peppers, rutabagas, summer squash, parsley, vegetable soup, and white corn • Greens: Swiss chard, beet greens, mustard greens, Dandelion greens, spinach, kale, collards, escarole • Potatoes, French fries, sweet potatoes • Tomato paste, canned • Beans: baked, black, white, great northern, navy, pink
Nuts	• Almonds, cashews, peanuts, peanut butter, pecans, sesame seeds
Beverages	• Chocolate/chocolate-containing beverages (cocoa, Ovaltine, chocolate and soy milk, lattes, etc.) • Tea, instant coffee, colas, carob ice cream
Starches	• Grits, barley, cornmeal, buckwheat, lentil, and potato soup • Whole wheat products: breads, pastas, tortillas, wheat germ, wheat bran and bran cereal, cream of wheat, shredded wheat
Other	• Tofu and soy products, miso, black olives, chocolate and chocolate ice cream, pepper (> 1 tsp per day), poppy seed, turmeric
Alcohol	• Draft beer

Source: Parrish, C.R., *A Patient's Guide to Managing a Short Bowel*, 3rd ed., Universal Wilde, Westwood, MA, 2015. Available at no cost at: www.shortbowelsupport.com. With permission.

Fat Restriction

Fat restriction is recommended in those SBS patients with a colon remaining to reduce free fatty acids in the intestinal lumen and lower oxalate absorption. A low-fat, high-complex-carbohydrate diet supplemented with medium-chain triglycerides was shown to be associated with less oxalate absorption and reduced urinary excretion of oxalate [78].

Salt Intake

A reduction in sodium intake may reduce recurrent stone formation [79]; however, this may not be feasible in SBS patients with end-jejunostomies and high sodium loss. High sodium intake leads to increased renal sodium excretion and hypercalciuria [80]. In patients with documented hypercalciuria, it is generally advised to limit daily sodium intake to less than 2 g/day (about 87 mmoL/day) [79]. A reduction in salt, however, may not be suitable for many SBS patients since increased sodium intake is linked to increased intestinal fluid absorption.

Protein Intake

A diet rich in animal protein results in aciduria and increased urine calcium excretion, which is associated with stone formation [81]. The metabolism of amino acids results in the generation of hydrogen ions, which, in turn, leads to calcium release from bone and an increase in urinary calcium [82]. Therefore, a reduction in dietary animal protein consumption may reduce stone formation. Excess of dietary protein, especially from meat, is a risk factor for uric acid stones, in particular by lowering urine pH and increasing uric acid excretion [83]. In general, uric acid stone formers are counseled to consume a diet with protein in the amount of 0.8–1.0 g/kg daily.

Citrate

Citrate as the potassium salt has been shown to effectively inhibit recurrent calcium stones in patients with hypercalciuria [84]. Citrate inhibits the nucleation, growth, and aggregation of calcium oxalate crystals. Metabolic acidosis or acid loading (e.g., excess of amino acids) leads to an increase in citrate reabsorption and a decrease in renal citrate excretion. Citrate forms soluble complexes with calcium and lowers calcium oxalate and phosphate supersaturation. The basis of therapy for hypocitraturia is correction of any underlying disorder that reduces urine citrate (e.g., acidosis, acid load, or hypokalemia). Neutralization of the acid load and systemic pH correction with oral potassium citrate or bicarbonate supplementation or the addition of acetate in the PN may be beneficial [85]. Potassium citrate can effectively prevent stone recurrence or dissolve existing calculi. Sodium citrate or sodium bicarbonate can be used in patients intolerant of potassium salts. The maximal oral recommended dosage is 60 mEq/day; however, treatment can be initiated with 30–40 mEq/day. Alkali supplements may be beneficial in raising urinary citrate levels, but they may also raise urine pH, thereby worsening calcium phosphate supersaturation. Urine pH should be monitored often and the alkali dose titrated to maintain urinary pH above 6.1 but less than 7.0 to avoid calcium phosphate stones. In individuals who are intolerant to these supplements, orange or grapefruit juice may be used due to both citraturic and alkalinizing effects [86].

Calcium Intake

Restriction of dietary calcium can reduce the urinary excretion of calcium; however, severe dietary restriction of calcium causes hyperoxaluria and loss of bone. Urinary calcium excretion is also influenced by other dietary components, including sodium, potassium, protein, and refined carbohydrates. A lower incidence of oxalate stone formation has been demonstrated in association with consumption of adequate amounts of calcium [87,88]. Ingested calcium binds to intestinal oxalate and reduces oxalate absorption. It has been shown that the organic form of calcium reduces oxalate absorption in the colon without a corresponding increase in calcium absorption. Use of calcium supplements (e.g., 500–1000 mg of calcium carbonate or citrate antacid at the end of each meal) can reduce oxalate absorption in the gut lumen.

Importantly, renal stones may be also promoted by excessive dietary calcium intake. Increasing dietary calcium or giving a high load of calcium in PN will increase urinary calcium excretion. Patients with calcium phosphate stones are typically hypercalciuric, and lowering urine calcium level is a priority by adjusting calcium intake.

Magnesium Intake

Magnesium supplementation leads to increased concentrations of magnesium in urine and inhibits nucleation and growth of calcium oxalate crystals [89]. Magnesium can be adjusted in the PN formula to raise the urine magnesium concentration; however, the potential benefits of magnesium supplementation have been recently questioned because of its hypercalciuric effects [90]. Additionally, oral magnesium salts may worsen diarrhea in SBS patients, lead to dehydration, and aggravate stone formation.

Cholestyramine

Cholestyramine, 2–4 g with each meal, is an effective oxalate binder and has been shown in SBS patients to decrease urinary oxalate excretion [49]. Its use is limited, however, by poor palatability and interference with absorption of some medications and vitamins. In addition, binding bile acids in the setting of SBS, where bile acid deficiency is common, may further impair fat absorption and worsen steatorrhea. Furthermore, long-term use of cholestyramine was not found to be beneficial in SBS patients [91]. Other bile acid binders have not been studied in SBS patients with renal stones.

Fiber

Fiber supplementation has been suggested as a means to reduce the risk of renal stones by shortening small bowel transit time, thereby limiting oxalate exposure to absorbing mucosa surface. However, fiber was shown to be poorly tolerated and ineffective for prevention of stone formation in both healthy individuals and patients with SBS [92,93].

Bile Acid Supplementation

Natural conjugated bile acid replacement has been shown in case reports to significantly reduce urinary oxalate excretion [94,95]. The presumed mechanism underlying the benefit is improved fat absorption, which may also improve the overall nutritional status of SBS patients. A concern, however, with the use of bile acids in SBS is that at high concentrations of dihydroxy bile acids, inhibition of colonic sodium chloride and water absorption may occur and lead to increased fecal water output. Furthermore, bile acid supplements are not available for commercial use.

Xanthine Oxidase Inhibitors

For patients with hyperuricosuria refractory to diet modification, xanthine oxidase inhibitors such as allopurinol should be considered. The potential side effects of allopurinol, including rash, gastrointestinal upset, and transaminitis, may limit its use [96]. The novel xanthine oxidase inhibitor febuxostat has a more favorable safety profile and improved bioavailability and is more potent than allopurinol [97]. Further study of its use in SBS is warranted.

Probiotics

Probiotics have the potential for treatment and prevention of oxalate stones by lowering oxalate absorption and urinary excretion. The multiorganism probiotic VSL#3 was studied in 11 healthy volunteers for 4 weeks after ingestion of 80 mg oxalate [98]. Those individuals who were high oxalate absorbers at baseline had a particularly marked probiotic-induced reduction in oxalate absorption. The results suggest that VSL#3 has the potential to reduce gastrointestinal oxalate absorption and decrease the risk of kidney stones. Other studies have shown that the administration of selected oxalate-degrading probiotics may reduce the intestinal absorption of oxalate and be beneficial in preventing renal stone formation [99]. More clinical data are needed to confirm this innovative approach to prevent oxalate stones in patients with SBS.

SUMMARY

Patients with SBS are at risk for uric acid and oxalate renal stone formation; those with colon-in-continuity are at risk for oxalate stones. Factors other than altered bowel anatomy that may contribute to the development of stones include insufficient fluid consumption/dehydration and excessive intake of stone-provoking foods. Specific factors such as the stone size, location, and type will dictate how aggressively to manage. In patients with symptomatic calculi, a variety of techniques are available to assist in stone removal. Observation is a reasonable approach in asymptomatic patients with small calculi without evidence of obstruction. Preventing new stone formation is the focus of management in most patients and will, to some degree, depend upon the composition of the stone. Dietary recommendations should be tailored to the SBS patient's remaining bowel anatomy and dietary habits. Avoidance of chronic dehydration is critical. A variety of treatments may correct the underlying metabolic defects responsible for stone formation and should be considered.

REFERENCES

1. Nightingale JM et al. Colonic preservation reduces need for parenteral therapy, increases incidence of renal stones, but does not change high prevalence of gallstones in patients with a short bowel. *Gut* 1992;33:1493–1497.
2. Dray X et al. Incidence, risk factors, and complications of cholelithiasis in patients with home parenteral nutrition. *J Am Coll Surg* 2007;204:13–21.
3. Thompson JS. The role of prophylactic cholecystectomy in the short bowel syndrome. *Arch Surg* 1996;131:556–560.
4. Roslyn JJ et al. Parenteral nutrition induced gallbladder disease: A reason for early cholecystectomy. *Am J Surg* 1984;63:148–158.
5. Manji N et al. Gallstone disease in patients with severe short bowel syndrome dependent on parenteral nutrition. *JPEN J Parenter Enteral Nutr* 1989;13:461–464.
6. Tavill AS, Cooksley WE. Biochemical aspects of liver disease. In: Elkeles RS, Tavill AS, eds. *Biochemical Aspects of Human Disease*. Oxford: Blackwell Scientific Publications, 1983, pp. 290–362.
7. Nightingale JM. Hepatobiliary, renal and bone complications of intestinal failure. *Best Pract Res Clin Gastroenterol* 2003;17:907–929.
8. Kelly DA. Preventing parenteral nutrition liver disease. *Early Hum Dev* 2010;86:683–687.
9. Roslyn JJ et al. Increased risk of gallstones in children receiving total parenteral nutrition. *Pediatrics* 1983;71:784–789.
10. Roslyn JJ et al. Gallbladder disease in patients on long-term parenteral nutrition. *Gastroenterology* 1983; 84:148–154.
11. Utili R et al. Cholestatic effects of *Escherichia coli* endotoxin on the isolated perfused rat liver. *Gastroenterology* 1976;70:248–253.
12. Pitt HA et al. Parenteral nutrition induces calcium bilirubinate gallstones. *Gastroenterology* 1983; 84:1274.
13. Cano N et al. Ultrasonographic study of gallbladder motility during total parenteral nutrition. *Gastroenterology* 1986;91:313–317.
14. Messing B et al. Does total parenteral nutrition induce gallbladder sludge formation and lithiasis? *Gastroenterology* 1983;84:1012–1019.
15. Diehl AK. Epidemiology and natural history of gallstone disease. *Gastroenterol Clin North Am* 1991;20:1–19.
16. Bigg-Wither GW et al. Effects of long term octreotide on gall stone formation and gall bladder function. *BMJ* 1992;304:1611–1612.
17. van Liessum PA et al. Postprandial gallbladder motility during long term treatment with the long-acting somatostatin analog SMS 201–995 in acromegaly. *J Clin Endocrinol Metab* 1989;69:557–562.
18. Craig RM et al. Severe hepatocellular reaction resembling alcoholic hepatitis with cirrhosis after massive small bowel resection and prolonged total parenteral nutrition. *Gastroenterology* 1980;79:131–137.
19. Stanko RT et al. Development of hepatic cholestasis and fibrosis in patients with massive loss of intestine supported by prolonged parenteral nutrition. *Gastroenterology* 1987;92:197–202.
20. Ito Y, Shils ME. Liver dysfunction associated with long-term total parenteral nutrition in patients with massive bowel resection. *JPEN J Parenter Enteral Nutr* 1991;15:271–276.

21. Chan S et al. Incidence, prognosis, and etiology of end-stage liver disease in patients receiving home total parenteral nutrition. *Surgery* 1999;126:28–34.
22. Luman W, Shaffer JL. Prevalence, outcome and associated factors of deranged liver function tests in patients on home parenteral nutrition. *Clin Nutr* 2002;21:337–343.
23. Langrehr JM et al. Hepatic steatosis due to total parenteral nutrition: The influence of short gut syndrome, refeeding, and small bowel transplantation. *J Surg Res* 1991;50:335–343.
24. Nightingale JMD. Physiological consequences of major small intestinal resection in man and their treatment. MD Thesis, University of London, 1993, p. 294.
25. Thompson JS. Reoperation in patients with the short bowel syndrome. *Am J Surg* 1992;164:453–456.
26. Messing B et al. Gallstone formation during total parenteral nutrition: A prospective study in men. *Gastroenterology* 1984;86:1183 (abstract).
27. Spagnuolo MI et al. Urosodeoxycholic acid for treatment of cholestasis in children on long-term total parenteral nutrition: A pilot study. *Gastroenterology* 1996;111:716–719.
28. Al-Hathlol K et al. Ursodeoxycholic acid therapy for intractable total parenteral nutrition-associated cholestasis in surgical very low birth weight infants. *Singapore Med J* 2006;47:147–151.
29. Byrne MF, Murray FE. Gallstones. In: Nightingale JMD, ed. *Intestinal Failure.* San Francisco, CA: Greenwich Medical Media, 2001, pp. 213–226.
30. Kelly DA. Preventing parenteral nutrition liver disease. *Early Hum Dev* 2010;86:683–687.
31. Capron JP et al. Metronidazole in prevention of cholestasis associated with total parenteral nutrition. *Lancet* 1983;1:446–447.
32. Lambert JR, Thomas SM. Metronidazole prevention of serum liver enzyme abnormalities during total parenteral nutrition. *JPEN J Parenter Enteral Nutr* 1985;9:501–503.
33. Hutton SW et al. The effect of sphincterotomy on gallstone formation in the prairie dog. *Gastroenterology* 1981;81:663–667.
34. Teitelbaum DH et al. Use of cholecystokinin-octapeptide for the prevention of parenteral nutrition-associated cholestasis. *Pediatrics* 2005;115:1332–1340.
35. Sitzmann JV et al. Cholecystokinin prevents parenteral nutrition induced biliary sludge in humans. *Surg Gynecol Obstet* 1990;170:25–31.
36. Teitelbaum DH et al. Use of cholecystokinin to prevent the development of parenteral nutrition-associated cholestasis. *JPEN J Parenter Enteral Nutr* 1997;21:100–103.
37. Nealon WH et al. Intravenous amino acids stimulate human gallbladder emptying and hormone release. *Am J Physiol* 1990; 259:G173–G178.
38. Zoli G et al. Promotion of gallbladder emptying by intravenous amino acids. *Lancet* 1993;341:1240–1241.
39. Shirohara H et al. Effects of intravenous infusion of amino acids on cholecystokinin release and gallbladder contraction in humans. *J Gastroenterol* 1996;31:572–577.
40. Wu ZS et al. Rapid intravenous administration of amino acids prevents biliary sludge induced by total parenteral nutrition in humans. *J Hepato-Biliary-Pancr Surg* 2000;7:504–509.
41. Kalfarentzos F et al. Gallbladder contraction after administration of intravenous amino acids and long-chain triacylglycerols in humans. *Nutrition* 1991;7:347–349.
42. Tomson CRV. Nephrocalcinosis and nephrolithiasis. In: Nightingale JMD, ed. *Intestinal Failure.* San Francisco, CA: Greenwich Medical Media, 2001, pp. 227–242.
43. Scales CD Jr et al. Prevalence of kidney stones in the United States. *Urol Dis Am Eur Urol* 2012;62:160–165.
44. Teichman JM. Clinical practice. Acute renal colic from ureteral calculus. *N Engl J Med* 2004;350:684.
45. Bennett RC, Jepson RP. Uric acid stone formation following ileostomy. *Aust N Z J Surg* 1966;36:153–158.
46. Kennedy HJ et al. The health of subjects living with a permanent ileostomy. *Q J Med* 1982;51:341–357.
47. Christl SU, Scheppach W. Metabolic consequences of total colectomy. *Scand J Gastroenterol* 1997;222(Suppl):202–204.
48. Clarke AM, McKenzie RG. Ileostomy and the risk of urinary uric acid stones. *Lancet* 1969;23:395–397.
49. Bushinsky DA et al. Nephrolithiasis. In: Brenner BM, ed. *The Kidney.* Philadelphia, PA: W.B. Saunders, 2012, pp. 1455–1507.
50. Stauffer JQ, Humphreys MH. Hyperoxaluria with intestinal disease. *N Engl J Med* 1972;287:412.
51. Stauffer JQ et al. Acquired hyperoxaluria with regional enteritis after ileal resection. Role of dietary oxalate. *Ann Intern Med* 1973;79:383–391.
52. Earnest DL et al. Hyperoxaluria in patients with ileal resection: An abnormality in dietary oxalate absorption. *Gastroenterology* 1974;66:1114–1122.
53. Glew RH et al. Nephropathy in dietary hyperoxaluria: A potentially preventable acute or chronic kidney disease. Frequency, risk factors, and adverse sequelae of bone loss in patients with ostomy for inflammatory bowel diseases. *World J Nephrol* 2014;3:122–142.

54. Argenzio RA et al. Intestinal oxalate-degrading bacteria reduce oxalate absorption and toxicity in guinea pigs. *J Nutr* 1988;118:787–792.
55. Vaidyanathan S et al. Hyperoxaluria, hypocitraturia, hypomagnesiuria, and lack of intestinal colonization by *Oxalobacter formigenes* in a cervical spinal cord injury patient with suprapubic cystostomy, short bowel, and nephrolithiasis. *Scientific World Journal* 2006;6:2403–2410.
56. Okombo J, Liebman M. Probiotic-induced reduction of gastrointestinal oxalate absorption in healthy subjects. *Urol Res* 2010;38:169–178.
57. Finch AM et al. Urine composition in normal subjects after oral ingestion of oxalate-rich foods. *Clin Sci (Lond)* 1981;60:411–418.
58. Chadwick VS et al. Mechanism for hyperoxaluria in patients with ileal dysfunction. *N Engl J Med* 1973;289:172–176.
59. Hatch M, Freel RW. The roles and mechanisms of intestinal oxalate transport in oxalate homeostasis. *Semin Nephrol* 2008;28:143–151.
60. Fairclough PD et al. Effect of sodium chenodeoxycholate on oxalate absorption from the excluded human colon—Mechanism for "enteric" hyperoxaluria. *Gut* 1977;18:240–244.
61. Rudman D et al. Hypocitraturia in patients with gastrointestinal malabsorption. *N Engl J Med* 1980;303:657–661.
62. Smith LH et al. Acquired hyperoxaluria, nephrolithiasis, and intestinal disease. Description of a syndrome. *N Engl J Med* 1972;286:1371–1375.
63. Hofmann AF et al. Acquired hyperoxaluria and intestinal disease. Evidence that bile acid glycine is not a precursor of oxalate. *Mayo Clin Proc* 1973;48:35–42.
64. Pak CY et al. A simple test for the diagnosis of absorptive, resorptive and renal hypercalciurias. *N Engl J Med* 1975;292:497–500.
65. Norman DA et al. Jejunal and ileal adaptation to alterations in dietary calcium: Changes in calcium and magnesium absorption and pathogenetic role of parathyroid hormone and 1,25-dihydroxyvitamin D. *J Clin Invest* 1981;67:1599–1603.
66. Hallson PC et al. Magnesium reduces calcium oxalate crystal formation in human whole urine. *Clin Sci (Lond)* 1982;62:17–19.
67. Hallson PC et al. Effects of Tamm-Horsfall protein with normal and reduced sialic acid content upon the crystallization of calcium phosphate and calcium oxalate in human urine. *Br J Urol* 1997;80:533–538.
68. Johnson CM et al. Renal stone epidemiology: A 25-year study in Rochester, Minnesota. *Kidney Int* 1979;16:624–631.
69. Heneghan JP et al. Helical CT for nephrolithiasis and ureterolithiasis: Comparison of conventional and reduced radiation-dose techniques. *Radiology* 2003;229:575–580.
70. Patlas M et al. Ultrasound vs CT for the detection of ureteric stones in patients with renal colic. *Br J Radiol* 2001;74:901–904.
71. Springhart WP et al. Forced versus minimal intravenous hydration in the management of acute renal colic: A randomized trial. *J Endourol* 2006;20:713–716.
72. Coll DM et al. Relationship of spontaneous passage of ureteral calculi to stone size and location as revealed by unenhanced helical CT. *AJR Am J Roentgenol* 2002;178:101–103.
73. Teichman JM. Clinical practice. Acute renal colic from ureteral calculus. *N Engl J Med* 2004;350:684–693.
74. Segura JW et al. Ureteral Stones Clinical Guidelines Panel summary report on the management of ureteral calculi. The American Urological Association. *J Urol* 1997;158:1915–1921.
75. Preminger GM et al. 2007 guideline for the management of ureteral calculi. Nephrolithiasis Guideline Panel. *J Urol* 2007;178:2418.
76. Borghi L et al. Urinary volume, water and recurrences in idiopathic calcium nephrolithiasis: A 5-year randomized prospective study. *J Urol* 1996;155:839–843.
77. Meschi T et al. Body weight, diet and water intake in preventing stone disease. *Urol Int* 2004;72(Suppl 1):29–33.
78. Andersson H, Jagenburg R. Fat-reduced diet in the treatment of hyperoxaluria in patients with ileopathy. *Gut* 1974;15:360–366.
79. Borghi L et al. Comparison of two diets for the prevention of recurrent stones in idiopathic hypercalciuria. *N Engl J Med* 2002;346:77–84.
80. Breslau NA et al. The role of dietary sodium on renal excretion and intestinal absorption of calcium and on vitamin D metabolism. *J Clin Endocrinol Metab* 1982;55:369–373.
81. Reddy ST et al. Effect of low-carbohydrate high-protein diets on acid-base balance, stone-forming propensity, and calcium metabolism. *Am J Kidney Dis* 2002;40:265–274.

82. Robertson WG et al. The effect of high animal protein intake on the risk of calcium stone-formation in the urinary tract. *Clin Sci (Lond)* 1979;57:285–288.
83. Asplin JR. Uric acid stones. *Semin Nephrol* 1996;16:412–424.
84. Barcelo P et al. Randomized double-blind study of potassium citrate in idiopathic hypocitraturic calcium nephrolithiasis. *J Urol* 1993;150:1761–1764.
85. Preminger GM et al. Prevention of recurrent calcium stone formation with potassium citrate therapy in patients with distal renal tubular acidosis. *J Urol* 1985;134:20–23.
86. Goldfarb DS, Asplin JR. Effect of grapefruit juice on urinary lithogenicity. *J Urol* 2001;166:263–267.
87. Lemann J Jr et al. Urinary oxalate excretion increases with body size and decreases with increasing dietary calcium intake among healthy adults. *Kidney Int* 1996;49:200–208.
88. Curhan GC et al. A prospective study of dietary calcium and other nutrients and the risk of symptomatic kidney stones. *N Engl J Med* 1993;328:833–838.
89. Li MK et al. Effects of magnesium on calcium oxalate crystallization. *J Urol* 1985;133:123–125.
90. Bonny O et al. Mechanism of urinary calcium regulation by urinary magnesium and pH. *J Am Soc Nephrol* 2008;19:1530–1537.
91. Caspary WF et al. "Enteral" hyperoxaluria. Effect of cholestyramine, calcium, neomycin, and bile acids on intestinal oxalate absorption in man. *Acta Hepatogastroenterol (Stuttg)* 1977;24:193–200.
92. Kelsay JL, Prather ES. Mineral balances of human subjects consuming spinach in a low-fiber diet and in a diet containing fruits and vegetables. *Am J Clin Nutr* 1983;38:12–19.
93. Hiatt RA et al. Randomized controlled trial of a low animal protein, high fiber diet in the prevention of recurrent calcium oxalate kidney stones. *Am J Epidemiol* 1996;144:25–33.
94. Emmett M et al. Conjugated bile acid replacement therapy reduces urinary oxalate excretion in short bowel syndrome. *Am J Kidney Dis* 2003;41:230–237.
95. Gruy-Kapral C et al. Conjugated bile acid replacement therapy for short bowel syndrome. *Gastroenterology* 1999;116:15–21.
96. Kenny JE, Goldfarb DS. Update on the pathophysiology and management of uric acid renal stones. *Curr Rheumatol Rep* 2010;12:125–129.
97. Goldfarb DS et al. Randomized controlled trial of febuxostat versus allopurinol or placebo in individuals with higher urinary uric acid excretion and calcium stones. *Clin J Am Soc Nephrol* 2013;8:1960–1967.
98. Siva S et al. A critical analysis of the role of gut *Oxalobacter formigenes* in oxalate stone disease. *BJU Int* 2009;103:18–21.
99. Mogna L et al. Screening of different probiotic strains for their in vitro ability to metabolize oxalates: Any prospective use in humans? *J Clin Gastroenterol* 2014;48(Suppl 1):S91–S95.

8 Metabolic Bone Disease in Adults with Short Bowel Syndrome

Lynn R. Mack and Fedja A. Rochling

CONTENTS

KEY POINTS

- The identification of metabolic bone disease should be a primary concern when evaluating the patient with short bowel syndrome (SBS).
- Vitamin D deficiency and metabolic bone disease are common in SBS.
- Bone density measurement should be an integral tool of the long-term management of SBS patients, in combination with the FRAX tool.
- Vitamin D and calcium status should be corrected before any further pharmacological treatment of osteoporosis is considered.
- Insurance coverage creates a significant obstacle for osteoporosis treatment and high-dose vitamin D replacement.
- A proactive and collaborative management approach to metabolic bone disease by endocrinologists and gastroenterologists is recommended.

INTRODUCTION

Metabolic bone disease (MBD) is present in up to 50% of patients at the time of initiation of parenteral nutrition (PN) and commonly develops after initiation of PN, resulting in a prevalence of about 80% in patients affected by short bowel syndrome (SBS) requiring PN. The lifelong process of bone development and bone homeostasis is coupled with repair and maintenance and depends on the interplay of osteoblasts and osteoclasts, while being coordinated by hormonal and paracrine signaling pathways. Genetic, mechano-response-related, endocrine-metabolic, and nutritional determinants impact bone homeostasis. In this chapter, we review the components of the key pathways in bone health among the bone, intestine, and kidneys and follow this with a discussion of the approach to diagnosing and managing MBD in the context of the adult patient with SBS [1–3]. This chapter concludes with a brief synopsis of our suggested approach to the maintenance of bone health in SBS.

BONE COMPOSITION

Bone consists of mineral in two forms, hydroxyapatite and amorphous calcium phosphate, together with type I collagen and water. In adults, normal bone is made up of compact (cortical) bone as the outer layer (80% of bone mass in adult humans) and trabecular (spongy) bone (the other 20%). The bone matrix is made up of 90% type I collagen, which is impregnated with calcium and phosphorus (hydroxyapatite) (Figure 8.1) [4]. Three main cell types are present in human bone and include osteoblasts, osteoclasts, and osteocytes. Osteoblasts, the principal bone-forming cells, are modified

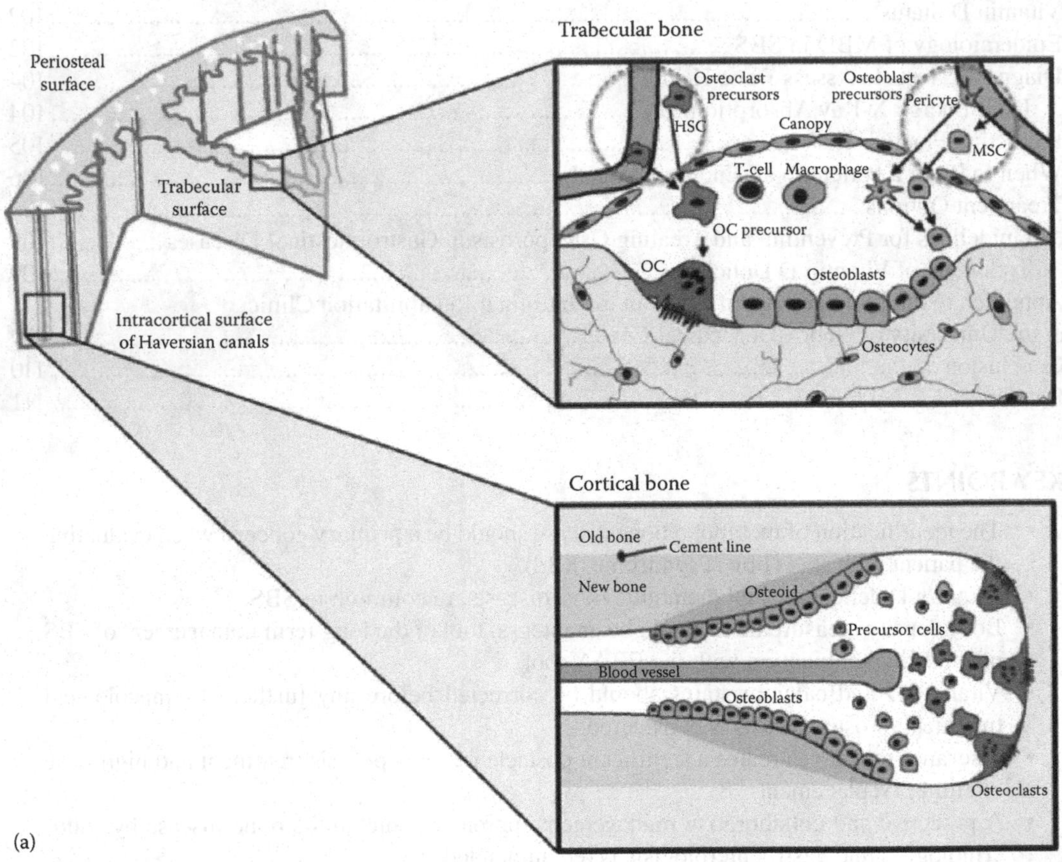

FIGURE 8.1 **(See color insert.)** Osteoblast, osteoclast, and osteocyte interaction—the bone remodeling unit. (a) Remodeling is initiated within the bone remodeling compartments (BRCs) at points beneath the canopy of cells lining the trabecular bone (upper panels) and within the cortical bone haversian canals (lower panels). Osteoclasts (OCs) are formed from hemopoietic precursors (HSC) supplied by marrow and the bloodstream. Precursors of osteoblasts come from MSCs in the marrow, from blood and from pericytes, and differentiate within the bone metabolic unit (BMU) through the osteoblast precursor stage to fully functional synthesizing osteoblasts and to osteocytes. Lining cells may also differentiate into active osteoblasts. *(Continued)*

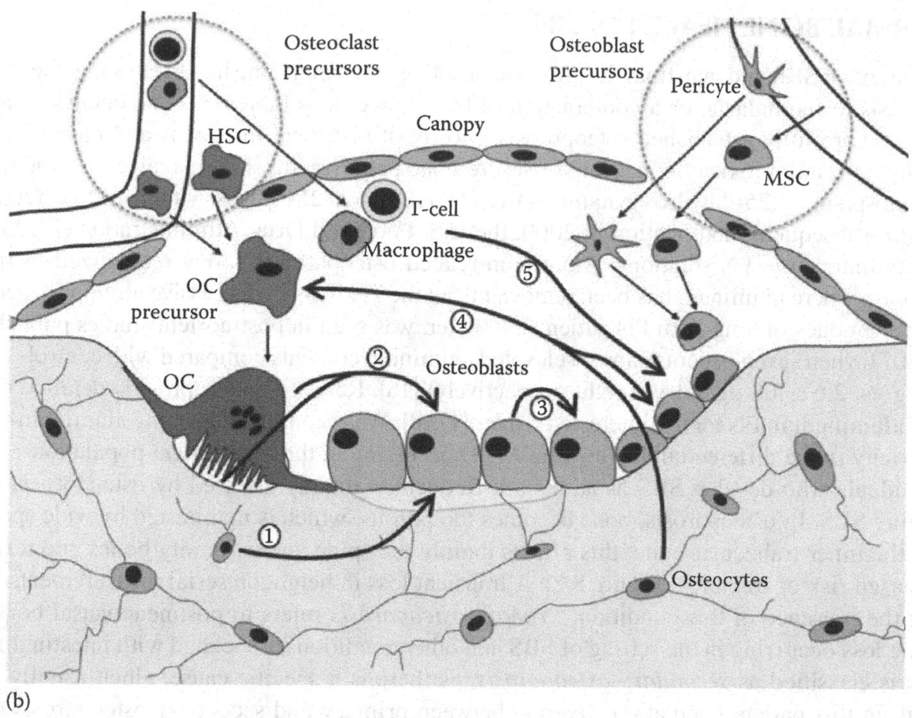

FIGURE 8.1 (CONTINUED) **(See color insert.)** Osteoblast, osteoclast, and osteocyte interaction—the bone remodeling unit. (b) Intercellular communication pathways within the BMU that comprise the remodeling process. (1) Stimulatory and inhibitory signals from osteocytes to osteoblasts (e.g., oncostatin M [OSM], parathyroid hormone–related protein [PTHrP], and sclerostin). (2) Stimulatory and inhibitory signals from osteoclasts to osteoblasts (e.g., matrix-derived transforming growth factor beta [TGF-β] and insulin-like growth factor-1 [IGF-1], secreted cardiotrophin [CT]-1, semaphorin-4D [Sema4D], and sphingosine-1-phosphate [S1P]). (3) Signaling within the osteoblast lineage (e.g., ephrinB2 and ephrin type-B receptor [EphB4], semaphorin-3A [Sema3a], PTHrP, OSM). (4) Stimulatory and inhibitory signals between the osteoblast and osteoclast lineages (e.g., RANKL, semaphorin-3B [Sema3B], wingless-type MMTV integration site family member 5A [Wnt5a], and OPG). (5) Marrow cell signals to osteoblasts (e.g., macrophage-derived OSM, T-cell-derived interleukins, and RANKL).

fibroblasts that originate from common pluripotent mesenchymal stem cells (MSCs). The differentiation of osteoblasts results in bone matrix production and bone apposition, which is also called bone formation. Osteoblasts account for 3–4% of resident bone cells and can undergo (1) apoptosis, (2) transformation into inactive osteoblasts called bone-lining cells, or (3) terminal differentiation into osteocytes. Osteocytes are star-shaped cells that account for 90–95% of all bone cells. Osteocytes play a key role in mechanotransduction [5]. Osteoclasts are multinucleated cells that are derived from pluripotent hematopoietic precursors of the macrophage lineage.

Bone formation and reabsorption involve essentially three stages. In the first stage, common pluripotent MSCs develop into osteo/chondroprogenitor cells, while osteoprogenitor cells (a.k.a., pre-osteoblasts) differentiate into osteoblasts. Osteoblast activity can be assessed by measuring serum bone-specific alkaline phosphatase and osteocalcin. In the second stage, osteoblast-dependent regulation of osteoclastogenesis occurs through the secretion of receptor activator of nuclear factor κB ligand (RANKL) and osteoprotegerin (OPG). Osteoclast activity can be assessed by measuring specific products of collagen degradation such as urinary excretion of pyridinoline and deoxypyridinoline. In the third stage, osteoclast activity occurs through cell-autonomous regulation. Osteoclasts function to facilitate bone resorption and arise as a result of fusion of 10 to 20 individual blood-borne mononuclear cells [6–10].

ABNORMAL BONE HEALTH IN SBS

In the context of SBS and intestinal failure, we can define abnormal bone health as being due to either osteoporosis, osteomalacia, or a combination of both processes (Table 8.1). Osteopenia represents the stage before fully established osteoporosis. Mostly of historical interest is a clinical syndrome caused by aluminum toxicity consisting of severe bone pain, fractures, hypercalcemia, and normal serum phosphate, 1,25-dihydroxyvitamin D (1,25OHD), and 25-hydroxyvitamin D (25OHD). In 1986, with subsequent modification in 2000, the U.S. Food and Drug Administration (FDA) mandated aluminum-free PN solutions. Aluminum-related osteopathy is rarely recognized in routine clinical care where aluminum has been removed from the PN [11–15]. Excessive aluminum accumulation in the bones of long-term PN patients, however, was seen in postmortem studies published as late as 2014 when seven patients showed elevated aluminum contents compared with controls (32.0 ± 18.7 μg/g vs. 2.6 ± 1.8 μg/g dry weight, respectively) [16]. Recent reviews provide detailed discussions of aluminum in PN for the interested reader [17,18]. We recommend keeping aluminum-related bone toxicity in the differential diagnosis of MBD occurring in the SBS patient population.

Individuals who develop SBS as adults are frequently already affected by osteoporosis before developing SBS. In osteoporosis, bone becomes too porous, which is manifested by wide spaces or gaps in the inner trabecular bone; this affects mainly the spine and extremity bones and results in an increased risk of fractures (Figure 8.2). A transient loss in height on serial measurements would support the presence of this condition. *Primary osteoporosis* refers to postmenopausal bone loss. The bone loss occurring in the setting of SBS and other conditions associated with intestinal failure patients is classified as *secondary osteoporosis*, as there is a specific cause, albeit usually multifactorial, in this patient population. Overlap between primary and secondary osteoporosis occurs

TABLE 8.1
Definition of Osteopenia and Osteoporosis by Bone Mineral Density (BMD)

	BMD	T-Score
Normal	Within 1 standard deviation (SD) of the mean level for a young-adult reference population	T-score at −1.0 and above
Osteopenia	Between 1.0 and 2.5 SDs below that of the mean level for a young-adult reference population	T-score between −1.0 and −2.5
Osteoporosis	2.5 SDs or more below that of the mean level for a young-adult reference population	T-score at or below −2.5
Severe or established osteoporosis	2.5 SD or more below that of the mean level for a young-adult reference population with fractures	T-score at or below −2.5 with one or more fractures

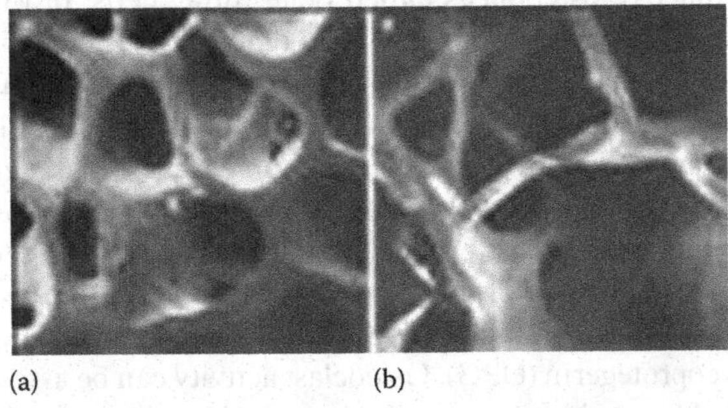

FIGURE 8.2 Photographs of normal bone and osteoporotic bone. Low-power scanning electron micrographs of iliac crest biopsies from a 44-year-old healthy male (a) and a 47-year-old female with osteoporotic compression fracture (b).

commonly in adult SBS patients (e.g., a postmenopausal woman with osteopenia or osteoporosis who sustains bowel loss which leads to secondary osteoporosis) [2]. The presence and severity of osteopenia and osteoporosis are determined most commonly by measurement of bone density using dual-energy x-ray absorptiometry (DXA; previously called DEXA scan).

In osteomalacia, the osteoid is insufficiently mineralized with low phosphorous and calcium as a consequence of vitamin D deficiency irrespective of the cause. While a bone density assessment can be abnormal in osteomalacia, it is not needed to make the diagnosis. Instead, the diagnosis is generally based on clinical suspicion in the setting of bone pain, bone tenderness, fractures, muscle weakness, gait anomalies, appropriate laboratory and radiology findings, and, occasionally, bone histomorphometry (bone biopsy using a trephine and obtained from the anterior iliac crest with subsequent tetracycline labeling) in patients at risk. Osteomalacia has been reported in patients with prior gastric surgeries for obesity, peptic ulcer disease, and cancer [19]. Bhambri et al. [20] reported on increases in bone mineral density (BMD) at the femoral neck and lumbar spine on 26 patients with frank osteomalacia, two of whom had malabsorptive syndromes, whose low 25OHD levels were corrected. Bone loss at the forearm (cortical site) appeared irreversible. Osteoporosis and osteomalacia are compared in Table 8.2.

TABLE 8.2
Comparison of Clinical Features, Risk Factors, and Diagnostic Tests between Osteoporosis and Osteomalacia

	Osteoporosis	Osteomalacia
Clinical findings	Decreased bone mass Painless If compression fracture, pain may occur and be worsened by activity; relieved by rest	Defective mineralization Muscle weakness—proximal muscles Muscle wasting Hypotonia Discomfort with movement Bone pain—lower spine, pelvis, lower extremities Pain made worse by activity Pain worse at night Bone tenderness Waddling gait Sine curvature changes in advanced disease
Risk factors	Menopause, sedentary, hereditary	Lack of sunlight, dietary, liver disease, renal disease
25 Vitamin D	Normal	Low <15 ng/mL in 100%
Calcium	Normal	Low in 27–38% of patients
Phosphorus	Normal	Low
Alkaline phosphatase	Normal	Up in 95–100% of patients
PTH	No change	Up
Urinary calcium		Low in 87% of patients
Bone biopsy	No utility	Tetracycline labeled bone biopsy Prolonged mineralization lag time Widened osteoid seams Increased osteoid volume
DXA	Abnormal (see text) BMD reduced by definition	Abnormal (see text) BMD reduced in some
X-ray	Fractures from minimal trauma	Looser's zone-pseudofractures Fissures Narrow radiolucent lines Loss of vertebral body trabeculae Loss of concavity of vertebral bodies

VITAMIN D STATUS

The World Health Organization (WHO) defines vitamin D insufficiency as serum 25OHD below 20 ng/mL (50 nmol/L) [21,22]. Others define vitamin D deficiency as serum 25OHD level below 20 ng/mL and vitamin D insufficiency as less than 30 ng/mL (75 nmol/L) [23]. A reason for the differing definition is the finding that serum parathyroid hormone (PTH), which is inversely related to serum 25OHD, decreases as serum 25OHD increases and reaches a plateau at a serum 25OHD of approximately 30 ng/mL (75 nmol/L) [24]. Many authorities suggest, therefore, that vitamin D-replete status should be considered a serum 25OHD level of 30 ng/mL or greater (75 nmol/L or greater) [25,26].

Treatment of vitamin D deficiency in healthy individuals may be accomplished with over-the-counter vitamin D. The commonly available forms of vitamin D supplements are cholecalciferol (vitamin D_3) and ergocalciferol (vitamin D_2). A meta-analysis of seven randomized trials evaluating serum 25OHD concentrations after supplementation with cholecalciferol versus ergocalciferol showed that cholecalciferol increased 25OHD more efficiently than ergocalciferol did [27]. Most experts therefore recommend supplementation with vitamin D_3 over vitamin D_2; however, vitamin D_2 is generally covered by insurance as it is considered a medication, while vitamin D_3 is classified as a medical food.

In general, for healthy patients, each 1000 IU daily of vitamin D3 increases the 25OHD level by 10 ng/dL over 8 to 12 weeks (alternatively, each 100 units of vitamin D3 increases the 25OHD level by 0.7 to 1.0 ng/dL over 8 to 12 weeks) [28–30]. Patients with malabsorption, as in SBS, are not able to absorb vitamin D efficiently. Therefore, even with the use of high-dose oral vitamin D supplementation (e.g., 10,000 to 50,000 IU daily or more of either vitamin D_2 or vitamin D_3), there is often minimal improvement in the vitamin D level [31–33]. Those patients who remain deficient on high doses of oral vitamin D may be treated with a vitamin D metabolite such as calcitriol 0.25 to 0.5 µg per day, although caution is needed as it may cause hypercalcemia.

Calcitriol will enhance the intestinal absorption of calcium and, in turn, lower intact PTH, thus helping resolve the compensatory hyperparathyroidism associated with vitamin D deficiency. This can then help reduce bone loss but will not alter the 25OHD level. As such, monitoring of patients on calcitriol should include checking calcium, phosphorus, and intact PTH [34].

Outside the United States, calcidiol is available and is considered best for those with liver disease as it does not require hepatic hydroxylation to the bioactive form, which is impaired in patients with liver disease [35]. Injectable vitamin D is also an option; however, there are no FDA-approved formulations in the United States. Nevertheless, some centers compound their own injectable preparations [36].

Alternatively, or in addition to vitamin D supplementation, sun or sunlamp exposure is another option. Artificial ultraviolet B (UVB) radiation exposure from tanning beds effectively increases 25OHD levels; however, caution is needed given the lack of defined exposure limits and the concern for skin cancer formation [37]. It is reassuring that psoriasis patients exposed to UVB 100 times or more over a 5-year period had the same rate of skin cancer as the general population [38]. Chandra and colleagues [39] showed that in patients with cystic fibrosis or SBS, exposure to a commercially available home UVB lamp twice weekly for 3 to 6 minutes each time depending on skin type for 8 weeks significantly improved 25OHD levels. In a randomized controlled pilot study at our institution, weekly exposure using the same UVB lamp in SBS patients showed a 38% increase in 25OHD levels after 12 weeks and a concomitant reduction in intact PTH [40].

EPIDEMIOLOGY OF MBD IN SBS

An estimated 10 million people over the age of 50 in the United States have osteoporosis of the hip, with another 33.6 million over the age of 50 being affected by osteopenia. Worldwide, 200 million people are thought to have osteoporosis, with the majority (80%) being postmenopausal women [22]. The prevalence of MBD in patients on home PN is anywhere between 40% and 100% [41]. Over the last three decades, the knowledge of MBD in SBS has evolved. Table 8.3 provides a chronological synopsis of the relevant studies from Europe and North America.

TABLE 8.3
Summary of Studies of Metabolic Bone Disease in Patients with Short Bowel Syndrome

Topic	Country	Pts	Etiology of SBS	Ref.
Prospective study calcium and bone metabolism	Canada 1980	16	5 Crohn's disease 3 CIIP 6 bowel resection 2 other	[14]
Painful osteomalacia	United States 1980	11	4 radiation enteritis 4 Crohn's disease 1 CIIP 2 other	[13]
Prospective study of MBD due to reduced bone formation; no osteomalacia	France 1984	7	No data	[42]
Study of calcium, phosphate, bone GLA protein, and vitamin D prior to PN initiation	United States 1986	25	No data	[43]
Osteomalacia study compared with MBD seen in 1980 study	United States 1986	13	2 Crohn's disease 1 CIIP 5 radiation enteritis 5 other	[15]
Impact of aluminum deposition on MBD	United States 1987	26	No data	[44]
Urinary calcium loss in long-term PN	United States 1988	17	No data	[45]
Long-term PN associated with ongoing bone loss	Israel 1990	10	No data	[46]
Prospective follow-up shows bone loss continues while on PN	Denmark 1994	15	13 Crohn's disease 2 ulcerative colitis	[47]
Vitamin D withdrawal during PN can increase lumbar bone density	Canada 1995	No data	No data	[48]
Diurnal regulation of calcium and PTH occurs during PN	United States 2000	6	2 Crohn's disease 1 bowel resection 1 radiation enteritis 2 mesenteric ischemia	[49]
Prevalence and severity of BMD in long-term PN	Italy 2002	165	48 IBD 65 mesenteric ischemia 18 dysmotility 6 extensive disease 6 fistula	[41]
Prevalence of MBD in SBS	France 2003	88	16 IBD 23 radiation enteritis 23 mesenteric ischemia 4 Gardner disease 4 CIIP 5 bowel resection 4 volvulus	[50]
Annual decline in BMD is moderate while on PN	Denmark 2004	75	35 Crohn's disease No data on other	[51]
Prevalence and risk factors for MDD and impact of pamidronate	Canada 2006	11	No data	[52]

Note: CIIP, chronic idiopathic intestinal pseudoobstruction; GLA protein, serum bone GLA protein also called BGP or osteocalcin; IBD, inflammatory bowel disease; PN, parenteral nutrition.

The etiology of MBD in patients with SBS is multifactorial, including traditional risk factors such as female gender, advancing age, low body weight (body mass index [BMI] <25), glucocorticoid use, hypogonadism, excessive alcohol consumption (three units per day or more; one unit = 12 oz of beer = 5 oz of wine = 1 oz of hard liquor), tobacco smoking, family history, and physical inactivity [53]. Specific PN-related factors that may contribute include the following [54]:

- Aluminum contamination (eliminated around 1986 with the removal of casein hydrolysates); aluminum reduces PTH secretion and 1,25OHD [55]
- Amino acid infusions exceeding 2 g/kg/day; may lead to enhanced calciuresis and subsequent bone loss
- Hypophosphatemia; adversely affects renal tubular calcium absorption
- Chronic metabolic acidosis; impairs vitamin D metabolism, which worsens enteric calcium absorption
- Vitamin D toxicity; can increase bone resorption, causing bone loss and hypercalcemia [14,56]
- Hypomagnesemia; reduces PTH secretion, which results in reduced renal calcium absorption and reduced 1,25OH production, which causes further reduction in enteric calcium and magnesium absorption (positive feedback loop)

DIAGNOSTIC TESTS TO ASSESS BONE HEALTH

In addition to blood and urine studies, there are a number of technologies that provide a quantitative and qualitative assessment of bone health. Three tests are currently in use in clinical practice: (1) DXA scan, which is the preferred test in adults; (2) the Fracture Risk Assessment Tool (FRAX score), which is an online fracture risk assessment tool that integrates DXA scan and clinical parameters; and (3) microstructure-based scanning using quantitative computed tomography (CT), advanced CT imaging, and magnetic resonance imaging (MRI), which are available only in specialized centers [57]. Table 8.4 shows tests used in most contemporary clinical practices, while Table 8.5 indicates tests used mainly in clinical research that may enter clinical practice in the future. Evidence supporting the clinical utility of these newer technologies in patients with SBS is limited.

Dual-Energy X-Ray Absorptiometry

DXA scanning of the spine and hips is the standard of care for the initial diagnosis and subsequent long-term follow-up of patients with osteoporotic MBD. DXA does involve exposure to ionizing radiation; however, DXA-related radiation exposure is similar to that associated with an intercontinental flight across the United States. Nevertheless, the total personal lifetime accumulation of ionizing radiation due to diagnostic tests should be considered when deciding on the most appropriate test to pursue [58,59].

DXA measures bone mineral content (BMC) in grams and bone area (BA) in square centimeters, then calculates BMD in grams per centimeter squared by dividing BMC by BA. BMD is then interpreted by comparisons with a young-adult reference population (T-score) and with a patient's age-matched peers (Z-score). The T-score is the value used for the diagnosis of osteoporosis. It is calculated by subtracting the mean BMD of a young-adult reference population from the patient's BMD and dividing by the standard deviation (SD) of the young-adult population. The Z-score is a comparison of a patient's BMD with a population of peers. It is calculated by subtracting the mean BMD of an age-, ethnicity-, and sex-matched reference population from the patient's BMD and dividing by the SD of the reference population. The WHO began using T-scores to classify and define BMD in 1994. A T-score of less than −1 to −2.5 is defined as osteopenia, while a T-score of −2.5 or lower is defined as osteoporosis [60]. The spine and hip are the preferred sites

TABLE 8.4
Tests to Assess Bone Health and Evaluation of Secondary Osteoporosis in Clinical Practice

Clinical Setting	Specific Test
Labs in all patients at the initial intake visit	• CBC • Chemistry panel • Liver panel • TSH, T4 • 25 (OH) Vitamin D • PTH • Total testosterone, LH, FSH
Labs in selected patients at the initial intake visit	• Serum protein electrophoresis • Serum immunofixation • Tissue transglutaminase • Iron panel, ferritin • Homocysteine • Prolactin • Tryptase • Urine methylhistamine • UPEP • Urinary free cortisol • Urinary histamine • 24-hour urine calcium collection
Bone density	• DXA
Fracture risk	• FRAX

Note: CBC, complete blood count; FSH, follicle stimulating hormone; LH, luteinizing hormone; TSH, thyroid-stimulating hormone; T4, thyroxine.

to measure in the absence of a fragility fracture when using DXA. The specific sites for measurement are the lumbar spine, total hip, or femoral neck. The 33% radius—a mid-forearm reading available on most DXA scanners—may be used if the hip or spine cannot be measured or the patient has hyperparathyroidism or has a weight that exceeds the limit of the DXA table. DXA is currently considered the best means to monitor changes in BMD over time due to low radiation exposure, low cost, and good reproducibility [60,61]. While the BMD measured in grams per centimeter squared on different manufacturers' scanners are not directly comparable, the T-scores that are obtained may be compared [62]. For the most accurate results, patients should be measured on the same scanner.

PREDICTING FRACTURE RISK

The FRAX tool is a WHO-sponsored, country-specific fracture risk tool that combines BMD at the femoral neck or total hip with a group of validated and weighted clinical risk factors for fracture that are independent of BMD. FRAX allows for the prediction of the risk of hip fracture and major osteoporotic fractures (spine, hip, and forearm) in previously untreated men and women aged 40 to 90 years. FRAX is accessible online and is available as desktop and iPhone applications (available at http://www.shef.ac.uk/FRAX). The FRAX score calculates a person's 10-year risk of a major osteoporotic fracture (spine, hip, or wrist) and hip fracture separately. If the major fracture risk is 20% or greater, treatment with a prescription osteoporosis medication is recommended. If the hip fracture risk is 3% or more, treatment with a prescription osteoporosis medication is recommended.

TABLE 8.5
Tests Primarily Reserved for Research Use to Assess Bone Health and Evaluation of Secondary Osteoporosis

Research Setting	Specific Test
Bone formation marker	• Serum bone-specific alkaline phosphatase • Osteocalcin • Aminoterminal propeptide type I procollagen
Bone resorption marker	• Serum C-telopeptide • Urinary N-telopeptide
Bone turnover	• Histomorphometry
Bone turnover	• PTH • Bone alkaline phosphatase • Sclerostin
Mineralization	• Histomorphometry • Spectroscopy
Microfractures	• Histology • Confocal microscopy
Matrix composition	• Infrared spectroscopy • Raman spectroscopy
Microarchitecture	• Histomorphometry • HR-pQCT • HR-MRI • Micro MRI • Micro CT

Note: HR, high resolution; pQCT, peripheral quantitative computed tomography.

WHEN TO REFER A PATIENT TO AN ENDOCRINOLOGIST

If bone density testing shows osteopenia or osteoporosis and there is uncertainty about whether to prescribe an osteoporosis medication, or the patient shows a significant decline in bone density on a prescription osteoporosis treatment, then referral to an endocrinologist should be considered. If there is difficulty with vitamin D repletion, consideration may be made to referring to an endocrinologist. In addition, patients with osteoporosis-related fractures should be considered for referral. Given the complexity of care in SBS combined with the presence of one or more of these issues, most SBS patients may benefit from an evaluation by an endocrinologist.

TREATMENT OPTIONS

The primary goals of any therapy for MBD are fracture prevention and risk reduction, thereby resulting in a reduction in morbidity and mortality with secondary benefits of reduced direct and indirect healthcare costs. The treatment of osteoporosis involves primarily two groups of drugs: (1) antiresorptive drugs such as bisphosphonates, estrogen agonist/antagonists (formerly known as selective estrogen receptor modulators), and RANKL antibodies, and (2) anabolic drugs that stimulate bone formation. In the following discussion, we review the currently available therapies, provide a focused approach to their use in SBS, and briefly describe treatments in development [63,64]. Table 8.6 provides a summary of the treatment options currently approved for use in the United States and European Union.

TABLE 8.6
Drug Therapies Available for Osteoporosis (Approved and Off-Label)

Drug	Trade Name (United States)	Trade Name (EU)	Class	Route, Dose, and Frequency	FDA Approved for Osteoporosis	EMA Approved for Osteoporosis
Alendronate	Fosamax Binosto	Adrovance	Bisphosphonate	10 mg p.o. daily 70 mg p.o. weekly	Yes	Yes
Alendronate plus D		Fosavance	Bisphosphonate	70 mg + D p.o. weekly	Yes	Yes
Ibandronate	Boniva	Boniva	Bisphosphonate	2.5 mg p.o. daily, 150 mg p.o. monthly, or 3 mg IV every 3 months	Yes	Yes
Risedronate	Actonel Altevia (delayed release)		Bisphosphonate	5 mg p.o. daily, 35 mg p.o. weekly, 150 mg p.o. monthly	Yes	No data
Zoledronic acid	Reclast Zometa	Aclasta Zolendroic Acid Teva	Bisphosphonate	5 mg IV once yearly	Yes	Yes
Calcitonin	Fortical Miacalcin Generic	No data		200 IU intranasally once a day	Yes	No data
Calcitonin	Miacalcin	No data		100 IU SQ qod	Yes	
Estrogen					Yes	
Raloxifene	Evista	Evista Optruma Raloxifene Teva	Estrogen agonist/ antagonist	60 mg p.o. daily	Yes	Yes
Conjugated estrogen/ bazedoxifene	Duavee	Conbriza	Tissue-selective estrogen complex	0.45–20 mg p.o.	Not for treatment, but for prevention	Yes

(*Continued*)

TABLE 8.6 (CONTINUED)
Drug Therapies Available for Osteoporosis (Approved and Off-Label)

Drug	Trade Name (United States)	Trade Name (EU)	Class	Route, Dose, and Frequency	FDA Approved for Osteoporosis	EMA Approved for Osteoporosis
PTH1-34 (Recombinant)	Teriparatide Forteo	Forteo	Parathyroid	20 μg SQ daily	Yes	Yes
Denusomab	Prolia Xgeva (for bone metastasis)	Prolia	RANKL	60 mg SQ every 6 months	Yes	Yes
Calcitriol	Rocaltrol Vectical		Vitamin D analog	Hypocalcemia 0.5 μg p.o. q day	No	No data
Genistein		No data	Isoflavone	54 mg	No	No data
Etidronate	Generic	No data	Bisphosphonate	Paget's disease 5–10 mg/kg per day for 6 months, hypercalcemia 20 mg/kg daily for 30 days	No	No data
Pamidronate	Generic	No data	Bisphosphonate	Hypercalcemia 90 mg intravenously	No	No data
Tiludronate	Skelid	No data	Bisphosphonate	Paget's disease 400 mg p.o. q day for 3 months	No	No data
Sodium fluoride					No	No data
Strontium ranelate		Osseor Protelos		2 g daily p.o.	No	Yes

Note: EMA, European Medicines Agency; FDA, Food Drug Administration.

Guidelines for Preventing and Treating Osteoporosis in Gastrointestinal Diseases

In 2002, the American Gastroenterological Association provided guidelines for evaluating and treating osteoporosis in inflammatory bowel disease (IBD), celiac disease, and postgastrectomy states [65]. Patients with IBD who had undergone surgery with ostomy creation were not included. The authors pointed out that there was a paucity of therapeutic intervention studies specifically aimed at bone health in gastrointestinal diseases. Little has changed since that time, with most available data for the management of bone health in gastrointestinal diseases being in IBD and primarily case reports in SBS. The bisphosphonates oral alendronate, oral risedronate and intravenous pamidronate have been studied in small trials of patients with Crohn's disease and ulcerative colitis with intact bowel who were not receiving steroids, showing improvement in the spine and hip bone density after 1 year of exposure to these bisphosphonates. These studies, however, were too small and the duration was too short to show fracture reduction [66].

Approximately 0.6% of oral bisphosphonates are absorbed when taken on an empty stomach in those with a normal length of bowel. The poor absorption is attributed to very poor lipophilicity, which prevents transcellular transport across epithelial barriers, so they must be absorbed via the paracellular route, which is best in the upper part of the small intestine [67]. Therefore, those with SBS would be expected to have essentially no absorption of oral bisphosphonates. For this reason, intravenous administration of bisphosphonates is preferred when this class of medication is selected for use.

Treatment of Vitamin D Deficiency

There are no guidelines on the replacement of calcium in SBS. Guidelines from the National Osteoporosis Foundation (NOF.org) and Institute of Medicine (iom.edu) suggest that individuals in the general population under the age of 50 take 1000 mg/day of calcium and those over the age of 50 take 1200 mg/day, with most of this from dietary sources (e.g., milk, cheese, yogurt). In SBS patients with unreliable absorption of nutrients, calcium supplements will generally be necessary. Calcium carbonate comes in a form that may be chewed or swallowed. Calcium citrate is preferred in those who also take acid blocking medication since the citrate form does not require acid to be present for absorption, while the carbonate form does require acid for absorption.

A common practice for vitamin D repletion in SBS is to start with vitamin D_2 or vitamin D_3 50,000 IU weekly with the selection of the type of vitamin D determined in the United States by insurance coverage. However, if the patient has failed prior weekly intervention, then daily replacement with 50,000 IU of either vitamin D_2 or vitamin D_3 is indicated. After the initiation of vitamin D replacement, 25OHD levels are then tested 8 to 12 weeks later to determine adequacy of replacement with adjustment of the dose of vitamin D as needed [36].

Anecdotally, some or our patients have required up to 300,000 IU daily, so cost considerations become important. As discussed previously, alternatives to oral vitamin D_2 and D_3 supplementation include use of oral calcitriol (or calcidiol), UVB exposure, or injectable vitamin D, where available. For those SBS patients on PN who are candidates for the glucagon-like peptide 2 (GLP-2) analog teduglutide (see Chapter 24), consideration of its use should be given in an attempt to enhance vitamin D absorption. Jeppesen and colleagues [68] studied 11 patients with SBS, where 7 had intestinal failure and 4 had intestinal insufficiency. After administration of native GLP-2 subcutaneously three times daily, a significant improvement in 25OHD levels was seen after both 1 and 2 years [68].

APPROACH TO THE MANAGEMENT OF MBD IN THE INTESTINAL REHABILITATION CLINIC AT THE UNIVERSITY OF NEBRASKA MEDICAL CENTER

All patients seen in our Intestinal Rehabilitation Clinic, including those with SBS, undergo an initial assessment followed by longitudinal follow-up of bone health. Table 8.7 describes the general

TABLE 8.7
Bone Health Management Approach at University of Nebraska Medical Center

	Initial Visit	Follow-Up Year 1	Follow-Up Year 2	Interval Thereafter
Height, weight, BMI	Yes	Yes	Yes	Yes
Review of compliance with treatment plan review	Yes	Yes	Yes	Yes
Lifestyle factor review	Smoking cessation, alcohol intake assessment, weight-bearing exercise	Smoking cessation	Smoking cessation	Smoking cessation
Labs	Yes	Yes	Yes	Yes
DXA	Yes	No	Yes	Every 2 years
FRAX score	Yes	No	No	No
Fall risk assessment	Yes	Yes	Yes	Yes
Assessment of intervention cost and insurance coverage	Yes	Yes	Yes	Yes

approach used in our clinic, although deviation may occur in selected circumstances. Treatments provided attempt to be evidence based but are restricted by formulary guidelines. Furthermore, the ability of patients to meet the sometimes significant copay and deductible mandates imposes additional challenges to their treatment.

The initiation of therapy implies that a baseline assessment of bone health has been performed and that longitudinal imaging (DXA scan) and laboratory studies (comprehensive metabolic panel, magnesium, phosphorus, 25OHD, and PTH levels) will be completed to monitor effectiveness. Following the correction of vitamin D status, single-drug therapy typically involves zoledronic acid or denosumab, with a preference for zoledronic acid as it is now generic and readily covered by most insurance carriers. Zoledronic acid and denosumab are injectable, thus requiring no gut absorption, and have been shown to reduce the risk of both spine and hip fracture. Zoledronic acid should not be used in patients with a glomerular filtration rate <35 mL/min/1.73 m^2. In those with impaired renal function, denosumab would be the preferred alternative to zoledronic acid since it does not require renal dose adjustment. Both zoledronic acid and denosumab may cause hypocalcemia, although this effect tends to be more pronounced with denosumab. Hence, patients with SBS who are not fully vitamin D replete with borderline hypocalcemia and hypomagnesemia may be at risk for hypocalcemia when given either zoledronic acid or denosumab that necessitates replacement with intravenous calcium. Therefore, serum calcium and magnesium should be normalized and the 25OHD level should be >30 ng/mL before either zoledronic acid or denosumab is given. Teriparatide is reserved for those patients with severe osteoporosis who are willing to administer a daily injection for up to 2 years; its use should be avoided in those with prior skeletal irradiation due to the risk of osteosarcoma in this setting. Given its expense, the common difficulty in obtaining insurance coverage, and lack of evidence supporting specific hip fracture reduction, it would best be kept as a later treatment option. Combination therapy with teriparatide and denosumab has been reported in the treatment of primary osteoporosis; however, given the significant expense of using both agents and lack of fracture reduction data in any group, this should be considered experimental [48,64].

CONCLUSION

MBD is commonly present in adults at the time of SBS development, with an increasing incidence afterward. Significant morbidity from MBD can occur in the form of both fractures and bone pain.

Concurrent muscle loss in the setting of protein-calorie malnutrition adds to the problem. SBS patients need to be managed proactively at the time of their initial diagnosis. Consultation with an endocrinologist should be considered for optimal management of these complex patients. The diagnosis is most commonly based on results from a DXA scan and the fracture risk can be individually determined using the FRAX score. Challenges in the treatment of MBD in patients with SBS relate, in part, to the poor absorption of orally administered medications. This creates the need for alternative routes of administration. The presence of chronic kidney disease, a not uncommon condition in the SBS patient, often precludes the use of established drugs such as bisphosphonates. The high cost of many of the medications and supplements necessary to treat MBD presents another management challenge. Physicians need to recognize that formulary restrictions and rising copay burdens present their SBS patients with obstacles when already faced with a costly disease. Further research that focuses on the prevalence of MBD, fracture risk, efficacy of current and novel treatments, and cost-effectiveness of the diagnostic and treatment options in the SBS population is needed [69].

REFERENCES

1. Remer T et al. Dietary protein's and dietary acid load's influence on bone health. *Crit Rev Food Sci Nutr* 2014;**54**:1140–1150.
2. Shoback D, Sellmeyer D, and Bikle DD. Metabolic bone disease. In: *Greenspan's Basic & Clinical Endocrinology*, 9th ed. Gardner DG, Dolores Shoback M, eds. New York: McGraw-Hill Lange, 2011.
3. Barrett KEB et al. *Ganong's Review of Medical Physiology*, 24th ed. New York: McGraw-Hill Lange, 2012, Chapter 21, pp. 377–390.
4. Clarke B. Normal bone anatomy and physiology. *Clin J Am Soc Nephrol* 2008;**3**(Suppl 3):S131–S139.
5. Rochefort GY et al. Osteocyte: The unrecognized side of bone tissue. *Osteoporos Int* 2010;**21**:1457–1469.
6. Manolagas SC. Corticosteroids and fractures: A close encounter of the third cell kind. *J Bone Miner Res* 2000;**15**:1001–1005.
7. Capulli MR et al. Osteoblast and osteocyte: Games without frontiers. *Arch Biochem Biophys* 2014;**561**:3–12.
8. Kim JH, Kim N. Regulation of NFATc1 in osteoclast differentiation. *J Bone Metab* 2014;**21**:233–241.
9. Delmas PD et al. Urinary excretion of pyridinoline crosslinks correlates with bone turnover measured on iliac crest biopsy in patients with vertebral osteoporosis. *J Bone Miner Res* 1991;**6**:639–644.
10. Boyle WJ et al. Osteoclast differentiation and activation. *Nature* 2003;**423**:337–342.
11. Klein GL et al. Aluminum and TPN-related bone disease. *Am J Clin Nutr* 1992;**55**:483–485.
12. Klein GL et al. Aluminum as a factor in the bone disease of long-term parenteral nutrition. *Trans Assoc Am Physicians* 1982;**95**:155–164.
13. Klein GL et al. Bone disease associated with total parenteral nutrition. *Lancet* 1980;**2**:1041–1044.
14. Shike M et al. Metabolic bone disease in patients receiving long-term total parenteral nutrition. *Ann Intern Med* 1980;**92**:343–350.
15. Shike M et al. Bone disease in prolonged parenteral nutrition: Osteopenia without mineralization defect. *Am J Clin Nutr* 1986;**44**:89–98.
16. Kruger PC et al. Excessive aluminum accumulation in the bones of patients on long-term parenteral nutrition: Postmortem analysis by electrothermal atomic absorption spectrometry. *JPEN J Parenter Enteral Nutr* 2014;**38**(6):728–735.
17. Gura KM. Aluminum contamination in parenteral products. *Curr Opin Clin Nutr Metab Care* 2014;**17**:551–557.
18. Hernandez-Sanchez A et al. Aluminium in parenteral nutrition: A systematic review. *Eur J Clin Nutr* 2013;**67**:230–238.
19. Basha B et al. Osteomalacia due to vitamin D depletion: A neglected consequence of intestinal malabsorption. *Am J Med* 2000;**108**:296–300.
20. Bhambri R et al. Changes in bone mineral density following treatment of osteomalacia. *J Clin Densitom* 2006;**9**:120–127.
21. WHO. Prevention and management of osteoporosis. *World Health Organ Tech Rep Ser* 2003;**921**:1–164.
22. Bone health and osteoporosis: A report of the surgeon general. In: *Bone Health and Osteoporosis: A Report of the Surgeon General*. Rockville, MD: Department of Health and Human Services, 2004. Available at http://www.niams.nih.gov/Health_Info/Bone/SGR/surgeon_generals_report.asp. Accessed February 4, 2016.

23. Holick MF. Vitamin D deficiency. *N Engl J Med* 2007;**357**:266–281.
24. Gallagher JC, Sai AJ. Vitamin D insufficiency, deficiency, and bone health. *J Clin Endocrinol Metab* 2010;**95**:2630–2633.
25. Dawson-Hughes B et al. IOF position statement: Vitamin D recommendations for older adults. *Osteoporos Int* 2010;**21**:1151–1154.
26. Holick MF et al. Evaluation, treatment, and prevention of vitamin D deficiency: An Endocrine Society clinical practice guideline. *J Clin Endocrinol Metab* 2011;**96**:1911–1930.
27. Tripkovic L et al. Comparison of vitamin D2 and vitamin D3 supplementation in raising serum 25-hydroxyvitamin D status: A systematic review and meta-analysis. *Am J Clin Nutr* 2012;**95**:1357–1364.
28. Vieth R. Critique of the considerations for establishing the tolerable upper intake level for vitamin D: Critical need for revision upwards. *J Nutr* 2006;**136**:1117–1122.
29. Heaney RP et al. Human serum 25-hydroxycholecalciferol response to extended oral dosing with cholecalciferol. *Am J Clin Nutr* 2003;**77**:204–210.
30. Gallagher JC et al. Dose response to vitamin D supplementation in postmenopausal women: A randomized trial. *Ann Intern Med* 2012;**156**:425–437.
31. Koutkia P et al. Treatment of vitamin D deficiency due to Crohn's disease with tanning bed ultraviolet B radiation. *Gastroenterology* 2001;**121**:1485–1488.
32. Haderslev KV et al. Vitamin D status and measurements of markers of bone metabolism in patients with small intestinal resection. *Gut* 2003;**52**:653–658.
33. Leichtmann GA et al. Intestinal absorption of cholecalciferol and 25-hydroxycholecalciferol in patients with both Crohn's disease and intestinal resection. *Am J Clin Nutr* 1991;**54**:548–552.
34. Gallagher JC et al. Combination treatment with estrogen and calcitriol in the prevention of age-related bone loss. *J Clin Endodrinol Metab* 2001;**86**(8):3618–3628.
35. Lim LY et al. Vitamin D deficiency in patients with chronic liver disease and cirrhosis. *Gastroenterol Rep* 2012;**14**:67–73.
36. Roger Warndahl RP. *Compounding Vitamin D by Mayo Clinic Pharmacy.* Rochester, MN: Mayo Clinic, 2015.
37. Osmancevic A et al. Vitamin D production after UVB exposure—A comparison of exposed skin regions. *J Photochem Photobiol B* 2015;**143**:38–43.
38. Osmancevic A et al. The risk of skin cancer in psoriasis patients treated with UVB therapy. *Acta Derma Venereol* 2014;**94**(4):425–430.
39. Chandra P et al. Treatment of vitamin D deficiency with UV light in patients with malabsorption syndromes: A case series. *Photodermatol Photoimmunol Photomed* 2007;**23**:179–185.
40. Makhija C et al. Treatment of vitamin D deficiency in intestinal rehabilitation clinic patients with portable ultraviolet-B lamp. THR-251 Endocrine Society's 97th Annual Meeting and Expo, March 5–8, 2015, San Diego. *Endocrine Reviews* 2015;**36**(2). Available at http://press.endocrine.org/doi/abs/10.1210/endo-meetings.2015.BCHVD.13.THR-251#sthash.EqPQT2CM.dpuf.
41. Pironi L et al. Prevalence of bone disease in patients on home parenteral nutrition. *Clin Nutr* 2002;**21**:289–296.
42. de Vernejoul MC et al. Multifactorial low remodeling bone disease during cyclic total parenteral nutrition. *J Clin Endocrinol Metab* 1985;**60**:109–113.
43. Epstein S et al. Bone and mineral status of patients beginning total parenteral nutrition. *JPEN J Parenter Enteral Nutr* 1986;**10**:263–264.
44. Lipkin EW et al. Heterogeneity of bone histology in parenteral nutrition patients. *Am J Clin Nutr* 1987;**46**:673–680.
45. Lipkin EW et al. Mineral loss in the parenteral nutrition patient. *Am J Clin Nutr* 1988;**47**:515–523.
46. Foldes J et al. Progressive bone loss during long-term home total parenteral nutrition. *JPEN J Parenter Enteral Nutr* 1990;**14**:139–142.
47. Staun M et al. Bone mineral content in patients on home parenteral nutrition. *Clin Nutr* 1994;**13**(6):351–355.
48. Verhage AH et al. Increase in lumbar spine bone mineral content in patients on long-term parenteral nutrition without vitamin D supplementation. *JPEN J Parenter Enteral Nutr* 1995;**19**(6):431–436.
49. Goodman WG et al. Altered diurnal regulation of blood ionized calcium and serum parathyroid hormone concentrations during parenteral nutrition. *Am J Clin Nutr* 2000;**71**:560–568.
50. Cohen-Solal M et al. Osteoporosis in patients on long-term home parenteral nutrition: A longitudinal study. *J Bone Miner Res* 2003;**18**:1989–1994.
51. Haderslev KV et al. Assessment of the longitudinal changes in bone mineral density in patients receiving home parenteral nutrition. *JPEN J Parenter Enteral Nutr* 2004;**28**:289–294.

52. Raman, M et al. Metabolic bone disease in patients receiving home parenteral nutrition: A Canadian study and review. *JPEN J Parenter Enteral Nutr* 2006;**30**(6):492–496.
55. Ott SM et al. Aluminum is associated with low bone formation in patients receiving chronic parenteral nutrition. *Ann Intern Med* 1983;**98**:910–914.
53. Nanes MS, Kallen CB. Osteoporosis. *Semin Nucl Med* 2014;**44**:439–450.
54. Jeejeebhoy KN. Metabolic bone disease and total parenteral nutrition: A progress report. *Am J Clin Nutr* 1998;**67**:186–187.
56. Selby PL et al. Vitamin D intoxication causes hypercalcaemia by increased bone resorption which responds to pamidronate. *Clin Endocrinol (Oxf)* 1995;**43**(5):531–536.
57. Link TM. Osteoporosis imaging: State of the art and advanced imaging. *Radiology* 2012;**263**:3–17.
58. Radiological Society of North America. Radiation Dose in X-Ray and CT Exams. 2015. Cited February 3, 2015. Available from: http://www.radiologyinfo.org/en/safety/index.cfm?pg=sfty_xray#part3.
59. Njeh CF et al. Radiation exposure in bone mineral density assessment. *Appl Radiat Isot* 1999;**50**:215–236.
60. ICSD. 2013 ISCD official position—Adult. 2013. Cited January 20, 2015. Available from: http://www.iscd.org/official-positions/2013-iscd-official-positions-adult/.
61. El Maghraoui A, Roux C. DXA scanning in clinical practice. *QJM* 2008;**101**:605–617.
62. Hui SL et al. Universal standardization of bone density measurements: A method with optimal properties for calibration among several instruments. *J Bone Miner Res* 1997;**12**:1463–1470.
63. Watts NB et al. American Association of Clinical Endocrinologists medical guidelines for clinical practice for the diagnosis and treatment of postmenopausal osteoporosis. *Endocr Pract* 2010;**16**(Suppl 3): 1–37.
64. Cosman F et al. Clinician's guide to prevention and treatment of osteoporosis. *Osteoporos Int* 2014;**25**(10):2359–2381.
65. Bernstein CN et al. AGA technical review on osteoporosis in gastrointestinal diseases. *Gastroenterology* 2003;**124**:795–841.
66. Rodriguez-Bores L et al. Basic and clinical aspects of osteoporosis in inflammatory bowel disease. *World J Gastroenterol* 2007;**13**:6156–6165.
67. Lin JH. Biphosphonates: A review of their pharmacokinetic properties. *Bone* 1996;**18**(2):75–84.
68. Jeppesen PB et al. Short bowel patients treated for two years with glucagon-like peptide 2: Effects on intestinal morphology and absorption, renal function, bone and body composition, and muscle function. *Gastroenterol Res Pract* 2009;**2009**:Article ID 616054. Available at http://www.hindawi.com/journals/grp/2009/616054. Accessed May 22, 2015.
69. Rachner TD et al. Osteoporosis: Now and the future. *Lancet* 2011;**377**(9773):1276–1287.

9 Clinical and Nutritional Assessment in the Patient with Short Bowel Syndrome

Denise Konrad and Betsy Gallant

CONTENTS

KEY POINTS

- Assessment of the patient with short bowel syndrome (SBS) requires a careful and detailed history and physical examination.
- Determining the SBS patient's remaining gastrointestinal (GI) anatomy is the cornerstone of the initial assessment.
- In addition to GI anatomy, the clinical and nutritional assessment should include documentation of medical/surgical history, medication profile, dietary and beverage practices, nutrition support history, as well as patient goals and concerns.
- A thorough assessment of the SBS patient is invaluable in the development of the optimal treatment plan.

INTRODUCTION

Short bowel syndrome (SBS) is defined as a compromised ability to absorb nutrients and fluids arising from a shortened length of remaining bowel [1]. The optimal management of SBS requires a skilled, experienced, and resourceful multidisciplinary team to meet the challenging goal of maximizing the use of the remaining gastrointestinal (GI) tract. The aim of this chapter is to recognize the key clinical and nutritional factors to assess in patients with SBS. It should act as a reference to key topics discussed in greater detail in the chapters that follow to help guide clinicians through the initial and follow-up appointments.

DEFINING GI ANATOMY

One of the first areas to assess in the patient with suspected or known SBS is the remaining small bowel length and segments of the small bowel that remain, whether the ileocecal valve is intact, how much of the colon remains, and whether it is in continuity with the small intestine. A determination of functional capacity and whether any active disease processes such as Crohn's disease, *Clostridium difficile* infection, or the presence of radiation enteritis that may contribute to the patient's clinical picture is also necessary. The presence and location of an enterostomy, enterocutaneous fistula, enteral tube, or peritoneal drain are important to note.

The normal small bowel ranges in length from 260 to 800 cm [2]. Small bowel length is measured in centimeters starting at the ligament of Treitz, also known as the duodenjejunal flexure, and ends at the ileocecal valve. The length of colon remaining is typically represented as a percentage of what remains (i.e., >50% or <50%); which segment remains is also valuable to note: ascending, transverse, or descending. Each section of the small bowel and colon play an important role in the absorption of nutrients, electrolytes, and/or fluids (see Chapter 3) (Table 9.1 [1]).

The quality, length, and segments of bowel remaining are important factors in terms of the potential for intestinal adaptation and ultimately portend significant prognostic information in the SBS patient with respect to the eventual restoration of enteral autonomy. For example, three anatomical configurations that have been shown to increase the risk of a patient requiring permanent parenteral support are as follows [3]:

- <100 cm of total small bowel proximal to a stoma or enterocutaneous fistula
- <65 cm of jejunum anastomosed to the colon, resulting in the loss of the ileocecal valve
- <30 cm of small bowel, including the ileocecal valve and terminal ileum anastomosed to the colon

TABLE 9.1
Fluid and Nutrition Absorption

Location	Length (cm)	Fluid or Nutrients Absorbed
Duodenum	25–30	Amino acids Carbohydrates Iron Folate
Jejunum	160–200	Carbohydrates Fatty acids Fat-soluble vitamins (A, D, E, K) Folate Sodium Fluid
Ileum	Up to 300	Vitamin B_{12} (food-bound only) Sodium Fluid Bile acids
Colon	150	Electrolytes Fluid Medium-chain triglycerides Bile acids (small amount)

Source: Jeejeebhoy, K., *CMAJ*, 166, 1297–1302, 2002.

The ileum has the ability to adapt when jejunum is removed. Unfortunately, the opposite is not true. If the colon remains in continuity, the patient is less likely to require parenteral support as the colon avidly absorbs fluid and electrolytes. In addition, colonic bacteria ferment undigested carbohydrates and soluble fiber into short-chain fatty acids. This process, known as carbohydrate salvage, provides additional energy and further enhances sodium and water absorption, as well as stimulates mucosal adaptation in the large intestine [4]. Patients experience severe malabsorption when >100 cm of terminal ileum is lost due to the important role of this bowel segment in the enterohepatic circulation of bile salts. When unabsorbed bile salts enter the colon, the caustic nature of these salts stimulates electrolyte and water secretion, exacerbating diarrhea. Additionally, bile salt deficiency leads to fat and fat-soluble vitamin malabsorption and increases the total volume of stool/ostomy output in the form of steatorrhea [1]. Finally, when the ileum is resected, the hormonal (e.g., peptide YY and glucagon-like peptide-1) feedback mechanism known as the "ileal brake" is lost, which, under normal circumstances, would decrease gastric hypersecretion and motility as well as peristalsis in the upper GI tract [5].

DETERMINE REMAINING GI ANATOMY

Despite the importance of this information, it is often challenging to determine a patient's remaining bowel anatomy, particularly when multiple surgeries have been performed (and in more than one institution no less!). There are a variety of ways to determine the remaining bowel anatomy. Ideally, operative reports will make note of how much of the bowel is remaining, the segment of bowel that was removed, and the apparent health of the remaining bowel. Unfortunately, it is more common for operative reports to note how much was resected, but not necessarily which bowel segment or the length that is remaining. If the operative reports are not available or lack this information, a barium contrast small bowel follow through (SBFT) can be ordered to *estimate* bowel length; an opisometer is a measuring instrument that can be used for this purpose. An SBFT also provides information regarding transit time and other structural information, including strictures and bowel dilatation [6]. A three-dimensional reconstructed abdominal computed tomography (CT) scan may also provide this information, presuming it was done since the patient's last operation. CT enterography (CTE) combines a CT scan with large volumes of oral contrast to image the small bowel, is highly sensitive in evaluating small bowel disorders, and is increasingly being used to assess the small bowel because it is noninvasive and accurate. CTE has been shown to be more effective at detecting strictures than SBFT.

Once a patient's GI anatomy has been determined, it is helpful to keep it at the top of the patient's clinic note in the electronic medical record each time they return to clinic for quick reference. For example:

> 58 year-old man with SBS as a result of multiple resections for Crohn's disease.
> *GI anatomy*: 60 cm jejunum past the ligament of Treitz anastomosed to midtransverse colon.

MEDICAL AND SURGICAL HISTORY

Other historical information that is useful in the management of patients with SBS includes medical and surgical history. Treatment plans need to be individualized for each patient and must consider all these factors to be successful. Knowledge of the underlying disease that led to SBS, such as Crohn's disease, mesenteric ischemia, and abdominal trauma, along with any other comorbidities, including diabetes, cardiac disease, hepatic failure, renal disease, or cancer, is important. Similarly, a history of underlying mucosal disease, enterocutaneous fistulae, intestinal strictures, chronic obstruction, radiation enteritis, or bouts of chronic dehydration will aid in patient management. Finally, a determination of psychological, social, and economic factors that may affect treatment plans is important to consider, as management of SBS often includes a specialized diet and a variety of medications that can become expensive and overwhelming.

Obtaining a surgical history is vital; however, access to operative reports may be limited, especially if performed several years ago or at an outside institution. The number and type of operations performed, along with the indication (i.e., obstruction, stricture, active disease, enterocutaneous fistula, and trauma), should be noted. Also note whether the gallbladder has been removed, or if the patient had (or still has) any external drains, stoma, feeding tubes, enterocutaneous fistula, or wounds present.

MEDICATIONS AND SUPPLEMENTS

Document all medications and oral supplements that an SBS patient is taking, including prescription and over-the-counter. Inquire about dose, timing, form (especially delayed- or sustained-release), frequency, and route of delivery. Be sure to query the patient about any over-the-counter medications or supplements, but also record the specific agents being used, including herbal, prebiotics or probiotics, protein powders, fiber, vitamins, and minerals, all of which are common in this patient population. Finally, it is very important to periodically do a "total pill count," as some patients may end up taking an unwieldy number of medications over the course of the day. Not only is this a lot to expect of patients, but also the volume of fluid required to take numerous medications as well as the osmotic load some of them contain may work against the very goals of decreasing stool output. Consider when, perhaps, a stronger medication requiring fewer pills would be beneficial to the patient. Also, periodically reassess their clinical need for certain medications as circumstances may have changed such that a medication is not needed anymore (e.g., antihypertensive or cholesterol-lowering agent in a patient who has lost a substantial amount of weight compared with their pre-morbid body weight).

MALNUTRITION IN SBS

Malnutrition from undernutrition is common in SBS. Multiple factors contribute to the risk of malnutrition in SBS, including the shortened length of the remaining bowel, rapid intestinal transit, time elapsed since resection and intestinal adaptation that may have occurred, presence of small intestinal bacterial overgrowth, bile salt deficiency causing maldigestion, GI symptoms limiting oral intake, and alterations in the diet [7]. Patients with SBS may also have chronic inflammation from the underlying disease process that caused their SBS. Inflammation is now recognized as an important underlying risk factor for malnutrition and may thwart attempts at anabolism due to its catabolic effects which increase mortality risk [8,9].

WEIGHT CHANGE HISTORY

Determining weight change involves obtaining a detailed weight history, accurately measuring the patient's current weight, and adjusting for any factors that might falsely contribute to weight gain or loss. The medical record should be used to confirm weight information provided by the patient and caregiver whenever possible as self-reported weight data may not be accurate or available (e.g., if the patient is intubated and on mechanical ventilation, has an altered mental status, or caregiver is unavailable) [10]. Besides loss of muscle and subcutaneous fat, sources of weight loss include amputation, removal of a cast or other medical device that contributes to body weight, and removal of a body organ (e.g., intestinal resection). Additionally, it is crucial to take into consideration fluid status (dehydration or fluid retention/overload) to accurately determine weight change. In patients with SBS, a sudden weight loss of >1 kg (2.2 lb) per day for two or more consecutive days is likely related to dehydration. Fluid overload can mask weight loss and should also be considered (1 L = 1 kg).

Obtaining accurate weights in hospitalized patients is necessary to develop and monitor individualized nutrition care plans but continues to be a challenge in most institutions. The scale used to measure body weight should be accurate and regularly calibrated. Standing scales are more accurate than bed scales and should be used whenever possible. If a bed scale is used, it should be set at zero prior to each use to ensure an accurate weight. Ideally, the person would be weighed on the same scale, wearing the same amount of clothing, and at the same time of day. Weight change over a period of time is reported as a percentage of weight change from the patient's baseline or usual body weight [11].

When assessing changes in body weight, the clinician should determine the following:

- Usual body weight prior to illness and when the patient last weighed that amount
- If the weight change was intentional; if so, method used to lose weight
- Signs or symptoms of dehydration, including lightheadedness, dizziness, dry mouth, excessive thirst, poor skin turgor, low urine output (< 1 L/24 hours), cramping in the extremities, tachycardia (>100 beats/minute or 10–20 beats/minute increase from baseline), hypotension, orthostasis, and elevated blood urea nitrogen (BUN) and creatinine
- History of kidney stones or admissions for dehydration
- Signs or symptoms of fluid overload such as rapid weight gain without change in dietary intake, localized or generalized edema, dyspnea, crackles identified when evaluating breath sounds, distended neck veins, change in medication or organ failure

ORAL DIET AND FLUID HISTORY

The goal of diet modification in conjunction with medication therapy is to decrease or avoid the need for home parenteral fluids and parenteral nutrition (PN). A careful and complete diet history (or ideally diet records kept by the patient prior to the clinic visit) will aid the clinician in targeting which areas are in need of attention as well as may be contributing to stool/ostomy output. Patients should be specifically asked about the use of dairy products, fruit juices, soda, as well as any liquid nutritional supplements (e.g., Ensure, Boost, or store brand equivalent), or instant breakfast-type drinks. It is not uncommon for SBS patients to report to a clinic having been told by a well-meaning clinician to start drinking Ensure or an equivalent type product in response to weight loss; unfortunately, this often acts to increase stool output due to its hypertonic nature. Use of other sugars or consumption of highly osmotic agents in foods and beverages also needs to be investigated. How one asks the question may make the difference in a patient's success with the diet. For example, if patients are asked to tell them about all the things they eat, many patients will not consider liquids as something that they "eat." Having patients bring a 2- to 3-day diet record of all the food and fluid they consume to every clinic visit until they stabilize (or the clinician is sure the patient knows what they are doing) is prudent. Estimation of energy, protein, and fluid needs can be helpful to the managing clinician and patient alike; examples are shown in Tables 9.2 [12,13] and 9.3 [14].

Included in the assessment of diet and fluid intake should be whether the patient has used any oral rehydration solutions (ORSs). Discuss with the patients which ones have they tried, how much they drink, and how (i.e., whether sipped slowly throughout the day—the preferred approach—or ingested in large volumes in one sitting). Many patients may find the ORS unpalatable due to the salty flavor. Mixing with sugar-free flavoring and keeping the ORS drink cold often improves palatability. If the patient is still unable to tolerate the ORS, consider decreasing the salt content (if homemade)—as long as their output is controlled, a slightly suboptimal version of ORS is better than the hypotonic (water) or hypertonic (juice and soft drink) alternatives. Encouragement in ORS use at each clinic visit is also helpful to enhance its use.

TABLE 9.2
Estimated Energy and Protein Requirements

Energy	Protein
Mifflin St. Jeor [12]	Healthy adults:
Men: 9.99 × weight (kg) + 6.25 × height (cm) – 4.92 × age + 5	0.8 g/kg/day actual weight
Women: 9.99 × weight (kg) + 6.25 × height (cm) – 4.92 × age – 161	Metabolically-stressed:
	1.2–2.0 g/kg/day actual weight [13]

Note: Method of choice at the Cleveland Clinic.

TABLE 9.3
Age- and Weight-Based Estimate of Fluid Requirements

Age Method[a]	mL/kg/day
16–30 years, active	40
20–55 years	35
56–75 years	30
>75 years	25

Source: Whitmire, S.J., in Gottschlich, M.M., Matarese, L.E., eds. *Contemporary Nutrition Support Practice. A Clinical Guide*, WB Saunders Company, Philadelphia, PA, 1998, 127–144.

[a] This is a good place to start for fluid needs but will need to account for the high losses of stoma and stool in the SBS patient population. Monitor for adequate urine output, BUN, creatinine, as well as signs and symptoms of dehydration.

NUTRITION AND PARENTERAL FLUID SUPPORT HISTORY

It is important to note if the patient is receiving or has previously received nutrition support, either parenteral and/or enteral, or intravenous hydration, and if so, the type, volume, and components of each as well as catheter/tube access for the same. Determine if there have been any catheter-related or feeding tube-related complications. In particular, knowledge of the frequency and severity of any catheter-related bloodstream infection (CRBSI) and any loss of central venous access sites is critical. Determine how long the catheter has been in place and what type of training they have received in terms of catheter/tube care. If the patient has a short-term catheter (i.e., peripherally inserted central venous catheter), consider changing to a long-term catheter (i.e., tunneled or subcutaneously implanted port) if it has been in place for more than 1 month and parenteral support needs are ongoing. An inquiry into the use of antibiotic or ethanol locks, which are being used more commonly to prevent CRBSI, is encouraged. Finally, an intimate knowledge and close working relationship with the home infusion provider, home health nurse, and the patient's other healthcare providers will enhance care.

INTAKE AND OUTPUT MEASUREMENTS

Patients should be asked to record 24-hour measurements of urine and stool volumes, as well as their body weight at least one to two times per week until stable. This information will augment the subjective information provided by the patient. To facilitate recording these measurements, a stool hat should be provided (Figure 9.1). Just as important is to give them a form to record this information (Figure 9.2). Occasionally, it may be helpful to determine whether the patient is a "net secretor" (stool output remains high even when the patient is nil per os [NPO; i.e., nothing by mouth]), as these patients do not respond as well to antidiarrheal agents and will require more in the way of antisecretory agents. There are a couple ways to obtain this information. One is to measure all oral fluid intake and subtract all stool output during a 24-hour period; that is, the so-called enteral balance. Another less commonly used method is to conduct a 24-hour stool/ostomy measurement while strictly NPO (and maintained on intravenous fluids—this is typically done in the hospital) [6]. Output that slows to <500–800 mL/day is suggestive of an osmotic diarrhea related to the foods and fluids ingested. If the output remains >800 mL in a 24-hour period, this is likely a secretory diarrhea. Table 9.4 [15] lists urine and stool output goals based on anatomy type. Those with jejunostomies may have a stool output of >4–6 L/day, in which case oral foods (and fluids especially) may need to be limited until the stool volume can be brought down to a manageable amount. An avoidance of strict NPO status due to the important trophic effects of foods is advised; however, it may be worthwhile to provide small amounts of food and liquid over the day. These patients will require PN to meet 100% of their nutrient needs during this time.

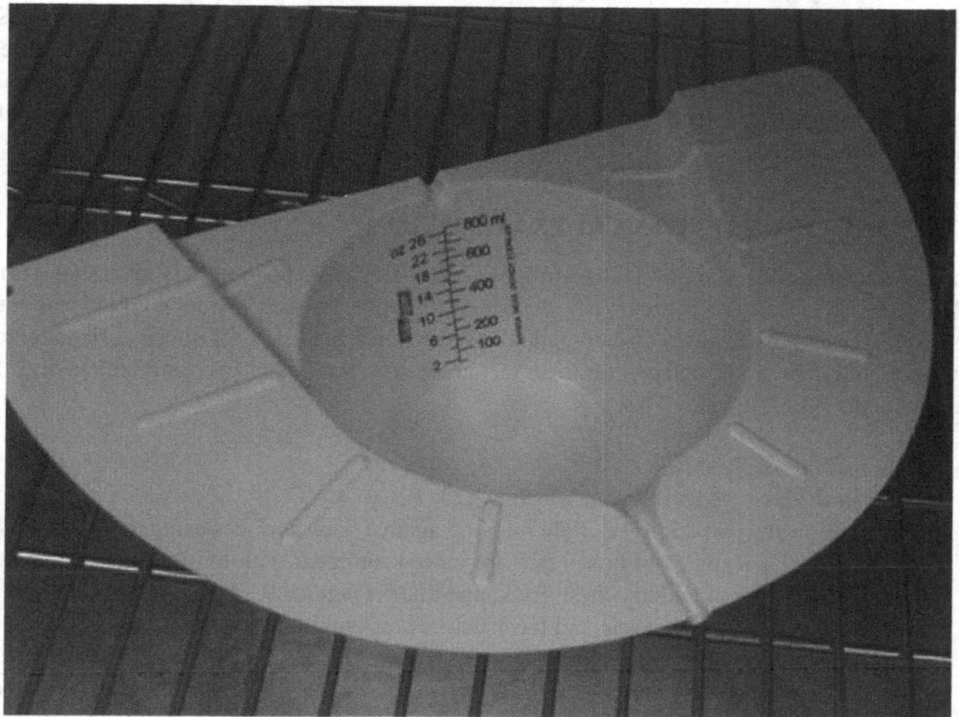

FIGURE 9.1 Stool hat for measuring stool/ostomy/urine output.

Date	Weight	Stool/Ostomy	Urine

FIGURE 9.2 Sample form to document intake and output for patient use.

TABLE 9.4
Goals of Urine and Ostomy Output/Day

Urine	Ostomy
• Jejunostomies without colon >1200 mL	• Colostomies: 200–600 mL
• Ileostomies without colon >1200 mL	• Ileostomies: 1200 mL
• Ileostomies with colon >1500 mL	• Jejunostomies: 1200–2000 mL

Source: Nightingale, J.M. et al., *Gut*, 55, iv1–iv2, 2006.

Improvement in the consistency of stool output may indicate improved absorption; however, weight gain and increased urine output may be more clinically meaningful. The Bristol stool form scale (http://www.ncbi.nlm.nih.gov/pubmedhealth/PMH0033428/) is commonly used to classify stool into seven types based on its appearance; this correlates well with colon transit time. At each clinic visit, the patient should describe any change in stool consistency, particularly with each change in antidiarrheal and/or antisecretory medications, to determine if the therapy is working. Ideally, consistency would be less watery and more paste-like with a brown color instead of green or yellow. The frequency of bowel movements should also be determined with a goal of increasing the length of time between eating to when the output begins. Finally, patients should be queried if their output is higher at any particular time of the day. For example, if they notice their output is greatest at night and affects their sleep, perhaps a higher dose or stronger gut-slowing agent before bed may be worthwhile.

NUTRITION-FOCUSED PHYSICAL EXAMINATION

The use of a nutrition-focused physical examination (NFPE) should be used in conjunction with the detailed historical information previously described to better assess a patient's nutritional status. The NFPE assesses muscle and fat wasting, fluid accumulation, and signs of micronutrient deficiencies (often found in areas of high cell turnover including skin, hair, nails, eyes and oral cavity). Tips for performing a NFPE are listed here.

Assess fat and muscle wasting:

- Start from the head and work your way down the body.
- Use inspection and palpation (i.e., light pressure against body surfaces using the finger tips) to assess any sharp angles of bones that are more prominent with loss of muscle and fat tissue such as arms, shoulders, chest, back, and knees (Figures 9.3 through 9.5).
- Evaluate whether current muscle and fat structure is normal for patient.
- For example, a normally thin patient who has marginal fat and muscle stores but no other symptoms of malnutrition is probably well nourished, while a previously obese patient who has had significant unintentional weight loss but still has adequate fat and muscle stores is probably malnourished.
- Assess both sides of your patient to determine whether wasting is symmetric.
- Symmetric/bilateral muscle and fat wasting is typically associated with malnutrition; unilateral wasting is typically a symptom of another medical issue.
- Account for age-related loss.
- Particularly in the orbital area and interosseous muscles of the hands as this may not be related to malnutrition.
- Account for gender differences in muscle mass.
- What may appear to be wasting on males may be normal in females. For example, clavicles are mildly prominent in females but should not be visible in males.

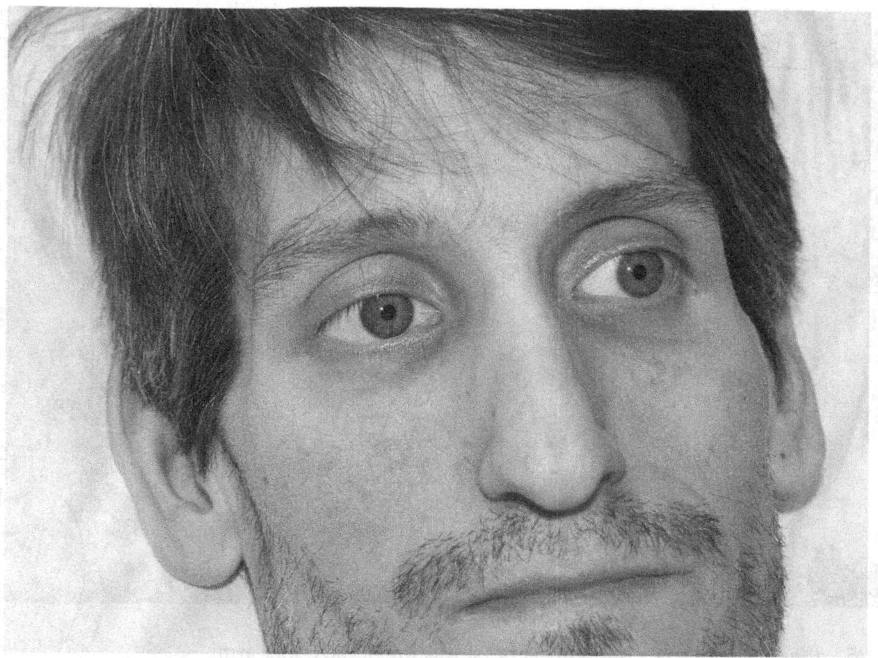

FIGURE 9.3 **(See color insert.)** Assessment of muscle wasting of temporal region and fat wasting of orbital region.

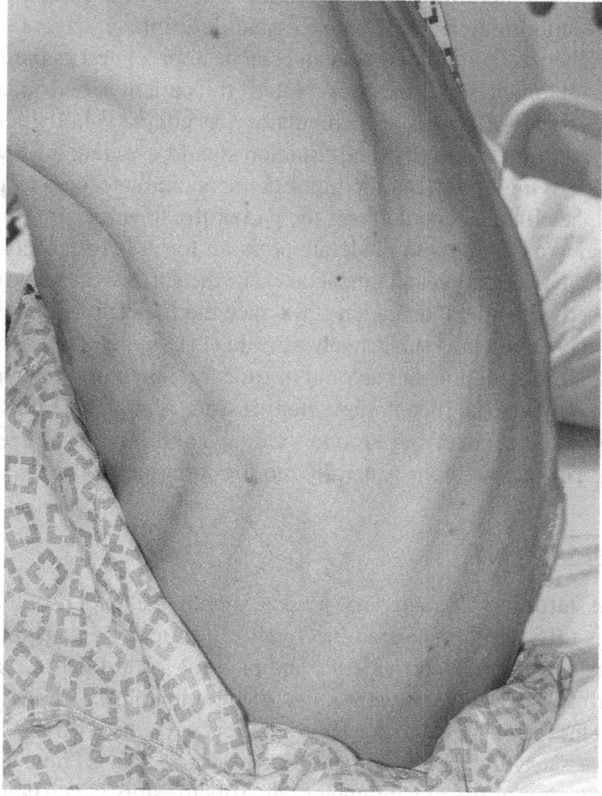

FIGURE 9.4 **(See color insert.)** Assessment of muscle wasting of scapula and fat wasting of thoracic area.

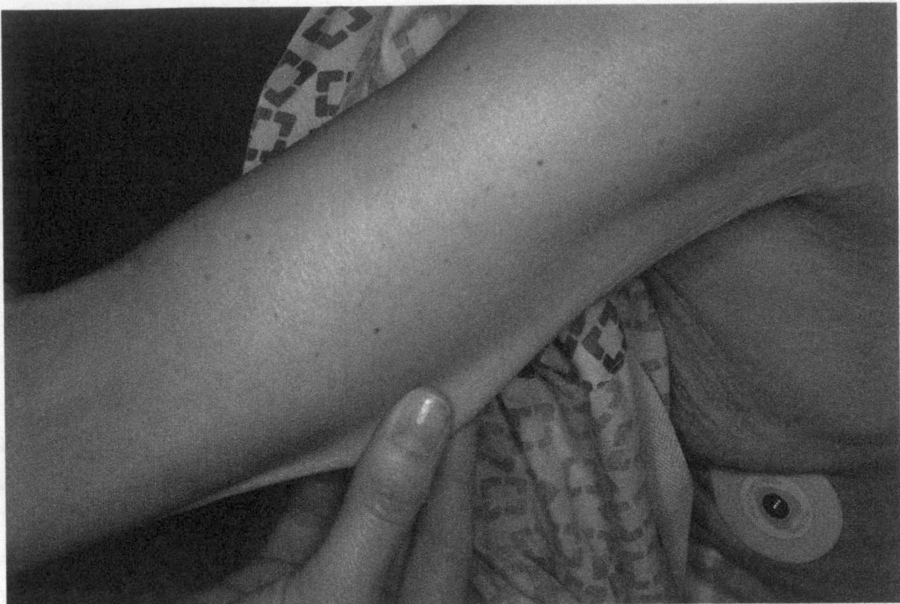

FIGURE 9.5 **(See color insert.)** Assessment of fat wasting of the upper arm.

FLUID ACCUMULATION

Fluid accumulation may be generalized or localized and should be assessed using both inspection and palpation. Fluid retention may result from excessive fluid intake, excess sodium intake, organ failure (i.e., heart, renal, hepatic) or malnutrition and can be appreciated as fluid accumulation in the extremities, face, neck, abdomen, hips, and back. Note if the patient is bedridden and lying with his or her head and feet elevated or if he or she is ambulatory, as edema is body position dependent and tends to pool at the lowest point of gravity. The clinician should evaluate for lower extremity edema starting at the foot and moving up toward the hip. Edema is characterized as pitting or nonpitting. To evaluate for edema, the clinician should press the pad of the fingertip or thumb on the area of the patient's body that is being assessed with moderate pressure for at least 5 seconds, then remove and observe for the depth of the indentation and time it takes for the surface of the skin to return to normal. Pitting edema is identified when the indentation stays once the fingertip is removed. Pitting edema is further categorized by most clinicians subjectively as mild (1+), moderate (2+), and severe (3+ to 4+) depending on the depth of indentation and amount of time the indentation persists (Figure 9.6) [16]. Nonpitting edema does not leave an indentation after pressure is applied. Fluid can also accumulate in the abdominal cavity (i.e., ascites) and around the lungs and heart (i.e., pleural and pericardial effusion, respectively). These conditions generally require imaging studies to detect.

FUNCTIONAL ASSESSMENT

A decline in functional status is a characteristic used as supportive evidence in the diagnosis of malnutrition; however, it is difficult to measure objectively, and it can be affected by multiple nonnutritional factors such as neurological, orthopedic, and psychological factors, as well as medications and frank deconditioning. A validated measurement of functional assessment is handgrip strength. A handgrip dynamometer may be used to compare a patient's results with the standards supplied by the manufacturer for one's age and gender to determine performance. Of note, body posture, the arm used, and the handle position of the dynamometer can affect results [17]. Handgrip strength can be used in underweight, normal-weight, and obese individuals [9].

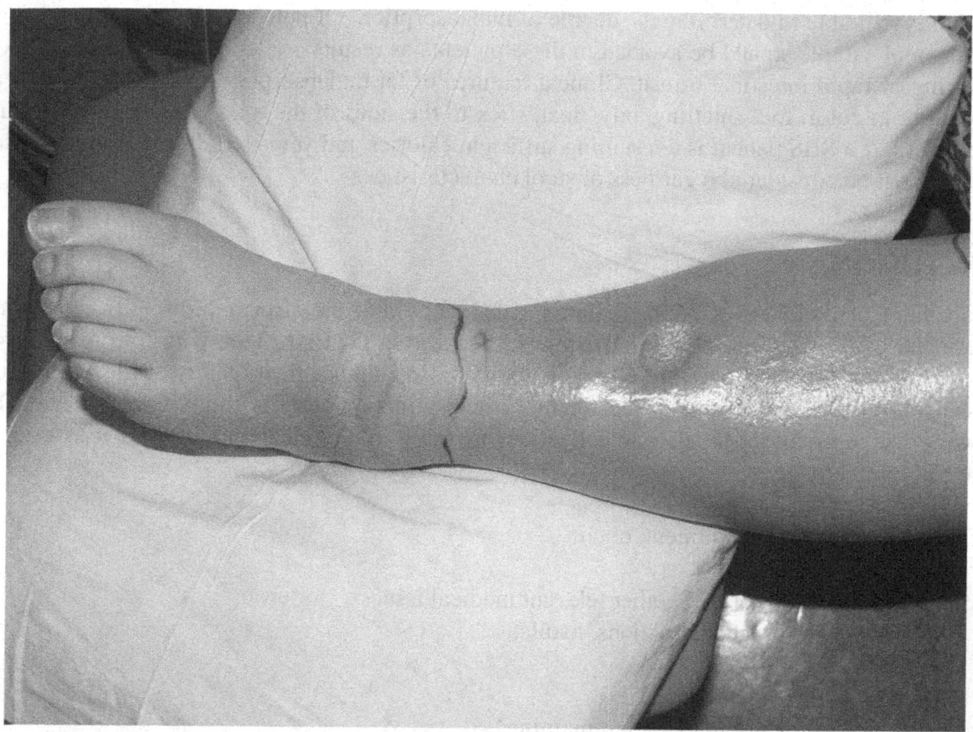

FIGURE 9.6 (See color insert.) Assessment of lower extremity edema with a thumb print indention.

LABORATORY VALUES

At the initial appointment, a comprehensive metabolic panel, complete blood count, magnesium, phosphorus, and a C-reactive protein (CRP), if an inflammatory or infectious process is suspected, should be obtained. If the CRP is normal, then the following laboratory tests should also be considered:

- Trace elements: copper, manganese, zinc, selenium
- B vitamins: specifically B_6 (if symptoms suggest deficiency) and B_{12}
- Fat-soluble vitamins: A, D, E, and prothrombin time (PT)/international normalized ratio (INR)
- Iron studies: iron, total iron binding capacity, and ferritin
- Other: methylmalonic acid (when ordering B_{12})

Long-term monitoring of laboratory values in patients receiving home PN is discussed further in Chapter 25.

Serum protein markers, specifically albumin and prealbumin, were at one time considered markers of nutritional status. They are no longer considered a reliable indicator of nutritional status, as there are a number of factors that alter the results and, as such, lack sensitivity and specificity [18].

A *quantitative* fecal fat test may be useful to determine the presence and extent of fat malabsorption [19] in those patients failing to thrive on oral/enteral intake. The results of this test can also be used to document the medical necessity for PN and may be required for patients with Medicare. During the test, the patient should consume (and document) adequate fat (e.g., 100 g/day) and collect the stool over a sufficient number of days (e.g., 2 or 3 days) for the test to produce accurate results. However, as long as the patient consumes a consistent known amount of fat, such as 50 g/day, the clinician is still able to determine the degree of malabsorption. Of note, a qualitative fecal fat on a random stool sample should be avoided in these patients as results are less reliable, particularly in the setting of rapid intestinal transit. Clinical features of fat malabsorption include stools that are bulky, light in color, foul-smelling, oily, float, stick to the sides of the toilet, and difficult to flush. Nonetheless, if a SBS patient is consuming sufficient calories and yet is still losing weight, malabsorption must be considered regardless of stool characteristics.

CONCLUSION

Management of patients with SBS requires a dedicated and creative multidisciplinary team to achieve the goal of preserving and utilizing the remaining GI tract. This will not only improve their nutritional status and overall well-being but will also enhance their quality of life. A thorough assessment of the SBS patient is invaluable in the determination of the optimal treatment plan. The following list summarizes the data to collect during the initial clinical and nutritional assessment of the SBS patient.

If possible, prior to appointment, obtain

- Medical history
    - Specific cause of SBS, other relevant medical issues
    - History of bowel obstructions, fistulae
    - Comorbid illnesses
- Surgical history
    - Bowel segments and length remaining
    - Presence of colon and continuity with small bowel
    - Presence of ileocecal valve
    - Enterocutaneous fistulae, obstructions, drains
- Nutrition support history
    - Parenteral nutrition/fluid use, enteral nutrition use
    - Central venous access, enteral access
    - Complications
- Social/psychiatric history
- Radiologic imaging
    - Length of bowel, transit time, structural features
- 3-day diet record of all food and beverages consumed
- Relevant lab work
    - Blood, stool, urine

At appointment, obtain

- Medication history and use
    - Medications tried in the past and response
    - Medications currently taking
        - Dosing, frequency
- Standing height, weight, and body mass index
- Weight history
    - Usual body weight, weight loss, percentage change from usual (and when weighed last)
- Physical assessment
    - Fat and muscle loss
    - Micronutrient deficiency signs (commonly found in rapid cell growth areas)
        - Oral cavity, hair, skin, nails, eyes
        - Fluid accumulation
        - Functional status changes

- Intake and output
  - Intake:
    - Oral diet and fluids
      - Foods and fluids currently eating
    - Enteral nutrition
      - Rate, duration, compliance with infusions
    - Parenteral nutrition and fluids
      - Duration, frequency, volume, calories, compliance with infusions
  - Output:
    - Stool/ostomy
      - Consistency, volume, frequency
    - Urine
      - Volume, color
    - Other
      - Drains, tubes, emesis, fistulas, wounds

REFERENCES

1. Jeejeebhoy K. Short bowel syndrome: A nutritional and medical approach. *CMAJ.* 2002;166(10):1297–1302.
2. Weser E. Nutritional aspects of malabsorption: Short gut adaptation. *Clin Gastroenterol.* 1983;12(2): 443–461.
3. Carbonnel F et al. The role of anatomic factors in nutritional autonomy after extensive small bowel resection. *JPEN J Parenter Enteral Nutr.* 1996;20:275–280.
4. Jeppesen PB et al. Colonic digestion and absorption of energy from carbohydrates and medium-chain fat in small bowel failure. *JPEN J Parenter Enteral Nutr.* 1999;23:S101–S105.
5. Maljaars PW et al. Ileal brake: A sensible food target for appetite control. *Physiol Behav.* 2008;95:271–281.
6. Parrish CR. The clinician's guide to short bowel syndrome. *Pract Gastroenterol.* 2005;31:67–106.
7. DiBaise JK et al. Part 1: Short bowel syndrome in adults—Physiological alterations and clinical consequences. *Pract Gastroenterol.* 2014;38(8):30.
8. White JV et al. Consensus statement: Academy of Nutrition and Dietetics and American Society for Parenteral and Enteral Nutrition: Characteristics recommended for the identification and documentation of adult malnutrition (undernutrition). *JPEN J Parenter Enteral Nutr.* 2012;36:275–283.
9. Norman K et al. Hand grip strength: Outcome predictor and marker of nutritional status. *Clin Nutr.* 2011;30:135–142.
10. Rowland ML. Self-reported weight and height. *Am J Clin Nutr.* 1990;52:1125–1133.
11. Blackburn GL et al. Nutritional and metabolic assessment of the hospitalized patient. *JPEN J Parenter Enteral Nutr.* 1977;1:11–22.
12. Mifflin MD et al. A new predictive equation for resting energy expenditure in healthy individuals. *Am J Clin Nutr.* 1990;51:241–247.
13. Mirtallo J et al. A.S.P.E.N safe practices for parenteral nutrition. *JPEN J Parenter Enteral Nutr.* 2004;28:S52–S57.
14. Whitmire SJ. Fluid and electrolytes. In: Gottschlich MM, Matarese LE, eds. *Contemporary Nutrition Support Practice. A Clinical Guide.* Philadelphia, PA: WB Saunders; 1998:127–144.
15. Nightingale JM et al. Guidelines for management of patients with a short bowel. *Gut.* 2006;55(Suppl. 4):iv1–iv12.
16. Grey Bruce Health Services. Assessment Chart for Pitting Edema; 2014. http://www.gbhn.ca/ebc/documents/ASSESSMENTOFPITTINGEDEMA.pdf. Accessed March 9, 2015.
17. Litchford MD. *Nutrition Focused Physical Assessment: Making Clinical Connections.* Greensboro, NC: CASE Software & Books, 2013.
18. Jensen GL. Inflammation as the key interface of the medical and nutrition universe: A proactive examination of the future of clinical nutrition and medicine. *JPEN J Parenter Enteral Nutr.* 2006;30:453–463.
19. Van de Kamer JH et al. Rapid method for the determination of fat in feces. *J Biol Chem.* 1949;177:347–355.

10 Diet Considerations in Short Bowel Syndrome

Rebecca A. Weseman and Laura E. Beerman

CONTENTS

KEY POINTS

- Determining the length, location, and continuity of the remnant bowel is the first step in the initial assessment of nutrition therapy in short bowel syndrome (SBS).
- Clear and full-liquid diets should be avoided in this population as they are high in osmolality unless they are modified to meet the needs of the SBS patient.
- Concentrated sweets cause fluid to be pulled into the bowel lumen, worsening watery diarrhea. Similarly, commercial oral liquid nutritional supplements should be avoided as they are high in sugar and contribute to osmotic overload/diarrhea.
- Four to six small meals/snacks consumed throughout the day may help to reduce stool output and promote better enteral absorption.
- Diet prescriptions should be tailored to modify usual intake based on patient's anatomy together with the provision of the supportive rationale for better acceptance of change and long-term compliance.

INTRODUCTION

Designing the optimal diet for the patient with short bowel syndrome (SBS) requires a detailed individualized assessment of the patient's gastrointestinal (GI) anatomy, including length remaining, segments present, the time that has elapsed since the last resection, and whether the intestinal tract is in continuity or if an end-jejunostomy is present. This information is important for designing individualized diet therapy and education plans. The ultimate goal of nutrition therapy and education in SBS is to achieve independence from parenteral nutrition (PN) or intravenous (IV) fluids along with the removal of the central venous catheter. While this goal may not be realistic for all patients, a reduction in parenteral support is often achievable, while simultaneously maintaining fluid homeostasis and reducing malabsorption. Maintenance of the patient's goal weight and adequate hydration requires regular, periodic assessment of dietary changes, caloric intake, and review of appropriate oral fluids [1]. This chapter is designed to provide a practical step-by-step approach to the assessment and education of the SBS patient with the goal of enhancing their nutritional freedom and quality of life.

STEP 1: ASSESS REMAINING BOWEL ANATOMY

Short bowel patients will fall into one of three bowel anatomy types: terminal jejunostomy, jejunocolonic, and jejunoileocolonic. An end-jejunostomy is the most challenging SBS bowel anatomy to restore enteral autonomy as a consequence of the physiological differences of the jejunum compared with the ileum and colon. This includes the limited potential for jejunal adaptation and the more permeable jejunal epithelium that results in higher ostomy output due to greater fluid shifts across the mucosa [2–4]. In contrast, the ileum has greater adaptive potential and tighter intercellular junctions with reduced permeability and active transport and uptake of sodium chloride, leading to a net increase in fluid and electrolyte absorption. The colon also undergoes adaptation after massive small bowel resection and is able to salvage substantial energy from malabsorbed carbohydrates due to the fermentative actions of its microbial inhabitants. It also has the tightest intercellular junctions, thereby playing an important role in the absorption of fluid in the SBS patient. Indeed, those SBS patients with at least a portion of colon remaining tend to have the best prognosis [5,6].

Both functional and structural changes (i.e., intestinal adaptation) occur to the small and large intestines after intestinal resection that result in mucosal growth and the potential for enhanced absorptive function (see Chapter 4) [4]. Intact luminal nutrients, started as soon as possible after bowel resection, are one of the most potent stimulators of intestinal adaptation [4].

DIFFERENCES IN DIET BASED ON REMAINING BOWEL ANATOMY

Diet plays an important role in optimizing energy intake and lowering stool output in SBS. Because the SBS population is small and heterogeneous in remaining bowel anatomy and underlying disease responsible, available evidence that guides diet therapy today is limited primarily to small studies and the clinical experience of those working extensively with these patients. Nevertheless, the data that are available have provided a solid base for diet therapy in practice today at many intestinal failure centers.

Supportive Diet Evidence for Patients with an End-Jejunostomy

SBS patients with an end-jejunostomy are encouraged to consume 40–50% of their daily energy intake in complex carbohydrates (CHO), 20% in protein, and up to 40% in fat content. The evidence for this breakdown comes from the following:

- Using a randomized, crossover design, Woolf et al. [7] evaluated the effect of a high-fat (60% fat kcal) diet compared with that of a low-fat (20% fat kcal) diet on stool output and energy absorption in eight SBS patients, five of whom had an end-jejunostomy. Although the fecal fat excreted was three times higher when receiving the high-fat diet, the proportion of ingested fat absorbed was not different and no differences were noted in the absorption of calcium, magnesium, or zinc.

- In another study using a randomized, crossover design, Nordgaard [8] compared the effect of a high-fat (60% fat kcal) diet with that of a low-fat (20% kcal) diet on stool volume and energy absorption in six patients with an end-jejunostomy ranging in length from 100 to 250 cm. Dietary energy absorption was approximately 50% during both study periods and did not differ based on amount of fat ingested; stool water and dry weight were not different.
- Ovesen et al. [9] compared three isocaloric, isonitrogenous diets in five stable patients with an end-jejunostomy varying in length from 35 to 125 cm. The three diets were as follows:
  1. Low fat (30% kcal), high complex carbohydrate (55% kcal)
  2. High fat (60% kcal with polyunsaturated/saturated fat ratio of 1:4), low carbohydrate (25% kcal)
  3. High fat (60% kcal with polyunsaturated/saturated fat ratio of 1:1), low carbohydrate (25% kcal)

  They found that increasing the amount of fat resulted in an increase in diarrhea; however, changing the ratio of polyunsaturated to saturated fat had no clear effect (beneficial or detrimental) on absorption. In addition, neither the amount nor the type of fat consistently influenced the volume of jejunal output. Although sodium and potassium concentration of effluent remained constant, the higher fat diet was associated with an increased loss of divalent cations (e.g., calcium, magnesium, copper, and zinc).

Based on the reported evidence, therefore, a fat-restricted diet offers no appreciable benefit in SBS patients without a colon regarding energy, fluid, or monovalent electrolyte absorption. Furthermore, a positive linear relationship appears to exist, in that more fat is absorbed when more is ingested.

Without a colon, fewer oxalates are absorbed. Restriction of oxalate is therefore generally unnecessary in those with an end-jejunostomy. Furthermore, supplementation of the diet with medium-chain triglycerides (MCTs; see section on MCTs) does not seem to confer benefit to those without a colon; in fact, supplementation with MCTs was shown to *decrease* carbohydrate and protein absorption in those without a colon and is not recommended in this setting [10].

Supportive Diet Evidence for Patients with Colon-in-Continuity

It is recommended that SBS patients with at least a portion of colon ingest a diet consisting of 50–60% as complex carbohydrates (CHO), < 30% of total energy intake as fat, and 20% as protein of high biologic value [8,11,12].

The rationale for the emphasis on complex CHO and limited fat use in patients with even a segment of colon is as follows:

1. A diet lower in fat has been associated with improved outcomes when compared with a higher-fat diet in SBS patients with colon-in-continuity, including an increase in both nutrient and mineral absorption, while reducing sodium and fluid losses [8,13,14].
   - Andersson [13] compared a 100 g/day vs. 40 g/day fat diet in 13 patients with either resected (mean length, 90 cm) or diseased (not SBS patients) distal ileum; only 1 had an ileostomy. To compensate for the energy loss caused by the reduction in fat, protein- and carbohydrate-rich foods were increased (diets were not isocaloric, however). A reduction in water and sodium excretion was observed on the low-fat diet; an increase in total body potassium and weight maintenance was noted in all but one patient despite the lower daily energy intake on the low-fat diet.
   - In a follow-up study to the Andersson study, 9 of 13 patients who had previously participated took part in another comparative study of a diet containing 100 g/day vs. 40 g/day fat [14]. As in the first study, protein- and carbohydrate-rich foods were increased to

account for the energy loss caused by the decrease in fat calories (diets were not isocaloric). Higher quantities of calcium, magnesium, and zinc were absorbed in those receiving the low-fat diet. The authors did concede, however, that the lower-fat diet contained a higher percentage of these nutrients also.

- In a 4-day, crossover nutrient balance study, Nordgaard [8] investigated differences in energy and nutrient absorption when changing from a high-fat (60% kcal), low-carbohydrate (20% kcal) to a low-fat (20% kcal), high-carbohydrate (60% kcal) diet in 16 SBS patients (10 with colon-in-continuity and 6 with end-jejunostomy). The high-carbohydrate, low-fat diet group was found to have reduced energy loss in the stool and a concomitant increase in energy absorption from 49% to 69%. Mineral output was not evaluated.

2. The colon, capitalizing on fermentation of unabsorbed carbohydrates into absorbable short-chain fatty acids (SCFAs) by resident bacteria within its lumen, salvages up to an additional 1000 calories per day when small bowel length is reduced [8,11,15–18].
3. Fat malabsorption increases the risk for enhanced oxalate absorption in the colon that may result in calcium oxalate kidney stone formation [19,20]. Twenty-five percent of SBS patients with <200 cm of jejunum anastomosed to the colon have a tendency to develop symptomatic kidney stones; in some, oxalate nephropathy will lead to significant chronic kidney disease [19]. Implementation of an oxalate-restricted diet is sometimes necessary to avoid oxalate stone formation, particularly for those with a history of kidney stones (see section on oxalate).

Tables 10.1 through 10.3 [21,22] provide specific diet recommendations for SBS patients based on the remaining bowel anatomy type, suggested food selections, and a sample meal plan based on remaining bowel anatomy.

TABLE 10.1
Diet Summary Based on Anatomy

Diet Component	End-Jejunostomy/Ileostomy	Colon-Segment-in-Continuity
Meals/snacks	• Five to six or more smaller meals/snacks per day • Chew foods *really* well!	• More than five smaller meals/snacks per day
Carbohydrates	• ~50% complex CHO/avoid simple sugars, including – Fructose, high-fructose corn syrup, sugar alcohols such as sorbitol, etc. – Lactose (up to 20 g over the day)	• 50%+ complex CHO/avoid simple sugars, including – Fructose, high-fructose corn syrup, sugar alcohols such as sorbitol, etc. – Lactose (up to 20 g over the day)
Fat	• 30–40%; encourage fats containing high essential fatty acid content • MCT not beneficial	• <30% fat; encourage fats containing high essential fatty acid content • Some MCT can be beneficial
Protein	• 20–30%; high biological value	• 20–30%; high biological value
Fiber	• Usual intake—limit if too high	• Encourage soluble; 5 to 10 g/day (see the "Fiber" section)
Oxalate	• No restriction	• Limit, but first ensure adequate urine output of >1 L daily
Salt	• Increase intake by salting foods, or using high sodium food choices	• Usual intake
Fluids	• ORS/high-sodium fluids; total fluid restriction may be necessary in some (and IV fluids given)	• ORS may be necessary in some; total fluid restriction may be necessary in some (and IV fluids given)

Source: Adapted from Parrish, C.R. et al., *Pract. Gastroenterol.*, 38, 40, 2014.

TABLE 10.2
Early Postresection Diet Progression

Recommended	Foods to Avoid
Sugar-free clear liquids—small amounts only • Weak tea, broth, oral rehydration solutions, sugar-free gelatin *made without* sugar alcohols such as sorbitol	Standard clear liquid diets • Sugar-containing gelatin • Fruit juices and fruit-flavored sugar-containing beverages
Low-fat, low-sugar, low-lactose full liquid • Low-fat broth-type soups • Cooked cereal • Low-fat, sugar-free yogurt • Sugar-free pudding	Standard full-liquid diets • Cream soups • Ice cream, sherbet, puddings • Standard commercial nutritional supplements containing sugar
Meat, fish, poultry • Tender chicken, turkey, fish, canned tuna, ground lean beef, pork loin • Egg, tuna, or ham salad • Lean deli meats: turkey, roast beef, and ham	Meat, fish, poultry • Tough cuts of meat, fried meats, unground cuts of beef or pork • Shrimp, tough connective tissue • Fried fish and meats • Fatty cuts of beef, pork, or canned fish packed in oils • Salami or high fat deli meats
Protein sources • Cottage cheese 1–2%; eggs; egg whites; low-fat, low-sugar yogurt without seeds; low-fat cheese; tofu; natural smooth peanut butter	Protein sources • Limit egg yolks to three to four per week • Seeds, nuts
Starches • Cream of wheat or rice, refined oatmeal • Low-fiber cold cereals • White rice, pasta, noodle dishes • White bread (especially dense calorie types such as potato bread and cottage bread, dinner rolls, bagels, English muffins, low-fat, low-fiber crackers) • Peeled and boiled potatoes, winter squash • Pretzels, rice cakes, low-sugar plain cookies such as shortbread type or vanilla wafers	Starches • Whole-grain breads or rolls • Brown, wild rice • High-fiber cereals, granola • Popcorn • Beans (kidney, pinto, navy, garbanzo)
Vegetables • Soft, well-cooked green beans, young-tender peas, peeled carrots, beets, asparagus tips	Vegetables • All raw vegetables • Cauliflower, broccoli, mushrooms, salads, water chestnuts, corn, mixed vegetables, lima beans, edamame, celery, green and red pepper
Fruits • Canned fruits in natural juice or water packed (applesauce, peaches, pears) • Ripe banana • Limit all fruits to two (1/2 cup servings/day)	Fruits • All fruit juices • All fresh fruits • Dried fruits (raisins, dates, figs, coconut) • Skins of fruits
Fats • Limit to 2–3 teaspoons per meal or snack • Safflower, soybean, sunflower oils or margarines with high essential fatty acids	Fats • Sauces made with butter, cream, whole milk, or high-fat cheeses • Caution with high-fat salad dressings

TABLE 10.3
Differences in Food Selection Based on Anatomy (Sample 2200 Calorie Meal Plan)

Patients without Colon	Patients with Some Colon
Breakfast	Breakfast
	1 cup oatmeal
2 scrambled eggs	2 scrambled eggs
1 English muffin or 2 slices toast	1 English muffin or 2 slices toast
6 oz lactose-free nonfat milk (if allowed)	6 oz lactose-free nonfat milk (if allowed)
1 tablespoon margarine	
1 teaspoon diet jelly (use sparingly)	1 teaspoon diet jelly (use sparingly)
4 oz coffee (if allowed)	4 oz coffee (if allowed)
Morning snack	Morning snack
1 slice bread	1 slice bread
2 tablespoons peanut butter	1 tablespoon peanut butter
1/2 banana	1 banana
Lunch	Lunch
4 oz turkey breast	4 oz turkey breast
1 hoagie roll	1 hoagie roll
2 teaspoons mayonnaise	1 oz cheese
2 oz cheese	2 slices tomato
2 slices tomato	
Afternoon snack	Afternoon snack
6 crackers	12 crackers
2 oz cheddar cheese	2 oz cheddar cheese
	2 oz deli ham
Dinner	Dinner
4 oz grilled salmon	4 oz grilled salmon
1 large baked sweet potato	1 large baked sweet potato
1 tablespoon butter	1 small dinner roll
	1 teaspoon butter
Evening snack	Evening snack
8 animal crackers	16 animal crackers

Source: Parrish, C.R. et al., *Pract. Gastroenterol.*, 39, 40, 2014. With permission.
Note: Beverage choices and amount should be individualized for each patient.

STEP 2: PERFORM INDIVIDUALIZED ASSESSMENT OF INTAKE AND OUTPUT

After massive intestinal resection, four clinical stages have been described [23]; an awareness of the clinical stage will guide the appropriate diet prescription.

- Stage 1 (immediately after resection) typically includes the first 7–10 days and involves stabilization of the critical illness, resolution of the postoperative ileus, and aggressive fluid and electrolyte replacement. During this time, PN may be initiated, and oral foods and fluids may be resumed as GI function and output allow. Clear and full-liquid diets should generally be avoided in this patient population due to their high osmolality and the propensity to result in an osmotic diarrhea and aggravation of stool output. Once the GI tract is deemed "operational," very small amounts of specific clear liquids (see Table 10.2) or oral rehydration solution (ORS) for one to two meals is allowed with fairly quick progression to soft solids following early recovery after surgery (ERAS) guidelines [24].
- Stage 2 (1–3 months after resection) is characterized by a shift of emphasis from fluid and electrolyte balance to nutrition support. In this stage, full PN support along with continued optimization of large fluid and electrolyte losses is stressed. Diarrhea can be severe during this period, and enteral absorption limited, although with the use of an appropriate diet, a gradual increase in oral tolerance with reduction in stool losses can be seen [25].

- Stage 3 (1–2 years after resection) is the period of greatest intestinal adaptation. During this stage, PN, enteral tube feedings, and/or IV fluids may be used in conjunction with an oral diet to meet the SBS patient's nutritional and fluid requirements. Emphasis on the appropriate modified SBS diet based on the remaining bowel anatomy, as described previously, should be aggressively implemented along with aggressive use of antisecretory and antimotility medications and concomitant tapering of PN. It is during this stage that most PN weaning will occur. Frequency, volume, and consistency of stools and stool pattern should be evaluated in relationship to meal consumption, type of oral fluids, and volume of fluids taken orally or intravenously. Some individuals with SBS may report having infrequent stools daily; however, the actual volume may be excessive [26]. Fluid considerations in the SBS patient are imperative and considered to be the "often forgotten nutrient."
- Stage 4 (>2 years after resection) is considered a state of relative equilibrium where no further improvement or adaptive changes occur. Nevertheless, with aggressive management, some patients are able to be weaned from PN during this stage. It is important to remember that periodic assessment of food and oral fluid intake, urine output, and stool/ostomy output not only provides the clinician with objective measurements to monitor effectiveness of interventions but also identifies areas for improvement. In addition, it affords patients with an opportunity to participate in their care by reinforcing to the patients the importance of adequate hydration and diet, thereby enlisting further compliance from the patients.

STEP 3: DESIGNING THE DIET PRESCRIPTION AND EDUCATING THE PATIENT ON THE RATIONALE FOR ENHANCED COMPLIANCE AND PATIENT EMPOWERMENT

When patients begin eating after extensive intestinal resection, they will need to be encouraged to follow an optimized SBS diet designed to achieve the maximum enteral absorption possible. This extremely important step requires intensive diet education and counseling specific for their bowel anatomy and should include the rationale for the necessary diet changes. Ultimately, this will lead to greater patient self-management and compliance with their SBS diet [27,28] as they witness direct evidence of its effects, including reduced stool frequency, improved stool consistency and fluid balance demonstrated by improved urine output and a decrease in the side effects of dehydration, and an overall sense of improved well-being. As individuals gain confidence that their diet and oral fluid choices aid in regaining their premorbid health status, they generally become increasingly empowered with the ability to comply with the burden of dietary modifications and fluid restrictions [29].

GENERAL GUIDELINES

The goals of diet therapy are to enhance absorption and decrease stool burden by

- Consuming intact, whole nutrients
- Decreasing the particle size presented to the upper gut (chewing foods well)
- Avoiding hyperosmolar foods/fluids (simple sugars/sugar alcohols/fruit juices, etc.) that create osmotic drag and pull more fluid into the bowel adding more volume to stool output
- Eating meals slowly and with increased frequency to distribute nutrients to accommodate the decreased surface area in an effort to improve nutrient to cm of mucosa contact time and utilization

A balanced diet including protein, CHO, and fats high in essential fatty acids (EFAs) is important to provide satiety and adequate calories. Importantly, as patients with SBS absorb only about two-thirds of their usual intake, energy ingestion will need to be increased up to 50–75% over their usual requirements to compensate for the associated malabsorption [30–32]. Fortunately, SBS patients typically develop adaptive hyperphagia, which facilitates an increase in energy consumption and net nutrient absorption [30]. From the individualized daily calorie goal, all meals and snacks should be reasonably balanced and evenly distributed as much as possible throughout the day.

Too much food, however, as well as excessive fat or carbohydrate intake at any meal, can increase stool volume. Therefore, not only the type of food but also the quantity at each meal/snack must be taken into consideration. Working closely with the SBS patient to design an appropriate diet that is individualized to their food preferences and tolerances within the guidelines of the SBS diet will have a positive influence on enteral absorption. The use of a food record can be very helpful and should be maintained early on and any intolerance noted so the diet can be modified accordingly. It is important to start the diet planning with what the patient normally eats and adjust only those food items that require changing to bring the diet into compliance with SBS diet guidelines (see Tables 10.1 and 10.2). Focusing on all the food items they cannot have often sets the stage for a sense of further loss of control in these patients.

Because food is often central to social, family, and religious events, SBS patients trying to follow an appropriate diet may feel left out. As such, quality of life issues also need to be considered and discussed with these patients. Such issues include dining out on an SBS diet [29,33], meal preparation, and recipe modification. While an appropriate SBS diet prescription does not guarantee the optimal clinical response, an optimal diet requires education, reinforcement, and long-term follow-up to aid in influencing a positive response to this intervention [29]. The goal is to improve the quality of life and give the patient a restored sense of control. Quality of life has been shown to be improved when the necessary diet education is obtained from a center of excellence that specializes in treating the patient with SBS [33–36].

Calories

The cornerstone of the dietary management in SBS is to establish the optimal calorie goal for the individual, along with the fluid intake to allow for maximal enteral absorption, without contributing to excessive losses of micronutrients and diarrhea leading to weight loss and dehydration [37]. In the early postresection period, the patient should be encouraged to sip small amounts of an isotonic ORS and empirically restrict food to 500 calories/day initially to avoid exacerbating stool losses [38]. As patients stabilize, most will absorb only about two-thirds as many calories as compared with their pre-SBS state. Ultimately, a hyperphagic diet of 50–75% more calories (up to 60 calories/kg/day in some patients) than they normally consumed prior to intestinal resection may be required to sustain their weight [30–32]. Some patients will not have difficulty eating this increased quantity of food to meet their level of calorie intake, while others may find this challenging and overwhelming, particularly as the food selections have been modified (especially with reduction of simple sugars to avoid osmotic effects). There is also an increased cost associated with this increased food requirement that also needs to be considered. Limiting oral fluids at meal times, in an attempt to reduce gastric dumping, may allow the patient to consume more calories at meals without exacerbating stool output. Oral fluids can then be sipped between the five to six meals spread throughout the day [39,40].

Supplemental Enteral Feedings

Nocturnal enteral/tube feedings are a good option for some SBS patients as they take advantage of the absorptive capabilities of the GI tract at a time when it is not normally in use. Enteral nutrition should be considered in those patients who cannot meet their energy needs beyond what they can consume orally during the daytime and those patients whose output is too high when they try to do so (see Chapter 14).

Carbohydrates

CHO such as potatoes, rice, and pasta should provide between 40% and 60% of the calories as these are well tolerated, with reported absorption of two-thirds to three-fourths of the amount consumed

[32,39,40]. Complex CHO also reduces the osmotic load compared with simple carbohydrates or concentrated sweets, which will generate a high osmotic load and lead to greater stool output. In particular, fruit juices and sweetened fruit drinks should be avoided. Even canned, no-sugar-added fruits and peeled fresh fruits should be limited as they also may exacerbate stool output. Finally, in those patients who seem refractory to dietary manipulation, a review of the fermentable oligosaccharide, disaccharide, monosaccharide, and polyols (FODMAP) content of their diet (and medications) may be worthwhile [41]. FODMAPs are highly osmotic, in addition to highly fermentable by gut bacteria. FODMAPs draw fluid into the lumen of the bowel, further aggravating stool volume and causing symptoms such as gas, bloating, and abdominal distension. They are found in certain foods, some enteral formulas (as fructooligosaccharides), and many liquid medications for flavorings, including sugar alcohols (e.g., sorbitol, mannitol, and xylitol) [42]; their effect can be additive over the day.

Lactose

Dairy products can provide a good source of calcium and calories to those who enjoy them. Twenty grams of lactose over the course of a day is generally well tolerated, even in patients with SBS [43]. Yogurt, cheese, and limited amounts of milk typically do not exacerbate stool losses. Some SBS patients may try reduced lactose dairy products; however, it is important to note that some patients experience worsening stool output using low-lactose products as the disaccharide lactose is cleaved into two monosaccharides, thereby increasing the osmolality of the product.

Fiber

Soluble fiber, in the form of pectin, has been studied in SBS patients with remaining colon [15]. This indigestible, noncellulose fiber is fermented by colonic bacteria to form SCFAs. In adults with normal bowel length and colon, it is estimated that SCFA oxidation contribute 5–15% of total energy absorbed (up to 1000 calories/day) [8,11,16–18]. Soluble fiber is highly fermentable and results in greater production of SCFAs compared with other fibers such as wheat bran, psyllium, and oats [15]. It also may act to slow gastric emptying. In patients with a colon segment who are able to consume excessive calories (i.e., hyperphagia) in an effort to overcome their malabsorption (and without driving their stool output too high), soluble fiber supplementation in the form of oatmeal, oat bran, ground flax seeds, blueberries, carrots, etc., results in a higher production of SCFAs than insoluble fibers do. The use of soluble fiber requires further study, however, as patients may complain of increased gas, bloating, and abdominal distention, especially in those plagued with small bowel bacterial overgrowth. Furthermore, in some patients, fiber may worsen diarrhea.

Protein

Eighty-one percent of ingested protein is readily absorbed in the small intestine; 80–100 g protein/day has been suggested for patients with SBS [32]. High biological value protein such as beef, pork, chicken, turkey, fish, eggs, and dairy is preferred. Consumption of dried beans and legumes may be met with variable success; one-half cup servings of bean or split pea soup can be successfully incorporated into the diet. A protein source should be included in all meals and snacks consumed daily by the SBS patient in the attempt to achieve an optimal protein intake.

Fat

As the length of the small bowel decreases, consumption of dietary fat requires increased consideration due to the intricacy of its absorption [32]. Excessive fat intake may lead to steatorrhea, resulting in increased stool volume and fat-soluble vitamin loss. In those with a colon segment remaining, fat should be kept to <30% of calories to reduce the risk of developing calcium oxalate kidney stones [19].

In patients with an end-jejunostomy, fat content can be increased up to 40% of calorie intake, thereby improving both the calorie content and palatability of the diet [29,44].

Essential Fatty Acids

EFAs are needed for human growth and development [38]. EFAs, including linoleic, arachidonic and alpha-linolenic, are polyunsaturated fatty acids that are not synthesized by the body. Linolenic acid is the precursor to arachidonic acid, a polyunsaturated, omega-6 EFA. Alpha-linolenic acid is a polyunsaturated, omega-3 EFA. Deficiency may occur in the setting of SBS, where fat malabsorption is common, or in those on a very-low-fat diet. Symptoms of EFA deficiency may develop in as little as 2–4 weeks. Clinical signs of EFA deficiency include excessively dry, flakey, or red patchy skin [25]. The diagnosis of EFA deficiency is usually based on the determination of the triene–tetraene ratio. A ratio >0.2 is considered consistent with EFA deficiency; however, clinical features typically do not become evident until the ratio is >0.4 [45]. The EFA panel generally needs to be sent to a reference laboratory, is expensive, and usually takes 7–10 days for results to return; therefore, prevention is the preferred approach. Healthy adults require 4% of total calories as EFA, while in those deficient in EFA, requirements increase to 8–10% of total calories [46]. EFAs are found in vegetable oils such as sunflower, corn, and soybean oil (see Table 10.4 [47]). To achieve an adequate intake, 1–2 teaspoons of these oils may be needed at each meal and snack, depending on the other fat sources consumed.

Medium-Chain Triglycerides

MCTs are thought by some to be a panacea for use in patients with fat malabsorption, as, unlike long-chain fat, they can be absorbed directly across the small bowel and colonic mucosa. Their benefit, however, is not so clear-cut. In a study in patients with SBS, replacement of long-chain triglyceride (LCT) with MCT in patients with an end-jejunostomy resulted in a negative effect on the absorption of carbohydrate and nitrogenous substances [17]. In contrast, patients with a preserved colon had improvement in fat absorption, resulting in a net gain in total energy absorption. Hence, those with a colon seem to derive a preferential benefit from MCT use.

Importantly, MCT derived from coconut oil contains both MCT and LCT (66% MCT, 44% LCT). Hence, coconut oil should not be used interchangeably with MCT oil. MCT contains 8.3 calories per gram vs. 9 calories per gram in LCT. MCT should be used in moderation, as ingestion of large amounts of MCT decreases the absorption of LCT, thereby increasing stool fat loss [48,49]. Furthermore,

TABLE 10.4
EFA Content of Common Oils

Vegetable Oil	g EFA/ teaspoon (tsp)	Kcal EFA/tsp	No. of tsp to Meet 4% EFA/1000 Calories
Almond	0.9	7.8	5.0
Canola	1.5	13.3	3.0
Corn	2.7	24.3	1.7
Flaxseed	3.3	29.7	1.4
Olive	0.5	4.5	8.9
Soybean	2.9	26.0	1.5
Sunflower	3.3	29.6	1.4
Walnut	3.2	28.8	1.4
Wheat germ	3.1	27.9	1.4

Source: McCray, S. et al., *Pract. Gastroenterol.*, 35, 12, 2011. With permission.
Note: 100 g oil = 20 tsp; 5 g = 1 tsp oil.

excess MCT oil has been associated with crampy abdominal pain, abdominal distension, nausea, emesis, bloating, and diarrhea [50]. Finally, it is important to note that MCT does not contain EFA, so those receiving supplemental MCT on a very-low-fat diet will require a source of EFA.

Oxalates

When >100 cm of terminal ileum has been resected, the enterohepatic circulation of bile acids is disrupted to such a degree that the liver is unable to maintain sufficient bile acid production, leading to bile acid deficiency and reduced micelle formation, resulting in fat malabsorption and steatorrhea. In the setting of fat malabsorption, dietary calcium is preferentially bound to unabsorbed fatty acids instead of oxalate, leading to increased absorption of the now free oxalate, particularly in the colon. Oxalate is then excreted in the urine, raising the potential for oxalate kidney stones, a risk increased in the setting of marginal hydration that occurs commonly in SBS. Calcium oxalate kidney stones develop in nearly 25% of patients with SBS with remaining colon-in-continuity [19]. Maintaining hydration and good urine output is the best defense against kidney stones of any kind. Without this, compliance even with an oxalate-restricted diet will be ineffective in preventing them. Once a patient develops an oxalate stone, urine output expectation should increase to >1500 mL daily. Oral calcium citrate supplements administered with meals can be used to bind luminal oxalate reducing the risk for calcium oxalate renal stones [51]. Diet counseling should include education on high-oxalate foods to avoid (see Table 10.5 [52]). Oxalate restriction is not necessary in SBS patients with a terminal jejunostomy.

Salt

In the SBS patient with an end-jejunostomy, maintaining sodium homeostasis can be challenging, especially in those patients who may have, for years, been told to restrict sodium in their diets. Consumption of salty food along with an ORS should be encouraged in these patients [33]. Those

TABLE 10.5
Foods and Beverages High in Oxalates

Food	Examples
Fruits	• Apricots, figs, rhubarb, kiwi fruit
Vegetables	• Artichoke, green and wax beans, beets, raw red cabbage, celery, chives, eggplant, endive, leeks, okra, green peppers, rutabagas, summer squash, parsley, white corn, vegetable soup
	• Greens: Swiss chard, beet greens, mustard greens, Dandelion greens, spinach, kale, collards, escarole
	• Potatoes, french fries, sweet potatoes
	• Tomato paste, canned
	• Beans: baked, black, white, great northern, navy, pink
Nuts	• Almonds, cashews, peanuts, peanut butter, pecans, sesame seeds
Beverages	• Chocolate/chocolate containing beverages (cocoa, Ovaltine, chocolate, and soy milk, lattes, etc.)
	• Tea, instant coffee, colas, carob ice cream
Starches	• Grits, barley, cornmeal, buckwheat, lentil and potato soup
	• Whole-wheat products: breads, pastas, tortillas, wheat germ, wheat bran and bran cereal, cream of wheat, shredded wheat
Other	• Tofu and soy products, miso, black olives, chocolate and chocolate ice cream, pepper (>1 tsp per day), poppy seed, turmeric
Alcohol	• Draft beer

Source: Parrish, C.R., *A Patient's Guide to Managing a Short Bowel*, 3rd ed., Universal Wilde, Westwood, MA, 2015. With permission.

with an end-jejunostomy lose water and sodium from their stoma even when they take nothing by mouth and tend to be net secretors (net secretors are patients who lose more from the stoma than they take in by mouth; absorbers are those whose output is less than their oral intake). The sodium concentration of the effluent in either group of patients is about 90 mmol/L. The secretors are in constant negative sodium balance of up to 400 mmol/day depending on the total volume of stool lost [53]. Both will benefit from high-sodium foods or an oral sodium supplement to maintain balance, although net secretors will often require supplemental IV sodium-containing fluids in addition to sipping an ORS throughout the day [54].

Fluid/Hydration Selection

Fluid selection is integral to the SBS diet and overall patient success. It is a common mistake for patients to drink excessive amounts of hypotonic (and at times hypertonic) fluids in an attempt to quench their thirst and compensate for ostomy losses only to worsen dehydration with accelerated fluid and electrolyte losses. ORSs are typically good choices for SBS patients; however, palatability and cost can be limiting factors. Hypotonic fluids of water, tea, coffee, and sugar-free carbonated beverages should be limited, particularly in those SBS patients without a colon. Hypertonic/hyperosmotic fluids containing high sugar or fructose content will draw fluid into the bowel due to the high osmotic load and should be avoided regardless of the SBS bowel anatomy. Chapter 11 provides details on this important aspect of the care of the SBS patient.

STEP 4: PATIENT SELF-MONITORING

The final step in designing the diet prescription for the patient with SBS and providing recommendations for long-term therapy is to focus on educating patients on how to remain in control of their nutritional status. They will need to learn key clinical parameters to monitor so they are able to discern their "new normal." When their clinical status changes, this new awareness may lead them to seek advice and assessment early. Patients with SBS tend to be motivated and learn quickly what is normal for them and ultimately know what they should be looking for so they can seek assistance before severe problems occur. Table 10.6 outlines key areas of self-monitoring.

CONCLUSION

Selecting and tailoring the appropriate composition of the oral diet for each individual SBS patient based upon the remaining bowel anatomy are important to optimize clinical outcomes and decrease dependence on parenteral support. Along with appropriate oral fluids, optimal calorie intake, and nutrient composition, providing patient education and monitoring can lead to an improvement in

TABLE 10.6
Patient Self-Monitoring

Parameter	Rationale
Weight and trends	Adequate oral calories to allow for maintenance
Fluid intake and type	Prevention of dehydration or renal compromise
Urine output/volume	Goal is minimum of 1 L per day
Stool output/volume/frequency	Diet compliance for optimal enteral absorption

quality of life and enhance the possibility of achieving restoration of nutritional autonomy in these patients. The following is a list of diet resources for clinicians caring for these patients.

- University of Virginia Health System GI Nutrition website: http://www.ginutrition.virginia.edu
  Under the Patient Education Materials link
    Short bowel diet information
    Oral rehydration solutions
    Meal plan
    Snack ideas
- Parrish, C.R., *A Patient's Guide to Managing a Short Bowel*, 3rd ed., Universal Wilde, Westwood, MA, 2015:1–66. Available free at http://www.shortbowelsupport.com.
- Oley Foundation: http://www.oley.org (800/776-OLEY)

REFERENCES

1. Bizari L et al. Anthropometric food intake differences and applicability of low cost instruments for the measurement of body composition in two distinct groups of individuals with short bowel syndrome. *Nutr Hosp* 2014;30(1):205–212.
2. Nightingale JM et al. Jejunal efflux in short bowel syndrome. *Lancet* 1990;29;336(8718):765–768.
3. Tappenden KA. Pathophysiology of short bowel syndrome: Considerations of resected and residual anatomy. *JPEN J Parenter Enteral Nutr* 2014;38(1 Suppl):14S–22S.
4. Tappenden KA. Intestinal adaptation following resection. *JPEN J Parenter Enteral Nutr* 2014;38 (1 Suppl):23S–31S.
5. Carbonnel F et al. The role of anatomic factors in nutritional autonomy after extensive small bowel resection. *JPEN J Parenter Enteral Nutr* 1996;20(4):275–280.
6. Amiot A et al. Determinants of home parenteral nutrition dependence and survival of 268 patients with non-malignant short bowel syndrome. *Clin Nutr* 2013;32(3):368–374.
7. Woolf GM et al. Diet for patients with short bowel: High fat or high carbohydrate? *Gastroenterology* 1983;84:823–828.
8. Nordgaard I et al. Colon as a digestive organ in patients with short bowel. *Lancet* 1994;343(8894):373–376.
9. Ovesen L et al. The influence of dietary fat on jejunostomy output in patients with severe short bowel syndrome. *Am J Clin Nutr* 1983;38:270–277.
10. Jeppesen PB et al. The influence of a preserved colon on the absorption of medium chain fat in patients with small bowel resection. *Gut* 1998;43:478–483.
11. Nordgaard I et al. Importance of colonic support for energy absorption as small-bowel failure proceeds. *Am J Clin Nutr* 1996;64:222–231.
12. Kles KA et al. Short-chain fatty acids impact on intestinal adaptation, inflammation, carcinoma, and failure. *Gastroenterology* 2006;130(Suppl 2):S100–S105.
13. Andersson H. Fat-reduced diet in the symptomatic treatment of patients with ileopathy. *Nutr Metab* 1974;17:102–111.
14. Hessov I et al. Effects of a low-fat diet on mineral absorption in small-bowel disease. *Scand J Gastroenterol* 1983;18:551–554.
15. Atia A et al. Macronutrient absorption characteristics in humans with short bowel syndrome and jejuno-colonic anastomosis: Starch is the most important carbohydrate substrate, although pectin supplementation may modestly enhance short chain fatty acid production and fluid absorption. *JPEN J Parenter Enteral Nutr* 2011;35(2):229–240.
16. Bond JH et al. Colonic conservation of malabsorbed carbohydrate. *Gastroenterology* 1980;78:444–447.
17. Jeppesen PB et al. Colonic digestion and absorption of energy from carbohydrates and medium-chain fat in small bowel failure. *JPEN J Parenter Enteral Nutr* 1999;23(5 Suppl):S101–S105.
18. Royall D et al. Evidence for colonic conservation of malabsorbed carbohydrate in short bowel syndrome. *Am J Gastroenterol* 1992;87:751–756.
19. Nightingale JMD et al. Colonic preservation reduces need for parenteral therapy, increases incidence of renal stones, but does not change high prevalence of gallstones in patients with a short bowel. *Gut* 1992;33(11):1493–1497.

20. Rudman D et al. Hypocitraturia in patients with gastrointestinal malabsorption. *N Engl J Med* 1980;303(12):657–661.
21. Parrish CR et al. Part III: Hydrating the adult patient with short bowel syndrome. *Pract Gastroenterol* 2015;39(2):10.
22. Parrish CR et al. Part II: Nutrition therapy for short bowel syndrome in the adult patient. *Pract Gastroenterol* 2014;38(10):40.
23. Pullan JM. Massive intestinal resection. *Proc R Soc Med* 1959;52:31–37.
24. Thiele RH et al. Standardization of care: Impact of an enhanced recovery protocol on length of stay, complications, and direct costs after colorectal surgery. *J Am Coll Surg* 2015;220(4):430–443.
25. Thompson JS et al. Current management of the short bowel syndrome. *Surg Clin North Am* 2011;91(3):493–510.
26. Whelan K et al. Assessment of fecal output in patients receiving enteral tube feeding: Validation of a novel chart. *Eur J Clin Nutr* 2004;58(7):1030–1037.
27. Culkin A et al. Improving clinical outcome in patients with intestinal failure using individualized nutritional advice. *J Hum Nutr Diet* 2009;22:290–298.
28. Steiger E. Guidelines for pharmacotherapy, nutritional management, and weaning parenteral nutrition in adult patients with short bowel syndrome: Introduction. *J Clin Gastroenterol* 2006;40(Suppl 2):S73–S74.
29. Byrne TA et al. Clinical observations: Beyond the prescription: Optimizing the diet of patients with short bowel syndrome. *Nutr Clin Pract* 2000;15(6):306–311.
30. Crenn P et al. Net digestive absorption and adaptive hyperphagia in adult short bowel patients. *Gut* 2004;53:1279–1286.
31. Jeppesen PB et al. Intestinal failure defined by measurements of intestinal energy and wet weight absorption. *Gut* 2000;46(5):701–706.
32. Woolf GM et al. Nutritional absorption in short bowel syndrome. Evaluation of fluid, calorie, and divalent cation requirements. *Dig Dis Sci* 1987;32(1):8–15.
33. Wall EA. An overview of short bowel syndrome management: Adherence, adaptation, and practical recommendations. *J Acad Nutr Diet* 2013;113(9):1200–1208.
34. Gilchrist PN et al. Dietary compliance in the short bowel syndrome. *JPEN J Parenter Enteral Nutr* 1984;8(3):315–316.
35. Kelly DG et al. Short bowel syndrome: Highlights of patient management, quality of life, and survival. *JPEN J Parenter Enteral Nutr* 2014;38(4):427–437.
36. Winkler MF et al. The meaning of food and eating among home parenteral nutrition-dependent adults with intestinal failure: A qualitative inquiry. *J Am Diet Assoc* 2010;110(11):1676–1683.
37. DiBaise JK et al. Intestinal rehabilitation and the short bowel syndrome: Part 2. *Am J Gastroenterol* 2004;99(9):1823–1832.
38. Byrne TA et al. The role of diet and specific nutrients. In: Matarese LE, Steiger E, Seidner DL, eds. *Intestinal Failure and Rehabilitation: A Clinical Guide*. Boca Raton, FL: CRC Press;2005:129–147.
39. Jeejeebhoy KN. Short bowel syndrome: A nutritional and medical approach. *CMAJ* 2002;166(10):1297–302.
40. Byrne TA et al. A new treatment for patients with short bowel syndrome. *Ann Surg* 1995;222(3):243: 244–255.
41. Barrett JS et al. Dietary poorly absorbed, short-chain carbohydrates increase delivery of water and fermentable substrates to the proximal colon. *Aliment Pharmacol Ther* 2010;31(8):874–882.
42. Wolever TMS et al. Sugar alcohols and diabetes: A review. *Can J Diabet* 2002;26(4):356–362.
43. Marteau P et al. Do patients with short-bowel syndrome need a lactose-free diet? *Nutrition* 1997;13:13–16.
44. Byrne TA et al. Growth hormone, glutamine, and an optimal diet reduces parenteral nutrition in patients with short bowel syndrome: A prospective, randomized, placebo-controlled, double-blind clinical trial. *Ann Surg* 2005;242(5):655–661.
45. Gramlich L et al. Essential fatty acid deficiency in 2015: The impact of novel intravenous lipid emulsions. *JPEN J Parenter Enteral Nutr* 2015;39(1 Suppl):61S–66S.
46. Hamilton C et al. Essential fatty acid deficiency in human adults during parenteral nutrition. *Nutr Clin Pract* 2006;21(4):387–394.
47. McCray S et al. Nutritional management of chyle leaks: An update. *Pract Gastroenterol* 2011;35(4):12.
48. Bach AC et al. Medium-chain triglycerides: An update. *Am J Clin Nutr* 1982;36:950–962.
49. Jensen GL et al. Dietary modification of chyle composition in chylothorax. *Gastroenterology* 1989;97(3):761–765.
50. Ruppin DC et al. Clinical use of medium chain triglycerides. *Drugs* 1980;20(3):216–224.
51. Buchman AL. Etiology and initial management of short bowel syndrome. *Gastroenterology* 2006;130(2 Suppl 1):S5–S15.

52. Parrish CR. *A Patient's Guide to Managing a Short Bowel*, 3rd ed. Westwood, MA: Universal Wilde; 2015:1–66.
53. Lennard-Jones JE. Oral rehydration solutions in short bowel syndrome. *Clin Ther* 1990;12(Suppl A):129–137.
54. Nightingale JM et al. Oral salt supplements to compensate for jejunostomy losses: Comparison of sodium chloride capsules, glucose electrolyte solution, and glucose polymer electrolyte solution. *Gut* 1992;33(6):759–761.

11 Maintaining Hydration in the Short Bowel Patient

Bethany E. Blalock and Carol Rees Parrish

CONTENTS

KEY POINTS

- Inadequately treated, the dehydrated patient with short bowel syndrome may suffer fatigue, weight loss, nephrolithiasis, electrolyte abnormalities, and, if continued unchecked, potentially irreversible kidney damage.
- Detecting dehydration in this special population is more challenging since the usual laboratory parameters are not reliable markers of hydration status.
- Initial assessment should always include a 24-hour measurement of fluid intake and output.
- Oral rehydration therapy can be an inexpensive and very effective intervention in some patients.
- Occasionally, long-term parenteral fluid support will be needed, particularly in the patient with a high-output end-jejunostomy.

INTRODUCTION

The achievement of adequate fluid balance, or euvolemia, is a major challenge for many patients with short bowel syndrome (SBS); failure to achieve this balance is a leading source of morbidity. In the first weeks and months after a massive intestinal resection, achieving euvolemia is a major goal. Clinicians must first and foremost understand how to detect dehydration in this special population for whom the usual laboratory parameters may not reliably reflect hydration status [1]. This can be particularly challenging in patients who do not have an ostomy, since losses cannot be reliably estimated based on number of stools. Further, clinicians must be savvy in fluid management, which is more nuanced than a "just add water" approach in the setting of altered gastrointestinal (GI) anatomy. Although the small intestine and colon undergo a period of adaptation during the first 1 to 2 years after resection, the voluminous diarrhea (and attending fluid and electrolyte loss) experienced particularly in patients without a colon will continue for life if not appropriately managed. Increased stool output not only significantly impairs quality of life but also creates a number of serious comorbidities. Inadequately treated, the dehydrated SBS patient will suffer fatigue and weight loss and may develop nephrolithiasis, electrolyte abnormalities, and, if continued unchecked, potentially irreversible kidney damage [2,3].

In this chapter, we will provide a brief overview of the physiology of fluid maintenance along the GI tract, with a focus toward what makes SBS patients unique, followed by a brief discussion on the role of parenteral fluids in the management of early stages of SBS. Next, we will explain how to assess fluid status in this challenging patient population. We will close by offering suggestions for meeting fluid needs via the enteral route, whether by mouth, gastrostomy tube, or both. In this regard, we will discuss the use of oral rehydration therapy (ORT) and provide a number of suggested resources for clinicians and patients.

PHYSIOLOGY OF FLUID MAINTENANCE IN SBS

SBS is a condition that entails several different bowel anatomies. As such, the approach to hydrating the individual patient must be tailored to what remains of his or her particular GI tract. This is because the regional capacity to preserve water varies throughout the entire GI tract, including the colon, whose major role is to reabsorb water and sodium. In addition to the average 2 L of oral fluid consumed each day, this intake is diluted by an additional 4 L of endogenous fluid secreted into the intestinal lumen in response [4]. The components of this endogenous fluid include about 0.5 L of saliva, 2 L of gastric secretions, and 1.5 L of biliary and pancreatic secretions. Hence, a total of 6 L of chyme passes the duodenojejunal flexure each day [5]. Under normal conditions, the colon resorbs 90% of the fluid it encounters daily. Compared with the transverse colon and beyond, the ascending colon is most efficient at reclaiming water, and therefore, the degree of fluid losses after a resection will depend on which part, if any, of the colon is preserved [4]. Unfortunately, in the setting of SBS, the ascending colon is often resected.

Similarly, the ileum is very efficient at reabsorbing much of the water that is secreted into the more proximal gut. Sodium absorption—and, by extension, water absorption, since water follows sodium—is accomplished in the GI tract in part via passive diffusion down the concentration gradient. This occurs more so in the jejunum than in the rest of the bowel because the intercellular junctions in the jejunum are "leaky," and hence, jejunal contents can only be iso-osmolar with plasma. Thus, water and small molecules move much more freely into and out of the jejunal lumen—about nine times more so than in the ileum [4]. As a result, the loss of ileum is associated with less concentrated stools as compared with a similar length of lost jejunum [4]. Table 11.1 outlines the approximate expected output depending on type of resection undergone and the remaining bowel anatomy.

In the absence of a colon, patients may experience net secretion, in which losses of water and sodium outstrip gains (i.e., stool output > fluid intake). In the setting of an end-jejunostomy in which less than 100 cm of jejunum remains, stomal output not uncommonly exceeds 4 L per day [6]. For this reason, these SBS patients are at highest risk of chronic sodium depletion and dehydration.

TABLE 11.1
Typical 24-Hour Stool/Ostomy Output by Resection Type

Type of Resection	Typical Daily Output (mL)
Normal stool output	200
Colostomy	200–600
Ileostomy	
• Immediately postoperative	1200
• Average	750
Jejunostomy	Up to 6000

PARENTERAL FLUIDS

Most patients will require parenteral fluids in the early stages after major bowel resection; in most, this will not remain the case permanently. This is because the first 6–12 months postresection are characterized by a period of intense intestinal adaptation during which the physiology of the altered GI anatomy is changing to cope with diminished absorptive capacity (see Chapter 4). However, decreased absorptive surface is not the only factor that contributes to fluid and electrolyte losses. In the setting of extensive small bowel and colon resection, hormonal (e.g., glucagon-like peptide-1, peptide YY) feedback mechanisms that regulate intestinal transit, as well as others that effect gastric acid and bicarbonate secretion, are often disrupted, leading to excessive fluid and electrolyte losses that may be very difficult to control. Thus, at least during this early phase, even though macronutrient absorption may be sufficient, parenteral fluid support might still be necessary for some patients whose new bowel anatomy simply will not allow them to "stay ahead" of dehydration.

Clinicians caring for these patients should establish a urine output goal of at least 1 L daily [3,7,8]; short of this and the patient risks nephrolithiasis and even significant kidney injury over time [2,3]. Although many patients will be able to eventually wean from parenteral fluids and/or nutrition, some will continue to require supplemental parenteral fluids indefinitely. Patients with <100 cm small bowel proximal to an end-jejunostomy will frequently lose more fluid in their stool than they take in (a.k.a., net secretors), often well over 2 L daily [9]. Adding insult to injury, the addition of even more enteral fluids only exacerbates stool losses [4]. This is particularly true if the ingested fluids are not isotonic (unfortunately, this means most beverages), except the ones designed for this particular purpose, as we will explain momentarily.

In the home setting, parenteral fluid support is usually administered either at night or during the day as 1–3 L of half-normal saline, normal saline, or lactated ringers over 3 to 12 hours daily as needed depending on the patient's lifestyle and other factors. Other additives may be included in the fluid if needed, such as dextrose (if a small number of additional calories are needed to meet or maintain goal weight), sodium bicarbonate (if metabolic acidosis is persistent), electrolytes (most commonly magnesium and potassium), or vitamins and minerals (if deficiencies are known or clinically suspected). Of course, many SBS patients require parenteral nutrition (PN) support for some or all of their nutritional needs. In that case, PN is typically administered nocturnally to free them from pump encumbrance during the day. Among these PN-dependent patients, however, additional daytime parenteral fluids may still be needed to prevent dehydration and kidney injury during the warmer months of the year or in hotter climates where insensible losses are greater. Also, home PN bags typically only hold up to 4 L, so if a patient requires more, he or she will need to have parenteral fluid "chasers" during the day while off of PN.

ASSESSING HYDRATION STATUS IN SBS

If parenteral fluids are prescribed to be given "as needed," how do patients or their care provider know when these are needed? In other words, what signs and symptoms indicate inadequate hydration? Whereas serum sodium, blood urea nitrogen (BUN), creatinine, and other electrolytes quickly become hemoconcentrated in the setting of intravascular volume depletion/dehydration in people with normal GI anatomy, this is not always the case in those with SBS. Only after several days of poor hydration, when the SBS patient is significantly volume depleted, do these numbers start to indicate a problem [1]. This occurs because decreased renal blood flow and/or decreased serum sodium activates the renin–angiotensin–aldosterone system, causing a cascade of activity that ultimately leads to, among other things, increased reabsorption of sodium and water and the maintenance of blood volume. Thus, the kidneys do an exquisite job of maintaining blood volume even when total body water is being significantly depleted via GI losses. As a result, the BUN to creatinine ratio will belie dehydration and patients and clinicians must learn to rely on other markers of hydration status, the most important of which are urine output and swift change in weight in combination with an assessment for standard signs and symptoms of dehydration (Table 11.2).

TABLE 11.2
Sign and Symptoms of Dehydration

Sign	Symptom
Excessive and/or persistent thirst	Ostomy/stool output more than 2000 mL per day
Dry mouth	Ostomy/stool output in excess of total fluids consumed
Skin tenting	Urine output less than 1000–1200 mL per day
Fatigue, especially persistent	Reduced frequency of urination
Orthostatic hypotension	Dark urine color
Rapid weight loss	Declining kidney function

Initial assessment should include a 24-hour measurement of *fluid intake*, including all food, beverage, and parenteral fluid intake, and *fluid output*, including total urine and stool/ostomy output. Adequate hydration is generally considered to be achieved when urine output is greater than 1 L daily and urine sodium concentration is greater than 20 mEq/L [3,7,8]; lower values indicate that fluid and sodium, respectively, are being excreted in the stool before they can be absorbed and that the kidney is attempting to compensate for the loss of sodium by increasing its resorption. A stool hat, which can be used for both stool and urine measurement, is an essential "tool of the trade" for anyone caring for SBS patients. For patients who can easily measure their stool output via their ostomy appliance, a good practice is to specifically ask the size of their appliance and how many times they empty their appliance in a 24-hour period, or "per day *and* per night;" otherwise, they may inadvertently leave out nocturnal volume.

In addition to total daily urine output and urine sodium, serial weights are imperative in the assessment of hydration status in SBS patients. Not only do longer-term trends help signal nutritional compromise, but also daily weight changes can indicate the need for supplemental fluids, whether they be taken by mouth (unless this drives their output too much), feeding tube, or intravenously. Recalling that a liter of water weighs 1 kg, patients can readily tell from their home scale, when used daily under the same conditions (e.g., first thing in the morning, after voiding, and before eating or drinking), that they are "a quart low" if their weight is about 2 lb off from the day before or from its usual range.

In the hospital setting, "strict I's and O's" and daily weights are critical to track in this patient population, just as much so as daily basic metabolic panel. A dedicated standing scale is recommended whenever feasible, as is the buy-in of bedside nurses who may not be familiar with the special importance that these simple measurements have in SBS patients.

Finally, as time for hospital discharge nears, it is particularly important that, whenever possible, all parenteral fluids be consolidated into the PN prescription to mimic the home setting, preferably for at least 2 days before leaving. Unfortunately and not uncommonly, a patient has been discharged to home on the PN solution that has been running up until discharge in the hospital, but without the *second* IV that has been running at 100 mL/hour all along, only to return dehydrated in a few days because the PN did not provide adequate hydration.

HYDRATING THE SBS PATIENT

For patients with SBS, the world of fluids may seem reminiscent of the lines from the *Rime of the Ancient Mariner*: "Water, water, everywhere, Nor any drop to drink." Indeed, excessive thirst is not uncommon because while stool or ostomy output can sometimes be voluminous, many SBS patients will find that drinking more fluids only drives a vicious cycle of increased output that leads to more dehydration and thirst. It is difficult for some patients to grasp the concept that what they drink does not automatically stay in their bodies, or that the fluid has to get into their bloodstream to be able to make urine. A typical scenario is the patient who complains of an "unquenchable thirst" despite drinking liter after liter of (inappropriate) fluids such as water, sports drinks, soda, and tea and snacking on popsicles in between.

Many commonly consumed beverages, including water and sports drinks, are considered inappropriate in certain SBS bowel anatomies as they are quite low in or devoid of sodium (hypotonic). As such, ingestion leads to an influx of sodium and, thus, more water into the lumen of the proximal small bowel (since water follows sodium), leading to an increase in both sodium and fluid losses. Normally, this water would be reabsorbed by the distal small bowel and colon, but in SBS, particularly those with end-jejunostomies, the distal small bowel and proximal colon are often missing. Similarly, hyperosmolar/hypertonic fluids such as sodas and fruit juices also draw water into the lumen to equilibrate the solute load and, once again, the water is ultimately lost as osmotic diarrhea, particularly if the patient is without a colon. The tonicity of a number of common beverages is listed in Table 11.3 [10–13].

Thus, SBS patients with polydipsia must be thoroughly educated to understand that more is not better when it comes to drinking fluids. To bring stool or ostomy output under control and to demonstrate to patients that what they drink adds to their total stool output, a 24-hour trial of *zero (or near zero)* oral or enteral fluids and only recommended solid foods is suggested. Parenteral fluids to cover losses and maintain urine output of at least 1 L daily may be required during this time to

TABLE 11.3
Approximate Osmolality of Common Beverages

Beverage	mOsm/kg
Hypotonic Fluids (<300 mOsm/kg)	
Water, purified	0–28
Iced tea, sugar free	13–44
Coffee, black, no sugar	28–53
Sugar free soda, lemonade, punch, or Kool-Aid	13–44
Hypertonic Fluids (>300 mOsm/kg)	
Malted milk	940
Ice cream	1905
Eggnog	695
Fruited yogurt	870
Sherbet	1225
Popsicle	720
Ensure/Boost	590/640
Ensure Plus/Boost Plus	680/720
Resource Breeze	750
Enteral formulas	250–700
Prune juice	1265
Grape juice	865
Apple juice	685
Orange juice	615
Tomato juice	595
Punch with sugar	450
Broth	445
Flavored gelatin	735
Sugar sweetened beverages (soda, energy drinks, etc.)	535–1110

Source: Bell, S. et al., *Nutr. Clin. Pract.*, 2, 241–244, 1987, Parrish, C.R., *Nutr. Clin. Pract.*, 18, 76–85, 2003; Dini, E. et al., *Invest. Clin.*, 45, 323–235, 2004; Parrish, C.R, DiBaise, J., *Pract. Gastroenterol.* 39, 10, 2015. Available at http://www.ginutrition.virginia.edu. With permission.

prevent and/or correct dehydration. Patients are often surprised to find relief from their thirst with a 1.5-L fluid *restriction*, along with temporary parenteral fluids to maintain euvolemia [6].

Not all SBS patients struggle to the same extent to tolerate conventional oral fluids and maintain good hydration. This usually relates to their remaining bowel anatomy. Those with a colon are usually able to handle ingestion of hypotonic beverages because they have adequate reabsorption of water and sodium, so output is not exacerbated [14]. In the absence of a colon, however, more sodium is usually needed in fluids to avoid aggravating diarrhea. As a general guideline, about 5 g of additional table salt is needed per liter of stool lost (5 g table salt = 90 mEq sodium = 2 g sodium = ~1 teaspoon table salt).

ORAL REHYDRATION THERAPY

Patients who lack a colon frequently have a difficult time maintaining euvolumia due to their compromised ability to reabsorb water and electrolytes; SBS patients with end-jejunostomies have the hardest time maintaining their hydration because of regional differences in water movement and sodium absorption in the proximal versus distal small bowel, as discussed previously.

Enterocytes transport sodium and glucose (or galactose) across the apical membrane (the side that faces the lumen) together via a sodium-glucose linked transporter protein (SGLT). Both molecules—one sodium and either one glucose or one galactose—must be present in correct proportion to ensure absorption of water. This is because hundreds of water molecules flow into the epithelial cell along with each sodium molecule, but the SGLT protein will not move anything at all unless glucose or galactose is also present. This process is unidirectional [15]. Oral fluids known as oral rehydration solutions (ORSs) have been designed with these proportions in mind and are discussed in more detail in the following.

This stimulation of sodium and water absorption by way of the sodium-glucose cotransport system is the basis for the use of ORSs, which contain all three ingredients (i.e., water, sodium, and carbohydrate source) in the correct proportions. For maximum jejunal absorption, the ratio of carbohydrate to sodium should be 1:1 [14], and the concentration of sodium should be close to 90–120 mEq/L [16], although some newer reduced-osmolarity formulas have less and may be more palatable. In general, solutions with sodium >90 mEq/L are unpalatable regardless of efforts to flavor. In this way, sodium losses are replaced and water absorption is promoted. ORS has been used very successfully worldwide to treat acute (usually infectious) diarrheal illness and has also been shown to work well in SBS patients [17–20]. Its use has even liberated some SBS patients from reliance on supplemental parenteral fluids. Table 11.4 [21] provides a comparison of commercially available ORSs.

Although difficult to predict, ORT does not seem to provide benefit in all SBS patients, even those with an end-jejunostomy. For some, these solutions may even worsen stool output [18], particularly if they are taken in large boluses during meals rather than sipped throughout the day and ingested judiciously during meals. Some patients will need up to 2 or 3 L daily. A reasonable rule of thumb is to start with 500–1000 mL per day and titrate the volume as needed based on urine output, weight, and other signs and symptoms of hydration status. If stool or ostomy output increases in the absence of a net increase in urine, the therapy should be discontinued. In contrast, if it does seem to work well, it can be continued as long as the patient is willing to adhere to this type of therapy.

Some patients are not willing to use ORT because they find it unpalatable and/or they cannot afford the commercial products. To improve compliance with this cost-effective and low-risk therapy, ORS can be frozen into ice cubes or popsicles, and a variety of different homemade recipes can be tried (Table 11.5). Another consideration would be to administer ORS through a gastrostomy tube [20], which is a particularly appealing option if the only other choice is to begin use of parenteral fluids. Importantly, sports drinks and other electrolyte-enhanced beverages should not be used as a substitute for ORS in the SBS setting because they generally contain too much carbohydrate and not enough sodium and will therefore worsen diarrhea. At the end of the day, some patients are just not going to accept ORT. In these cases, it is best to simply suggest alternatives to beverages that are known offenders and will most certainly drive stool/ostomy output. Table 11.6 provides suggestions that may help guide advice.

TABLE 11.4
Commercially Available Oral Rehydration Solutions

Solution	Glucose (g/L)	Sodium (mEq/mg per Liter)	Potassium (mEq/mg per Liter)	Citrate (mEq/mg per Liter)	Osmolarity (mOsm/L)	Calories per Liter	Manufacturer
WHO packet	20	90/2070	20/780	30	330	152	Jianas Brothers
Reduced osmolarity	13.5	75/1725	20/780	30	245	126	
Rehydralyte	25	75/1725	20/780	30	310	172	Abbott Nutrition
Pedialyte	25	45/1035	20/780	30	250	100	
EquaLyte	25	78/1794	22/858	30	305	172	
Parent's Choice Pediatric electrolyte	20	45/1035	20/780	n/a	262	100	Walmart
CeraLyte 70	40	70/1610	20/780	30	<260	160	CeraLyte
CeraLyte 90	40	90/2070	20/780	30	<275	160	
DripDrop	33	58/1330	20/780	160/251	235	130	DripDrop

Source: Parrish, C.R. *A Patient's Guide to Managing a Short Bowel, 3rd Edition*, Universal Wilde, Westwood, MA, 2015. Available at no cost at http://www.shortbowelsupport.com.
Note: WHO, World Health Organization.

TABLE 11.5
Homemade Oral Rehydration Solution Recipes

Solution	Ingredients	Directions
Sugar and salt water	1 quart water 3/4 teaspoon salt 6 teaspoons sugar Crystal Light to taste (optional)	Mix all ingredients in a large pitcher until dissolved.
World Health Organization Reduced Osmolality ORT (Home Solution)	1/2 teaspoon table salt 1/4 teaspoon Morton salt substitute (use with caution in those with hyperkalemia) 1/2 teaspoon baking soda 2 tablespoons table sugar Add tap water to make 1 L Nutrasweet or Splenda (optional)	To a 1-L container, add about one-half the needed water. Add the dry ingredients, stir or shake well; add water to make a final volume of 1 L. Add artificial sweetener of choice if desired. Best if chilled. Sip as directed. Discard after 24 hours.
Gatorade G2	4 cups Gatorade G2 (or one 32-oz bottle) 1/2 teaspoon table salt	Mix ingredients together and shake or stir until dissolved.
Chicken broth A	4 cups water 1 dry chicken broth cube 1/4 teaspoon salt 2 tablespoons sugar	Mix ingredients together and shake or stir until dissolved.
Chicken broth B	2 cups liquid broth 2 cups water 2 tablespoons sugar	Mix ingredients together and shake or stir until dissolved.
Tomato juice	2 1/2 cups tomato juice 1 1/2 cups water	Mix ingredients together and shake or stir until dissolved.
Rice cereal	1/2 cup dry, precooked baby rice cereal 2 cups water 1/4 teaspoon salt	Combine ingredients and mix until well dissolved and smooth. Refrigerate. Solution should be thick, but pourable and drinkable.

Source: For more homemade "oral rehydration-like" solutions using alternative beverage bases, see Parrish, C.R., *A Patient's Guide to Managing a Short Bowel, 3rd edition*, Universal Wilde, Westwood, MA, 2015. Available at no cost at http://www.shortbowelsupport.com.

TABLE 11.6
Oral Fluid Options for Patients with Short Bowel Syndrome

Best Fluid Choices	Fluids Worth Trying Sparingly	Fluids That Will Increase Stool Output
Oral rehydration solutions	G2 Gatorade or other sports drink equivalents	Too much water
Ceralyte "jello"	Milk (1% or 2% may be better)	Fruit juice
	Broth or broth-based soups	Fruit drinks
	Diet sodas	Kool-Aid
	Diluted grape, orange, or pineapple juice	Coffee and tea
	1/2 strength flavored gelatin	Sweet tea
	Water, in small amounts	Ensure/Boost, etc.
		Soda
		Alcohol

Source: Parrish, C.R., DiBaise, J., *Pract. Gastroenterol.*, 39, 10, 2015. Available at http://www.ginutrition.virginia.edu. With permission.

CONCLUSION

Hydrating the SBS patient can present a major challenge, yet failure to do so adequately is a major source of morbidity in this population. Potential consequences of perpetual dehydration include failure to thrive, nephrolithiasis, and irreversible kidney damage. Furthermore, the cost to the patient in terms of quality of life is difficult to fully capture. Clinicians must be skilled in assessing hydration status since SBS patients do not always present with the usual laboratory abnormalities when they are mildly or even moderately behind on hydration. While some SBS patients may require long-term parenteral fluids and/or PN, many will only need parenteral fluids in the early period postresection and, perhaps, intermittently thereafter. It is important to remember that it may be possible to achieve euvolemia with avoidance of certain types of oral fluids and use of other types, although this is less likely in end-jejunostomy patients. ORT can be an inexpensive and effective treatment for maintaining hydration in some SBS patients.

REFERENCES

1. Nightingale JM. Management of a high-output jejunostomy. In: *Intestinal Failure*. Ed., Nightingale JM. London: Greenwich Medical Media, 2001, pp. 375–92.
2. Banerjee A et al. Acute renal failure and metabolic disturbances in the short bowel syndrome. *QJM*. 2001;95:37–40.
3. Lauverjat MA et al. Chronic dehydration may impair renal function in patients with chronic intestinal failure on long-term parenteral nutrition. *Clin Nutr.* 2003;25:75–81.
4. Lennard-Jones JE. Review article: Practical management of the short bowel. *Aliment Pharmacol Ther.* 1994;8:563–77.
5. Nightingale JM. The medical management of intestinal failure: Methods to reduce the severity. *Proc Nutr Soc*. 2003;62(3):703–10.
6. Hughes S et al. Care of the intestinal stoma and enterocutaneous fistula. In: *Intestinal Failure*. Ed., Nightingale JM. London: Greenwich Medical Media, 2001, pp. 53–63.
7. DiBaise JK et al. Strategies for weaning parenteral nutrition in adult patients with short bowel syndrome. *J Clin Gastroenterol*. 2006;40S:94–8.
8. O'Neil M et al. Total body sodium depletion and poor weight gain in children and young adults with an ileostomy: A case series. *Nutr Clin Pract*. 2014;29:397–401.
9. Nightingale JM et al. Jejunal efflux in short bowel syndrome. *Lancet*. 1990;336(8718):765–8.
10. Bell S et al. Osmolality of beverages commonly provided on clear and full liquid menu. *Nutr Clin Pract.* 1987;2:241–4.
11. Parrish CR. Enteral feeding: The art and the science. *Nutr Clin Pract*. 2003;18:76–85.
12. Dini E et al. Osmolality of frequently consumed beverages. *Invest Clin*. 2004;45:323–35.
13. Parrish CR, DiBaise J. Part III: Hydrating the adult patient with short bowel syndrome. *Pract Gastroenterol*. 2015;39(2):10. Available at http://www.ginutrition.virginia.edu.
14. Kelly DG et al. Oral rehydration solution: A "low-tech" oft neglected therapy. *Nutr Issues Gastroenterol.* 2004;28:51–62.
15. Lin R et al. D-Glucose acts via sodium/glucose cotransporter 1 to increase NHE3 in mouse jejunal brush border by a Na+/H+ exchange regulatory factor 2-dependent process. *Gastroenterology*. 2011;140:560–71.
16. Rodrigues C et al. What is the ideal sodium concentration of oral rehydration solutions for short bowel patients? *Clin Sci*. 1988;74:69.
17. Nightingale JM et al. Oral salt supplements to compensate for jejunostomy losses: Comparison of sodium chloride capsules, glucose electrolyte solution, and glucose polymer electrolyte solution. *Gut*. 1992;33:759–61.
18. Newton CR et al. Effect of different drinks on fluid and electrolyte losses from a jejunostomy. *J R Soc Med*. 1985;78:27–34
19. Beaugerie L et al. Isotonic high-sodium oral rehydration solution for increasing sodium absorption in patients with short bowel syndrome. *Am J Clin Nutr.* 1991;53:769–72.
20. Nauth J et al. A therapeutic approach to wean total parenteral nutrition in the management of short bowel syndrome: Three cases using nocturnal enteral rehydration. *Nutr Rev*. 2004;62:221–31.
21. Parrish CR. *A Patient's Guide to Managing a Short Bowel, 3rd Edition*. Westwood, MA: Universal Wilde, 2015:1–66. Available at no cost at http://www.shortbowelsupport.com.

12 Vitamins
Supplementation and Monitoring

Elizabeth A. Wall

CONTENTS

KEY POINTS

- The segment and length of bowel resected, intestinal transit time, residual bowel disease, diet, pharmacotherapies, psychosocial situations, growth, and aging all influence vitamin supplementation requirements in the short bowel syndrome (SBS) patient.
- The key to effective management of vitamin levels in SBS is to accurately assess physical and biological markers for baseline concentrations, develop a comprehensive and practical vitamin supplementation plan, educate patients and caregivers on the importance of adherence to prescribed vitamin supplementation regimens, and routinely monitor response to therapy.
- Frequent monitoring and adjustments are required during bowel adaptation, periods of growth, and with any clinical changes that impact nutrient absorption.

INTRODUCTION

Vitamins are defined chemicals that are essential for cellular metabolism, hematopoietic processes, and hormonal regulation of a myriad of physiologic functions [1,2]. Vitamins are categorized based on their solubility in either water or fat solvents. Water-soluble vitamins, with the exception of vitamin B_{12}, are absorbed either by passive diffusion or sodium-dependent transport throughout the intestine, particularly in the upper intestine. Fat-soluble vitamins are absorbed in the jejunum and ileum but require bile salts to form mixed micelles, which facilitate the transport of fat into the enterocyte. Vitamin absorption in those with short bowel syndrome (SBS) is influenced by the segment and condition of their remnant bowel, diet, and pharmaceutical therapies. In addition, acute inflammatory or infectious processes can alter serum vitamin transport protein concentrations and vascular permeability that, in turn, yield factitious vitamin levels [1,3]. Therefore, it is imperative that clinicians caring for patients with SBS have knowledge of the length, health, and specific segments of intestine remaining; medications the patient is taking, including supplements; and an understanding of the factors that alter vitamin assay results to develop a care plan for vitamin supplementation and monitoring.

This chapter will focus on the vitamins most difficult for those with SBS to absorb. Since each patient with SBS is unique with respect to bowel length, transit time, absorptive capacity, and underlying disease process, there are limited data available for standardization of care. Therefore, the recommendations made are based on scientific evidence where available, accepted practice guidelines, and clinical experience focusing on established principles of human anatomy and physiology. Discussion of common practice issues, including signs and symptoms of vitamin deficiencies, with standard recommendations and clinical pearls will be included to assist clinicians in providing safe and effective care to patients with SBS.

FAT-SOLUBLE VITAMINS

The fat-soluble vitamins A, D, E, and K are found in foods of both plant and animal origins and are absorbed in sufficient amounts in a normal intestinal tract by those who eat adequate and balanced diets. They are absorbed along with dietary fats and require bile salts to form micelles, which allow for absorption into the enterocyte, incorporation into chylomicrons, and transportation to target cells. Extensive small bowel resections involving the distal ileum modify fat and fat-soluble vitamin absorption by disruption of the enterohepatic circulation of bile salts. Depletion of bile salts has a cascade effect on fat-soluble vitamin absorption by reducing micelle formation, causing fat malabsorption and leading to reduced efficiency of fat-soluble vitamin absorption. Similarly, resection or bypass of the duodenum (although uncommon), such that normal bile and pancreatic enzyme mixing with chyme is disrupted, or rapid intestinal transit can result in fat and fat-soluble vitamin malabsorption. Some medications used to relieve diarrhea can worsen fat malabsorption. For example, bile salt sequestrants may be used after limited resection of the terminal ileum, when the colon is in continuity, to bind bile salts and prevent colonocyte irritation that results in sodium and water secretion, further aggravating diarrhea [4]. While these medications relieve choleretic diarrhea, they deplete bile salts and worsen fat and fat-soluble vitamin malabsorption in those with more extensive small bowel resections [5]. Finally, patients with known fat malabsorption may limit dietary fat intake to help manage steatorrhea, subsequently reducing intake of fat-soluble vitamins, which, over time, leads to depletion of vitamin stores [6].

At some point, most patients with SBS will require repletion of one or more fat-soluble vitamin deficiencies [7,8]. Most oral preparations of fat-soluble vitamins require the normal pathway of micelle and chylomicron formations for absorption and transportation. Thus, it is recommended to take fat-soluble vitamins with a meal or snack that includes some dietary fat. Water miscible preparations of fat-soluble vitamins, such as AquADEK, Vita4life ADEK· and Bariatric Advantage dry vitamins, are available and have been used with mixed success to replete and maintain fat-soluble vitamin levels in patients with malabsorption [9,10]. Patients with SBS who receive parenteral nutrition (PN) support that includes multivitamins are often able to maintain normal fat-soluble vitamin levels without oral supplements, except vitamin D. Table 12.1 details the contents of currently available adult and pediatric intravenous (IV) multivitamin (MVI) preparations. If MVIs are taken only intermittently, either because of days off PN infusions or drug shortages, then patients should take oral MVI supplements daily or at least on days without PN MVI in an effort to maintain serum concentrations and stores.

Fat-soluble vitamins are stored in varying concentrations and have potential for toxicity with severe consequences if excess vitamins are ingested and absorbed over time. Therefore, cautious supplementation and monitoring of patients receiving fat-soluble vitamin supplements can prevent deficiency as well as toxicity and potential harm to the patient. The following sections will discuss pertinent information for each of the fat-soluble vitamins as it relates to SBS.

TABLE 12.1
Commercially Available IV MVI Preparations

	Infuvite Adult (10 mL)	MVI Adult (10 mL)	MVI 12 (10 mL)	Infuvite Pediatric (5 mL)	MVI Pediatric (5 mL)
Vitamin A (IU)	3300	3300	3300	2300	2300
Vitamin D (IU)	200	200	200	400	400
Vitamin E (IU)	10	10	10	7	7
Vitamin K (μg)	150	150	0	200	200
Vitamin C (mg)	200	200	200	80	80
Thiamine (mg)	6	6	6	1.2	1.2
Riboflavin (mg)	3.6	3.6	3.6	1.4	1.4
Niacin (mg)	40	40	40	17	17
Pyridoxine (mg)	6	6	6	1	1
Pantothenic acid (mg)	15	15	15	5	5
Biotin (μg)	60	60	60	20	20
Folic acid (μg)	600	600	600	140	140
B_{12} (μg)	5	5	5	1	1

Vitamin A

Vitamin A (retinol) is necessary for vision, bone growth, immune function, and differentiation of epithelial and nerve tissues [1]. It can also reverse the negative effects of corticosteroids on wound healing [11]. Clinical signs of vitamin A deficiency, such as night blindness, are listed in Table 12.2. Dietary vitamin A is consumed in the form of retinol or provitamin A (carotenoids, mainly β-carotene). When consumed as part of the diet, vitamin A is liberated from food by pancreatic and digestive enzymes, incorporated into micelles, and then absorbed by enterocytes. After absorption and incorporation into chylomicrons, vitamin A is transported through the lymphatics to the liver, where it is transferred to retinol binding protein (RBP) and transthyretin. Protein-bound retinol is transported to target tissues, and any excess is stored in the liver (main site), adipose tissue, eyes, lungs, and kidneys [1].

RBP is synthesized in the liver in response to retinol absorption and therefore provides a good indication of vitamin A bioavailability. Protein malnutrition, zinc deficiency, hepatic failure, or inflammation can reduce hepatic production of transport proteins and limit bioavailability of vitamin A [12]. Serum and plasma levels of retinol remain near normal until body stores are depleted. It is recommended to check retinol levels after resolution of acute illness or protein malnutrition as low plasma retinol levels may be factitious and related to decreased transport protein levels versus a sign of true vitamin deficiency [13]. Measurement of inflammatory markers such as C-reactive protein (CRP) and retinol at the same time can help decipher true deficiency versus inflammatory suppression of transport proteins. Because RBP and transthyretin are excreted by the kidneys, patients with decreased renal clearance are at risk of hypervitaminosis A and potential toxicity. Patients with hepatic failure cannot mobilize vitamin A stores as a result of decreased synthesis of RBP, and therefore, serum levels may be low when stores are plentiful.

The recommended dietary intake (RDI) for vitamin A can be found in Table 12.3 [14]. Vitamin A is found primarily in animal foods high in fat, such as liver, cheese, butter, and high-fat fish. Plant-based carotenoids are found in red, orange, green, and yellow plant pigments and are converted into active forms of vitamin A shortly after absorption. Patients with SBS often have difficulty absorbing sufficient amounts of vitamin A and carotenoids due to fat malabsorption and dietary restriction of fat and many plant-based foods [6]. However, absorption is improved if vitamin A or carotenoids are taken with foods that contain a small amount of fat. Daily supplementation in excess of the RDI may

TABLE 12.2
Clinical Findings of Vitamin Deficiency and Toxicity

	Deficiency	Toxicity
Vitamin A	• Night blindness • Vision loss • Xerophthalmia • Bitot's spots • Follicular hyperkeratosis • Scaling skin • Growth retardation (children)	Acute • Seizures • Drowsiness • Nausea • Vomiting • Diplopia Chronic • Alopecia • Dry skin, desquamation • Skeletal pain and bone fractures • Increased intracranial pressure-nausea, vomiting, headache
Vitamin D	• Secondary hyperparathyroidism • Metabolic bone disease—osteopenia, osteoporosis, osteomalacia, rickets (children)	• Hypercalcemia
Vitamin E	• Ataxia • Peripheral neuropathy • Skeletal myopathy • Visual changes • Increase platelet aggregation • Hemolytic anemia • Bronchopulmonary dysplasia (premature infants)	• Hemorrhage
Vitamin K	• Increased bleeding time—elevated PT or INR • Ecchymosis • Hemorrhage	Not reported
Vitamin B_{12}	• Macrocytic anemia, leukopenia, thrombocytopenia • Peripheral neuropathy, autonomic neuropathy • Cognitive decline, reduced vibratory sense, personality and mood changes, delirium • Anorexia and weight loss • Malabsorption • Glossitis	Not reported
Folate	• Megaloblastic anemia, leukopenia, thrombocytopenia • Glossitis, stomatitis	Not reported

be needed to maintain normal retinol levels [15]. Table 12.3 also lists vitamin A supplementation guidelines, including maintenance doses for those with SBS.

High-dose vitamin A supplementation can pose harm to patients if given in one excessively high dose (300,000 IU in children or 660,000 IU in adults) or in moderately high daily doses (as low as 1500 IU/kg/d in children or 25,000 IU to 50,000 IU/d in adults) over several months [15,16].

Vitamin D

Vitamin D is best known for its effect on calcium absorption and bone mineralization (see Chapter 8), although vitamin D receptors have also been identified on nonskeletal cells throughout the body. This discovery has led to the understanding that vitamin D also modulates immunity, autoimmune diseases, glucose metabolism, cardiovascular diseases, and musculoskeletal function [2,17]. There

TABLE 12.3
Vitamin Reference Ranges and Dosing Recommendations for Patients with SBS

	Reference Ranges	RDI Upper Limit (UL)	Repletion and Maintenance Dosing Recommendations	Clinical Considerations
Vitamin A	Serum retinol (µg/dL) Deficiency, <10.0 Normal levels: 0–6 years, 11.3–64.7 7–12 years, 12.8–81.2 13–17 years, 14.4–97.7 ≥18 years, 32.5–78.0 Excess, >120.0	Retinol activity equivalents (RAE)[a] (µg/d) 0–3 years, 600 4–8 years, 900 9–13 years, 1700 14–18 years, 2800 ≥19 years, 3000 Pregnancy ≤18 years, 2800 ≥19 years, 3000	Vitamin A *Repletion* (oral or IM injection) Infants, 7500–15,000 IU/d × 10 d, then 5000–10,000 IU oral × 2 months 1–8 years, 17,500–35,000 IU/d × 10 d, then 5000–10,000 IU oral × 2 months Adults (>8 years) 100,000 IU/d × 3 d, then 50,000 IU/d × 14 d, then 10,000–20,000 IU/d × 2 months *Maintenance* (oral) Infants, 600–2000 IU/d 1–8 years, 2000–3000 IU/d Adults (>8 years), 5000–10,000 IU/d	• Serum levels decrease in malnutrition, hepatic failure, zinc deficiency, acute illness, and inflammation. Check CRP if question of inflammation. • Close monitoring in patients with cholestasis and renal insufficiency. • Teratogenic risk with supplementation during pregnancy, do not supplement >RDI.
Vitamin D	25(OH)D (ng/mL) Severe deficiency, <10 Mild deficiency, 10–19 Optimum, 20–50 Excess, >80	Vitamin D (IU/d) ≤1 year, 1000 >1 year, 2000	Vitamin D_2 or D_3 (oral) *Repletion* <1 year, 2000 IU/d >1 year, 6000–10,000 IU/d *Maintenance* <1 year, 200–1000 IU/d >1 year, 3000–6000 IU/d *Traditional adult therapy* 50,000 IU/1–7 × per week	• Cholecalciferol (D_3) is recommended over ergocalciferol (D_2). • Daily supplementation will be needed. • Monitor for hypercalcemia. • Avoid large doses with hyperphosphatemia to prevent soft tissue calcification. • Monitor levels closely in patients with renal impairment. • Unreliable results when measured during inflammation; check CRP. • Consider oral calcium supplements in conjunction with D. • Liquid form may improve absorption in those difficult to replete.

(*Continued*)

TABLE 12.3 (CONTINUED)
Vitamin Reference Ranges and Dosing Recommendations for Patients with SBS

	Reference Ranges	RDI Upper Limit (UL)	Repletion and Maintenance Dosing Recommendations	Clinical Considerations
Vitamin E	α-Tocopherol (mg/L) Deficiency Neonates, <2.0 >3 months, <3.0 Normal 0–17 years, 3.8–18.4 ≥18 years, 5.5–17.0 Excess, >40	α-Tocopherol (mg/d) <1 year, ND 1–3 years, 200 4–8 years, 300 9–13 years, 600 14–18 years, 800 ≥19 years, 1000	Vitamin E (oral) *Repletion/maintenance* <1 year, 40–50 IU/d 1–3 years, 80–150 IU/d 4–8 years, 100–200 IU/d >8 years, 200–400 IU/d	• Avoid supplementation in neonates due to risk of necrotizing enterocolitis. • Elevated levels with mild to moderate inflammation; check CRP. • High doses can induce vitamin K deficiency and increase risk of hemorrhage. • Higher doses of supplements may be needed in patients receiving omega-6 IV fat emulsions. • Calculate ratio of α-tocopherol/(TChol + TG) if lipid levels are low.
Vitamin K	PT, 9.5–13.8 seconds INR, 0.8–1.2 Phylloquinone (ng/mL), ≥18 years, 0.10–2.20 PIVKA-II (ng/mL), <7.5	RDA (μg/d) (no determined UL) 0–6 months, 2 7–12 months, 2.5 1–3 years, 30 4–8 years, 55 9–13 years, 60 14–18 years, 75 Males ≥19 years, 120 Females ≥19 years, 90	Phytonadione *Repletion* INR > 10, then 2.5–10 mg IM injection *Maintenance* Oral—per RDAs	• Caution with repletion in patients on warfarin therapy.

(Continued)

TABLE 12.3 (CONTINUED)
Vitamin Reference Ranges and Dosing Recommendations for Patients with SBS

	Reference Ranges	RDI Upper Limit (UL)	Repletion and Maintenance Dosing Recommendations	Clinical Considerations
Vitamin B_{12}	Vitamin B_{12} (ng/L) Deficiency, <150 Indeterminate, 150–400 Sufficient, >400 MMA (nmol/mL) Normal, ≤4 B_{12} deficiency, >4	Cobalamin RDA (μg/d) (no determined UL) 0–6 months, 0.4 7–12 months, 0.5 1–3 years, 0.9 4–8 years, 1.2 9–13 years, 1.8 ≥14 years, 2.4	Cyanocobalamin *Repletion* (oral or SQ injection) Children—100 μg/d × 10–14 d, then 100 μg/wk × 3 months Adults—1 mg/d × 7, then 1 mg/wk × 4 wk *Maintenance* Children—oral or SQ injection 100 μg/month Adults—oral 1–2 mg/d or SQ injection 1 mg/month	• Blood levels can remain normal when tissue stores are depleted. • Monitor MMA levels with repletion especially in patients with small bowel bacterial overgrowth. • SBS patients with >50–60 cm terminal ileum resection will require lifelong supplementation.
Folate	Folate (μg/L): Deficiency, <4 Normal, >4 Red cell folate (ng/mL): Normal, 150–450 Homocysteine (μmol/L): Normal, ≤13	Folate (μg/d) ≤1 year, ND 1–3 years, 300 4–8 years, 400 9–13 years, 600 14–18 years, 800 ≥19 years, 1000	Folate *Repletion* (oral, injection, IV) Infant, 0.1 mg/d <4 years, 0.3 mg/d >4 years, 0.8 mg/d *Maintenance* Per UL guidelines	• Check B_{12} level, homocysteine, and MMA levels prior to supplementing folic acid. • Serum folate reflects recent dietary intake, whereas red cell folate reflects long-term folate availability.

Source: Dietary Reference Intakes: Vitamins. Institute of Medicine Website. http://www.iom.edu/~/media/Files/Activity%20Files/Nutrition/DRIs/DRI_Vitamins.pdf. Published 1998; Lacy, C.F. et al., *Drug Information Handbook: A Comprehensive Resource for All Clinicians and Healthcare Professionals*, 21st ed., Lexi-Comp, Hudson, OH, 2012; Mayo Clinic, Mayo Medical Laboratories, *Interpretive Handbook*, http://www.mayomedicallaboratories.com/interpretive-guide/index.html. Published 1995.

Note: IM, intramuscular; ND, not determined; SQ, subcutaneous.

[a] Conversion: 1 RAE = 1 μg retinol, 1 μg retinol = 3.33 IU.

are two forms of vitamin D, vitamin D_3 (cholecalciferol) and vitamin D_2 (ergocalciferol) [18,19]. Both forms of vitamin D require double hydroxylation for activation; first, 25-hydroxyvitamin D [25(OH)D] is formed in the liver and then the kidney produces the active form 1,25-dihydroxyvitamin D (calcitriol). As such, hepatic and renal dysfunction can prevent conversion of D_2 and D_3 into active calcitriol. 25(OH)D is the primary form of vitamin D and is found circulating, bound to vitamin D transport protein as well as in adipose tissue, the main storage site for vitamin D. Calcitriol is produced as needed to maintain normal serum calcium and phosphate balance by hormonal regulation of the intestine, kidney, and parathyroid. It also regulates cellular differentiation and antiproliferation of nonskeletal cells [18].

Vitamin D deficiency is prevalent in the general population, but particularly in patients with malabsorption, including SBS, and those with inadequate oral intake or limited sun exposure. Table 12.2 describes clinical consequences related to vitamin D deficiency. Physical symptoms of severe vitamin D deficiency include bone pain, myalgias, weakness, and falls. The effects of vitamin D deficiency on nonskeletal tissue is unknown but may impair immunity and glucose control and increase risk of certain types of cancers, including breast, colon, and prostate [20,21].

Serum 25(OH)D level is the best indicator of vitamin D status, although controversy exists over the optimum level for disease prevention. The Institute of Medicine cites serum levels of 25(OH)D >20 ng/mL to be sufficient to prevent secondary hyperparathyroidism and metabolic bone disease [22]. Other experts consider the optimal range to be 30–80 ng/mL [20,23]. Patients with malabsorption related to SBS may be unable to attain 25(OH)D levels >30 ng/mL; a more realistic goal for these patients may be 20–30 ng/mL. Of note, there is evidence that 25(OH)D levels may be affected by acute inflammation [24]; however, the clinical importance of this finding remains unclear. Indirect measures of vitamin D status include serum levels of alkaline phosphatase and parathyroid hormone, 24-hour urine calcium excretion, and bone mineral density scan (dual-energy x-ray absorptiometry). Laboratory findings suggestive of vitamin D deficiency include normal or elevated alkaline phosphatase, elevated parathyroid hormone, and low 24-hour urine calcium excretion. Serum calcium and phosphate levels will remain normal until bone demineralization is severe.

Endogenous synthesis of vitamin D_3 by exposure of the arms and legs (without sunscreen) to ultraviolet (UV) B light, from the sun or a UV lamp, for 5 to 30 minutes can produce about 3000 IU vitamin D_3 [25,26]. However, for patients living in latitudes above the 35th parallel, cutaneous exposure to UVB irradiation is often insufficient for maintenance of optimal 25(OH)D levels. Food sources of vitamin D_3 are fatty fish and eggs. Vitamin D_2, derived from plants, is used to enrich foods such as milk, yogurt, cereals, and orange juice [21]. The RDI for vitamin D can be found in Table 12.3. As SBS patients are often deficient in vitamin D, doses higher than traditional dosing are common and most often needed for life. Given unreliable absorption on any given day, relying on a single 50,000 IU dose weekly may be risky. Daily dosing, divided in some, increases the chances of normalizing serum levels, depending upon the health and length of the remnant bowel and the degree of fat malabsorption [20,27]. Use of liquid forms may improve absorption. Both forms of vitamin D are available as oral supplements, although comparisons of cholecalciferol (vitamin D_3) and ergocalciferol (vitamin D_2) on 25(OH)D concentrations have shown vitamin D_3 to be more effective with respect to producing more rapid elevation in 25(OH)D levels [19,28,29]. Hypervitaminosis D is possible, although unlikely, in those with SBS.

Vitamin E

Vitamin E refers to a group of four tocopherols, with α-tocopherol as the most biologically active component. α-Tocopherol is a potent antioxidant that protects against oxidation of the polyunsaturated fatty acid (PUFA) component of cell membranes. During periods of oxidative stress, vitamin E donates hydrogen atoms to lipid peroxide free radicals to form a stable lipid hydroperoxide molecule [30,31]. The vitamin E radical is then reduced back to vitamin E by receiving a hydrogen atom from vitamin C [31,32]. Like the other fat-soluble vitamins, α-tocopherol is most efficiently absorbed when taken with fatty foods, as it requires bile salts for micelle formation and passage into enterocytes. Once absorbed, it is incorporated into chylomicrons and transported through the body in chylomicrons and phospholipids rather than on specific transport proteins [32]. Vitamin E is found in all cell membranes with the main storage site being adipose tissue, but it is also stored in liver and muscle tissues.

The process of recycling α-tocopherol helps to maintain adequate cellular levels despite limited absorption of the nutrient (<50% of oral intake is absorbed) [32]. However, in SBS patients, chronic fat malabsorption and PN infusions with IV PUFA lipid emulsion are risk factors associated with vitamin E deficiency [6,33,34]. Clinical signs of vitamin E deficiency are listed in Table 12.2 [12,35,36]. Populations at highest risk of developing clinically significant vitamin E deficiency are premature infants, those with steatorrhea, and patients with oxidative stress from injury or illness. Vitamin E toxicity is rare, although case reports in humans and studies in animal models have linked high-dose vitamin E with coagulopathy, hepatic failure, and neutrophil dysfunction [12,35].

Fasting plasma and serum levels of α-tocopherol reflect body stores of vitamin E. Table 12.3 describes age-based reference ranges [37]. Unlike vitamins A and D, mild to moderate inflammation increases vitamin E concentrations, while severe inflammation (i.e., CRP >80 mg/L) decreases vitamin E levels [13]. This is thought to occur because vitamin E is transported on lipoproteins, which are elevated during acute illness and inflammation rather than acute phase reactant proteins that are inversely related to inflammation. Reduced vitamin E concentrations are also seen when total circulating lipids are low. In this case, a ratio of α-tocopherol to total cholesterol can be useful to assess for deficiency; a ratio of >0.8 mg α-tocopherol/(cholesterol + triglyceride) suggests adequate vitamin E concentrations [12,32].

Vitamin E is found in foods with plant-based oils, including vegetable oils, margarines, and salad dressings, and foods that contain whole grains, nuts, seeds, and legumes. See Table 12.3 for vitamin E RDIs. Patients with SBS who receive PN with soybean-based IV fat emulsion and standard parenteral MVI dosing are at risk for developing vitamin E deficiency because the predominance of ω-6 fatty acids in the soybean oil increases lipid peroxidation rates, which can deplete serum vitamin E concentrations [38]. Therefore, PN-dependent patients require careful monitoring of serum α-tocopherol levels, and oral supplementation of vitamins E (and C to reduce vitamin E radicals back to the active form of vitamin E) may be needed. Table 12.3 also lists vitamin E repletion doses for all ages. Daily doses greater than 400 IU increase the risk of hemorrhage, particularly in patients receiving concomitant anticoagulation therapy.

Vitamin K

Vitamin K is a group of compounds that participate in the serum clotting cascade by activating factors II (prothrombin), VII, IX, and X as well as proteins S and C. Vitamin K also activates osteocalcin to regulate bone remodeling and mineralization. Phylloquinone (K_1 from plants) and menaquinones (K_2 from bacteria) are the biologically active forms of vitamin K. As is the case with other fat-soluble vitamins, dietary fat and bile acids facilitate absorption of vitamin K. Phylloquinone and menaquinones are transported to target tissues on lipoproteins and chylomicrons. Phylloquinone derived from the diet has a relatively small body pool and high turnover rate, whereas menaquinones from enteric bacteria are stored in the liver and have a longer half-life to maintain normal clotting function during periods of fasting or low dietary intake [39].

Vitamin K deficiency is rare in the general population, with the exception of infants who are born deficient. Patients with SBS are at risk of developing vitamin K deficiency, although it is less common than other fat-soluble vitamin deficiencies [40]. Vitamin K deficiency is often seen in SBS patients with severe malnutrition not taking daily MVI supplements or adhering to strict diet and medication regimes. Vitamin K deficiency may develop due to low dietary intake of foods high in vitamin K, poor absorption, and use of antibiotics to treat small intestinal bacterial overgrowth. Table 12.2 lists the hallmark signs of vitamin K deficiency. Clinical signs of vitamin K deficiency often develop with the start of antibiotic therapy in patients with marginal stores. Fasting serum phylloquinone levels reflect true circulating vitamin K and can be used to measure depletion and repletion, but not stored vitamin K [41,42]. Prothrombin time (PT) and international normalized ratio (INR) are, however, more commonly used to monitor vitamin K functional status rather than to measure vitamin K levels. Clinically significant vitamin K deficiency can lead to life-threatening hemorrhage and requires urgent repletion; the response to vitamin K repletion can be gauged by INR or PT levels. If long-term repletion of vitamin K is necessary, then serum phylloquinone and PIVKA-II (proteins induced by vitamin K absence; an assay used to measure inactive vitamin K-dependent clotting factors more sensitive than PT or INR) levels can be monitored over time [41].

Dietary phylloquinones are present in green vegetables, plant-based oils, and nutritional supplements. Bacteria in the intestine produce menaquinones, which can supply as much as 50% of the vitamin K requirement; the contribution may be higher in patients taking gastric acid suppression medications and those without colon-in-continuity or with bowel stasis [43,44]. Patients taking antibiotics for small intestinal bacterial overgrowth or those with rapid intestinal transit times will also produce less bacteria-derived vitamin K. If deficiency develops, SBS patients may require oral and/or parenteral supplementation. Most IV MVI preparations and many oral MVI preparations on the market contain a small amount of vitamin K. IV lipid emulsions also contain vitamin K—up to 300 μg phylloquinone/100 g soybean emulsion (e.g., Intralipid, Liposyn III, and Nutrilipid) [41]. Table 12.3 describes specific, age-based recommendations for vitamin K intake.

Vitamin K toxicity is unreported. The major concern with respect to vitamin K supplementation is for patients receiving warfarin anticoagulation therapy. Warfarin is a vitamin K antagonist that inhibits vitamin K activation of the clotting factors to prevent thrombosis. The effectiveness of warfarin can be altered by vitamin K intake and absorption as well as genetic factors that affect metabolism [37]. Stable warfarin dosing is accomplished with steady vitamin K intake. Patients with SBS receiving warfarin require stable daily dosing of vitamin K from an oral MVI or daily infusion of MVI and lipid emulsion. If a patient on warfarin infuses PN less frequently than daily or pharmaceutical supply shortages prohibit use of daily MVI additives, then MVI supplementation should be taken by the oral route only to avoid wide fluctuations in serum vitamin K levels. Our experience is that 150 μg phytonadione in some adult MVIs is enough to inhibit the anticoagulation effects of warfarin; thus, periodic monitoring of PT/INR is warranted when patients receive both MVI and warfarin therapies. Alternatively, MVI-12 is vitamin K-free and can be added to PN so as not to influence the patient's vitamin K status and warfarin dosing.

WATER-SOLUBLE VITAMINS

The water-soluble vitamin family is composed of the B vitamins and vitamin C. These vitamins dissolve in aqueous solutions and are easily absorbed throughout the small intestine by passive diffusion or sodium-dependent transport mechanisms. Absorption of water-soluble vitamins remains adequate as long as the remnant jejunum or ileum is healthy. In cases of near total enterectomy, where only the duodenum remains, or if the remaining small bowel is diseased, then SBS patients are at risk of developing water-soluble vitamin deficiencies. Rapid intestinal transit or altered dietary composition may necessitate water-soluble vitamin supplementation in doses >100% of the RDI. Also, utilization of chewable, gel cap, or liquid preparations may improve nutrient absorption. In most SBS cases, oral or parenteral MVI supplementation will meet or exceed water-soluble vitamin requirements. The exception is vitamin B_{12}, which is absorbed primarily in the ileum and must be supplemented if the distal ileum is resected, bypassed, or diseased (e.g., Crohn's disease).

VITAMIN B_{12}

Vitamin B_{12} (cyanocobalamin, cobalamin, B_{12}) is needed for normal hematopoiesis, maintenance of gut epithelium, and neurological functions. It also serves as a coenzyme required for metabolic reactions, such as synthesis of DNA nucleotides, methyl group transfers as in the case of the folate-dependent conversion of homocysteine to methionine, and the conversion of methymalonyl coenzyme A (CoA) to succinyl CoA to produce methylmalonic acid (MMA) [35,45]. Absorption of food-bound B_{12} is complex, requiring multiple steps. First, hydrochloric acid and gastric pepsin release the vitamin from food in the stomach, where it binds to R-protein (known as haptocorrin or transcobalamin I). In the small intestine, pancreatic enzymes release the B_{12} from R-protein. Then, free B_{12} binds with intrinsic factor (IF) in the duodenum and the B_{12}–IF complex travels to the ileum, where it binds to the IF receptor cubilin and B_{12} is absorbed by active transport. The highest B_{12} binding affinity is in the distal 60 cm of the ileum. IF-mediated absorption of B_{12} is efficient; up to 75% of ingested B_{12} is absorbed, but it is limited by IF saturation and the viability or continuity of the distal ileum [44]. Additionally, synthetic B_{12} is absorbed by passive diffusion throughout the GI tract, although this pathway is much less efficient compared with the IF-mediated pathway. SBS patients unable to absorb B_{12} via the IF-mediated pathway may be able to maintain normal B_{12} levels by ingestion of B_{12} in doses of 1000–2000 μg daily.

Once B_{12} is absorbed, it is transported on transcobalamin II transport protein in the portal circulation to the liver and target tissues. B_{12} is excreted in the bile and conserved through enterohepatic circulation; thus, whole-body turnover of B_{12} is minimal. Under normal conditions, hepatic stores allow for several years (about 3 years) of poor absorption before adults develop clinical signs of deficiency.

B_{12} deficiency in patients with SBS is assumed to be related to malabsorption of dietary B_{12} rather than inadequate dietary intake or pernicious anemia (i.e., antibodies against parietal cells and/or IF). In the setting of SBS, the risk of developing B_{12} deficiency increases when the distal ileum is resected, bypassed, or diseased. In addition, gastric acid suppression limits B_{12} release from food, and enteric bacteria compete for uptake of unbound B_{12} in the gut [46]. B_{12} deficiency can affect the nervous system, hematopoietic processes, and the gastrointestinal tract, as listed in Table 12.2 [45]. Neurological symptoms can be irreversible if the deficiency is not identified and treated quickly.

Assessment of B_{12} status may require several assays and differentiation in patients with SBS as serum B_{12} levels are highly variable and can yield false-negative results [47,48]. In fact, serum B_{12} levels remain normal at the expense of tissue depletion. Since B_{12} and folate are connected metabolically and clinically, assessment of both vitamin levels along with intermediate metabolites of B_{12} and folate can help identify the source of deficiency and properly direct repletion therapy. B_{12} is required for the conversions of homocysteine to methionine and methymalonyl–CoA to succinyl–CoA, but folate participates only in the conversion of homocysteine to methionine. If B_{12} is deficient, then both homocysteine and MMA are caught in their respective metabolic pathways and levels increase, but if folate is deficient, only homocysteine levels rise. If the B_{12} is <150 ng/L, then deficiency exists and therapeutic repletion is indicated. However, if the serum B_{12} is in the range of 150 ng/L to 400 ng/L, then the patient may have subclinical deficiency [49]. In this situation, an MMA level is needed to identify a deficiency state; if the MMA level is >0.4 nmol/mL, then B_{12} deficiency is confirmed [37].

Dietary sources of B_{12} are animal products or plant foods contaminated with microorganism-derived cobalamin. Vegans and babies born to, or receiving breast milk from, vegan mothers are at high risk of B_{12} deficiency and require daily supplementation. After surgical resection of the terminal ileum, patients will require lifelong pharmacologic supplementation of B_{12}. High-dose oral or subcutaneous injection, which is reported to be less painful than intramuscular injection, is effective at maintaining normal serum levels in this setting [8,31,50–52]. Patients with gastrectomy or gastrojejunostomy or those patients taking potent gastric acid suppression medications require routine monitoring of B_{12} levels and, possibly, supplementation. Table 12.3 lists recommended intake of cobalamin for repletion and maintenance. Toxicity from B_{12} is unreported, although serum levels can be elevated during periods of inflammation, liver disease, and after B_{12} injections [53].

Folic Acid

Folic acid (folate) functions as a coenzyme in DNA and amino acid metabolism. It participates in many metabolic pathways by contributing single carbon units [51]. Folate is required for normal hematopoietic and neurologic function. It is absorbed in the jejunum by a proton-coupled folate transporter. Zinc deficiency, alcohol consumption, and intestinal lumen pH >6 can limit folate absorption [12,51]. Patients with bypass or resection of the proximal jejunum are at risk of developing folate deficiency. Megaloblastic anemia is the main clinical manifestation of folate deficiency. It is rare in patients with SBS because dietary folate, found in enriched grain products, fruits, and vegetables, is easily absorbed in the proximal bowel and folate production by enteric bacteria is readily absorbed by the host.

The greatest issue regarding folate for SBS patients relates to B_{12} monitoring (discussed in detail previously). Serum folate levels typically reflect dietary intake of folate: normal folate concentration, ≥4 ng/mL, and deficient folate concentration, <2 ng/mL. Equivocal serum folate concentrations (2–4 ng/mL) can be evaluated with red blood cell folate, which is a better indicator of folate status over time, or assays of intermediate metabolites, such as homocysteine and MMA, to assess for true folate deficiency versus B_{12} deficiency [54]. Frequently, patients with SBS have high serum and red cell folate related to enrichment of folic acid in the U.S. food supply, use of MVI supplements, and enteric bacterial production. Although neither specific nor diagnostic, high folate levels are considered by some to be a sign of small intestinal bacterial overgrowth. Importantly, high doses of folic acid can mask B_{12} deficiency and worsen the neurological symptoms related to that deficiency, but actual folate toxicity is unreported. Table 12.3 provides dosing guidelines for folic acid repletion therapy in the rare case of deficiency.

ASSESSMENT AND MONITORING GUIDELINES

Assessment for Vitamin Deficiencies

Physical assessment for signs of vitamin deficiencies is an important part of every clinic visit for SBS patients. A head-to-toe inspection of the hair, eyes, mouth, skin, strength, and mental acuity will provide clues to the presence of clinical deficiencies and help determine whether or not measurement of vitamin levels is warranted (see Chapter 9). Patients with SBS who are nonadherent to prescribed vitamin supplements or are lost to follow-up by nutrition clinicians are at risk of developing multiple vitamin deficiencies. Deficiencies can also develop in PN-dependent patients during times of parenteral vitamin shortages [55,56], an all too common problem in recent years. Table 12.4 is a guide to key physical findings associated with the most common vitamin deficiencies found in SBS patients.

Each clinic visit should include a review and reconciliation of the vitamin supplementation profile to ensure correct dosing and patient adherence with prescribed supplements. Over time, patients can become complacent about, or resistant to taking, multiple medications to manage their SBS and perceive vitamins as optional supplements rather than essential nutrients. Other patients might not understand that vitamin supplementation is an integral part of the lifelong management of SBS and might not ask for prescription renewals. Ongoing patient education will help to minimize nonadherence to vitamin supplementation regimens. If a patient has developed physical signs of a vitamin deficiency or has stopped taking prescribed vitamin supplements, then (re)measurement of baseline vitamin levels prior to initiation of therapy is recommended. If inflammation is suspected from an underlying disease state or acute illness, then the addition of inflammatory markers (e.g., CRP) to the vitamin panel can help with interpretation of abnormal results. See Table 12.3 for clinical considerations related to dosing and monitoring vitamin levels in SBS.

TABLE 12.4
Signs of Vitamin Deficiency and Toxicity on Physical Examination

Area of Assessment	Physical Findings and Potential Vitamin Deficiency
Hair	• Alopecia—vitamin A toxicity or biotin deficiency • Corkscrew—vitamin C deficiency
Eyes	• Night blindness—vitamin A deficiency • Bitot's spots—vitamin A deficiency • Xerophthalmia—vitamin A deficiency • Ophthalmoplegia—thiamine deficiency
Mouth	• Cheilosis/angular stomatitis—riboflavin, niacin, and/or pyridoxine deficiency • Glossitis—riboflavin, niacin, pyridoxine, biotin, folate, and/or vitamin B_{12} deficiency • Bleeding gums—vitamin C or vitamin K deficiency
Skin	• Petechiae—vitamin C • Purpura, ecchymosis—vitamin C and/or vitamin K deficiency or vitamin E toxicity • Follicular hyperkeratosis—vitamins A and/or C deficiency • Seborrheic dermatitis—riboflavin, pyridoxine, and/or biotin deficiency • Scaling—vitamin A deficiency or toxicity • Desquamation of sun-exposed skin—niacin deficiency
Musculoskeletal	• Weakness and myalgia—vitamin D, vitamin E, thiamine, pyridoxine, and/or vitamin B_{12} deficiency; vitamin A toxicity • Tetany—vitamin D deficiency • Bone fractures—vitamin D deficiency
Nervous system	• Ataxia—vitamin E deficiency • Peripheral neuropathy—vitamins E or B_{12} deficiency • Depression—biotin deficiency • Dementia—niacin and/or vitamin B_{12} deficiency • Wernicke-Korsakoff syndrome—thiamine deficiency

Patients with SBS who present with severe malnutrition will likely have multiple vitamin deficiencies. It is important to obtain baseline vitamin levels before initiation of vitamin supplementation regimens. It is possible that some vitamin assays will not provide reliable results when transport proteins are depleted; in this case, vitamin repletion regimens should be based on physical findings suggestive of deficiencies, biochemical indices if judged reliable under the circumstance, and clinical gestalt. Initiation of multivitamins with 100% of the RDI, plus moderate repletion doses of vitamins thought to be deficient based on physical exam or laboratory assays, is a conservative and reasonable approach for several weeks to 1 month. Short-term, moderate supplementation regimens are unlikely to cause toxicity in most SBS patients. Once a patient's nutritional parameters improve, a reassessment of vitamin levels will help to develop a maintenance regimen. Exceptions to this rule are infants and pregnant patients, for whom vitamin repletion must be directed by biological measures of vitamin concentrations.

Monitoring Vitamin Levels

Current expert consensus and guidelines from the American Society for Parenteral and Enteral Nutrition support monitoring vitamin levels in patients with SBS. Specifically, measurement of baseline levels of the key vitamins (A, D, E, and B_{12}) with reassessment every 3 to 12 months depending on the presence of deficiency is recommended [31,51,57–59]. Infants and children who rely on adequate vitamin levels for growth and development require frequent monitoring every 3 to 6 months, whereas adults with stable bowel function and supplementation regimens require less frequent monitoring every (6 to 12 months) [57–59]. During periods of repletion with high-dose vitamin supplementation for deficiencies, frequent monitoring of serum levels every 4–8 weeks is appropriate until optimal levels are achieved. Thereafter, it is safe to monitor vitamin levels at intervals of 3 to 12 months. It is important to remember that patients with SBS can be dynamic and may require frequent adjustments and modification in their vitamin supplementation regimens. This is especially true in the first several years after bowel resection as the remnant bowel undergoes adaptation and/or PN supplementation is transitioned to exclusively enteral or oral support.

Monitoring vitamin levels in SBS patients with a concurrent active inflammatory process such as Crohn's disease is challenging due to ongoing inflammation that distorts the results of some vitamin assays [13]. It is helpful if prior vitamin levels, measured during times of quiescent disease, are available to determine if the patient has difficulty absorbing certain vitamins that should be replaced or supplemented in doses greater than 100% of the RDI. Close observation for clinical signs of vitamin deficiencies or toxicities, coupled with use of a daily MVI and additional dosing of specific vitamins found to be deficient, is a safe and efficacious approach to supplementation in this population.

CONCLUSION

Each patient with SBS provides a unique set of challenges for clinicians charged with optimizing their health. The site and length of bowel resected, intestinal transit time, residual bowel disease, diet, pharmacotherapies, psychosocial situations, and growth and aging all influence vitamin supplementation requirements. Keen attention to vitamin status will improve the health and well-being of patients with SBS and provide great satisfaction to the nutrition clinicians charged with their care.

REFERENCES

1. Ross AC. Vitamin A. In: *Modern Nutrition in Health and Disease.* 11th ed. Eds, Ross AC, Caballero B, Cousins RJ, Tucker KL, Ziegler TR. Baltimore, MD: Lippincott Williams & Wilkins, 2014, pp. 260–277.
2. Reichrath J et al. Vitamins as hormones. *Horm Metab Res.* 2007;39:71–84.
3. Fex GA et al. Serum concentrations of all-trans and 13-cis retinoic acid and retinol are closely correlated. *J Nutr Biochem.* 1996;7(3):162–165.
4. Hofmann AF et al. Cholestyramine and ileal resection. *N Engl J Med.* 1969;281:397–402.
5. Compston JE et al. Oral 25-hydroxyvitamin D_3 in treatment of osteomalacia associated with ileal resection and cholestyramine. *Gastroenterology.* 1978;74:900–902.
6. Luo M et al. Prospective analysis of serum carotenoids, vitamin A, and tocopherols in adults with short bowel syndrome undergoing intestinal rehabilitation. *Nutrition.* 2009;25:400–407.
7. Buchman AL et al. AGA technical review on short bowel syndrome and intestinal transplantation. *Gastroenterology.* 2003;124:1111–1134.
8. Matarese LE. Nutrition and fluid optimization for patients with short bowel syndrome. *JPEN J Parenter Enteral Nutr.* 2013;37(2):161–170.
9. Sundaram A et al. Nutritional management of short bowel syndrome in adults. *J Clin Gastroenterol.* 2002;34(3):207–220.
10. Howard L et al. Reversible neurological symptoms caused by vitamin E deficiency in a patient with short bowel syndrome. *Am J Clin Nutr.* 1982;36:1243–1249.
11. Hunt TK et al. Effect of vitamin A on reversing the inhibitory effect of cortisone on healing of open wounds in animals and man. *Ann Surg.* 1969;170(4):633–641.
12. Clark SF. Vitamins and trace minerals. In: *A.S.P.E.N. Adult Nutrition Support Core Curriculum.* 2nd ed. Eds, Mueller CM, Kovacevich DS, McClave SA, Miller SJ, Schwartz DB. Silver Spring, MD: American Society of Parenteral and Enteral Nutrition, 2012, pp. 121–151.
13. Duncan A et al. Quantitative data on the magnitude of the systemic inflammatory response and its effect on micronutrient status based on plasma measurements. *Am J Clin Nutr.* 2012;95:64–71.
14. Dietary Reference Intakes: Vitamins. Institute of Medicine Website. http://www.iom.edu/~/media/Files/Activity%20Files/Nutrition/DRIs/DRI_Vitamins.pdf. Published 1998. Updated 2011. Accessed February 12, 2015.

15. Lacy CF et al. *Drug Information Handbook: A Comprehensive Resource for All Clinicians and Healthcare Professionals.* 21st ed. Hudson, OH: Lexi-Comp, 2012.
16. Hathcock JN et al. Evaluation of vitamin A toxicity. *Am J Clin Nutr.* 1990;52:183–202.
17. Pittas AG et al. Role of vitamin D in adults requiring nutrition support. *JPEN J Parenter Enteral Nutr.* 2010;34:70–78.
18. Jones G. Vitamin D. In: *Modern Nutrition in Health and Disease.* 11th ed. Eds, Ross AC, Caballero B, Cousins RJ, Tucker KL, Ziegler TR. Baltimore, MD: Lippincott Williams & Wilkins, 2014, pp. 278–292.
19. Tripkovic L et al. Comparison of vitamin D_2 and vitamin D_3 supplementation in raising serum 25-hydroxyvitamin D status: A systematic review and meta-analysis. *Am J Clin Nutr.* 2012;95:1357–1364.
20. Kennel KA et al. Vitamin D deficiency in adults: When to test and how to treat. *Mayo Clin Proc.* 2010;85(8):752–758.
21. Bikle DD. Vitamin D metabolism, mechanism of action, and clinical applications. *Chem Biol.* 2014;21:319–329.
22. Institute of Medicine. Food and Nutrition Board. *Dietary Reference Intakes for Calcium and Vitamin D.* Washington, DC: National Academy Press, 2011.
23. Deluca HF. Vitamin D and the parenteral nutrition patient. *Gastroenterology.* 2009;137:S79–S91.
24. Bang UC et al. Variations in serum 25-hydroxyvitamin D during acute pancreatitis: An exploratory longitudinal study. *Endocr Res.* 2011;36(4):135–141.
25. Holick MF. Vitamin D deficiencies. *N Engl J Med.* 2007;357:266–281.
26. Chandra P et al. Treatment of vitamin D deficiencies with UV light in patients with malabsorption syndromes: A case series. *Photodermatol Photoimmunol Photomed.* 2007;23:179–185.
27. Holick MF et al. Evaluation, treatment and prevention of vitamin D deficiency: An Endocrine Society clinical practice guideline. *J Clin Endocrinol Metab.* 2011;96:1911–1930.
28. Logan VF et al. Long-term vitamin D_3 supplementation is more effective then vitamin D_2 in maintaining serum 25-hydroxyvitamin D status over the winter months. *Br J Nutr.* 2013;109:1082–1088.
29. Lehman U et al. Bioavailability of vitamin D_2 and D_3 in healthy volunteers, a randomized placebo-controlled trial. *J Clin Endocrinol Metab.* 2013;98:4339–4345.
30. Tappel AL. Vitamin E as the biologic lipid antioxidant. *Vitam Horm.* 1962;20:493–510.
31. Biesalski HK. Vitamin E requirement in parenteral nutrition. *Gastroenterology.* 2009;137:S92–S104.
32. Traber MG. Vitamin E. In: *Modern Nutrition in Health and Disease.* 11th ed. Eds, Ross AC, Caballero B, Cousins RJ, Tucker KL, Ziegler TR. Baltimore, MD: Lippincott Williams & Wilkins, 2014, pp. 293–304.
33. Estivariz CF et al. Nutrient intake from habitual oral diet in patients with severe short bowel syndrome living in the southeastern United States. *Nutrition.* 2008;24:330–339.
34. Yang CJ et al. High prevalence of multiple micronutrient deficiencies in children with intestinal failure: A longitudinal study. *J Pediatr.* 2011;159:39–44.
35. Greene HL et al. Guidelines for the use of vitamins, trace elements, calcium, magnesium, and phosphorus in infants and children receiving total parenteral nutrition: Report for the subcommittee on Pediatric Parenteral Nutrition Requirements from the Committee on Clinical Practice Issues of The American Society for Clinical Nutrition. *Am J Clin Nutr.* 1988;48:1324–1342.
36. Satya-Murti S et al. The spectrum of neurological disorders from vitamin E deficiency. *Neurology.* 1986;36:917–921.
37. Mayo Clinic. Mayo Medical Laboratories. *Interpretive Handbook.* http://www.mayomedicallaboratories.com/interpretive-guide/index.html. Published 1995. Updated 2015. Accessed March 4, 2015.
38. Pironi L et al. Lipid peroxidation and antioxidant status in adults receiving lipid-based home parenteral nutrition. *Am J Clin Nutr.* 1998;68:888–893.
39. Suttie JW. Vitamin K. In: *Modern Nutrition in Health and Disease.* 11th ed. Eds, Ross AC, Caballero B, Cousins RJ, Tucker KL, Ziegler TR. Baltimore, MD: Lippincott Williams & Wilkins, 2014, pp. 305–316.
40. Krzyzanowska P et al. Vitamin K status in patients with short bowel syndrome. *Clin Nutr.* 2012; 31:1015–1017.
41. Shearer MJ. Vitamin K in parenteral nutrition. *Gastroenterology.* 2009;137:S105–S118.
42. Booth SL et al. Determinants of vitamin K status in humans. *Vitam Horm.* 2008;78:1–22.
43. Suttie JW. The importance of menaquinones in human nutrition. *Ann Rev Nutr.* 1995;15:399–417.
44. Paiva SA et al. Interaction between vitamin K nutriture and bacterial overgrowth in hypochlorhydria induced by omeprazole. *Am J Clin Nutr.* 1998;68:699–704.
45. Carmel R. Cobalamin (vitamin B_{12}). In: *Modern Nutrition in Health and Disease.* 11th ed. Eds, Ross AC, Caballero B, Cousins RJ, Tucker KL, Ziegler TR. Baltimore, MD: Lippincott Williams & Wilkins, 2014, pp. 369–389.

46. Giannella RA et al. Competition between bacteria and intrinsic factor for vitamin B_{12}: Implications for vitamin B_{12} malabsorption in intestinal bacterial overgrowth. *Gastroenterology*. 1972;62:255–260.
47. Solomon LR. Cobalamine-responsive disorders in the ambulatory care setting: Unreliability of cobalamin, methylmalonic acid, and homocysteine testing. *Blood*. 2005;105(3):978–985.
48. Lindenbaum J et al. Diagnosis of cobalamin deficiency: II. Relative sensitivities of serum cobalamin, methylmalonic acid, and total homocysteine concentrations. *Am J Hematol*. 1990;34(2):99–107.
49. Stabler SP. Clinical practice. Vitamin B_{12} deficiency. *N Engl J Med*. 2013;268(2):149–160.
50. Tarleton S et al. Short bowel syndrome. In: *A.S.P.E.N. Adult Nutrition Support Core Curriculum*. 2nd ed. Eds, Mueller CM, Kovacevich DS, McClave SA, Miller SJ, Schwartz DB. Silver Spring, MD: American Society of Parenteral and Enteral Nutrition, 2012, pp. 511–522.
51. Kuzminski AM et al. Effective treatment of cobalamin deficiency with oral cobalamin. *Blood*. 1998;92(4):1191–1198.
52. Stover PJ. Folic acid. In: *Modern Nutrition in Health and Disease*. 11th ed. Eds, Ross AC, Caballero B, Cousins RJ, Tucker KL, Ziegler TR. Baltimore, MD: Lippincott Williams & Wilkins, 2014, pp. 358–368.
53. Da Silva L et al. Vitamin B_{12}: No one should be without it. *Pract Gastroenterol*. 2009;33(1):34–46.
54. Piyathilake CJ et al. A practical approach to red blood cell folate analysis. *Anal Chem Insights*. 2007;2:107–110.
55. Balint JP. Physical findings in nutritional deficiencies. *Pediatr Clin N Am*. 1998;45(1):245–260.
56. Heimburger DC. Nutrition assessment. In: *Handbook of Clinical Nutrition*. 4th ed. Eds, Heimburger DC, Ard JD. Philadelphia, PA: Mosby Elsevier, 2006, pp. 242–261.
57. Winkler M et al. Home nutrition support. In: *A.S.P.E.N. Adult Nutrition Support Core Curriculum*. 2nd ed. Eds, Mueller CM, Kovacevich DS, McClave SA, Miller SJ, Schwartz DB. Silver Spring, MD: American Society of Parenteral and Enteral Nutrition, 2012, pp. 639–655.
58. Wall E. An overview of short bowel syndrome management: Adherence, adaptation, and practical recommendations. *J Acad Nutr Diet*. 2013;113(9):1200–1208.
59. Mziray-Andrew CH et al. Nutritional deficiencies in intestinal failure. *Pediatr Clin N Am*. 2009; 56:1185–1200.

13 Management of Trace Elements in Short Bowel Syndrome

Joe Krenitsky

CONTENTS

KEY POINTS

- Patients with short bowel syndrome (SBS) are at risk for trace element deficiencies.
- Inappropriate trace element supplementation has the potential to create toxicity or deficiencies of other nutrients.
- Understanding individual gastrointestinal anatomy and absorption sites for trace elements is important in order to reduce the risk of deficiency in SBS.

INTRODUCTION

Patients with short bowel syndrome (SBS) are at risk for trace element deficiencies due to decreased absorption from dietary intake and increased losses in gastrointestinal (GI) fluids. Deficiencies generally occur when trace element status is not considered or GI losses are not addressed. Inadequate trace element status typically develops over time, with the potential for deficiency syndromes to be overlooked until symptoms are severe. In recent years, shortages of parenteral nutrition (PN) components have also contributed to cases of trace element deficiencies [1,2]. Deficiencies of trace elements can impair protein metabolism, slow growth and wound healing, compromise immune function, cause anemia, or even result in neuromuscular dysfunction. Inappropriate trace element supplementation can result in toxicity or create deficiencies of other trace elements.

GENERAL CONSIDERATIONS

As in all aspects of SBS management, elucidation of anatomy and consideration of the functionality of the remaining bowel are paramount. The type and degree of trace mineral disturbance and requirements will depend on the segment and length of existing bowel, route and adequacy of nutrition intake, and the volume of GI fluid losses. The proximal duodenum is the primary absorptive area for a number of trace elements; therefore, proximal bowel resections, fistulas, or procedures that result in enteral nutrients bypassing the duodenum pose a significant risk for the development of several trace element deficiencies. Intuitively, it may seem that patients with very short lengths of existing bowel would be at the greatest risk for deficiencies due to decreased absorption of dietary intake; however, patients with longer lengths of bowel may be at greater risk for some deficiencies due to secretion of trace elements into the GI fluids from the lumen [3]. Ongoing, large-volume losses of small bowel fluids are a significant risk factor in the development of several trace element deficiencies. See Table 13.1 for a summary of trace element considerations in SBS.

Compared with the macrominerals such as calcium, magnesium, or phosphorus, there is a greater potential for toxicity from excessive doses of trace elements. Parenteral administration of trace elements has a greater risk for toxicity than oral or enteral administration does because absorption control is bypassed. Organ dysfunction that impairs a primary route of excretion can also increase the likelihood of toxicity of some trace elements. Additionally, products that contain multiple trace elements for parenteral administration were formulated at a time when very limited information was available regarding requirements and parenteral dosing [4]. Subsequently, case reports of toxicity and other information have accrued over time, revealing that some trace elements have been dosed in excessive amounts in the multitrace element parenteral products [4]. Unfortunately, manufacturers have not been responsive to expert recommendations and reformulated trace element products have not been produced in the United States [4]. Table 13.2 [5] summarizes the multitrace element formulations currently available in the United States.

Although oral or enteral trace element administration may reduce the risk, the potential for toxicity remains. Furthermore, there is competition for absorption between a number of the trace elements; long-term enteral supplementation of trace elements can induce severe deficiency of those that share the same absorptive pathway [6,7].

MONITORING TRACE ELEMENT STATUS

Monitoring of trace element status is controversial, in part because whole blood and serum measurements do not always accurately reflect whole body stores. Blood levels may not decrease until a deficiency is advanced, so normal laboratory values do not necessarily exclude the possibility of a subclinical insufficiency that is in progression. Of additional importance is that the blood concentration of a number of trace elements is acutely decreased, while serum levels of some trace elements are increased, in response to infection, injury, or inflammation (Table 13.1). It has been theorized that the decrease in serum levels of some trace elements in response to infection or injury may serve as a protective mechanism, and supplementation in these settings may have undesirable consequences [8].

Despite these limitations, in patients with SBS, especially those with ongoing GI losses or who require long-term PN, monitoring trace element status can help prevent severe deficiency syndromes or toxicity. In individuals without active inflammation or infection, serum levels of trace elements can help distinguish between symptoms that may be related to a nutrient deficiency or other factors. An observational study of clinical practices involving long-term PN-dependent patients reported that trace elements were monitored yearly for nutrients lost in various GI secretions (zinc, selenium) and less than annually for nutrients with less commonly reported deficiency or toxicities (copper, chromium) [9].

ZINC

Zinc is an essential cofactor for more than 300 enzymes within the body, including those required for metabolism of carbohydrate, fat, and protein; clearance of reactive oxygen species; regulation of gene transcription; cell signaling; hormone release; and apoptosis [10,11]. Zinc is present in most body tissues and fluids, but there is very minimal storage of zinc in the liver and plasma and through

TABLE 13.1
Trace Element Considerations in SBS

	Risk of Deficiency in SBS	Risk of Toxicity	Effect of Stress on Lab Values	Lab Test	Clinical Considerations
Zinc	Increased	Minimal	Decreased	Serum zinc	Monitor copper and iron during long-term zinc supplementation
Copper	Increased (anatomy dependent)	Increased in PN	Increased	Serum copper	Monitor copper during long-term jejunal feeding
Iron	Moderate without blood loss	Risks with parenteral iron	Ferritin increased Iron decreased	Ferritin, % iron saturation	Parenteral supplementation may be required
Selenium	Increased	Minimal with standard doses	Decreased	Serum selenium	Monitor if duodenum bypassed
Manganese	Minimal	High risk with PN	Unchanged	Whole blood manganese	Risk for toxicity with PN
Chromium	Minimal	Increased with PN	Unchanged	Not recommended	Possible toxicity with PN
Molybdenum	Minimal	No	N/A	Not recommended	N/A
Iodine	Minimal	Minimal	Unchanged	Thyroid function tests	N/A

Note: N/A, not applicable.

TABLE 13.2
Currently Available Multitrace Element (MTE) Formulations in the United States

Trace Element	DRI	Parenteral FDA Guidelines	ASPEN Most Recent Proposal	MTE-4C (per 1 mL) American Regent	MTE-4 (per 3 mL) American Regent	MTE-5C (per 1 mL) American Regent	MTE-5 (per 3 mL) American Regent	Addamel N (per 10 mL) Fresenius Kabi
Chromium	20–35 μg	10–15 μg	Omit or <1 μg	10 μg	12 μg	10 μg	12 μg	10 μg
Copper	0.9 mg	0.5–1.5 mg	0.3–0.5 mg	1 mg	1.2 mg	1 mg	1.2 mg	1.3 mg
Fluoride	3–4 mg	Not routinely added	N/A	N/A	N/A	N/A	N/A	0.95 mg
Iodine	150 μg	Not routinely added	N/A	N/A	N/A	N/A	N/A	0.13 mg
Iron	8–18 mg	Not routinely added	N/A	N/A	N/A	N/A	N/A	1.1 mg
Manganese	1.8–2.3 mg	0.15–0.8 mg	0.055 mg	0.5 mg	0.3 mg	0.5 mg	0.3 mg	0.27 mg
Molybdenum	45 μg	2.5–5 mg	N/A	N/A	N/A	N/A	N/A	19 μg
Selenium	55 μg	20–60 μg	60–100 μg	N/A	N/A	60 μg	60 μg	0.13 mg
Zinc	8–11 mg	3–4 mg	3–4 mg	5 mg	3 mg	5 mg	3 mg	6.5 mg

Source: Pogatschnik, C., *Pract. Gastroenterol.* 38, 27, 2014. With permission.
Note: DRI, Dietary Reference Intake; N/A, not applicable.

tissue turnover [10,11]. Serum zinc is neither a sensitive nor specific indicator of overall zinc status [10,11]. Serum zinc can remain within normal limits until a deficiency is severe. Zinc is primarily bound to albumin and serum levels are decreased in response to physiologic stress, such as an infection or injury, which does not necessarily reflect a true zinc deficiency [10–12]. Even minor illness, with a C-reactive protein <15 mg/L, causes a 10% decrease in plasma zinc; more severe stress causes a 40–60% decrease in zinc levels [10,12]. Unfortunately, individual variability is high; therefore, it is not possible to make accurate adjustments based on degree of stress or albumin level [10,12].

Dietary zinc is primarily absorbed in the duodenum and proximal jejunum; however, there is also a possible role for the colon in zinc absorption [10,13]. Metallothionein-bound zinc within enterocytes enters luminal secretions during the normal turnover of enterocytes. Enterohepatic recycling of enteric zinc occurs and, as such, zinc is also excreted into bile [10]. Normal GI losses of zinc in healthy adults are 2–4 mg/day, but GI loss of zinc in subjects with mature ileostomies and full length of small bowel was between 6.4 and 7.8 mg/day [10,14]. The importance of zinc losses related to villus turnover was documented in a study of zinc requirements in PN-dependent patients [3]. Zinc losses in patients with "massive" small bowel resection were only 3.6 ± 0.29 mg/L of GI fluid compared with 15.2 ± 1.0 mg/L for patients with longer lengths of remaining small intestine [3]. The authors recommended adjustment of parenteral zinc provision by the addition of 17 mg/L of stool or ileostomy output or 12 mg/L of upper small bowel stoma or fistula losses [3].

Zinc deficiency can result in alopecia, delayed wound healing, dysgeusia, hypogonadism in males, and reduced growth rate in children [10,11]. Severe zinc deficiency can cause diarrhea, impair immune function, and result in skin rash similar to that seen in acrodermatitis enteropathica [10,15].

Recommendations for oral zinc in healthy individuals are 8–11 mg/day for adults, 11–13 mg/day during pregnancy and lactation, 2–3 mg/day for infants, and 3–8 mg/day for children [10,11]. Recommendations for parenteral zinc are 4 mg/day; most multiple trace element preparations in the United States provide between 3 and 5 mg per recommended daily dose [4]. In patients with increased GI losses, a positive zinc balance was achieved with 12 mg of parenteral zinc/day [3].

Patients with SBS who have intact proximal bowel and controlled transit time will generally respond appropriately to oral zinc supplements to balance increased GI losses. The coefficient for zinc absorption is approximately 30% of intake under normal conditions, which means that a patient who loses 2 L of small bowel fluids may need to take as much as 100 mg/day of additional elemental zinc (440 mg $ZnSO_4$) to balance losses [3,14]. Zinc absorption from grain-rich diets may be as low as 15–20% of intake because phytates and cereal fiber decrease zinc absorption [10,14].

Enteral zinc supplements compete for absorption with iron and copper [6,7]. If patients are maintained on oral zinc supplements to balance GI losses due to SBS, then clinicians should be vigilant for deficiencies of these other trace elements. Long-term oral/enteral zinc supplementation with doses greater than 50 mg/day have resulted in copper and iron deficiency; very high zinc intake from zinc-containing denture cream (such as Fixodent from Procter & Gamble; Poligrip from GlaxoSmithKline is now zinc-free) has resulted in severe copper deficiency [6,7,16]. Zinc is also excreted in the urine, and chronic high-dose zinc supplementation has been associated with increased incidence of urinary tract infections [17]. Toxicity from zinc is rare and generally only results from very large doses of parenteral zinc [18]. Nausea, vomiting, and diarrhea have been reported in acute zinc toxicity, and more chronic zinc excess results in copper deficiency [10,18].

Copper

Copper is an essential component of superoxide dismutase and enzymes that transfer iron from storage to bone marrow, catalyze collagen and elastin cross-linking, convert dopamine to norepinephrine, and synthesize serotonin and melanin, among other functions [19]. Dietary copper is absorbed in the duodenum and proximal jejunum [19]. Serum copper and ceruloplasmin, a major copper transport protein, are acute phase reactants and increase during physiologic stress, so a mild copper deficiency can be missed in hospitalized or ill patients [19]. A low serum copper, however, has positive predictive value and is more representative of a true deficiency.

Copper deficiency results in anemia that resembles iron deficiency but can also cause neutropenia and thrombocytopenia [20]. In severe deficiency, pancytopenia, neuropathy, and myeloneuropathy have been reported [21,22]. Copper deficiency was once considered rare; however, in recent years, a number of cases of severe copper deficiency have been reported after gastric bypass, PN without adequate trace element supplementation, and due to chronic high-dose zinc intake related to supplements or zinc-containing denture cream [1,23,24]. Copper deficiency has also been reported in patients with normal-length small bowel but fed via a jejunostomy tube due to the use of enteral formulas with marginal copper content being infused beyond the primary sites of copper absorption [25].

The recommended dietary allowance for healthy adults is 0.9 mg/day, 1 mg/day during pregnancy, and 1.3 mg/day during lactation [26]. A study of patients who were PN dependent and not taking food by mouth determined that copper balance was achieved with 0.3 mg/day [27]. Patients with diarrhea were reported to have increased copper losses and required 0.4–0.5 mg/day to achieve copper balance [27]. Adult PN multitrace element products contain 1 mg/day, so patients with increased GI losses who are receiving PN with standard trace element dosing should not require additional copper. However, patients with SBS who do not receive parenteral nutrients, for example, due to national shortages experienced in recent years or because of elevated serum levels, who receive high-dose chronic oral zinc administration, may require additional dietary copper or monitoring of copper status in non-physiologic stressed states.

The primary control of copper levels is through regulation of copper absorption, and the primary route for copper excretion is in bile [19]. Excessive parenteral copper can accumulate in the liver and other tissues and may result in copper toxicity. Patients who require long-term PN are at risk for copper overload due to the excess of copper provided in trace element formulations [4]. Owing to the biliary excretion of copper, patients with cholestasis probably have a reduced requirement for copper. One study reported copper balance with only 0.15 mg copper/day in PN of patients with cholestasis [27]. However, in an anecdotal report, severe copper deficiency resulted from removal of all copper from PN in a cholestatic patient, so copper should not be empirically removed without monitoring copper status [28].

Iron

The majority of iron in the body is incorporated into hemoglobin, with lesser amounts as a component of myoglobin and as a cofactor for enzymes. The primary control of iron status is through regulation of iron absorption. Iron is preferentially absorbed in the duodenum, and dietary iron absorption is enhanced in the presence of gastric acid, in part, due to conversion of ferric iron from food to the more readily absorbed ferrous form [4,29]. This is important to remember, as gastric resection and surgical or pharmacological interventions that persistently decrease gastric acid production can decrease iron absorption and result in iron deficiency. Iron status is most commonly determined by measuring ferritin level in the blood rather than simply measuring the iron level. The percentage transferrin saturation (iron divided by iron binding capacity) is also commonly used, since it serves as an indicator of iron that is available for erythropoiesis [30]. Ferritin is an intracellular iron storage protein that acts as a good indicator of iron stores in nonstressed individuals; however, ferritin is an acute-phase reactant and, as such, is increased in response to injury or illness [30–32]. In contrast, during physiologic stress, serum iron level is decreased [30–32]. In patients with physiologic stress such as inflammatory illness, infection, or injury, traditional lab indicators of iron deficiency have a very low sensitivity and specificity [31]. Bone marrow biopsy is considered the gold standard for diagnosis of iron deficiency in stressed patients but, due to inconvenience, pain, and expense, is very rarely utilized [31,32]. Soluble transferrin receptor, or the ratio of the soluble transferrin receptor to the log of the ferritin level, has been found to be a much more accurate indicator of true iron status of patients with physiologic stress or inflammatory response, but these labs have not been widely adopted, nor are they available at all facilities [31]. In practice, clinicians usually do not diagnose iron deficiency by labs alone. Lab results such as ferritin and percentage transferrin saturation are evaluated within the context of an individual patient's GI anatomy, nutrition history, and risk factors for iron deficiency, while considering the effects of stress on lab results.

Healthy adults can absorb from 2% to 23% of dietary iron, and absorption is up-regulated in the setting of iron deficiency [29]. Iron absorption is enhanced by coingestion with ascorbic acid (vitamin C) while excess dietary or supplemental zinc and calcium use decreases iron absorption. [29,33]. There is a greater reserve of iron in the body than most other trace elements, and in the absence of blood loss, there is minimal daily iron excretion in stool and skin. Iron requirements are not necessarily increased in SBS; however, patients with a history of inflammatory bowel disease can have increased risk for iron deficiency owing to chronic blood loss via the GI tract [4].

The recommended dietary allowance for iron in adults is 8 mg/day for men and postmenopausal women and 18 mg/day for women. Iron requirements increase to 27 mg/day during pregnancy and decrease to 9 mg/day during lactation [26]. Iron is one of the few nutrients with requirements that are not substantially different between children and adults, with recommended intakes between 7 and 11 mg/day for children, depending on age. Iron is not routinely provided in PN in the United States due to concerns regarding incompatibility with lipid emulsions and fear of anaphylactic reactions [34]. However, several European trace-element preparations contain 1–2 mg iron per dose and are routinely used, even with lipid-containing PN, without reported problems. Many patients who receive PN without substantial oral intake can go months or years without showing signs of an iron deficiency [4].

A complete guide to iron supplementation is beyond the scope and space limitations of this chapter, but some basic considerations follow. In the setting of iron deficiency, iron absorption is unregulated and increased dietary iron is absorbed. Traditionally, guidelines for oral iron supplementation recommend providing 100–200 mg of elemental iron daily in adults (3–6 mg/kg/day for children) in several divided doses per day [31,32]. However, there are limited randomized data that have investigated the optimal dosing strategy for oral iron supplementation, and several studies have demonstrated that lower iron doses may be as effective and better tolerated [31,34].

Oral iron supplements can cause GI side effects such as constipation and nausea, which may limit compliance [31,32]. Iron sulfate is the most common form used and also one of the least expensive iron supplements available, but iron sulfate has also been reported to have frequent GI side effects [31,32]. There are no high-quality data that have demonstrated superiority for one iron salt versus another in terms of efficacy in resolution of anemia, but if a patient has GI side effects with one form of iron, reducing the daily dose or changing to a different iron salt such as ferrous fumarate or iron gluconate may be helpful.

Failure to reverse iron deficiency with oral iron may be caused by factors beyond SBS that relate to either impaired absorption or ongoing iron loss that exceeds the supplementation. Examples include *Helicobacter pylori* infection, celiac disease, GI bleeding, acid suppressing medication use, prior gastric resection, or GI anatomy that bypasses the duodenum such as Roux-en-Y gastrojejunostomy [32]. Iron absorption and the release of iron from stores are decreased in states of injury, infection, or inflammation, and this decreased iron availability is believed to be a protective mechanism in acute injury or infection [31,32]. Providing parenteral iron can bypass the limitation of decreased iron absorption during stressed states, but the advisability of providing parenteral iron in stressed or inflammatory states remains an area of ongoing controversy and research [31,32].

Patients who are unable to absorb sufficient iron via the oral route due to SBS or inadequate contact of enteral nutrients with the duodenum can receive periodic iron infusions [35,36]. Older parenteral iron preparations, such as iron dextran, had the disadvantage of the risk of anaphylactic reactions associated with dextran [31]. Newer parenteral iron products, such as iron sucrose, are rarely associated with serious adverse events, but less serious infusion reactions (that are still concerning to patients) have been reported. Parenteral iron is usually administered in a supervised setting or infusion center rather than at home [31,32,36]. Because parenteral iron bypasses absorption through the gut and with no routine mechanism for excretion of excess, iron provided beyond needs can be deposited in hepatic, renal, and cardiac tissue [31]. If excess parenteral iron is provided over an extended period of time, iron deposition in the heart, liver, and/or kidney may be complicated by eventual organ failure [31].

Blood transfusion as a treatment of routine iron deficiency anemia is discouraged but may be indicated in severe iron deficiency anemia that results in cardiovascular symptoms [32,36]. It is helpful to remember that in patients who receive transfusion for other indications while hospitalized, every unit of packed cells provides approximately 200 mg of parenteral iron [32].

Selenium

Selenium plays a role in antioxidant systems, thyroid hormone metabolism, and immune regulation [37]. Selenium is primarily absorbed in the duodenum and is excreted in urine and stool. Thus, patients who have had surgical alterations that allow ingested nutrients to bypass the proximal bowel appear to have increased selenium requirements [37–39]. Serum selenium levels are decreased in sepsis or injury, but in unstressed patients, serum selenium levels can be useful to detect deficiency or excess [40]. Selenium deficiency can cause cardiomyopathy, macrocytosis, myopathy, altered pigmentation, and growth retardation and alopecia in children [37,38]. The recommended dietary allowance for selenium is 55 μg/day for adults and between 15 and 40 μg/day for infants and children [37].

Symptomatic selenium deficiency is uncommon outside of long-term PN use without adequate selenium supplementation. Due to the uncommon occurrence of selenium deficiency in non-PN-dependent patients, there are no controlled studies of oral selenium supplementation for selenium deficiency. Studies that have investigated supplemental selenium for disease prevention utilized doses of 50–200 μg/day, and the tolerable upper intake levels are 45–280 μg/day for children and 400 μg/day for adults [37]. Initial oral selenium doses of 50–200 μg/day may be a reasonable starting dose in deficient patients who are not PN dependent. Several cases of selenium deficiency were reported in SBS patients who received long-term PN that did not contain selenium [38,41,42]. Selenium absorption can be decreased in SBS, depending on the length and segment of the remaining bowel [37,41]. Although there is a degree of urinary conservation when intake or absorption is decreased, patients who cannot meet calorie and protein needs from an oral diet also likely need parenteral selenium [38,43]. Previous parenteral selenium recommendations were 20–60 μg/day, but more recent recommendations for adults were increased to 60–100 μg/day [4]. However, an observational study of long-term PN patients documented that even while receiving 70 μg of selenium per day, 40% of patients had a serum selenium concentration below the normal range [9]. Serum selenium is decreased in physiologic stress, so it is possible that some reports of selenium insufficiency were a reflection of patients with nonapparent stress response [9]. Pediatric multitrace elements in the United States do not generally provide selenium. Therefore, selenium must be added to PN separately to meet recommendations for 2 μg/kg/day for neonatal and pediatric patients [4].

While rare, excessive selenium intake can cause toxicity with symptoms that include diarrhea, fatigue, hair loss, joint pain, nail discoloration, and nausea. Acute selenium toxicity has been reported from use of dietary supplements that were formulated with excessive selenium [44].

Manganese

Manganese is a cofactor for several enzymes, including superoxide dismutase, and plays a role in bone formation [26,45]. Manganese is regulated through absorption and excreted primarily in bile. Therefore, patients with later-stage chronic cholestatic or biliary disorders and all patients who receive long-term PN with multitrace element preparations are at risk for manganese toxicity [45,46]. Manganese is widely distributed throughout the body, and manganese deficiency is virtually unknown outside of experimental conditions. A number of cases of manganese toxicity, however, have been reported [45,47]. Some cases of manganese toxicity have been reported as early as 2 weeks after the initiation of PN [47]. Excess manganese crosses the blood–brain barrier, accumulates in the globus pallidus, and is believed to alter catecholamine storage or metabolism [46,48]. Symptoms of manganese toxicity include tremor and altered gait that resemble Parkinson's disease, insomnia, headache, confusion, and memory disturbances [45,48].

Manganese is included as a component of parenteral multiple trace element preparations, and available evidence suggests that the products made in the United States with 500 μg/day provide approximately 10 times the necessary dose [4]. Patients who require long-term PN should have whole blood manganese checked after 3 months and periodically thereafter. Importantly, patients with cholestasis who receive PN require more frequent monitoring. If whole blood manganese is elevated, then multiple trace elements should be removed from the PN and parenteral zinc, copper, and selenium should be added back individually.

Chromium

Chromium facilitates the action of insulin as a component of glucose tolerance factor (trivalent chromium, niacin, cysteine, glycine, and glutamic acid) [26]. Dietary chromium is absorbed in the small intestine, and adults with normal chromium status absorb only 0.4–2.5% of ingested chromium [49]. Chromium status is regulated by absorption, and most of the absorbed chromium is excreted in the urine [26,49]. Chromium deficiency is extremely rare; the only known cases have been reported in patients receiving long-term PN without chromium [4,49]. Deficiency symptoms included peripheral neuropathy, weight loss, hyperglycemia with increased insulin requirements, and elevated plasma free fatty acid levels, which resolved with supplemental chromium [26,49]. Patients with SBS do not appear to be at particularly increased risk of chromium deficiency, as patients who are PN dependent receive chromium with the multiple trace element product and patients with SBS who are not PN dependent do not appear to be at risk for deficiency. As stated previously, chromium deficiency is extremely rare, and the only known cases have been in people who received long-term PN without chromium [49].

Chromium toxicity is a greater concern than deficiency in patients who receive long-term PN, especially in pediatric patients [4,49]. The chromium provided in multiple trace element formulations, combined with contamination of PN components during their manufacture, provides excessive chromium [4,49]. Patients receiving long-term PN may have elevated serum chromium, and increased tissue deposition of chromium has been reported [4,49]. Excessive serum chromium has been associated with compromised renal function in PN-dependent pediatric patients, and although no cases of overt chromium toxicity have been reported, tissue levels of chromium are elevated after extended PN use [49,50]. Routine monitoring of blood chromium is generally not recommended because the concentration of chromium in the serum is so minimal that an accurate measurement with the possibility of contamination in normal clinical settings makes the results unreliable [4].

Molybdenum and Iodine

Molybdenum is a cofactor for several enzymes, including xanthine dehydrogenase, aldehyde oxidase, and sulfite oxidase [26]. Patients with SBS do not appear to be at increased risk of molybdenum deficiency. There has been only a single case report of molybdenum deficiency in a patient on long-term PN. Symptoms included mental status and visual and cardiac alterations, which resolved after molybdenum supplementation [4]. Trace element preparations made in the United States do not contain molybdenum, but several products made outside of the United States include molybdenum at a dose of 20 μg/day [4]. It is generally thought that molybdenum contamination of PN components is adequate to prevent deficiency [4]. Plasma and urine tests are not useful indicators of molybdenum status; therefore, routine monitoring is not feasible or recommended [4].

Iodine plays an essential role in the synthesis of thyroid hormones [26]. Iodine is rapidly absorbed in the proximal bowel and is excreted in the urine [26]. Iodine deficiency is rare in areas of the world with widespread use of iodized salt, and patients with SBS who have an intact duodenum do not appear to be at increased risk of iodine deficiency. Iodine is not included in parenteral trace element preparations made in the United States but is included in several products produced outside the United States. There are no case reports of symptomatic iodine deficiency in adults receiving PN, but there is a report of hypothyroidism in a preterm infant with SBS who was PN dependent [51]. Iodine deficiency should be considered in PN-dependent patients who develop thyroid enlargement or hypothyroidism [4].

CONCLUSION

Patients with SBS, whether on or off PN, are at increased risk for a number of trace element derangements, particularly deficiencies. Due to interactions between trace elements, long-term supplementation can induce deficiencies of other elements. Parenteral trace element supplementation as part of PN carries the risk for toxicity of several trace elements. While periodic monitoring is advised, objective data on the optimal monitoring schedule for toxicities and deficiencies of trace elements remain scarce. Clinicians need to remain vigilant for signs of potential trace element deficiencies and toxicities and not become complacent regarding the nutrition status of long-term SBS patients.

REFERENCES

1. Palm E et al. Copper and zinc deficiency in a patient receiving long-term parenteral nutrition during a shortage of parenteral trace element products. *JPEN J Parenter Enteral Nutr.* 2015;39(8):986–989.
2. Davis C et al. Selenium deficiency in pediatric patients with intestinal failure as a consequence of drug shortage. *JPEN J Parenter Enteral Nutr.* 2014;38(1):115–118.
3. Wolman SL et al. Zinc in total parenteral nutrition: Requirements and metabolic effects. *Gastroenterology.* 1979;76(3):458–467.
4. Vanek VW et al. Novel Nutrient Task Force, Parenteral Multi-Vitamin and Multi-Trace Element Working Group; American Society for Parenteral and Enteral Nutrition (A.S.P.E.N.) Board of Directors. A.S.P.E.N. position paper: Recommendations for changes in commercially available parenteral multivitamin and multi-trace element products. *Nutr Clin Pract.* 2012;27(4):440–491.
5. Pogatschnik C. Trace element supplementation and monitoring in the adult patient on parenteral nutrition. *Pract. Gastroenterol.* 2014;38(5):27.
6. de Brito NJ et al. Oral zinc supplementation decreases the serum iron concentration in healthy schoolchildren: A pilot study. *Nutrients.* 2014;6(9):3460–3473.
7. Willis MS et al. Zinc-induced copper deficiency: A report of three cases initially recognized on bone marrow examination. *Am J Clin Pathol.* 2005;123(1):125–131.
8. Jonker FA et al. Anaemia, iron deficiency and susceptibility to infections. *J Infect.* 2014;69(Suppl 1): S23–S27.
9. Btaiche IF et al. Dosing and monitoring of trace elements in long-term home parenteral nutrition patients. *JPEN J Parenter Enteral Nutr.* 2011;35(6):736–747.
10. Livingstone C. Zinc: Physiology, deficiency, and parenteral nutrition. *Nutr Clin Pract.* 2015;30(3): 371–382.
11. Jeejeebhoy K. Zinc: An essential trace element for parenteral nutrition. *Gastroenterology.* 2009;137 (5 Suppl):S7–S12.
12. Galloway P et al. Effect of the inflammatory response on trace element and vitamin status. *Ann Clin Biochem.* 2000;37:289–297.
13. Gopalsamy GL et al. The relevance of the colon to zinc nutrition. *Nutrients.* 2015;7(1):572–583.
14. Sandström B et al. Apparent small intestinal absorption of nitrogen and minerals from soy and meat-protein-based diets. A study on human ileostomy subjects. *J Nutr.* 1986;116(11):2209–2218.
15. Lewandowski H et al. Kwashiorkor and an acrodermatitis enteropathica-like eruption after a distal gastric bypass surgical procedure. *Endocr Pract.* 2007;13(3):277–282.

16. Afrin LB. Fatal copper deficiency from excessive use of zinc-based denture adhesive. *Am J Med Sci.* 2010;340(2):164–168.
17. Johnson AR et al. High dose zinc increases hospital admissions due to genitourinary complications. *J Urol.* 2007;177(2):639–643.
18. Brocks A et al. Acute intravenous zinc poisoning. *Br Med J.* 1977;1(6073):1390–1391.
19. Shike M. Copper in parenteral nutrition. *Gastroenterology.* 2009;137(5 Suppl):S13–S17.
20. Chan LN et al. The science and practice of micronutrient supplementations in nutritional anemia: An evidence-based review. *JPEN J Parenter Enteral Nutr.* 2014;38(6):656–672.
21. Imataki O et al. Pancytopenia complicated with peripheral neuropathy due to copper deficiency: Clinical diagnostic review. *Intern Med.* 2008;47(23):2063–2065.
22. Yaldizli O et al. Copper deficiency myelopathy induced by repetitive parenteral zinc supplementation during chronic hemodialysis. *J Neurol.* 2006;253(11):1507–1509.
23. Jaiser SR et al. Copper deficiency myelopathy. *J Neurol.* 2010;257(6):869–881.
24. Prodan CI et al. Copper deficiency after gastric surgery: A reason for caution. *Am J Med Sci.* 2009;337(4):256–258.
25. Nishiwaki S et al. Predominant copper deficiency during prolonged enteral nutrition through a jejunostomy tube compared to that through a gastrostomy tube. *Clin Nutr.* 2011;30(5):585–589.
26. Institute of Medicine (US) Panel on Micronutrients. *Dietary Reference Intakes for Vitamin A, Vitamin K, Arsenic, Boron, Chromium, Copper, Iodine, Iron, Manganese, Molybdenum, Nickel, Silicon, Vanadium, and Zinc.* Washington, DC: National Academies Press, 2001.
27. Shike M et al. Copper metabolism and requirements in total parenteral nutrition. *Gastroenterology.* 1981;81(2):290–297.
28. Fuhrman MP et al. Pancytopenia after removal of copper from total parenteral nutrition. *JPEN J Parenter Enteral Nutr.* 2000;24(6):361–366.
29. Collings R et al. The absorption of iron from whole diets: A systematic review. *Am J Clin Nutr.* 2013;98(1):65–81.
30. Shander A et al. Iron deficiency anemia—Bridging the knowledge and practice gap. *Transfus Med Rev.* 2014;28(3):156–166.
31. Polin V et al. Iron deficiency: From diagnosis to treatment. *Dig Liver Dis.* 2013;45(10):803–809.
32. Camaschella C. Iron-deficiency anemia. *N Engl J Med.* 2015;372(19):1832–1843.
33. Scheers N. Regulatory effects of Cu, Zn, and Ca on Fe absorption: The intricate play between nutrient transporters. *Nutrients.* 2013;5(3):957–970.
34. Rimon E et al. Are we giving too much iron? Low-dose iron therapy is effective in octogenarians. *Am J Med.* 2005;118(10):1142–1147.
35. Hwa YL et al. Iron deficiency in long-term parenteral nutrition therapy. *JPEN J Parenter Enteral Nutr.* May 13, 2015. Epub ahead of print.
36. Avni T et al. The safety of intravenous iron preparations: Systematic review and meta-analysis. *Mayo Clin Proc.* 2015;90(1):12–23.
37. Rayman MP. Selenium and Human Health. *Lancet.* 2012;379(9822):1256–1268.
38. Shenkin A. Selenium in intravenous nutrition. *Gastroenterology.* 2009;137(5 Suppl):S61–S69.
39. Freeth A et al. Assessment of selenium in Roux-en-Y gastric bypass and gastric banding surgery. *Obes Surg.* 2012;22(11):1660–1665.
40. Sammalkorpi K et al. Serum selenium in acute infections. *Infection.* 1988;16(4):222–224.
41. Baptista RJ et al. Suboptimal selenium status in home parenteral nutrition patients with small bowel resections. *JPEN J Parenter Enteral Nutr.* 1984;8(5):542–545.
42. Yusuf SW et al. Cardiomyopathy in association with selenium deficiency: A case report. *JPEN J Parenter Enteral Nutr.* 2002;26(1):63–66.
43. Rannem T et al. The metabolism of [75Se]selenite in patients with short bowel syndrome. *JPEN J Parenter Enteral Nutr.* 1996;20(6):412–416.
44. MacFarquhar JK et al. Acute selenium toxicity associated with a dietary supplement. *Arch Intern Med.* 2010;170(3):256–261.
45. Hardy G. Manganese in parenteral nutrition: Who, when, and why should we supplement? *Gastroenterology.* 2009;137(5 Suppl):S29–S35.
46. Hollingsworth KG et al. *Globus pallidus* magnetization transfer ratio, T(1) and T(2) in primary biliary cirrhosis: Relationship with disease stage and age. *J Magn Reson Imaging.* 2009;29(4):780–784.
47. Fitzgerald K et al. Hypermanganesemia in patients receiving total parenteral nutrition. *JPEN J Parenter Enteral Nutr.* 1999;23(6):333–336.

48. Uchino A et al. Manganese accumulation in the brain: MR imaging. *Neuroradiology.* 2007;49(9): 715–720.
49. Moukarzel A. Chromium in parenteral nutrition: Too little or too much? *Gastroenterology.* 2009;137 (5 Suppl):S18–S28.
50. Howard L et al. Autopsy tissue trace elements in 8 long-term parenteral nutrition patients who received the current U.S. Food and Drug Administration formulation. *JPEN J Parenter Enteral Nutr.* 2007;31(5):388–396.
51. Clarridge KE et al. Hypothyroidism and iodine deficiency in an infant requiring total parenteral nutrition. *JPEN J Parenter Enteral Nutr.* 2014;38(7):901–904.

14 Enteral Feeding in Short Bowel Syndrome

Lore Billiauws, Emilie Latour Beaudet, and Francisca Joly

CONTENTS

KEY POINTS

- Enteral nutrition promotes spontaneous intestinal adaptation and may accelerate oral autonomy when administered in the early postresection phase.
- Enteral nutrition should be considered in selected short bowel patients when an adequate nutritional status cannot be achieved with oral nutrition alone in an attempt to avoid or transition off of parenteral nutrition.
- Enteral feeding may be considered in the setting of SBS for the maintenance or improvement of nutritional status, residual bowel function (adaptation), and quality of life.

INTRODUCTION

Short bowel syndrome (SBS) is a rare disease that results from surgical resection, congenital defect, or disease-associated loss of absorption and is characterized by the inability to maintain protein-energy, fluids, electrolytes, or micronutrient balance when on a conventionally accepted, normal diet [1,2]. Improving absorption is the priority of therapy [3]. SBS is the main cause of intestinal failure (IF) [4]. The primary pathophysiological mechanism of IF in the patient with SBS is the reduced intestinal absorptive surface area. The likelihood of developing SBS-IF depends upon the residual small bowel length, the presence of colon-in-continuity, and several "concomitant pathophysiological mechanisms" related to the anatomy, integrity, function, and adaptive potential of the small bowel remnant, as well as to the underlying clinical condition [5–7]. The minimal length of postduodenal remnant small bowel required to maintain hydration and/or nutrient balance by means of an oral diet and avoid parenteral nutrition (PN) dependence was reported to be ≥35 cm in jejunoileal anastomosis with an intact colon, ≥60 cm in a jejunocolic anastomosis, or ≥115 cm in an end-jejunostomy [8,9].

Enteral nutrition (EN) may be used when an adequate nutritional status cannot be achieved with oral nutrition alone in an attempt to avoid PN use. EN is also occasionally used to facilitate independence from PN when attempts to wean PN have stalled. Illustrating this is a study published in 1983 that reports two patients with a malabsorption syndrome secondary to Crohn's disease with SBS and weight loss refractory to conventional pharmacologic and dietary therapy who showed significant improvements (e.g., increased body weight, fat-free tissue mass, skeletal muscle, and fat) after initiating EN [10]. Around the same time, McIntyre and colleagues [11] reported five patients with SBS who received nocturnal EN via a nasogastric tube that the patients placed and removed by themselves each night and day, respectively. This treatment was found to be safe, effective at inducing weight gain in all cases, acceptable to the patients, and economical [11]. In this chapter, we will discuss the impact of EN on postresection intestinal adaptation and the practical aspects of EN use in SBS patients.

POSTRESECTION INTESTINAL ADAPTATION AND ENTERAL NUTRITION

Postresection intestinal adaptation is a spontaneous process that attempts to ensure a more efficient absorption of nutrients per unit length of the remaining bowel [5,6]. This occurs partly by increasing the absorptive area (structural adaptation) and/or by slowing the gastrointestinal transit (functional adaptation) and treating gastric hypersecretion. It is promoted by the presence of nutrients in the gut lumen, by pancreatic and biliary secretions, and by gut hormones produced mainly by the distal ileum and proximal colon (if still present) and usually takes place over 1 or 2 years. Mechanisms underlying enhancements in absorption include crypt cell hyperplasia, increased villus height, and crypt depth and upregulation of epithelial transporter proteins [12–15]. Several factors are important determinants in the adaptation process and, ultimately, clinical outcome [8,16]. These include the presence or absence of the colon, length of remaining small intestine, health of the remaining bowel, patient age, and presence of comorbid conditions. Moreover, it is well known that whole, intact enteral nutrients are crucial to optimize intestinal adaptation [17–20].

Evidence that luminal nutrients induce intestinal adaptation include the structural and functional gradient along the length of the healthy intestine with a trophic effect of the nutrients to the small intestinal mucosa, the atrophy and functional compromise induced by fasting and exclusive PN (i.e., reducing exposure to luminal nutrients negatively impacts the intestinal mucosa), and the enhanced capacity of the distal intestine after partial enterectomy [21]. The adaptive capacity of the residual ileum after a proximal resection is dependent upon enteral stimulation, and the mechanisms involved include a sensitive feedback system involving malabsorbed nutrients reaching the distal gastrointestinal tract, the commensal microbiota, and the resulting production of short-chain fatty acids (e.g., butyrate) [21]. Intestinal adaptation is further enhanced through the stimulation of humoral factors such as glucagon-like peptide-2, peptide YY, and epidermal growth factor.

ENTERAL NUTRITION

Indications in SBS

Enteral feeding may be considered in the setting of SBS for the maintenance or improvement of nutritional status, residual bowel function (adaptation), and quality of life [22]. As previously stated, EN may be used when an adequate nutritional status cannot be achieved with oral nutrition alone in an attempt to avoid or eliminate PN use. This may be of particular relevance in the setting of serious

PN-related complications such as the loss of vascular access sites or the development of chronic liver disease. EN results in greater adaptation and should be instituted to the extent possible [23–26].

Postoperative Period (Hypersecretion Phase)

Studies describing EN use in SBS patients are scarce. In one small study of SBS patients [27], continuous EN administered through a gastrostomy, jejunostomy, or nasogastric tube in the early postoperative period (first 14 days) with polysaccharides, medium-chain triglycerides (MCTs), and protein hydrolysates mixed with a high-viscosity tapioca suspension was well tolerated and provided a high-caloric intake with a decrease in fecal volume despite a regular increase in the infused enteral volume. In that study, there was no comparison with oral intake alone and data on absorption were not provided. Thus, even if PN is obligatory in the postoperative hypersecretory phase to guarantee adequate nutritional intake and fluid and electrolyte balance [22], enteral feeding should also be considered, especially in those who cannot begin taking food orally. In general, the introduction of EN can be considered when bowel activity has resumed, diarrhea is limited to less than 2000 mL/day, and hydration and electrolytes are stable [28]. Cosnes et al. compared oral nutrition and continuous gastric tube feeding delivered in a series of five patients 5 to 12 weeks after massive ileal resection [29]. A 35% reduction in steatorrhea was seen during tube feeding with use of a nonelemental solution.

Adaptation and Stabilization Phases

More recently, a study was conducted to test the hypothesis that continuous EN could improve intestinal absorption in SBS. EN administered through a nasogastric tube for 7 days was compared with a regular oral diet after the early (first days) or late (more than 6 months after surgery) postoperative period; a standard polymeric solution containing 21% protein, 18% long-chain triglycerides (LCTs), 13% MCT, and 48% carbohydrate without fiber was used [30]. EN was found to increase the mean percentage absorption of protein, lipid, and energy compared with oral feeding. In a third group administered combined feedings (oral and EN), the total enteral intake and net percentage absorption for protein, lipid, and total energy increased compared with oral feeding alone (Figure 14.1). This study demonstrated a significant increase in net macronutrient absorption during continuous EN compared with oral feeding in a heterogeneous but representative series of 15 short bowel patients after the postoperative period (3 to 130 months after last surgery). The net gains per day were clinically relevant and represented 280 kcal for lipid, 23 g for protein, and 125 kcal for carbohydrate and a total energy gain of 700 kcal per day.

Furthermore, EN was well tolerated in all patients, and the supplement of 1000 kcal/day did not result in a decrease in oral intake in the short-term. While encouraging, it is difficult to determine whether the significant absorptive gain of lipids and proteins induced by EN was due to the continuous mode of EN and/or of the difference in the type of macronutrients used with EN. The authors suggested that continuous EN accommodates the gastric and small intestinal motor disturbances related to SBS and improves intestinal absorption by increasing nutrient-to-mucosa contact time [31–33].

Currently, EN is recommended in postoperative SBS patients [5], yet in one recent report from a large home EN program in Canada, only 9 of the 727 patients on EN had SBS [34]. While EN tends to be used more commonly among children with SBS, given the results previously described, tube feeding should be considered as a potentially effective nutrition therapy in intestinal rehabilitation programs for adult SBS patients after the postoperative period. Continuous EN, in limited amounts, could be used to improve intestinal adaptation during the adaptation phase [22]. Moreover, continuous tube feeding can be recommended for patients with a low level of home PN dependence and in whom the expected gain with tube feeding could potentially allow them to wean completely from PN [30]. In practice, EN can be used when patients cannot meet their needs orally. EN administered

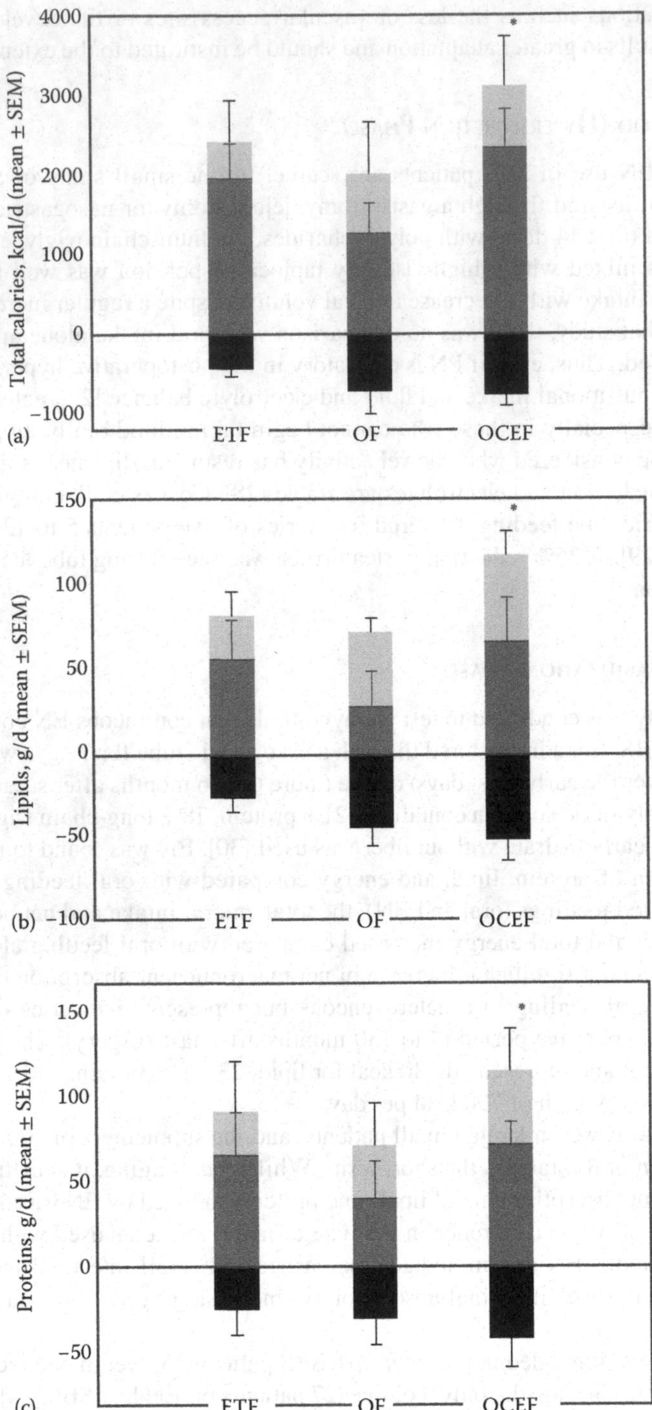

FIGURE 14.1 Net absorption for (a) total calories, (b) lipids, and (c) proteins during the three study periods. Intakes (in light gray) and losses (in black) are above and below the zero line, respectively, the dark gray being the net absorption (intake − losses). Total calories are expressed in kcal/d, and lipids and proteins, in g/d. *Total calories, fat, and protein intakes were significantly higher with OCEF than with OF and ETF ($P < 0.001$). ETF, exclusive tube feeding; OCEF, oral combined with tube feeding; OF, oral feeding. (Adapted from Joly, F. et al., *Gastroenterology*, 136, 824–831, 2009. With permission.)

nocturnally to deliver a portion of nutrients during a time that the GI tract is not in use should be considered in those not quite meeting their needs during daytime hours. With day and night feeding, it may be possible to meet the needs of some SBS patients and eliminate their requirement for any form of parenteral support [35]. A limiting factor for use of nocturnal EN in SBS, however, would be the potential for increasing stool output such that the patient might have to get up too often during the night to get adequate sleep.

MODALITIES OF ADMINISTRATION

Type of Enteral Feeding

According to a technical review, dietary macronutrient recommendations after the postoperative period depend upon the presence or absence of the colon: patients with a jejunocolic anastomosis should receive 30–35 kcal/kg per day of complex carbohydrates with soluble fibers, with 20–30% of caloric intake as fat in the form of MCTs and LCTs with intact protein (1.0–1.5 g/kg/day). In patients without a colon, there is no need for fiber supplementation; one study even showed an increase in fecal losses in patients with an ileostomy when guar gum was given [36]. In the end-jejunostomy short bowel patients, LCTs (which provide essential fatty acids) alone are recommended, with MCT being reserved for short bowel patients with a colon [5]. However, fat tolerance has to be evaluated individually [37]. Although dietary fat restriction may result in decreased fecal fat losses, there is no difference in the percentage of fat absorbed between high-fat/low-carbohydrate and low-fat/high-carbohydrate, isocaloric, and isonitrogenous diets [38]. Bosaeus showed a lower excretion of bile salts to the colon when a low-fat diet (versus medium-fat) is prescribed to patients after ileal resection and suggested that it could be an explanation of reduced diarrhea in these cases [39]. Because fat is energy-dense (9.0 kcal/g) when compared with carbohydrate (4.0 kcal/g), fat restriction may ultimately deprive the patient of a necessary source of energy [5]. In patients with a jejunostomy, the relative proportions of carbohydrate and fat are without significance [22]. However, if the colon is intact, the delivery of large amounts of complex carbohydrate can improve energy absorption up to 1000 additional calories per day through colonic bacterial fermentation of unabsorbed carbohydrates into absorbable short-chain fatty acids [40]. Patients with malabsorption are often able to compensate for the absorption deficit by increasing food and carbohydrate intake (hyperphagia) [41].

With regard to EN formula use in SBS, semidigested formulas are not superior to polymeric formulas, and there are no data to support the use of modified/supplemented formulas such as those containing glutamine or nucleotides [42]. Available evidence suggests that elemental and polymeric formulas are similar in terms of nutrient absorption and fluid and electrolyte loss [27,43]. Furthermore, polymeric diets are less costly and less hyperosmolar than elemental diets and are, generally, well tolerated.

Importantly, the more complex nutrients in polymeric formulas may enhance intestinal adaptation to a greater degree than elemental diets [44–46]. The mechanisms by which a complex diet may promote adaptation or an elemental diet may suppress adaptation are not well understood. It has been suggested that complex protein may protect certain endogenous or exogenous growth factors from destruction in the lumen by pancreatic or intestinal enzymes [47]. This would enable growth factors present in the lumen to maximally influence mucosal repair and regeneration. Another study showed that disaccharide infusion stimulates mucosal growth to a greater extent than monosaccharides do, suggesting that the functional work load of absorbing epithelium, including the "work of hydrolysis," plays an important role as a stimulus for intestinal adaptation [48].

Given these potential advantages, isotonic, polymeric enteral formulas are recommended for patients with SBS [49]. In the case of worsening diarrhea on a polymeric formula, a semielemental or elemental formula could be tried; however, the hypertonicity and total fat content of some semi-elemental products may limit their use in individual patients depending on their remaining bowel anatomy. Table 14.1 lists commonly used commercial EN formulas and selected nutritional contents.

The choice between regular (i.e., 1.0–1.2 kcal/mL) and high-energy (i.e., 1.5–2.0 kcal/mL) preparations will depend on the patient's needs; however, the greater osmolarity of high-energy enteral formulas may aggravate stool losses and the negative fluid balance that follows without nutritional gain. Commercial EN formulas are intentionally low in sodium content, and it may be necessary to introduce additional salt into the EN of short bowel patients with an end-jejunostomy [42,50] to make up for excess sodium loss in the stool (see Table 14.1). In these patients daily losses of sodium can be as high as 105 mEq (2430 mg) per liter of stool lost.

Enteral Feeding Access

Ideally, EN should be infused into the stomach, assuming it functions normally. Gastric feeding has many advantages, including ease of percutaneous access, buffering capacity of gastric acid, and protection against stress gastropathy [51]. Compared with feeding into the small intestine, feeding into the stomach has the advantage of slowing transit time through the gut by regulating flow across the pylorus; this may reduce the potential for diarrhea and enhance nutrient-to-mucosa contact time and, hence, absorption.

Enteral tubes can be placed transnasally or percutaneously via endoscopic, radiologic, or surgical methods. In the setting of SBS, it may be prudent to conduct a trial of feeding (e.g., for 4–7 days) via a nasogastric tube before proceeding to percutaneous gastrostomy insertion to ensure success of the regimen prior to placing more permanent access. As with other indications for EN, percutaneous access is recommended in the case of EN anticipated for >1 month. Thus, due to the sometimes poor tolerance of enteral feeding in SBS, a less invasive technique should be tried first. In some cases, however, a gastrostomy can be placed during the initial surgery that resulted in SBS or at the time of a planned elective surgery for another indication. Placement of a percutaneous gastrostomy tube may sometimes be technically difficult because of the altered anatomy and the presence of intra-abdominal adhesions [52]. Nevertheless, in most SBS patients, percutaneous access to the stomach can usually be obtained using either an endoscopic or a radiologic approach [51]. If these are unsuccessful or not feasible, surgical placement will be needed. Gastrostomy tube placement is associated with the same risks as patients with an intact gastrointestinal tract [53].

CONTRAINDICATIONS TO EN IN SBS

Complete mechanical obstruction is the only absolute contraindication to EN. Severe diarrhea or vomiting, enterocutaneous fistulae, and intestinal dysmotility, while presenting significant challenges, are not absolute contraindications. EN should not be used in the early postoperative period if there is a risk of peritonitis. When there is more than 2 L of stool/ostomy output per day, the use of EN is not recommended as stool output would be even higher [49].

SPECIAL CONCERNS OF ENTERAL FEEDING IN SBS

Coverage of EN Support

In the United States, coverage of enteral nutrition supplies including formula depends on the patient's insurance coverage. For Medicare to cover home EN, the beneficiary must have a permanent functional impairment of the gastrointestinal tract, so that enteral feeding is necessary and reasonable. The patient must also require EN for at least 3 months, which is Medicare's definition of "permanence." Therefore, SBS patients often meet these conditions. If so, the related enteral equipment, supplies, and nutrients may be covered under Medicare (who pays 80% of the charges) [54].

TABLE 14.1
Characteristics of Selected Commercial Enteral Formulas

Product	Maker	Calories/mL	Fat/L Total/ MCT (gm)	Na mEq/L	Na mEq/L with 1/2 Teaspoon Salt[a,b]	mOsm/kg	Total mOsm/kg w/Na Added[c]	Fiber or FOS +/–
				Polymeric				
Compleat	Nestle	1.0	40/0	43	95	340	444	+
Fibersource HN	Nestle	1.2	39/8.8	52	104	490	594	+
Glucerna 1.0 Cal	Abbott	1.0	54.4/0	40.4	92.4	355	459	+
Isosource HN	Nestle	1.2	39/8.8	49	101	490	594	–
Jevity 1 Cal	Abbott	1.0	34.7/7.0	40.4	92.4	300	404	+
Nutren 1.0	Nestle	1.0	38/9.5	38	90	370	474	–
Osmolite 1 Cal	Abbott	1.0	34.7/7.0	40.4	92.4	300	404	–
Promote	Abbott	1.0	26/5.0	43.5	95.5	340	444	–
Replete	Nestle	1.0	34/8.4	38.1	90.1	350	454	–
				Semielemental/Elemental				
Peptamen 1.5	Nestle	1.5	56/40	44.3	96.3	550	654	–
Peptamen Bariatric	Nestle	1.0	38/18.4	29	81	345	449	+
Peptamen Unflavored	Nestle	1.0	39/27.6	24.3	76.3	270	374	–
Perative	Abbott	1.3	37.3/15	45.2	97.2	460	564	+
Vital 1.0 Cal	Abbott	1.0	38/18	45.9	97.9	390	494	–
Vital High Protein	Abbott	1.0	23.2/11.6	60.8	112.8	353	457	–
Vital HN	Abbott	1.0	10.8/5.4	24.6	76.6	500	604	–
Vivonex RTH	Nestle	1.0	11.6/4.6	30	82	630	734	–

Source: Parrish, C.R. et al. *University of Virginia Health System Nutrition Support Traineeship Syllabus*, Charlottesville, VA, University of Virginia, 2013. With permission.

[a] 1/2 teaspoon = 52 mEq sodium.

[b] Goal is ~ 90–100 mEq/L in those patients with high jejunostomy/ileostomy loss [55].

[c] For 1 mEq of sodium, add 2 mOsm/kg to total osmolality (1 for Na and 1 for Cl), or total of 104 mOsm.

In a patient transitioning off of PN and on to enteral nutrition, both modalities can be covered under Medicare as long as the patient has required the PN for at least 3 months.

Diarrhea with Fluid-Electrolyte and Metabolic Disturbances

Increased fecal losses can be a problem of considerable consternation to SBS patients receiving EN resulting not only in impairment in quality of life but also fluid and electrolyte disturbances. In the absence of a colon, the loss of hormonal regulation of the gastrointestinal tract (due to lack of peptide YY and glucagon-like peptide 1) further contributes to the diarrhea from more rapid intestinal transit [55]. To enhance EN absorption, it is suggested that enteral feeding should be administered slowly, as opposed to rapidly using a bolus method, with a pump in a continuous or cyclic nocturnal or daytime schedule to increase the nutrient-to-mucosa contact time. Fluid and electrolyte balance should be monitored at the initiation of EN and periodically thereafter.

Metabolic problems, including deficiencies of electrolytes, micronutrients, or water, can occur in patients receiving EN. In SBS patients, hypokalemia, hypomagnesemia, and hypocalcemia are quite frequent and require periodic monitoring [56]. Special attention should also be given to sodium and magnesium intake because commercial EN formulas are generally low in sodium and magnesium content. Sodium and water loss are major problems for SBS patients with an end-jejunostomy. Chronic dehydration can become problematic and, in extreme instances, may lead to the development of recurrent nephrolithiasis and chronic kidney disease. Because of the high permeability of the jejunal epithelium, these patients may benefit from the addition of sodium chloride to their formula (Table 14.1) and/or the use of an oral rehydration solution, which can be administered through their feeding tube.

Unlike the patient with a normal digestive tract, the osmolarity of EN becomes a concern in the SBS patient. Stool/ostomy output can be aggravated not only by hypertonic formulas such as elemental products but also by the fructo-oligosaccharide (FOS) content of some formulas. Finally, significant, yet often overlooked, contributors are the liquid medications containing sugar alcohols such as sorbitol, mannitol, and xylitol that are given once enteral access is achieved [57–59].

Clogged Feeding Tubes

The occlusion of feeding tubes is a common and frustrating problem. Clogged feeding tubes are responsible for significant loss of delivery of EN and also increase risks and costs to patients in the event that the tube must be replaced [60]. Common factors that contribute to tube blockage include the instillation of medications, inadequate flushing with water, and use of a small-diameter tube. Whenever possible, it is best to use liquid medications; check with the patient's pharmacist for liquid equivalents. It is important to remember, however, that many liquid medications contain sorbitol, which can contribute to diarrhea and fluid loss in SBS. When a liquid formulation is not available, the medication should be finely crushed, mixed with water, and administered via a syringe to minimize the chance of tube blockage. Enteric-coated, sublingual, and sustained-release medications should not be crushed. Medications through the tube should be administered one at a time with 10–30 mL of water flush between each medication. Routine flushing with water is the single most effective preventive measure to maintain tube patency. Depending on the number of medications required, however, attention to the sheer volume of water (a hypotonic fluid) needed to take all the medications may be necessary to avoid exacerbating stool volume.

Clogs are best treated with a warm water flush using a 30- to 60-mL syringe to avoid excess pressure and tube breakage. Initially, the tube should be drained of all retained fluid above the clog. Then, 5–10 mL of warm tap water should be instilled and allowed to set for several minutes. Finally, gentle pressure should be applied with a syringe slowly in a back-and-forth milking fashion until the clog is free. Use of cola products, carbonated drinks, or fruit juices to declog a feeding tube is not recommended; the low pH of these liquids hardens the existing clog and precipitates remnants of any protein-based formula remaining in the tube. An alkalinized solution of non-enteric-coated pancreatic enzymes may be effective in unblocking enteral tubes. If these methods are unsuccessful, a variety of devices (e.g., brush or corkscrew device) can be inserted into the tube in an attempt to mechanically dislodge the blockage [60]. If the tube cannot be unclogged using these maneuvers, it will need to be replaced by a healthcare provider or caregiver who has received training to do this procedure.

Nutrient–Drug Interactions

Nutrient–drug interactions may be responsible for decreased absorption of some medications when administered via a feeding tube. It should be remembered that either the tube itself or enteral formula may alter medication bioavailability; therefore, the serum levels of medications requiring periodic assessment (e.g., phenytoin, theophylline, digoxin, lithium) should be carefully monitored.

In other situations, the location of the feeding tube needs to be considered before medications are given through the tube. For example, antacids infused into a jejunal tube will only provide an osmotic load, possibly causing diarrhea, while not achieving the desired neutralization of gastric content. Therefore, guidance of medication provision via a feeding tube by an experienced pharmacist is encouraged.

CONCLUSION

Enteral feeding may be considered in the setting of SBS for the maintenance or improvement of nutritional status, residual bowel function (adaptation), and quality of life. In SBS, polymeric EN formulas are not inferior to semidigested or elemental formulas and may enhance intestinal adaptation. The list below provides a summary of considerations when enterally feeding the SBS patient.

Summary recommendations for enteral feeding in SBS

- Feed into the stomach to slow transit through the gut, maximize surface area used, and recruit as many digestive processes as possible.
- Use standard polymeric, isotonic, or near-isotonic enteral products.
- Use an infusion pump for feedings, not bolus, to increase the nutrient-to-mucosa contact time to enhance maximal absorptive capability.
- Avoid hypertonic and fructo-oligosaccharide (FOS)-containing tube feeding.
- Avoid fiber-containing enteral products if the colon is absent.
- Avoid sugar alcohol-containing liquid medications.

REFERENCES

1. O'Keefe SJD et al. Short bowel syndrome and intestinal failure: Consensus definitions and overview. *Clin Gastroenterol Hepatol.* 2006;4(1):6–10.
2. Pironi L et al. ESPEN endorsed recommendations. Definition and classification of intestinal failure in adults. *Clin Nutr Edinb Scotl.* 2015;34(2):171–80.
3. Jeejeebhoy KN. Short bowel syndrome: A nutritional and medical approach. *CMAJ Can Med Assoc J.* 2002;166(10):1297–302.
4. Pironi L et al. Candidates for intestinal transplantation: A multicenter survey in Europe. *Am J Gastroenterol.* 2006;101(7):1633–43; quiz 1679.
5. Buchman AL et al. AGA technical review on short bowel syndrome and intestinal transplantation. *Gastroenterology.* 2003;124(4):1111–34.
6. Nightingale J et al. Guidelines for management of patients with a short bowel. *Gut.* 2006;55(Suppl 4):iv1–12.
7. Amiot A et al. Determinants of home parenteral nutrition dependence and survival of 268 patients with non-malignant short bowel syndrome. *Clin Nutr Edinb Scotl.* 2013;32(3):368–74.

8. Messing B et al. Long-term survival and parenteral nutrition dependence in adult patients with the short bowel syndrome. *Gastroenterology.* 1999;117(5):1043–50.
9. Carbonnel F et al. The role of anatomic factors in nutritional autonomy after extensive small bowel resection. *JPEN J Parenter Enteral Nutr.* 1996;20(4):275–80.
10. Heymsfield SB et al. Home nasoenteric feeding for malabsorption and weight loss refractory to conventional therapy. *Ann Intern Med.* 1983;98(2):168–70.
11. McIntyre PB et al. Nocturnal nasogastric tube feeding at home. *Postgrad Med J.* 1983;59(698):767–9.
12. Doldi SB. Intestinal adaptation following jejuno-ileal bypass. *Clin Nutr Edinb Scotl.* 1991;10(3):138–45.
13. Hines OJ et al. Up-regulation of Na+, K+ adenosine triphosphatase after massive intestinal resection. *Surgery.* 1994;116(2):401–7; discussion 408.
14. Hines OJ et al. Adaptation of the Na+/glucose cotransporter following intestinal resection. *J Surg Res.* 1994;57(1):22–7.
15. Joly F et al. Morphological adaptation with preserved proliferation/transporter content in the colon of patients with short bowel syndrome. *Am J Physiol Gastrointest Liver Physiol.* 2009;297(1):G116–23.
16. Joyeux H et al. [Short bowel syndromes in adults. Prognostic factors. Evaluation and treatment. Retrospective study. A propos of 80 cases]. *Chir Mém Académie Chir.* 1994–1995;120(4):187–92; discussion 193.
17. Briet F et al. Bacterial adaptation in patients with short bowel and colon in continuity. *Gastroenterology.* 1995;109(5):1446–53.
18. Levine GM et al. Small-bowel resection. Oral intake is the stimulus for hyperplasia. *Am J Dig Dis.* 1976;21(7):542–6.
19. Biasco G et al. Intestinal morphological changes during oral refeeding in a patient previously treated with total parenteral nutrition for small bowel resection. *Am J Gastroenterol.* 1984;79(8):585–8.
20. Crenn P et al. Net digestive absorption and adaptive hyperphagia in adult short bowel patients. *Gut.* 2004;53(9):1279–86.
21. Tappenden KA. Mechanisms of enteral nutrient-enhanced intestinal adaptation. *Gastroenterology.* 2006;130(2 Suppl 1):S93–9.
22. Lochs H et al. ESPEN guidelines on enteral nutrition: Gastroenterology. *Clin Nutr Edinb Scotl.* 2006;25(2):260–74.
23. Feldman EJ et al. Effects of oral versus intravenous nutrition on intestinal adaptation after small bowel resection in the dog. *Gastroenterology.* 1976;70(5 Pt 1):712–19.
24. Ford WD et al. Total parenteral nutrition inhibits intestinal adaptive hyperplasia in young rats: Reversal by feeding. *Surgery.* 1984;96(3):527–34.
25. Johnson LR et al. Structural and hormonal alterations in the gastrointestinal tract of parenterally fed rats. *Gastroenterology.* 1975;68(5 Pt 1):1177–83.
26. Morin CL et al. Role of oral intake on intestinal adaptation after small bowel resection in growing rats. *Pediatr Res.* 1978;12(4 Pt 1):268–71.
27. Levy E et al. Continuous enteral nutrition during the early adaptive stage of the short bowel syndrome. *Br J Surg.* 1988;75(6):549–53.
28. Sundaram A et al. Nutritional management of short bowel syndrome in adults. *J Clin Gastroenterol.* 2002;34(3):207–20.
29. Cosnes J et al. [Continuous enteral feeding to reduce diarrhea and steatorrhea following ileal resection (author's transl)]. *Gastroentérol Clin Biol.* 1980;4(10):695–9.
30. Joly F et al. Tube feeding improves intestinal absorption in short bowel syndrome patients. *Gastroenterology.* 2009;136(3):824–31.
31. Nightingale JM et al. Disturbed gastric emptying in the short bowel syndrome. Evidence for a 'colonic brake'. *Gut.* 199;34(9):1171–6.
32. Remington M et al. Abnormalities in gastrointestinal motor activity in patients with short bowels: Effect of a synthetic opiate. *Gastroenterology.* 1983;85(3):629–36.
33. Quigley EM et al. The motor response to intestinal resection: Motor activity in the canine small intestine following distal resection. *Gastroenterology.* 1993;105(3):791–8.
34. Cawsey SI et al. Home enteral nutrition: Outcomes relative to indication. *Nutr Clin Pract.* 2010;25(3):296–300.
35. Gong J et al. Role of enteral nutrition in adult short bowel syndrome undergoing intestinal rehabilitation: The long-term outcome. *Asia Pac J Clin Nutr.* 2009;18(2):155–63.
36. Higham SE et al. The effect of ingestion of guar gum on ileostomy effluent. *Br J Nutr.* 1992;67(1):115–22.
37. Ovesen L et al. The influence of dietary fat on jejunostomy output in patients with severe short bowel syndrome. *Am J Clin Nutr.* 1983;38(2):270–7.

38. Woolf GM et al. Diet for patients with a short bowel: High fat or high carbohydrate? *Gastroenterology*. 1983;84(4):823–8.
39. Bosaeus I et al. Low-fat versus medium-fat enteral diets. Effects on bile salt excretion in jejunostomy patients. *Scand J Gastroenterol*. 1986;21(7):891–6.
40. Nordgaard I et al. Colon as a digestive organ in patients with short bowel. *Lancet*. 1994;343(8894):373–6.
41. Cosnes J et al. Compensatory enteral hyperalimentation for management of patients with severe short bowel syndrome. *Am J Clin Nutr*. 1985;41(5):1002–9.
42. Forbes A. Short Bowel Syndrome. In: *Home Parenteral Nutrition*, Eds, Bozzetti F, Staun M, Gossum A. Wallingford: CABI. 2015:70–81. http://www.cabi.org/cabebooks/ebook/20143413850.
43. McIntyre PB et al. Patients with a high jejunostomy do not need a special diet. *Gastroenterology*. 1986;91(1):25–33.
44. Healey KL et al. Morphological and functional changes in the colon after massive small bowel resection. *J Pediatr Surg*. 2010;45(8):1581–90.
45. Bines JE et al. Influence of diet complexity on intestinal adaptation following massive small bowel resection in a preclinical model. *J Gastroenterol Hepatol*. 2002;17(11):1170–9.
46. Hua Z et al. Effects of polymeric formula vs elemental formula in neonatal piglets with short bowel syndrome. *JPEN J Parenter Enteral Nutr*. 2014;38(4):498–506.
47. Playford RJ et al. Effect of luminal growth factor preservation on intestinal growth. *Lancet*. 1993;341(8849):843–8.
48. Weser E et al. Intestinal adaptation. Different growth responses to disaccharides compared with monosaccharides in rat small bowel. *Gastroenterology*. 1986;91(6):1521–7.
49. Matarese LE. Nutrition and fluid optimization for patients with short bowel syndrome. *JPEN J Parenter Enteral Nutr*. 2013;37(2):161–70.
50. Nightingale JM et al. Oral salt supplements to compensate for jejunostomy losses: Comparison of sodium chloride capsules, glucose electrolyte solution, and glucose polymer electrolyte solution. *Gut*. 1992;33(6):759–61.
51. Valentine RJ et al. Does nasoenteral feeding afford adequate gastroduodenal stress prophylaxis? *Crit Care Med*. 1986;14(7):599–601.
52. Buchman AL. Use of percutaneous endoscopic gastrostomy or percutaneous endoscopic jejunostomy in short bowel syndrome. *Gastrointest Endosc Clin N Am*. 2007;17(4):787–94.
53. Lockett MA et al. Percutaneous endoscopic gastrostomy complications in a tertiary-care center. *Am Surg*. 2002;68(2):117–20.
54. Newton A et al. Understanding Medicare coverage for home enteral nutrition: A case-based approach. *Pract Gastroenterol*. 2013;37(5):10.
55. Scolapio JS et al. Gastrointestinal motility considerations in patients with short-bowel syndrome. *Dig Dis Basel Switz*. 1997;15(4–5):253–62.
56. DiBaise JK et al. Enteral access options and management in the patient with intestinal failure. *J Clin Gastroenterol*. 2007;41(7):647–56.
57. Halmos EP et al. Diarrhoea during enteral nutrition is predicted by the poorly absorbed short-chain carbohydrate (FODMAP) content of the formula. *Aliment Pharmacol Ther*. 2010;32(7):925–33.
58. Halmos EP. Role of FODMAP content in enteral nutrition-associated diarrhea. *J Gastroenterol Hepatol*. 2013;28(Suppl 4):25–8.
59. Barrett JS et al. Dietary poorly absorbed, short-chain carbohydrates increase delivery of water and fermentable substrates to the proximal colon. *Aliment Pharmacol Ther*. 2010;31(8):874–82.
60. Fisher C et al. Clogged feeding tubes: A clinician's thorn. *Pract Gastroenterol*. 2014;38(3):16–22.

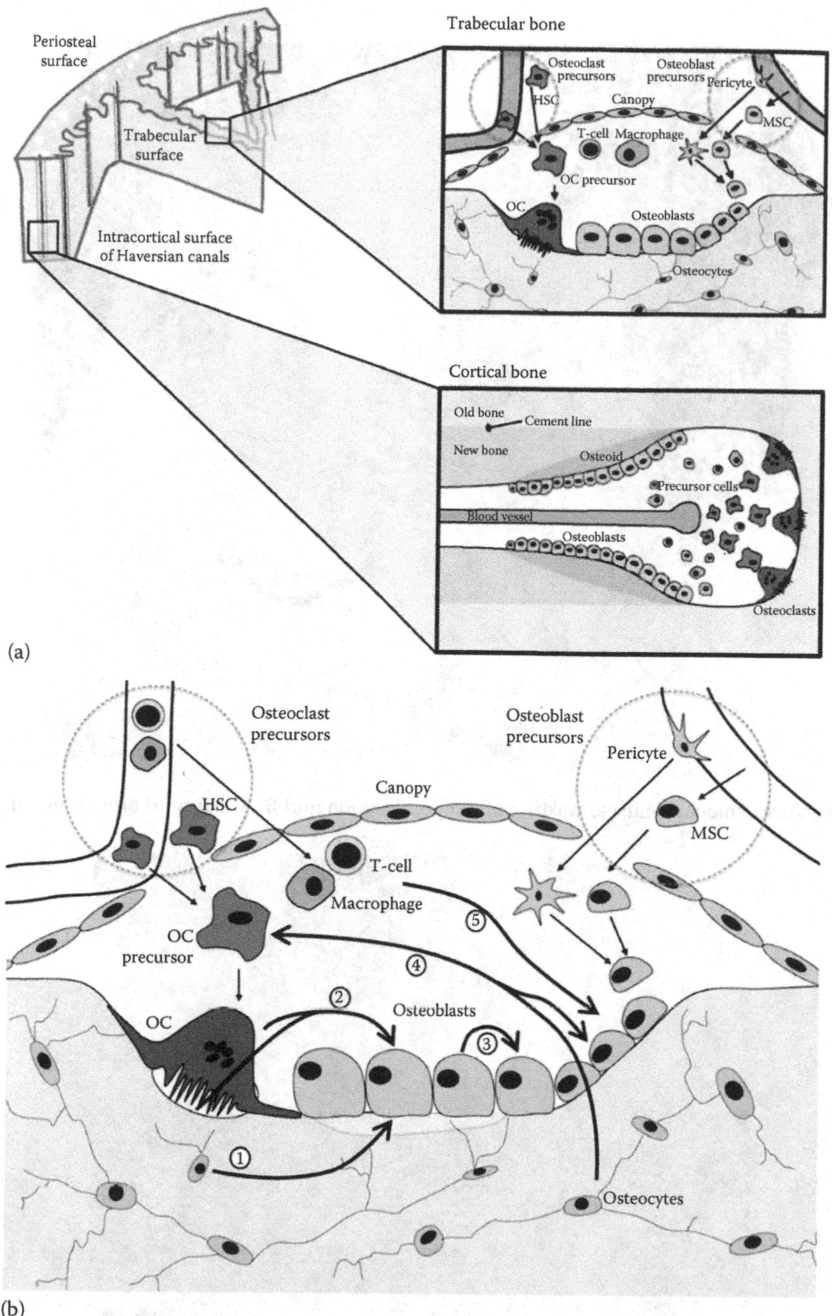

FIGURE 8.1 Osteoblast, osteoclast, and osteocyte interaction—the bone remodeling unit. (a) Remodeling is initiated within the bone remodeling compartments (BRCs) at points beneath the canopy of cells lining the trabecular bone (upper panels) and within the cortical bone haversian canals (lower panels). Osteoclasts (OCs) are formed from hemopoietic precursors (HSC) supplied by marrow and the bloodstream. Precursors of osteoblasts come from MSCs in the marrow, from blood and from pericytes, and differentiate within the bone metabolic unit (BMU) through the osteoblast precursor stage to fully functional synthesizing osteoblasts and to osteocytes. Lining cells may also differentiate into active osteoblasts. (b) Intercellular communication pathways within the BMU that comprise the remodeling process. (1) Stimulatory and inhibitory signals from osteocytes to osteoblasts (e.g., oncostatin M [OSM], parathyroid hormone–related protein [PTHrP], and sclerostin). (2) Stimulatory and inhibitory signals from osteoclasts to osteoblasts (e.g., matrix-derived transforming growth factor beta [TGF-β] and insulin-like growth factor-1 [IGF-1], secreted cardiotrophin [CT]-1, semaphorin-4D [Sema4D], and sphingosine-1-phosphate [S1P]). (3) Signaling within the osteoblast lineage (e.g., ephrinB2 and ephrin type-B receptor [EphB4], semaphorin-3A [Sema3a], PTHrP, OSM). (4) Stimulatory and inhibitory signals between the osteoblast and osteoclast lineages (e.g., RANKL, semaphorin-3B [Sema3B], wingless-type MMTV integration site family member 5A [Wnt5a], and OPG). (5) Marrow cell signals to osteoblasts (e.g., macrophage-derived OSM, T-cell-derived interleukins, and RANKL).

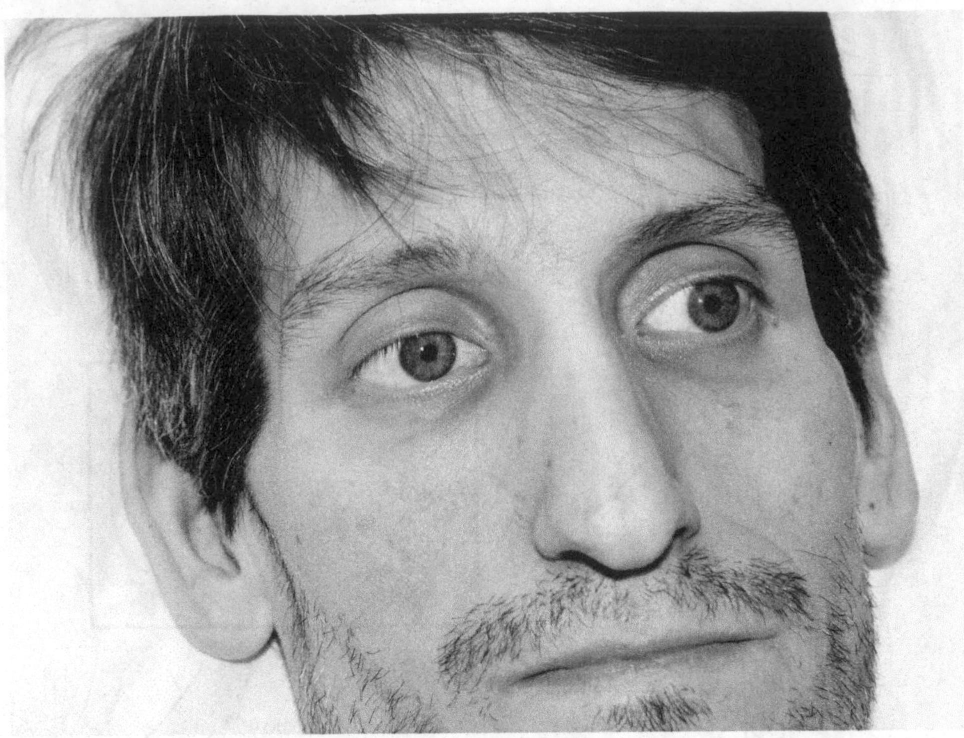

FIGURE 9.3 Assessment of muscle wasting of temporal region and fat wasting of orbital region.

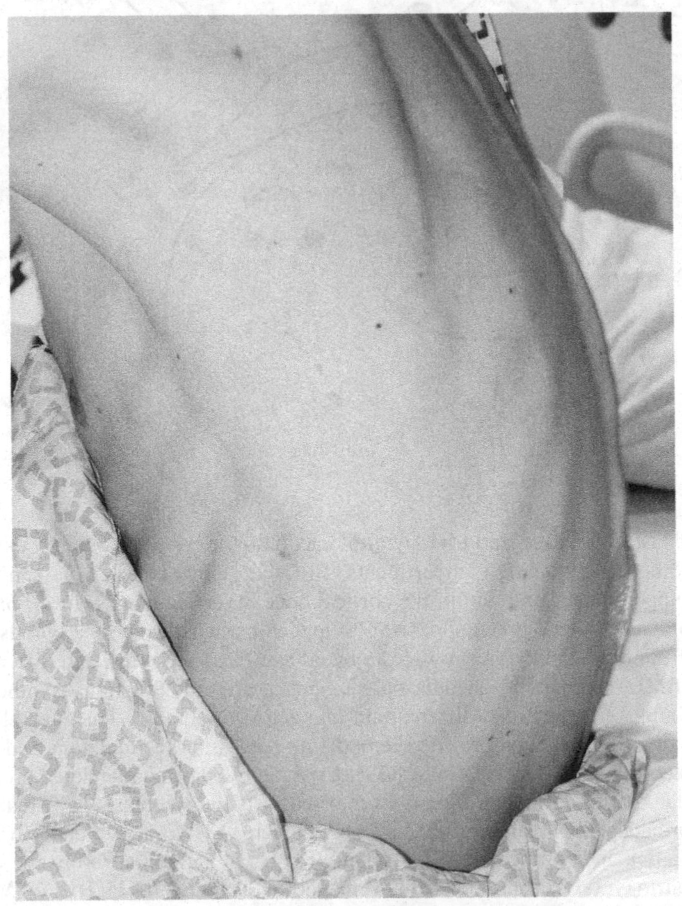

FIGURE 9.4 Assessment of muscle wasting of scapula and fat wasting of thoracic area.

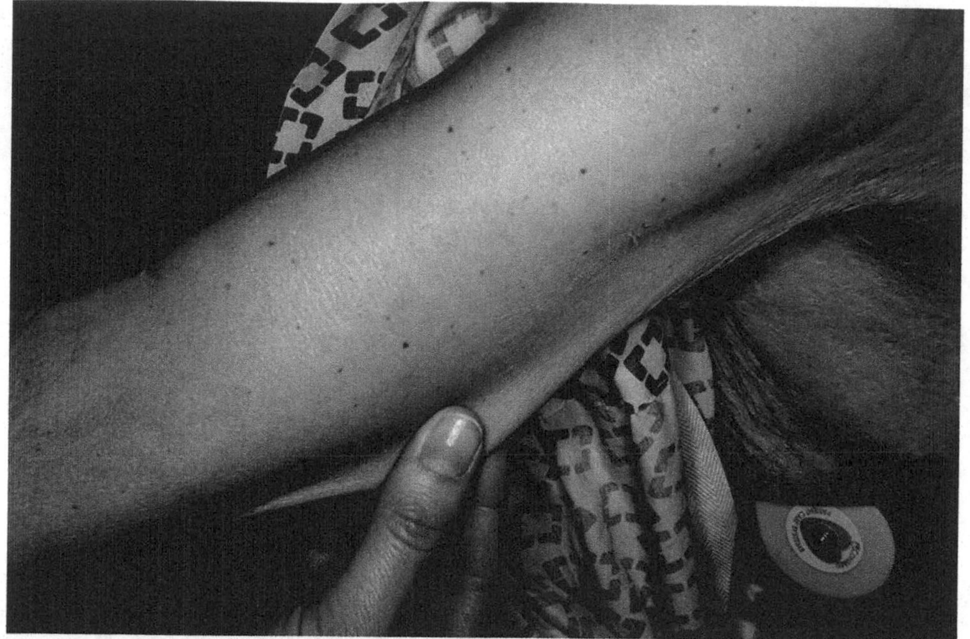

FIGURE 9.5 Assessment of fat wasting of the upper arm.

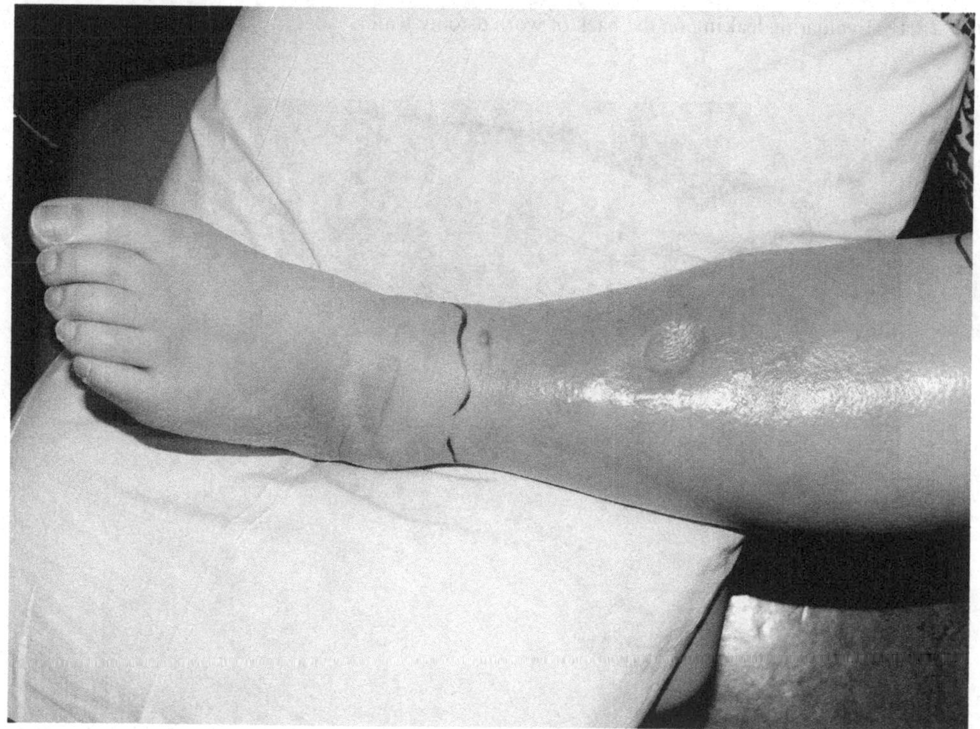

FIGURE 9.6 Assessment of lower extremity edema with a thumb print indention.

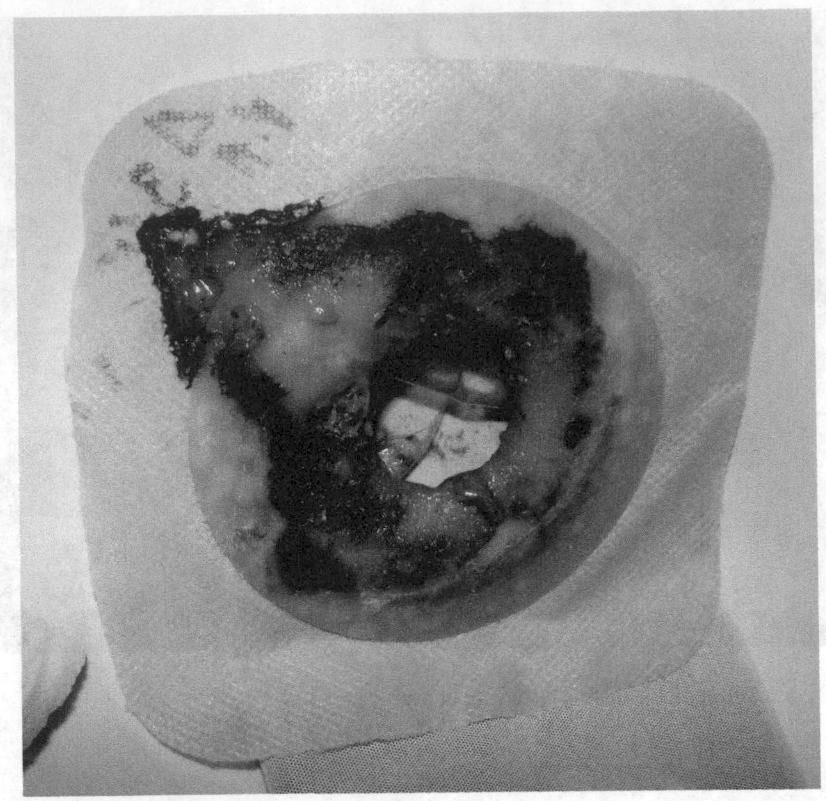

FIGURE 22.1 Evaluating leaking on the back of worn ostomy wafer.

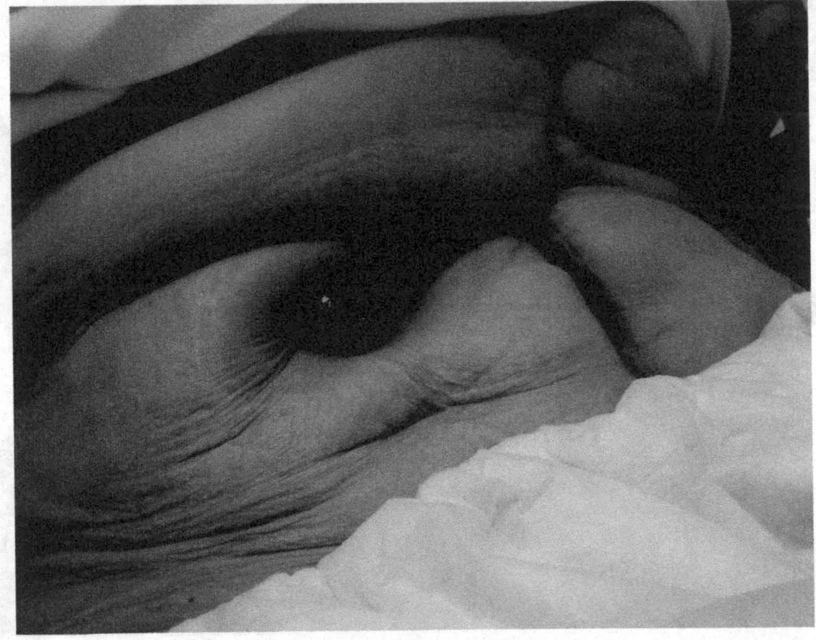

FIGURE 22.2 Stoma with deep peristomal skin creases.

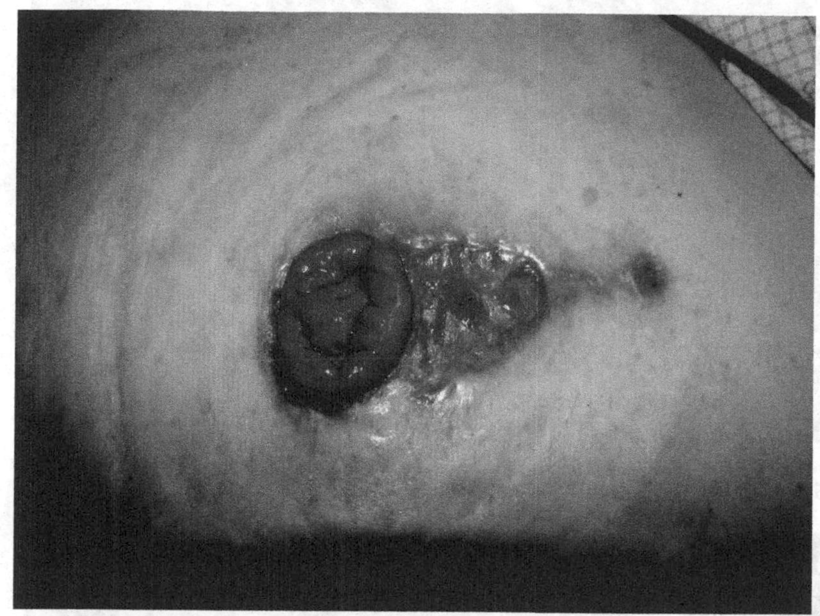

FIGURE 22.3 Stoma located near a scar.

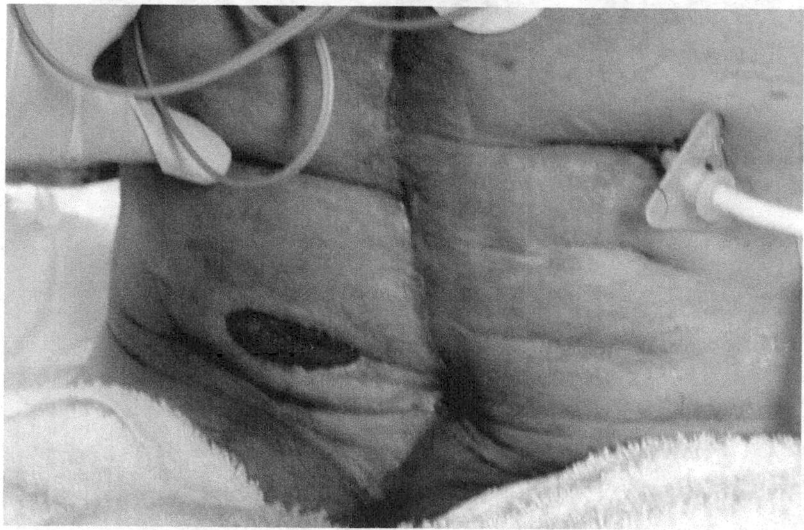

FIGURE 22.4 Stoma with low profile, crease, near fistula (distal midline); gastrostomy site with hypergranulation tissue.

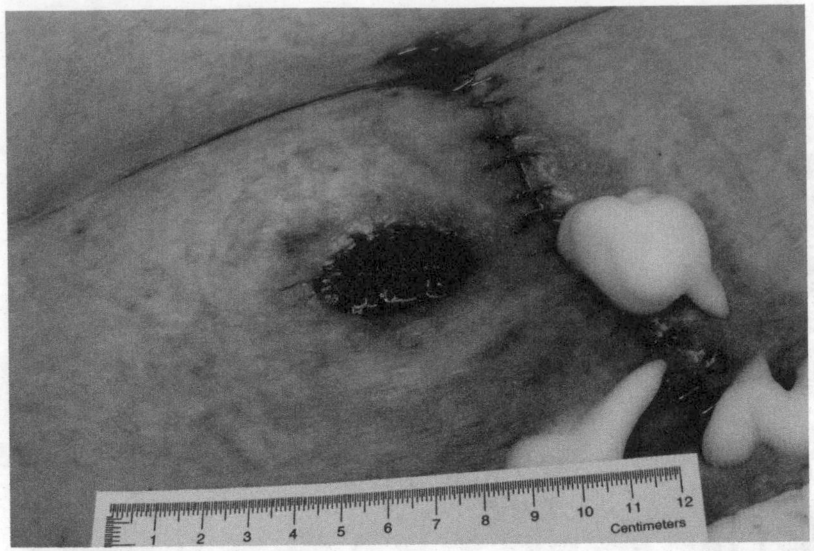

FIGURE 22.5 Stoma with low profile and skin level lumen.

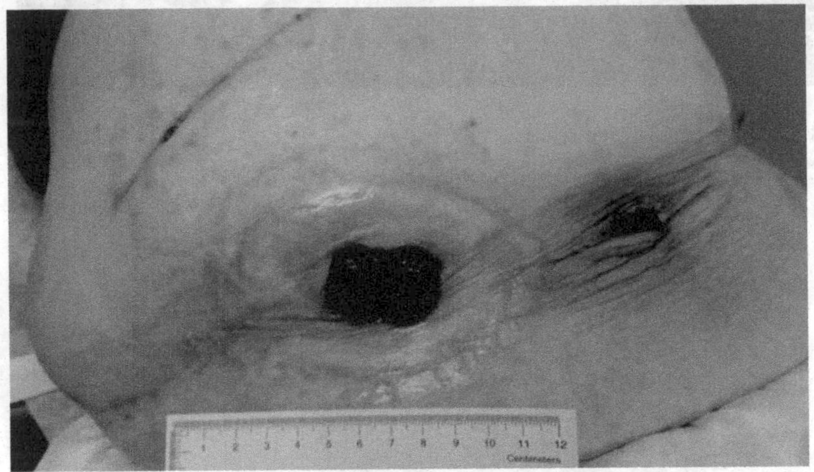

FIGURE 22.6 Stoma presentation with patient lying supine.

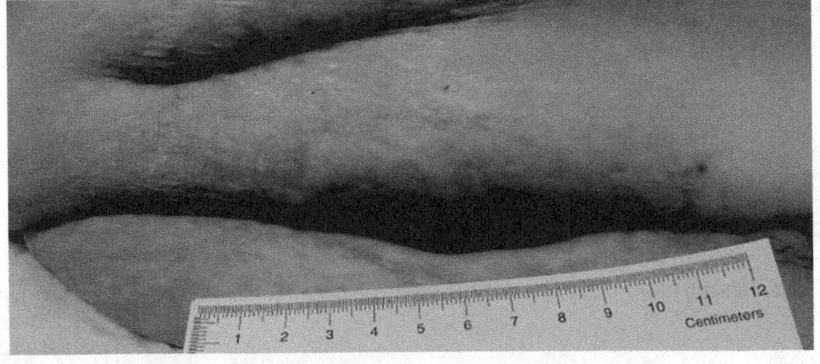

FIGURE 22.7 Stoma presentation with patient sitting upright.

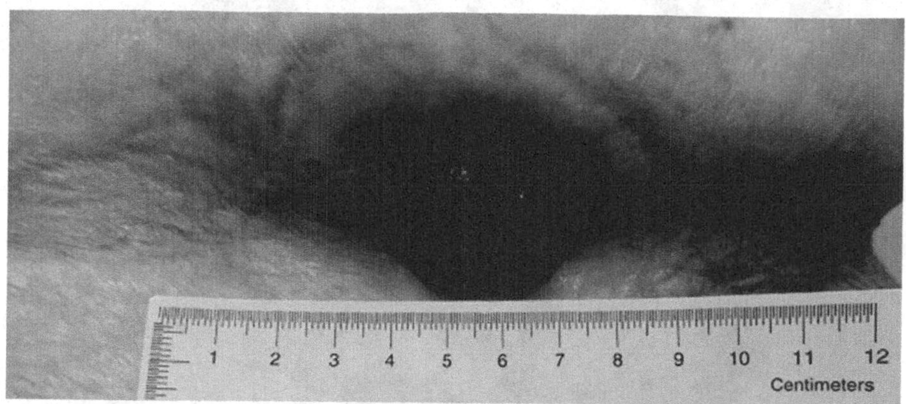

FIGURE 22.8 Stoma presentation with patient standing.

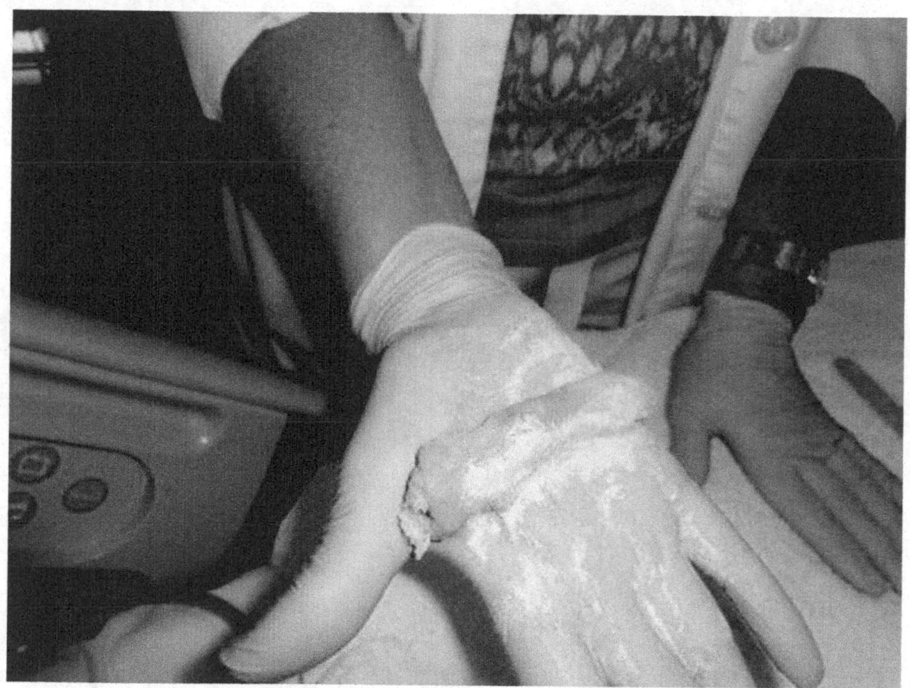

FIGURE 22.9 Combination of stoma paste and powder to create putty.

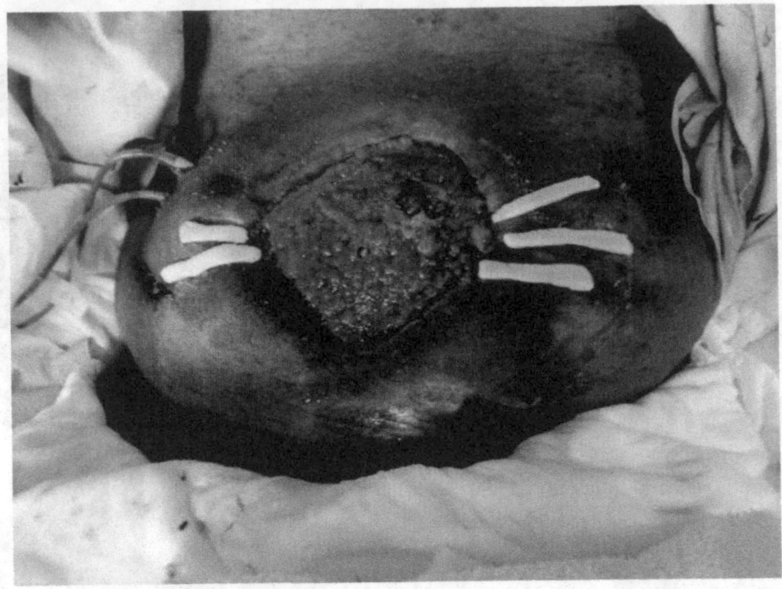

FIGURE 22.10 Filling in periwound creases with barrier product to even the plane for pouching.

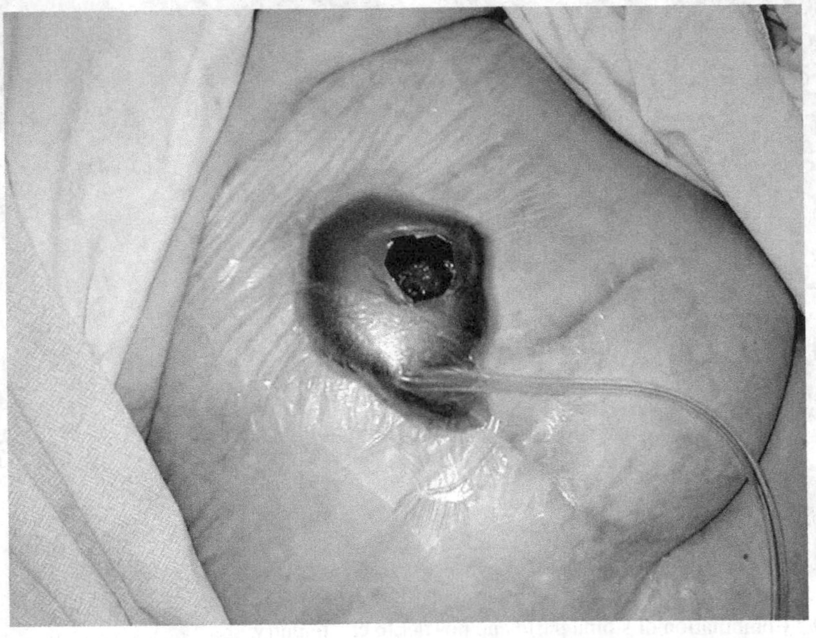

FIGURE 22.11 Negative pressure wound therapy for wound treatment with a fistula.

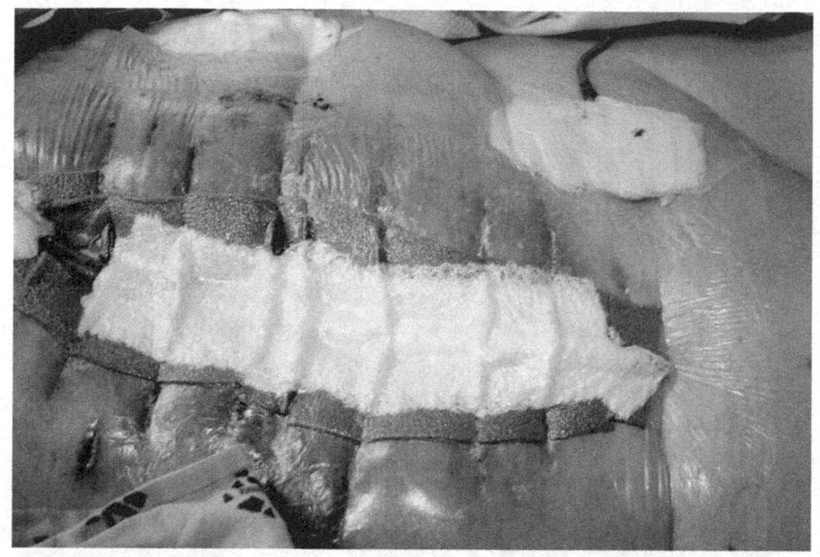

FIGURE 22.12 Custom-made fistula/wound management system connected to low intermittent suction.

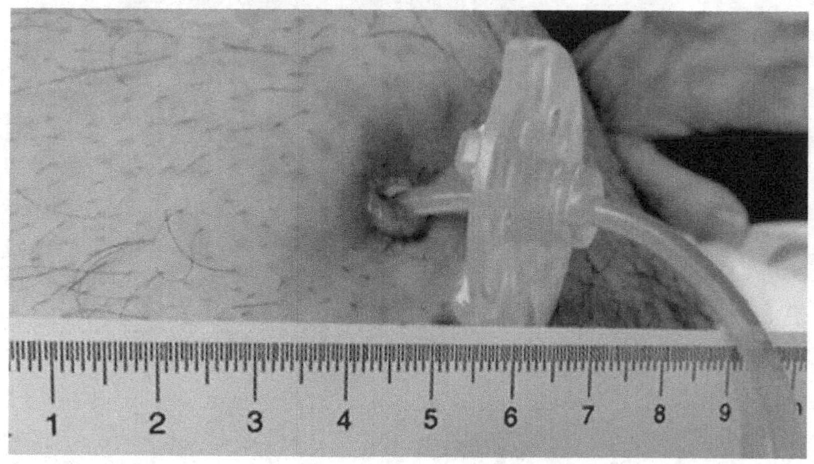

FIGURE 22.13 Gastrostomy tube mobility allowing hypergranulation tissue growth.

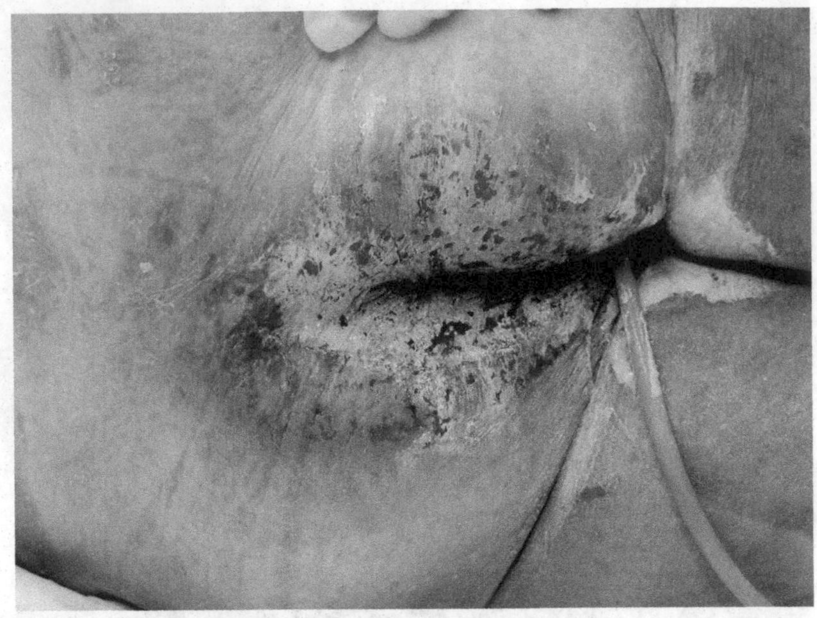

FIGURE 22.14 Severe fecal incontinence association dermatitis.

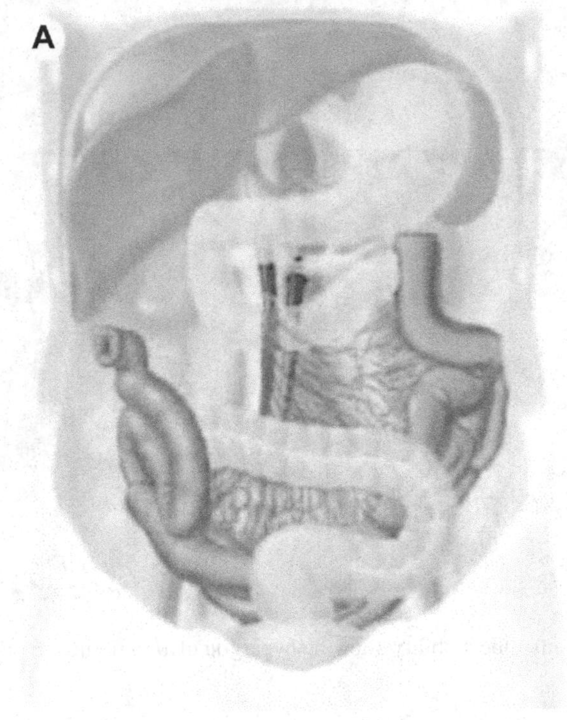

FIGURE 24.2 (A) Isolated intestinal graft. (*Continued*)

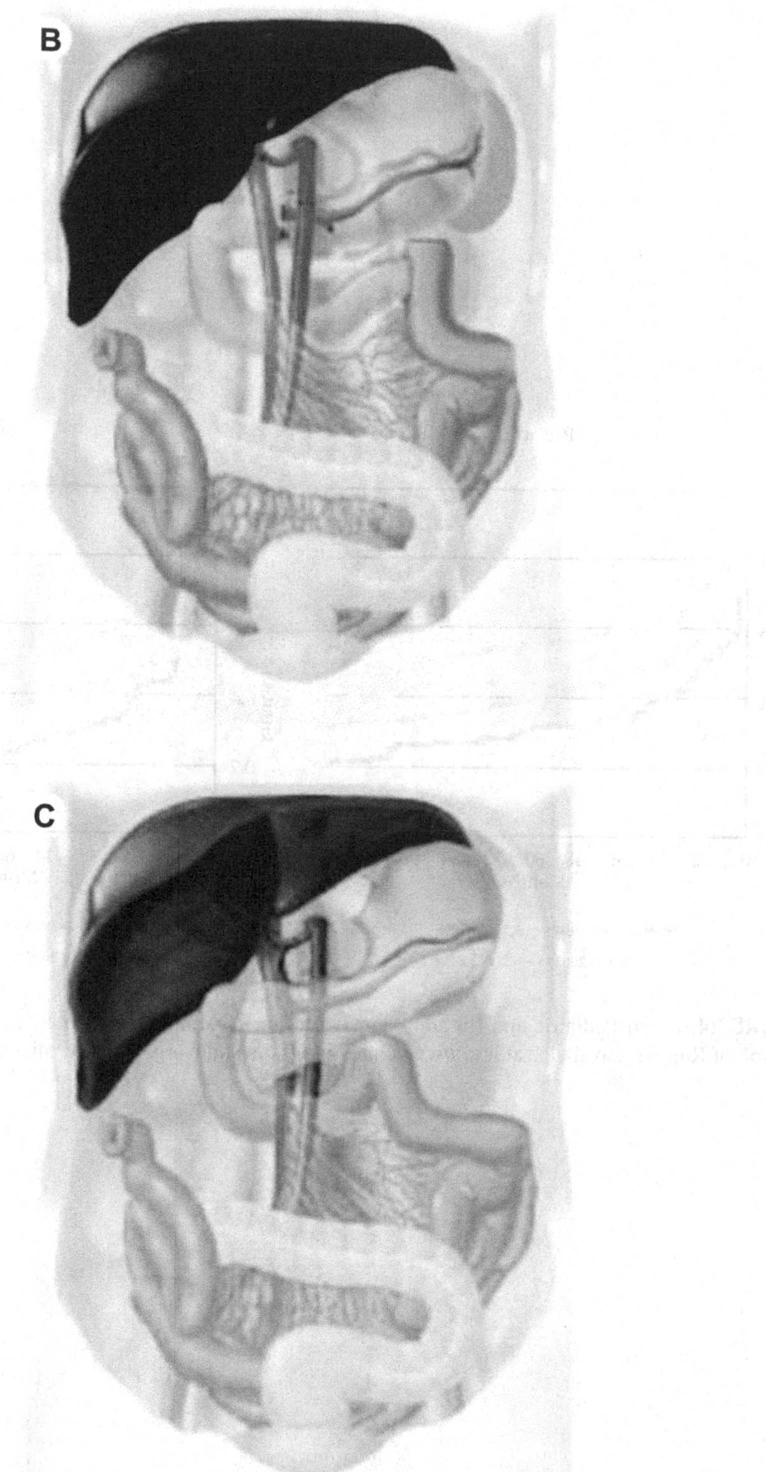

FIGURE 24.2 (CONTINUED) (B) Combined liver–intestinal graft. (C) Multivisceral graft. (From Fishbein, T.M. et al. *Gastroenterology*, 124, 1615–1628, 2003. With permission.)

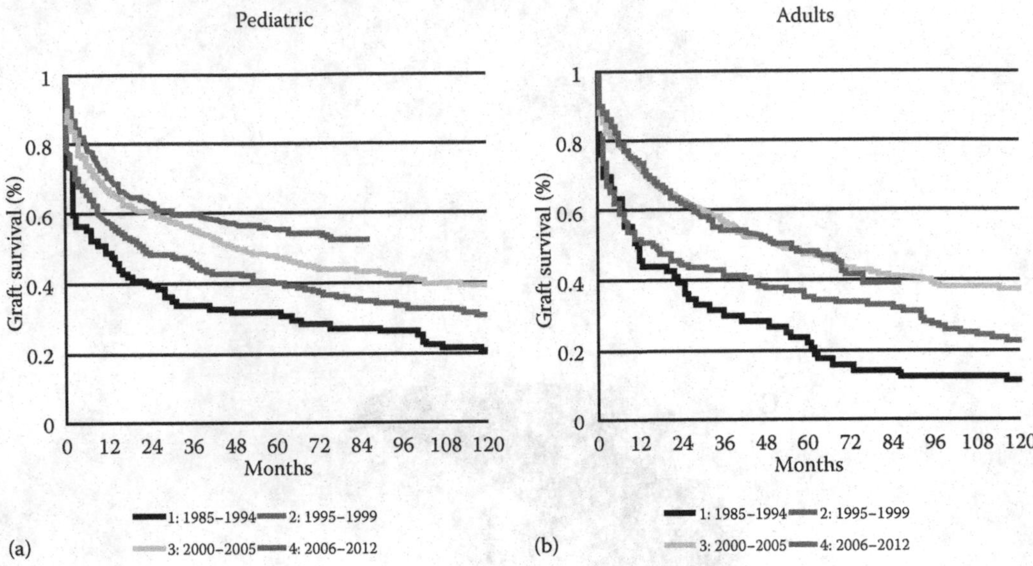

FIGURE 24.6 (a) Pediatric and (b) adult survival after intestinal transplantation by era. (From Intestinal Transplant Registry, available at http://www.intestinaltransplants.org. With permission.)

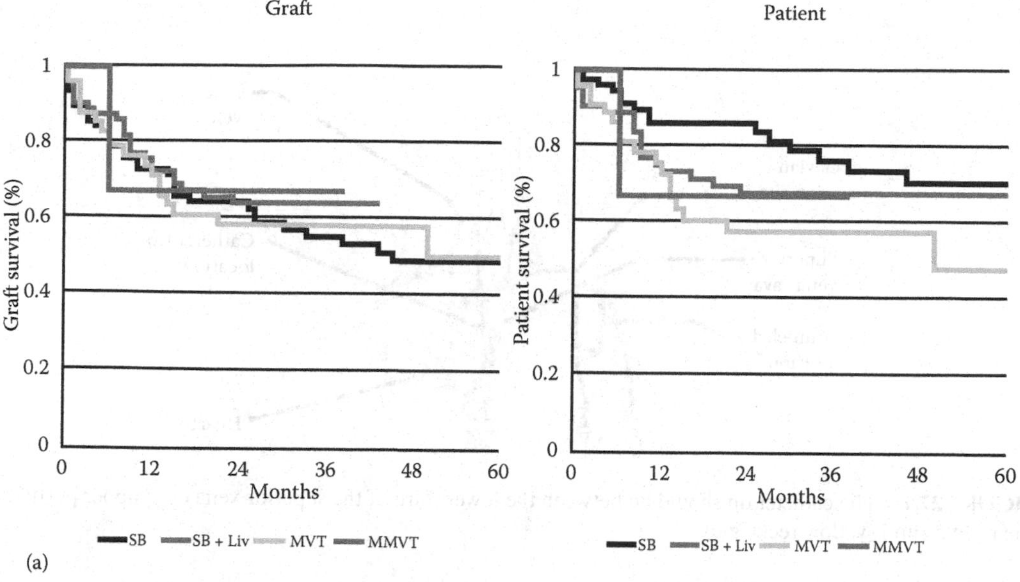

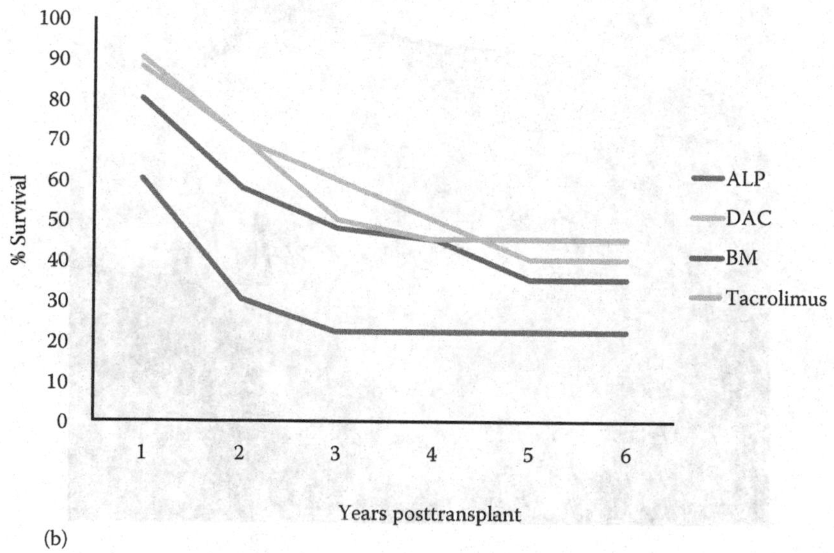

FIGURE 24.7 (a) Graft survival after intestinal transplantation by graft type (2008–2012). (b) Graft survival by induction agent. ALP, antilymphocyte product; BM, bone marrow; DAC, daclizumab. (From Intestinal Transplant Registry, available at http://www.intestinaltransplants.org. With permission.)

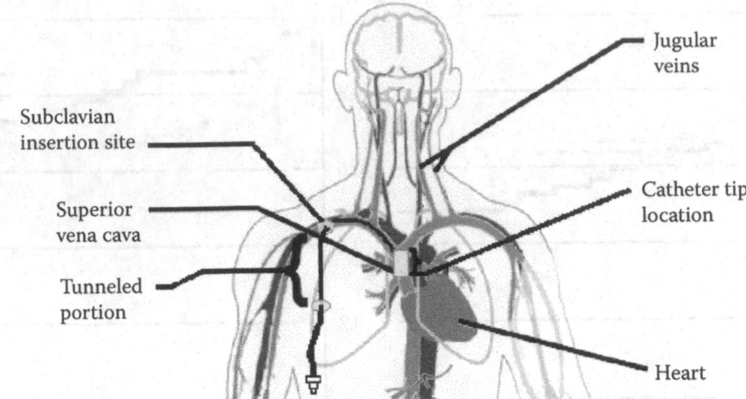

FIGURE 27.1 The catheter tip should be between the lower third of the superior vena cava upper portion of the right atrium (yellow rectangle).

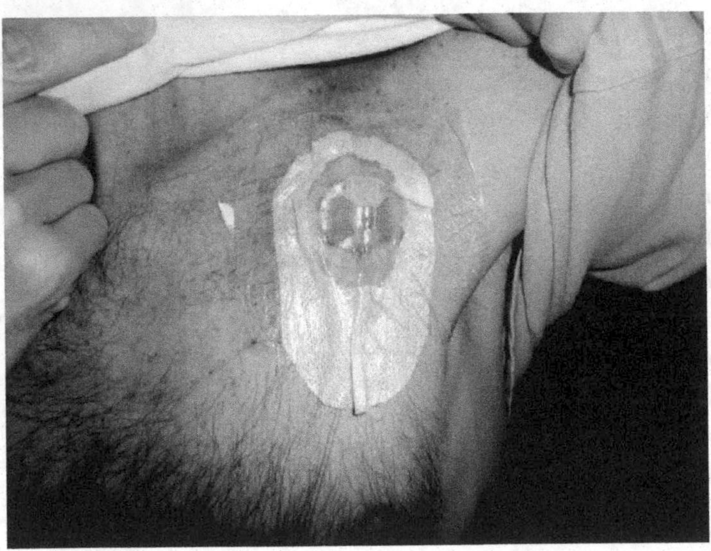

FIGURE 27.3 A subcutaneous port is accessed via an external needle.

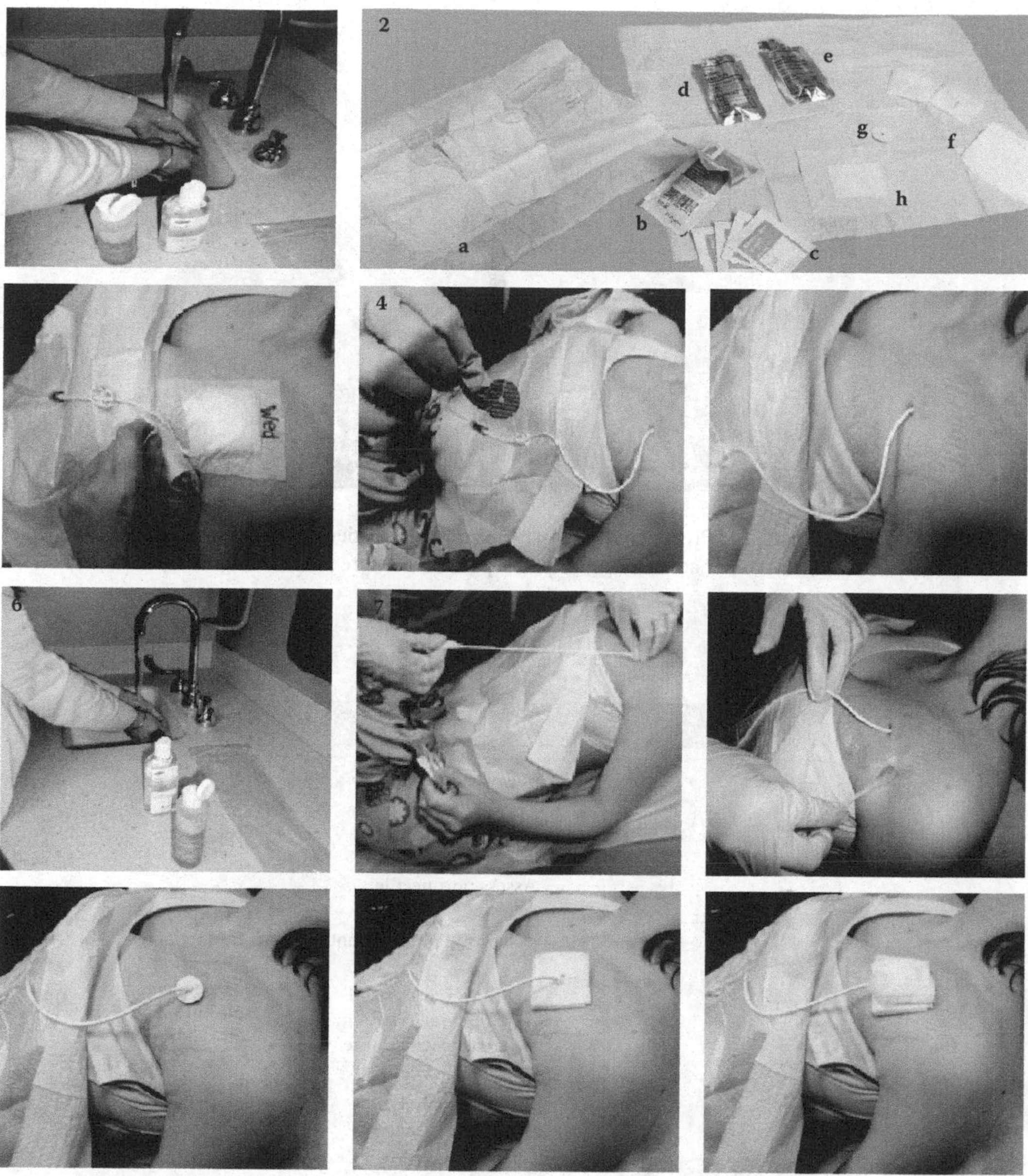

FIGURE 27.4 Procedure for dressing change. 1. Hands should be thoroughly scrubbed for 40–60 seconds with soap after CDC hand hygiene guidelines. 2. The materials necessary for the dressing change are organized on a clean surface and sterile sheet: a. sterile gloves, b. skin barrier film, c. alcohol wipes, d. alcohol swab, e. chlorhexidine or povidone-iodine swabs, f. gauze pads, and g. chlorhexidine gluconate (CHG) impregnated disk. 3. Remove dressing. 4. Remove CHG-impregnated disk. 5. Inspect and palpate exit site and tunnel. 6. Repeat hand-washing procedure, then don sterile gloves. 7. Clean line with 70% alcohol wipe. 8. Prep area by first lightly scrubbing with the chlorhexidine (or povidone-iodine) swabs provided no allergy or hypersensitivity to these, and use all three swabs, working in circular motions, beginning at the exit site and radiating out to clean the area. Then, repeat with the 70% alcohol swabs, allowing the area to dry in between. Apply the skin barrier film using the same technique. Allow film to dry. 9. Apply the CHG disk around the catheter, noting which side of the disk should contact the skin. 10. Apply the gauze pad with a hole for the catheter. 11. A second gauze pad is placed on top. *(Continued)*

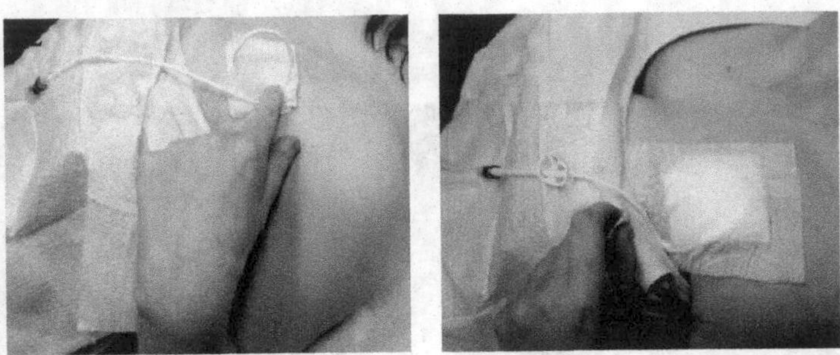

FIGURE 27.4 (CONTINUED) Procedure for dressing change. 12. Patient's finger holds back of the second dressing in place. 13. A final outer adhesive gauze pad is placed to secure the dressing.

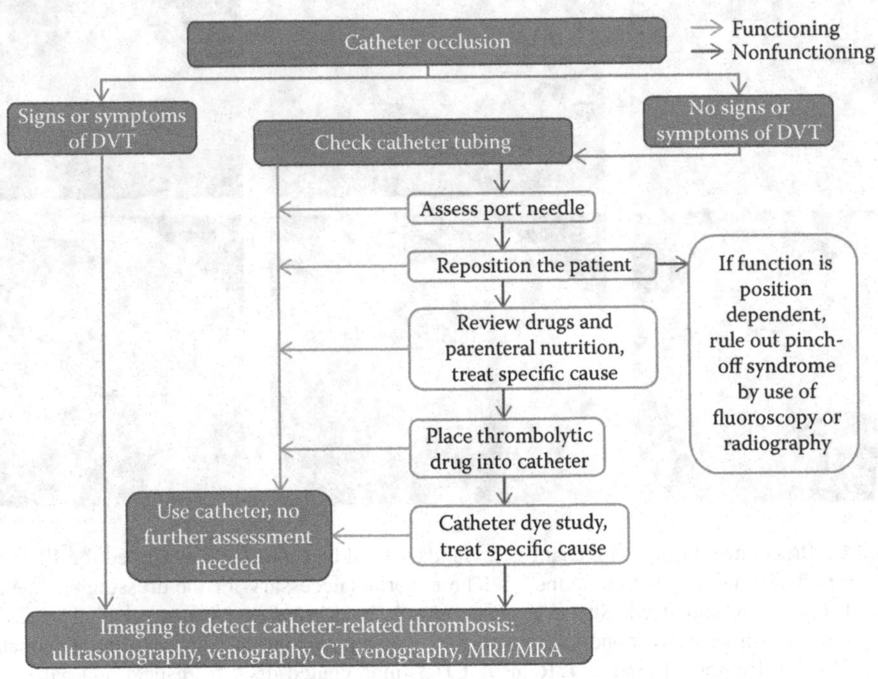

FIGURE 27.5 Clinical algorithm approach to catheter occlusion.

15 Parenteral Nutrition for Short Bowel Syndrome

Practical Aspects

Laura Matarese and Glenn Harvin

CONTENTS

KEY POINTS

- The primary goals for the use of parenteral nutrition (PN) in short bowel syndrome are to optimize nutritional status, prevent electrolyte and metabolic abnormalities, and preserve hepatic and renal function.
- Fluid and electrolyte composition of the PN must meet basal requirements as well as losses from ostomy effluent or diarrhea. The concentrations of all components must be consistent with the requirements for solution stability. The PN prescription must meet all vitamin and trace element requirements. Only those medications known to be stable in PN solutions should be added to the PN bag.
- The specific central venous access device will depend upon the length of therapy, nutrition requirements, goals of nutrition therapy, availability of central venous access sites, severity of illness, and fluid status.
- For short-term PN, typically provided in the hospital, a peripherally inserted central venous catheter or temporary nontunneled central venous catheter in the subclavian or internal

jugular vein is generally used. For those individuals requiring long-term PN, particularly in the home setting, a tunneled catheter or an implanted port is preferred.
- The patient who is receiving home PN should be monitored from both a clinical and biochemical standpoint.

INTRODUCTION

The goal of parenteral nutrition (PN), the administration of nutrients intravenously, is to maintain adequate fluid, electrolyte, and nutritional status in individuals who cannot absorb sufficient nutrients through the gastrointestinal (GI) tract. PN is a complex admixture of amino acids, dextrose, fat emulsion, sterile water, electrolytes, vitamins, and trace elements. PN is primarily indicated to provide nutrition to those patients whose GI tract is nonfunctional, inaccessible, or unsafe to use. The specific venous access will depend on the length of therapy, nutritional requirements, goals of nutrition therapy, availability of intravenous (IV) access sites, severity of illness, and fluid status. Provision of PN in any patient is complex; however, the provision of this therapy to individuals with short bowel syndrome (SBS) presents additional unique challenges. This chapter will focus on the specific issues associated with the provision of PN to individuals with SBS.

SBS AS AN INDICATION FOR PN

Intestinal failure occurs when GI function is inadequate to maintain the nutrition and hydration of the individual on a conventional diet [1,2]. SBS is the most common cause of intestinal failure. Patients with SBS typically experience severe diarrhea, steatorrhea, electrolyte disturbances, dehydration, nutrient deficiencies, malnutrition, and weight loss [2,3]. Conditions resulting in SBS include surgical resection due to Crohn's disease, malignancy, mesenteric vascular disease, trauma, postoperative catastrophes, and volvulus [3–5]. The end result is the same, an inability to digest and absorb sufficient nutrients to sustain bodily needs. Many patients with SBS will require long-term PN and/or IV fluids to maintain adequate fluid, electrolyte, and nutritional status. For these patients, PN, either in the short-term or permanently, is a life-saving therapy. The provision of PN to the SBS patient is associated with unique challenges due to the degree of malabsorption and presence of other complications associated with the underlying disease process.

CENTRAL VENOUS ACCESS

Once the decision is made to initiate PN, venous access will have to be established. Determination of the most appropriate venous access depends on several factors, including nutrient requirements of the patient, length of therapy, patient preference, ability of the patient/caregiver to manage or care for the device, and the availability of central venous access sites for cannulation. For short-term PN, typically provided in the hospital, a peripherally inserted central venous catheter (CVC) or a non-tunneled internal jugular and subclavian catheter is used. With any type of central venous access, it is important that the patient be able to see and reach the exit site to care for the catheter and connect the PN therapy. Extension tubing may be used to facilitate this access. For those individuals requiring long-term PN, particularly in the home setting, a tunneled catheter (e.g., Hickman, Broviac, or Groshong) or a subcutaneously implanted port may be used for access.

Since many patients with SBS will have an ostomy, it is important that the catheter be placed so that the proximal end is not directly over the ostomy, to reduce the risk of catheter-related infection. Again, the patient must be able to visualize the exit site to properly care for the catheter and connect the PN infusion. Correct catheter tip position is essential; the optimal location of the tip of a CVC is in the mid or distal superior vena cava adjacent to the right atrium to reduce the risk of catheter-related deep venous thrombosis. A retrospective study evaluated tunneled catheters in cancer patients and found that the incidence of venous thrombosis in patients with the catheter tip in the proximal superior vena cava was 41.7% compared with 5.3% in the mid and 2.6% in the distal portions [6]. This is a very important issue for patients with SBS as they are likely to require PN for long periods or even for life. Repeated thrombosis will ultimately result in vanishing sites of vascular access and is an indication for intestinal transplantation [5]. Chapter 27 reviews PN CVC-related concerns in more detail.

THE PN PRESCRIPTION

Designing the PN prescription for the patient with SBS requires consideration of numerous factors. The primary goals of PN are to optimize nutritional status and hydration, prevent electrolyte and metabolic abnormalities, and preserve hepatic and renal function. Optimizing nutritional status can be challenging in these patients as they are more susceptible to intestinal failure-associated liver disease (IFALD).

Patients with SBS will require PN in the initial postresection period until GI function returns and the patient is able to adequately consume an oral diet and fluids. Depending on the extent of the resection, some patients may be able to wean from PN during the period of intestinal adaptation, which may last 2–3 years [5]. Others may require partial or total PN long-term to maintain appropriate nutrition and hydration status.

FLUID AND ELECTROLYTES

The first step in designing the PN prescription is to determine fluid and electrolyte requirements. This is the most complicated aspect of writing the PN prescription in the SBS population as the PN must meet basal requirements and make up for losses from ostomy effluent or diarrhea. It is not unusual for these patients to require as much as 4 L of volume in the PN solution, especially if the patient has a high output jejunostomy. The SBS patient often presents at the time of initial evaluation with both clinical and biochemical signs of dehydration. They will typically experience thirst, which causes them to drink more by mouth, which then generally results in increased stool output, thus exacerbating the dehydration. The problem may be worsened further when they consume excess amounts of hyperosmolar and hypo-osmolar solutions. Although many SBS patients are PN dependent, most eat for pleasure. In some instances, oral fluid intake may need to be restricted to prevent excessive losses via the GI tract. Chapters 6 and 11 provide details on fluid and electrolyte problems affecting the SBS patient.

When making the transition from hospital to home, it should be remembered that fluid status in the hospital is maintained not only with PN but also with fluids from multiple sources, including IV medications and other supplemental IV fluids. These additional fluid volumes have to be considered when determining the final PN volume upon discharge. Some patients will also require supplemental IV fluids in addition to the PN to maintain hydration; this is especially the case when fluid requirements exceed the 4-L maximum volume of the PN bag. Another situation where additional IV fluids may need to be administered is during the summer months in hot weather locations, to compensate for increased insensible losses, particularly in active individuals.

Although attempts are generally made to cycle the PN infusion over a 12-hour period, it is not unusual to provide the PN over longer periods or even continuously to prevent periods of dehydration and damage to the kidneys. This approach often allows for better fluid utilization without fluid overload. If fluid status cannot be maintained with this approach, supplemental IV fluids such as normal saline can be infused when the patient is not on PN.

Determination of the electrolyte composition of the PN solution is dependent largely on the amount and source of GI losses (Table 15.1). For example, a patient with an ileostomy is likely to require more acetate to replace bicarbonate losses than would a patient with a colostomy. Accurate intake and output records are helpful in determining the GI losses and resulting electrolyte requirements.

TABLE 15.1
Volume and Electrolyte Content of Gastrointestinal Secretions

	Volume (mL/24 hours)	Na^+ (mEq/L)	K^+ (mEq/L)	Cl^- (mEq/L)	$HCO3^-$ (mEq/L)
Saliva	1500	10	26	10	30
	(500–2000)	(2–10)	(20–30)	(8–18)	–
Stomach	1500	60	10	130	–
	(100–4000)	(9–116)	(0–32)	(8–154)	
Duodenum	–	140	5	80	–
	(100–2000)	–	–	–	
Ileum	3000	140	5	104	30
	(100–9000)	(80–150)	(2–8)	(43–137)	–
Colon	–	60	30	40	–
Bile	–	145	5	100	35
	(50–800)	(131–164)	(3–12)	(89–180)	–
Pancreas	–	140	5	75	115
	(100–800)	(113–185)	(3–7)	(54–95)	–

Source: Whitmire, S.J., in: *Contemporary Nutrition Support Practice*, Matarese, L.E., Gottschlich, M.M., WB Saunders, Philadelphia, PA, 2003, p. 125. With permission.

Macronutrients

PN should provide sufficient energy to achieve and maintain a healthy body weight. Due to the heterogeneity of the SBS patient population, there are no specific recommendations for energy requirements. However, considering the severe malabsorption often experienced by these patients and their overall inability to maintain a healthy body weight, caloric requirements have been estimated at 32 kcal/kg/day [7,8]. Calories are derived mainly from carbohydrate in the form of dextrose and fat from IV lipid emulsions. Providing the optimal amount of calories to induce weight gain without damaging the liver can be difficult. Patients with SBS may require 2.5 to 6 g/kg/day of dextrose depending on the level of repletion required [7,8]. In long-term PN patients, it is recommended that IV lipids not exceed 1.0 g/kg/day [9]. For those individuals who are most susceptible to IFALD, it is best to provide the minimum level of total calories to support body weight and provide only enough lipid to meet requirements for essential fatty acids, approximately 1% to 2% of total calories derived from linoleic acid, and 0.5% from α-linolenic acid. In the SBS population, 1 to 1.5 g/kg/day of protein in the form of amino acids is generally required [7,10]. Overfeeding of any of the macronutrients, especially lipid, should be avoided to prevent complications [11,12].

PN Solution Stability

When designing the PN prescription, it is important to make certain that the concentrations of all components are such that the requirements for solution stability are met [13,14]. This is especially important for the patient receiving home PN since a 1-week supply is generally delivered by the home infusion provider and the solution instability increases over time. Strict adherence to these guidelines is mandatory.

When considering the stability of a total nutrient admixture (TNA) solution in which the dextrose, amino acids, and lipids are mixed together, there are several areas of immediate concern. The stability of a TNA is influenced by several factors: order of compounding, mixing technique, pH, buffer capacity of amino acids, concentration of electrolytes (including monovalents, divalents, and phosphates), addition of nonnutrient drugs, and storage conditions. Positively charged cations, commonly added to TNAs (e.g., Na^+, K^+, Ca^{2+}, and Mg^{2+}), are capable of destabilizing lipid injectable emulsions and may produce a fat embolism syndrome. Although others may be added (e.g., trace minerals), their amounts generally do not produce stability problems, with the exception of iron (Fe^{3+}), which can induce significant instability within 12–24 hours after compounding in amounts as low as 2 mg/L. As a rule, monovalents (Na^+, K^+) are the least destabilizing, with trivalent cations being most destabilizing (i.e., increase valence, increase destabilizing potential). The potential for dissociation and destabilization of lipid emulsions increases over time. Published stability data of macronutrients in soybean oil-based TNAs investigated over 24–48 hours at room temperature are listed in the following [14]:

Amino acids	≥4%
Dextrose	≥10%
Lipid	≥2%

The final concentration of lipids in TNA formulas affects destabilization. IV lipid emulsions are stable by virtue of a phospholipid coating and negative electrical charges surrounding each of the lipid particles, causing a repellent effect and preventing coalescence. High-lipid-concentration formulas tend to be more stable than low-concentration ones most likely due to the dilutional effect on the phospholipid emulsifier when the final concentration of lipid emulsion is low. A 2% solution is the minimum amount required to prevent destabilization of the lipid emulsion. Thus, a 2000-mL bag of PN should have a minimum of 40 g of lipid. If a 2.5% or 3% lipid concentration can be prescribed without impacting liver function, this would most likely reduce the risk even further, especially for the ambulatory bags, which must have a longer stability. In the hospital, concentrations of lipid less than 2% can be used if the lipid is infused separately via a Y-site adapter. Since use of a separate lipid infusion via a Y-site adapter requires administration via an additional infusion pump, this is discouraged in the ambulatory setting, where there is preference for TNAs designed for optimal patient safety and ease of usage. Lipids provide an excellent growth medium for bacteria and yeast. Therefore, lipid infusions provided separately in 2-in-1 formulations should preferably be infused over 12 hours to reduce the risk of infection and to promote adequate hepatic and systemic clearance. Lipids included in TNA formulations (i.e., 3-in-1 formulations) can be infused over 24 hours. Adherence to these guidelines should ensure a 24- to 48-hour stability of all PN solutions. This is clearly an important issue in the home PN population, where large volumes are often necessary due to extraordinary fluid requirements. Since many patients with SBS require large amounts of volume to maintain hydration status, this may require a minimal amount of fluid in the PN bag to meet stability requirements with additional IV fluids provided outside of the PN.

When using TNA therapy in the ambulatory setting, a dual-chamber bag that separates the lipids from the amino acid–dextrose–electrolyte mixture should be used whenever possible. In this way, the stability of the TNA coincides with the "activation" of the bag by the patient just prior to infusion, so that its "mix time" is commensurate with the cycled infusion (e.g., 8–16 hours) versus when premixed and provided with up to 2-week beyond-use times. Alternatively, if the home infusion company cannot provide dual-chamber bags, supplemental IV hydration fluids may be used in addition to the TNA formulation to meet fluid and electrolyte requirements. Additionally, no more than a 2-week supply should be dispensed to any home PN patient due to concerns about the stability of all additives over time.

Another major concern is with the potential to form an insoluble precipitate when calcium and phosphorus are added to the PN solutions. The most accurate method to check for calcium–phosphorus precipitation is with the use of a solubility curve.

Filtration during administration is recommended for all PN solutions to minimize the infectious risks from microbial contamination from multiple sources and to reduce the risk of air embolism and lethal embolic precipitates. A 0.2-μm filter should be used for 2-in-1 formulations, and a 1.2-μm filter, for 3-in-1 formulations. Note, the use of an in-line filter will not guarantee safety; strict adherence to compatibility limits is still necessary. If the TNA is unstable, the resulting incompatibility can expose the systemic circulation to potentially embolic large-diameter fat globules, since the filter does not completely trap the "flexible fat globules" from passing through a much smaller pore size (e.g., 1.2 μm), especially during a pump infusion and its associated pressures. These large-diameter fat globules can lodge in the pulmonary circulation, causing a capillary fat embolism, or they can pass on to the liver via the reticuloendothelial system, producing oxidative stress and injury to liver tissues. Additionally, exposure of unstable large-diameter fat globules to the permanent CVC has caused significant occlusions to the catheter in home PN patients.

PN Vitamins and Trace Elements

The PN prescription must meet all vitamin and trace element requirements. Serum vitamin and trace element levels should be measured as appropriate for all patients requiring long-term PN so that deficiencies can be identified and the prescription can be customized to meet the specific patient requirements. There are commercially available standard IV multivitamin and multitrace element preparations (Tables 15.2 and 15.3), but these do not meet the needs of patients with SBS requiring long-term PN who have existing deficiencies [15]. This is particularly important for those patients with excessive GI losses or for patients with hepatobiliary insufficiency who may develop deficiencies and/or excesses despite normal levels at the time of PN initiation [16]. Iron is not routinely added to the standard multitrace element preparations due to the potential for anaphylaxis, concerns of iron overload and ill-effects on the immune system, and the potential to destabilize the lipid emulsion in the 3-in-1 PN solutions. Thus, iron supplementation generally needs to be provided outside of the PN (or at least in non-lipid-containing PN solutions). Finally, there is a small amount of vitamin K in the multivitamin preparation. This amount is generally insufficient to affect anticoagulation therapy; however, coagulation parameters should be monitored in those PN-requiring individuals on anticoagulation therapy to ensure adequate dosing. Chapters 12 and 13 describe micronutrient deficiencies and toxicities in more detail.

TABLE 15.2
Adult Intravenous Multiple Vitamin Product Composition

Vitamin	Requirement and Product Dose
Ascorbic acid	200 mg
Retinol	1 mg (3300 USP units)
Ergocalciferol	5 μg (200 USP units)
Thiamine	6 mg
Riboflavin	3.6 mg
Pyridoxine	6 mg
Niacinamide	40 mg
Dexpanthenol	15 mg
DL-α-tocopherol acetate	10 mg (10 USP units)
Biotin	60 μg
Folic acid	600 μg
Cyanocobalamin	5 μg
Phylloquinone	150 μg

TABLE 15.3
Adult Intravenous Multiple Trace Element Composition[a]

	Requirement	Multitrace 4[b]	Multitrace 4 Concentrate[b]	Multitrace 5[b]	Multitrace 5 Concentrate[b]	Addamel N[c]
Zinc	2.5–5 mg	1 mg	5 mg	1 mg	5 mg	0.65 mg
Copper	0.3–0.5 mg	0.4 mg	1 mg	0.4 mg	1 mg	0.13 mg
Manganese	60–100 μg	0.1 mg	0.5 mg	0.1 mg	0.5 mg	0.027 mg
Chromium	10–15 μg	4 μg	10 μg	4 μg	10 μg	1 μg
Selenium	20–60 μg	–	–	20 μg	60 μg	3.2 μg
Iron		–	–	–	–	0.11 mg
Molybdenum		–	–	–	–	1.9 μg
Iodine		–	–	–	–	0.013 mg
Fluorine		–	–	–	–	0.095 mg

[a] Content per 1 mL.
[b] American Regent Products.
[c] Fresenius Kabi Products.

MEDICATIONS

Use of PN to deliver medications is generally not recommended due to potential drug–nutrient interactions, compatibility limitations, and the inability to readily adjust or discontinue the medication without discarding the PN [17]. However, for those medications that have been deemed safe to add to PN, delivery via PN can reduce nursing time and the risk of contamination due to decreased manipulation of the central line (Table 15.4). In addition, there is the added convenience of the patient not having to hang a separate IV medication or inject a separate medication into the PN solution.

TABLE 15.4
Medications Compatible in PN Solutions

Medication	Recommendation
Regular insulin	Only regular insulin can be added to PN. Insulin formulations such as NPH, Lente, Ultra Lente, Lispro, Aspart, and Glargine are not compatible in PN solutions and should never be added. A general initial dose of regular insulin is 1 unit of insulin/10 g of dextrose. See octreotide section in this table.
Histamine 2-receptor antagonists	Famotidine, ranitidine, and cimetidine can be added to the PN solution. Once added to the PN, other parenteral use of this class of drugs should be discontinued. Indications for use include peptic ulcer disease, gastroesophageal reflux disease (GERD), recent extensive small bowel resection with resultant hypergastrinemia, GERD-type symptoms due to ileus or bowel obstruction, and stress ulcer prophylaxis.
Octreotide	There are conflicting data in the literature regarding octreotide in PN solutions. Octreotide has been shown to be physically incompatible with insulin, rendering ineffective drug therapy of both insulin and octreotide when administered via PN. The addition of octreotide to PN should be evaluated carefully and on a case-by-case basis.
Corticosteroids	IV methylprednisolone and hydrocortisone can be added to PN.
Metoclopramide	Compatible in PN solutions; doses of 20 to 40 mg/day can be used.
Heparin	Heparin can be added to PN solutions to decrease thrombus formation at the catheter tip as long as the patient does not have heparin antibodies. The usual dose is 1 unit of heparin per 1 mL of PN solution.

Insulin

Regular human insulin is compatible and stable in PN solutions if needed; only regular human insulin can be added to PN. The advantage of adding insulin directly to the PN is that the insulin is titrated with the PN infusion, and because the half-life of regular insulin is only 5 minutes, stopping PN with insulin added is safe without the concern for rebound hypoglycemia. A regular schedule of glucose monitoring should be in place in those patients with insulin added to PN.

Histamine 2-Receptor Antagonists

Histamine 2-receptor antagonists are stable in PN solutions and are used to decrease gastric acid secretion, particularly in patients during the first 6–12 months after massive small bowel resections due to the presence of hypergastrinemia. Proton pump inhibitors are not compatible with PN solutions.

Octreotide

Octreotide is a somatostatin analog that is used to control hypersecretory states and severe diarrhea [18]. The standard dosage for octreotide is 100 μg, administered subcutaneously three times daily. According to the manufacturer, addition of this drug to PN solutions is prohibited; however, clinicians have been adding this to PN solutions for quite some time without complication [19]. The advantage to the patient is that it avoids intermittent and painful subcutaneous injections. The disadvantage, aside from potential incompatibility, is that the patient will only receive the drug during the PN infusion, which may last for only 12 hours. Considering the controversy, an alternative would be to give the patient a trial of subcutaneous octreotide injections, and if a benefit is seen and there are no adverse reactions, then use of a monthly long-acting depot form can be pursued. Caution should be exercised when administering octreotide during the period of greatest spontaneous intestinal adaptation, as some animal models have shown an inhibition in intestinal adaptation with the use of octreotide [20–23].

Corticosteroids

Corticosteroids such as IV methylprednisolone or hydrocortisone can be added to the PN for patients who cannot take oral corticosteroids.

Metoclopramide

Metoclopramide is a gastric prokinetic and antiemetic agent frequently used in the management of chronic nausea and gastric motility disorders. It is compatible in PN solutions. The usual dose is 20–40 mg/day. Caution is advised, however, as metoclopramide has many side effects with both short- and long-term use that must be considered, including the risk of tardive dyskinesia, which can be irreversible. A black box warning was issued early in 2009 for this drug by the U.S. Food and Drug Administration for this reason.

Heparin

From a compatibility standpoint, heparin may be added to PN solutions as a prophylaxis against catheter-related venous thrombosis, but it should never be added in doses required for use in full therapeutic anticoagulation. Additionally, heparin is contraindicated in patients with heparin-induced thrombocytopenia or active bleeding.

MONITORING OF PN

To ensure safe use of PN, the monitoring of laboratory data during initiation of PN in the hospital setting, prior to discharge home on PN (see the following list), and at defined intervals after discharge home on PN (see Chapter 25) is required.

Laboratory monitoring recommendations at time of hospital discharge on PN [24]*

Baseline labs
- Complete blood count/iron indices
- Comprehensive metabolic panel
- Magnesium, phosphorus
- Triglycerides
- Vitamin B_{12}, RBC folate, 25-OH vitamin D
- Trace elements as appropriate

PREPARATION FOR HOME PN

Many patients with SBS will require PN in the home setting. Once the decision is made to proceed with this therapy, the patient should be evaluated from a medical, nutritional, and psychosocial standpoint. From a medical standpoint, they must meet the Medicare criteria for permanent GI failure requiring therapy for at least 90 days. The patient should also be evaluated for placement of a CVC designed for long-term use. The PN solution will have to be stabilized, transitioned to an overnight infusion cycle in most instances, and adjusted so that all IV fluids are consolidated into the PN solution. Whenever possible, plans should be made to mimic the home regimen for at least 2 days prior to discharge. Teaching may be initiated in the hospital, but much of the teaching will occur in the home setting by a nurse employed by the home infusion company. Please refer to Chapter 25 for more details regarding home PN.

Stabilizing and Cycling of PN

In the hospital setting, PN is typically infused over a 24-hour period as it results in fewer metabolic complications such as electrolyte abnormalities or hyperglycemic/hypoglycemic events. Once a patient is stable and is expected to go home on PN, it is good to start the process early to increase his or her mobilization and time off the pump. In the home setting, it is generally advisable to cycle the PN over a shortened period of time ranging from 10 to 14 hours (although some patients may opt to run longer) to increase mobility and ease of care. Infusion of PN for only part of the day provides both metabolic and psychological benefits. Time without dextrose infusion allows the liver to mobilize stored glycogen and may decrease the incidence of IFALD and promote better nitrogen retention [24,25]. Additionally, the patient has a period of time unencumbered by the PN infusion, allowing the patient to assume as normal a lifestyle as possible. Cycling of the PN also creates a window of time to administer IV medications that are not compatible with PN in situations where IV access is limited.

It should be noted that PN cycling increases the risk for hyperglycemia and fluid overload. Tapering of the PN is a technique in which the rate of delivery of the PN solution is gradually increased or decreased at the beginning or end of the infusion period, respectively (home infusion pumps do this automatically). The rate of infusion is gradually increased over the first 1 to 2 hours (taper up) at the beginning of a cycle to avoid hyperglycemia and gradually decreased over 1 to 2 hours (tapered down) at the end of the cycle to minimize the risk of hypoglycemia [13,27,28].

The other caveat associated with PN cycling relates to potassium. Some SBS patients have extraordinary requirements for potassium. Potassium infusion should not exceed 10 mEq/hour in the home setting due to the absence of cardiac monitoring. This may necessitate the provision of oral potassium or a separate bag of IV fluids containing potassium to infuse when the PN is not running.

* See Chapter 25 for laboratory monitoring recommendations after discharge.

Special Considerations at Home

As described previously, the patient with SBS is at an increased risk for dehydration. As such, plans should be made to supply supplemental IV fluids to these patients who live in remote areas or areas where there are increased risks of severe weather such as hurricanes that may preclude a regularly scheduled delivery of PN solutions. These patients should maintain a supply (2 to 4 L) of standard IV fluids that have a long shelf-life in case of interrupted PN delivery. The hospital inpatient team will need to provide orders to the home care company detailing which labs are to be checked and how often after discharge. Finally, although not always done, it is extremely helpful to the home care company nutrition support specialist to receive a call from the inpatient clinician to provide details about the patient to avoid gaps in care.

REFERENCES

1. Hollwarth ME. Short bowel syndrome: Pathophysiological and clinical aspects. *Pathophysiology* 1999;6:1–19.
2. O'Keefe SJ et al. Short bowel syndrome and intestinal failure: Consensus definitions and overview. *Clin Gastroenterol Hepatol* 2006;4:6–10.
3. Thompson JS et al. Current management of the short bowel syndrome. *Surg Clin North Am* 2011;91:493–510.
4. Nightingale J et al. Small Bowel Nutrition Committee of the British Society of Gastroenterology. Guidelines for management of patients with a short bowel. *Gut* 2006;55(Suppl 4):iv1–12.
5. Buchman AL et al. AGA technical review on short bowel syndrome and intestinal transplantation. *Gastroenterology* 2003;124:1111–1134.
6. Cadman A et al. To clot or not to clot? That is the question in central venous catheters. *Clin Radiol* 2004;59:349–355.
7. Sundaram A et al. Nutritional management of short bowel syndrome in adults. *J Clin Gastroenterol* 2002;34:207–220.
8. Jeejeebhoy KN. Management of short bowel syndrome: Avoidance of total parenteral nutrition. *Gastroenterology* 2006;130:S60–S66.
9. Cavicchi M et al. Prevalence of liver disease and contributing factors in patients receiving home parenteral nutrition for permanent intestinal failure. *Ann Intern Med* 2000;132:523–532.
10. Buchman A. Total parenteral nutrition-associated liver disease. *JPEN J Parenter Enteral Nutr* 2002;26(Suppl 56):S43–S48.
11. Buchman A et al. Parenteral nutrition-associated liver disease and the role for isolated intestine and intestine/liver transplantation. *Hepatology* 2006;43:9–19.
12. Vanderhoof JA et al. Enteral and parenteral nutrition in the care of patients with short-bowel syndrome. *Best Pract Res Clin Gastroenterol* 2003;17:997–1015.
13. Ayers P et al. A.S.P.E.N. parenteral nutrition safety consensus recommendations. *JPEN J Parenter Enter Nutr* 2013;38:296–333.
14. Boullata JI et al. A.S.P.E.N. clinical guidelines: Parenteral nutrition ordering, order review, compounding, labeling and dispensing. *JPEN J Parenter Enter Nutr* 2014;38:334–337.
15. Howard L et al. Autopsy tissue trace elements in 8 long-term parenteral nutrition patients who received the current U.S. food and drug administration formulation. *JPEN J Parenter Enter Nutr* 2007;31:388–396.
16. Matarese LE. Nutrition interventions before and after adult intestinal transplantation: The Pittsburgh experience. *Pract Gastroenterol* 2010;34(11):11–26.
17. Trissel LA et al. Compatibility of medications with 3-in-1 parenteral nutrition admixtures. *JPEN J Parenter Enter Nutr* 1999;23:67–74.
18. O'Keefe SJ et al. Long-acting somatostatin analogue therapy and protein metabolism in patients with jejunostomies. *Gastroenterology* 1994;107:379–388.
19. Seidner DL et al. Can octreotide be added to parenteral nutrition solutions? Point–counterpoint. *Nutr Clin Pract* 1998;13:84–88.
20. Vanderhoof JA et al. Lack of inhibitory effect of octreotide on intestinal adaptation in short bowel syndrome in the rat. *J Pediatr Gastroenterol Nutr* 1998;26:241–244.
21. Seydel AS et al. Octreotide diminishes luminal nutrient transport activity, which is reversed by epidermal growth factor. *Am J Surg* 1996;172:267–271.

22. Bass BL et al. Somatostatin analogue treatment inhibits post-resectional adaptation of the small bowel in rats. *Am J Surg* 1991;161:107–111, discussion 111–112.
23. Sagor GR et al. Influence of somatostatin and bombesin on plasma enteroglucagon and cell proliferation after intestinal resection in the rat. *Gut* 1985;26:89–94.
24. Winkler, M. et al., in: *Adult Nutrition Support Core Curriculum*, 2nd ed., Mueller, C.M., ed. The American Society for Parenteral and Enteral Nutrition, Silver Spring, MD. 2012, p. 650.
25. Hwang TL et al. Early use of cyclic TPN prevents further deterioration of liver functions for the TPN patients with impaired liver function. *Hepatogastroenterology* 200;47:1347–1350.
26. Maini B et al. Cyclic hyperalimentation: An optimal technique for preservation of visceral protein. *J Surg Res* 1976;20:515–525.
27. Stout SM et al. Cyclic parenteral nutrition infusion: Considerations for the clinician. *Pract Gastroenterol* 2011;35(7):11.
28. Stout SM et al. Metabolic effects of cyclic parenteral nutrition infusion in adults and children. *Nutr Clin Pract* 2010;25:277–281.

16 Drug Delivery and Bioavailability in Short Bowel Syndrome

Lingtak-Neander Chan

CONTENTS

KEY POINTS

- In patients with short bowel syndrome, the intestine may have a reduced capacity to absorb drugs and other orally administered therapeutic compounds, such as micronutrients.
- Decreased oral absorption may adversely affect the efficacy of drug therapy and clinical outcomes.
- Oral bioavailability of drugs can be affected by different factors ranging from dosage form, drug formulation, the length and the health of the remaining gastrointestinal tract, and the magnitude of intestinal adaptation.
- When the patient is unable to adequately absorb drugs by the oral route, alternate routes of drug administration such as rectal, parenteral, and transdermal should be explored depending on feasibility, availability of drug formulations, safety and efficacy, and long-term affordability by the patient.

INTRODUCTION

One of the most important functions of the human intestine is to regulate the absorption of fluids, nutrients, and, since their advent, drugs. In patients with short bowel syndrome (SBS), the intestine may have a reduced capacity in absorbing drugs and other orally administered therapeutic compounds, such as micronutrients [1,2]. Decreased oral absorption may adversely affect the efficacy of drug therapy and clinical outcomes. These clinical outcomes are not limited to the bowel-related complications of SBS such as diarrhea and pain control but may also affect outcomes of other conditions such as hypertension and hypothyroidism. The purpose of this chapter is to discuss the process and factors that regulate oral drug absorption, how different drug formulations are affected by intestinal resection and SBS, and strategies that can be taken to optimize drug therapy in these patients.

METHODS OF DRUG DELIVERY

Oral Administration

The oral route is the most common route of drug administration because it provides the most convenient and affordable method of drug delivery. Tablets, capsules, solutions, and powder are the most commonly used oral dosage forms. The formulation of some drugs can be modified to alter the site along the intestine where the drug is released, which will affect the rate and extent of its absorption.

Despite being convenient and economical, the adequacy of and adherence to oral drug administration are limited by a number of host-related factors. Patients with dysphagia may have a difficult time swallowing pills or liquids. Those with nausea and vomiting may not be able to retain swallowed medications. Many oral tablets and liquids have an unpleasant taste, which can lead to nonadherence in some patient populations, especially infants and children. Pill burden and frequent dosing may also contribute to nonadherence [3]. For example, a patient with acute ulcerative colitis may need to take four to eight mesalamine capsules every 6 hours (and this may be just one of many medications a patient with SBS has to take).

The bioavailability of orally administered drugs may also be affected by the absorption process. After oral administration, drugs need to undergo disintegration and dissolution (except oral liquid) in the upper gastrointestinal (GI) tract and are subject to pre-systemic metabolism [4,5]. Pre-systemic metabolism, also known as first-pass metabolism, refers to the biotransformation of a drug by the body before it reaches systemic circulation. From the lumen of the GI tract, drug molecules enter the enterocyte through passive diffusion and/or transport-mediated processes to enter the hepatic portal vein, which takes the drug molecules to the liver before being distributed to the rest of the body by the systemic circulation. Common drug metabolizing enzymes, such as cytochrome P450 (CYP) 3A4 and uridine diphosphate glucuronosyltransferase 2B7, are present in the enterocytes [6,7]. Some drugs can therefore be metabolized by these enzymes as they enter the enterocytes, which may lead to lower systemic concentrations. Additionally, efflux transport proteins, such as P-glycoprotein (P-gp) and multidrug resistance–associated protein-2, act to transport compounds present in the enterocyte back into the GI tract lumen [8]. These efflux proteins are thought to serve as a protective mechanism from exposure to xenobiotics and other toxins present within the GI tract. Unfortunately, they may also adversely affect drug bioavailability. Furthermore, absorption can be altered by diet, nutrients, presence of inflammation, and other drug therapy (i.e., drug–drug interactions). For example, grapefruit juice inhibits intestinal CYP3A4, leading to increased oral absorption of certain drugs. Similarly, acute inflammation and acute phase reactions decrease the activity of CYP3A4, which may increase the bioavailability of certain drugs. In contrast, St. John's wort induces CYP3A4 and P-gp, which may decrease the bioavailability of some drugs [9–11].

CYP3A4 is expressed along the entire small intestine with a "crescendo–diminuendo" pattern such that the maximal relative amount of CYP3A4 is in the duodenum and proximal jejunum [6]. On the contrary, the expression of P-gp increases along the length of the human small intestine, with the lowest level of expression in the duodenum and the highest levels in the distal ileum [12,13]. These findings suggest that the impact of SBS on drug absorption can further be affected by the patient's GI tract anatomy, including the location, length, and health of the remaining intestine—important considerations in SBS.

Although the primary site of drug absorption is the proximal small bowel, data from animal research suggest that the intestinal adaption that occurs after bowel resection leads to an increase in mucosal protein expression and the number of crypts present [14]. These adaptive changes can be found in the remaining functional small bowel as well as in the colon [15,16]. In fact, a number of drugs can be absorbed in the colon, and the bioavailability through the colon can be enhanced by novel drug delivery systems and special formulations [17–20].

When the amount of drug absorbed from the GI tract becomes unreliable, unpredictable, or unattainable or when oral/enteral drug administration is not feasible (e.g., refractory vomiting or GI tract obstruction), nonoral methods of drug delivery should be considered. The most common routes of drug delivery other than the oral route include transdermal, parenteral (intravenous [IV], intramuscular [IM], or subcutaneous [SC]), and rectal administration. Although some drugs can also be delivered through less common routes such ocular, otic, intrathecal, intracerebroventricular, intraosseous, or epidural administration, these routes of administration generally provide local effects and are not a practical choice for patients with SBS. The choice of alternate route of drug delivery depends on a number of factors, which include (1) the availability of the formulation and dosage form, (2) the efficacy and the safety of the route of administration, and (3) the feasibility for the patient to self-administer the medication.

Parenteral Administration

Parenteral dosage forms are intended for administration as an injection or infusion. The most common types of parenteral administration include IV, SC, and IM injection. Compared with oral administration, the parenteral route is usually less convenient for the patient, involves higher risks (e.g., bleeding, bruises, infectious complications, and nerve injuries), is more expensive, and may not be feasible in some circumstances (e.g., lack of IV access, drug unavailable as a sterile product). Parenteral administration also offers some important benefits over other routes of administration, such as higher and more consistent bioavailability of drugs and relatively faster onset of action. More importantly, parenteral administration makes drug delivery possible when administration of drug through the GI tract is not feasible, such as active GI bleeding, bowel obstruction, or severe malabsorption. Specific considerations before administering a drug via IV or IM route are summarized in the following:

Safety factors to consider before administering a drug via IV route

- Can IV access be established safely in this patient?
- Is the drug available as a sterile, pyrogen-free product for IV administration?
- Is the osmolarity of the drug or final infusate safe for IV administration through the patient's available IV access?
  - General rule: <900 mOsm/L for peripheral IV line
- Should the drug be administered as an IV bolus or IV infusion?
- Is IV compatibility an issue?
  - Especially with the patient's existing IV and other parenteral products

Safety factors to consider before administering a drug as an IM injection

- Is the drug available as a sterile, pyrogen-free product for IM administration?
- Is the drug formulated for IM injection?
  - The presence of extreme pH and high osmolarity or the use of certain inactive ingredients may cause tissue necrosis.
- Does the patient have severe muscle wasting at a potential injection site?
- What is the volume to be injected IM?
  - Volume higher than 2 mL may cause pain and swelling in the site of injection.
- Is the patient coagulopathic?
  - Does the patient have clotting disorder?
- Using an ice pack or heating pad at the injection site may reduce pain but can also alter the blood flow to the injection site, which may change the rate of drug being distributed.

Malnutrition and wasting syndrome may be present in patients with SBS and may affect the safety of parenteral administration, especially IM injection. For example, patients with fat malabsorption syndrome or poor oral diet may have vitamin K deficiency, which can lead to coagulopathy. Administering IM injection to a patient with coagulopathy may cause severe bruising and excessive bleeding. Patients with severe muscle wasting and cachexia may have significantly reduced muscle mass in areas where an IM injection is typically administered, such as the deltoid muscle, the dorsogluteal muscle, and the gluteus medius muscle. Providing an IM injection in an area with limited muscle mass, especially with a large needle, can cause severe pain and, possibly, tissue damage. A physical exam should be performed in these patients to determine the safety and feasibility of delivering drugs via the IM route. Selection of the IM site should be partially determined by the volume of injection. Large-volume IM injections (3–5 mL) are generally better tolerated at the dorsogluteal site of adults and children older than 3 years of age [21]. To reduce pain at the injection site, some studies showed that the application of ice and manual pressure may be used [22,23]. One study suggests that the application of manual pressure to the injection site for 10 seconds before the procedure may help reduce the intensity of pain sensation in more than one-third of the patients [24]. If the 10-second manual pressure technique is adopted into routine procedures, the provider needs to practice good infection control techniques to minimize the risk of infection. Rotating the injection site may also reduce the likelihood of discomfort associated with IM and SC injections. Topical anesthetics that contain lidocaine or prilocaine can be considered to minimize pain associated with IM administration when necessary. Finally, injection site reactions can develop after IM or SC injections. Once again, rotation of the injection site may reduce the risk of these reactions. Patients should be advised to contact their provider as soon as possible if they experience serious injection site reactions such as swelling, bleeding, blistering, severe skin damage, or redness, tenderness, swelling, and itching that do not subside after 2 days.

Rectal Administration

Rectal administration of drugs can be a very practical and effective alternate route for drug administration in patients who have severe nausea and vomiting or who experience swallowing difficulties. The benefits of rectal route drug administration include easy application, requiring minimal educational efforts to the family and patient, and less expensive compared with the parenteral route. Additionally, patients can generally readily self-administer drugs using the rectal route without the assistance of others. Physical limitations associated with an infusion pump or other infusion devices are also avoided [25].

The drug absorption process from the rectum is similar to that through the oral route; however, the physiological parameters (e.g., pH, flow rate of epithelial fluid, electrolyte composition) differ substantially between the two sites [26]. With careful patient selection, rectal drug administration can achieve a fairly consistent bioavailability and predictable clinical responses. Indeed, there is some evidence to suggest that rectal administration of morphine, metoclopramide, ergotamine, and lidocaine may be associated with faster onset of action and higher bioavailability than oral administration is [26,27]. Partial avoidance of presystemic metabolism after rectal delivery of these drugs may be the explanation for the difference in bioavailability [26,28].

Besides suppositories, formulations such as tablets, solutions, and suspensions can all be absorbed in the rectum. Generally speaking, for a drug to be efficiently absorbed from the rectal mucosa, it needs to be mixed with at least 1–3 mL of fluid [26]. For crushed tablets or dry powder, rectal absorption can be improved by mixing with a small amount of water before administration. Drugs that are dissolved in aqueous or alcohol solutions are absorbed more rapidly and can achieve more complete absorption than in suspension or suppositories. Basic solutions are also better absorbed than acidic solutions [29]. A total fluid volume between 10 and 25 mL is generally well tolerated and retained by the patient without causing defecation urgency, whereas volumes of 80 mL and more can cause fecal urgency [26;30]. Importantly, rectal drug absorption is a mostly passive process and not facilitated by transport proteins. Drugs requiring active transport for optimal absorption will not be absorbed adequately with the rectal route. Table 16.1 summarizes drugs commonly used in patients with SBS that can also be administered rectally.

In many patients with SBS, chronic diarrhea is common. Unfortunately, diarrhea and hypersecretion that reaches the lower GI tract can decrease the reliability of the amount of drug being absorbed from the rectum. Therefore, rectal drug administration should be avoided in patients with diarrhea. The rectal route should also be avoided in patients with neutropenia, thrombocytopenia, anorectal disease (e.g., perianal abscess and fistula), and prior abdominoperineal resection [27]. Giving drugs rectally may cause local discomfort and flatulence and produce an uncomfortable sensation with the need to defecate. Rectal administration of oral syrup, such as carbamazepine, can also cause other complications such as skin irritation or infection due to the presence of sugars. In extreme cases, prolonged use of certain drugs, such as ergotamine and aspirin, may cause serious complications, including rectal ulceration, necrosis, and stenosis.

Transdermal Administration

Transdermal drug administration may involve the application of poultices, gels, ointments, creams, pastes, and adhesive skin patches to deliver drugs into the systemic circulation. The drug applied on the skin surface must effectively penetrate through the stratum corneum, a lipophilic membrane, to be absorbed in the dermis, where capillary blood flow can lead the drug into the systemic circulation [31]. Since the physiological function of the skin is to serve as a barrier for exposure to drugs and other xenobiotics, it is very difficult to optimize systemic drug therapy using the transdermal route. The role of most topical creams and ointments are limited to local effects, such as the treatment for neuromuscular pain, skin diseases, or local irritation/inflammation.

The adhesive transdermal drug delivery patch was first approved by the Food and Drug Administration in 1979 for scopolamine used to treat motion sickness [32]. Transdermal patches utilize either a drug reservoir or the drug is impregnated into the fabric of the patch. Upon applying the patch to the skin, the drug diffuses toward the skin tissue based on the concentration gradient. As a result, a second drug reservoir is established in the stratum corneum. As the drug molecules penetrate further into the skin, they are absorbed into the local capillary vasculature and, eventually, into the systemic circulation [33]. This reservoir-mediated absorption process results in a drug absorption rate that is gradual and slow. Therefore, the onset of action of drugs administered as a transdermal patch

TABLE 16.1
Commonly Used Drugs in Patients with SBS with Established Bioavailability after Rectal Administration

Analgesics	Antiemetics	Anti-Inflammatory	Anxiolytics
Acetaminophen[a]	Prochlorperazine[a]	Dexamethasone	Diazepam[b]
Morphine	Promethazine[a]	Hydrocortisone	Lorazepam
Hydromorphone	Chlorpromazine	Prednisolone	Midazolam
Oxycodone	Metoclopramide		
Codeine	Ondansetron		
Tramadol			

Source. Davis, MP et al., Palliative care per rectum, fast fact #257 for providers from the Center to Advance Palliative Care, http://www.capc.org/fast-facts/257-palliative-care-rectum/.

[a] Commercially available as rectal suppository.

[b] Commercially available as rectal gel.

is delayed. It is not unusual to take up to three patch applications to achieve steady-state plasma drug concentration. Therefore, transdermal patches are generally used for maintenance therapy and have no role in the acute management of symptoms. For example, a clonidine patch can be used as maintenance therapy for hypertension in patients with SBS; however, oral clonidine tablets should be used for immediate control of blood pressure [4]. Because a drug reservoir is formed in the stratum corneum, the drug may continue to have clinical effect for hours or even days after the patch is removed from the skin.

Although transdermal drug delivery is a viable option in patients with SBS, the number of drugs available as a transdermal patch is very limited. In addition, it is unclear whether the drug absorption rate from a transdermal patch is affected by the muscle wasting or dehydration. Similarly, the presence of edema may have a negative impact on drug bioavailability. The degree of adiposity affects the systemic availability of highly lipophilic drugs. As such, the efficacy of such formulations, such as fentanyl transdermal patch, may be lower in morbidly obese patients as the adipose tissue under the skin may serve as a reservoir for the drug and reduce the amount available in the systemic circulation. Remember that the presence of fever or concurrent use of heating pads causes vasodilatation and can increase the rate of drug absorption from the patch. Finally, some transdermal patches must be removed from the skin before the patient undergoes magnetic resonance imaging as the metal-containing component of the patch may catch fire during the procedure and cause burn injury [34,35].

ORAL DRUG FORMULATION AND BIOAVAILABILITY

Immediate-Release Oral Dosage Forms

As alluded to previously, medications in solid dosage forms, such as regular tablets, need to undergo disintegration and dissolution before absorption can take place. Disintegration refers to the process in which a solid dosage form is broken down into granules and fine particles that allow dissolution to take place. In most cases, disintegration takes place efficiently in the stomach in the presence of gastric acid along with the help of the churning and grinding action of the gastric antrum. Dissolution is the process by which a solute is dissolved into a liquid medium to form a solution. It is a key step to allow the active ingredient to be absorbed in the GI tract. Dissolution of the typical solid dosage forms, such as a regular tablet, capsule, or powder, can occur in the stomach, duodenum, or proximal jejunum. The dissolution rate may be more rapid at a specific pH, depending on the drug and the dosage form [4,36]. Based on these principles, impaired disintegration and dissolution of a regular tablet or capsule can occur with gastric, duodenal, or proximal jejunal resection or the presence of achlorhydria. Although it is less common for patients with SBS to have resections of the upper GI tract, concurrent antisecretory therapy with a proton pump inhibitor may decrease the dissolution of some drugs, which can then have a negative impact on oral bioavailability. In this situation, bioavailability may be optimized by the use of an oral liquid solution; however, this is specific to the drug. Importantly, in SBS patients with intact stomach, duodenum, and jejunum but with extensive resection of the ileum, changing from solid to liquid dosage form may not have a significant impact on bioavailability. In patients with partial resection of the jejunum or proximal ileum, although the rate of drug absorption may be altered, the overall extent of drug absorption appears to be preserved [37–39].

Delayed-Release and Enteric-Coated Tablets

Delayed-release tablets and enteric-coated tablets are formulated with an acid-resistant coating to delay disintegration and dissolution until the dosage form has passed through the stomach. The rationale is to prevent the active ingredient from being destroyed or deactivated by the low pH in the stomach and causing irritation to the gastric mucosa [40]. Although the onset of absorption is delayed, the rate of absorption of these formulations is similar to that of regular tablets. These formulations are not the same as extended-release formulations.

Time-Release Tablets

Time-release formulations, such as extended-release or controlled-release tablets, are formulated to make the active ingredient(s) available for absorption over an extended period of time after ingestion, especially in the small intestine [41,42]. The primary intention of time-release formulation is to decrease the frequency of drug dosing. In patients with SBS, the extent of drug absorption from time-released formulations may be reduced due to a shortened orocecal transit time. Higher doses or increased dosing frequency may be necessary in some cases, depending on the clinical response of patients.

Sublingual Formulations and Orally Disintegrating Tablets

Sublingual drug administration involves administering a drug under the tongue. Technically, a sublingual dosage form must be dissolved and well absorbed through the mucosal membranes lining the floor of the mouth to the systemic circulation without being swallowed. A true sublingual dosage form can be a good choice for patients with SBS with extensive GI malabsorption since the absorption process is completed in the mouth; however, only drugs with certain biochemical characteristics can be adequately absorbed in the oral and buccal mucosal tissues. In addition, the dosage form must be specifically formulated to allow rapid release and dissolution of the drug under the tongue to maximize absorption [43]. True sublingual dosage forms are also expensive to manufacture. The benefits of a sublingual formulation include convenience and rapid onset of action. There are only a few drugs that have been tested and are commercially available as true sublingual dosage forms that are adequately absorbed across the oral mucosa [44]. The classic example of a sublingually formulated drug is nitroglycerin sublingual tablet or spray, which is dissolved and rapidly absorbed under the tongue, with an onset of action within a few minutes to relieve chest pain. Other drugs demonstrating adequate absorption across the oral mucosa include fentanyl, morphine, zolpidem, and buprenorphine.

A drug or a supplement can be formulated as a tablet for sublingual administration but is not adequately absorbed in the oral mucosa. Instead, the tablet undergoes rapid dissolution in the mouth, which is then swallowed and follows the normal pattern of absorption from the GI tract [45,46]. This is what is referred to as an orally disintegrating tablet (ODT). ODTs are more convenient to administer compared with regular tablets as ODTs are easier to swallow and can be swallowed without the use of additional fluid or water. Since the absorption process for ODTs is the same as other oral dosage forms, however, these products offer no benefit over conventional oral dosage forms in terms of oral bioavailability and onset of action in patients with severe malabsorption and extensive small intestinal resection. As an example, the so-called sublingual vitamin B_{12} tablets are commonly ODTs formulated for sublingual administration, yet there is no evidence that vitamin B_{12} is optimally absorbed in the oral mucosa. Therefore, in patients with extensive small intestinal absorption with the exclusion of the terminal ileum, these vitamin B_{12} products will likely offer convenience, but not improved bioavailability compared with regular vitamin B_{12} tablets.

Oral Liquids

Oral liquid dosage forms may include oral solutions, suspensions, and syrups. These dosage forms do not require dissolution and can be readily absorbed in the GI tract. They are good choices for patients with swallowing difficulties or extensive gastric resection or those using a feeding tube for drug administration. However, some patients may not tolerate the taste or flavors of the oral liquid, which can lead to medication nonadherence. Nonabsorbable sugars (sugar alcohols), such as xylitol, mannitol, and sorbitol, are often added to the formulation to improve the taste. Unfortunately, these sugars can cause undesirable side effects in patients with SBS, such as bloating, flatulence, and osmotic diarrhea [47]. The risk of these adverse effects is proportional to the amount of sugar ingested. Therefore, patients taking multiple drugs containing sugar alcohols as a vehicle or requiring a large volume of oral liquid to meet dose requirements will experience more severe GI symptoms. Other disadvantages of oral liquid drugs include inconvenience due to their bulky packaging (e.g., large and heavy bottles), a requirement for more precise measuring of each dose, higher cost, and limited availability as commercial products with proven product quality and consistency.

ASSESSMENT AND MANAGEMENT OPTIONS FOR DRUG MALABSORPTION IN SBS

The magnitude of drug malabsorption in patients with SBS is influenced by the length, location, and health of the remaining functional bowel and the formulation of the oral drug administered. In patients with resection between the stomach and the proximal jejunum, the likelihood of experiencing drug malabsorption is low since the absorptive function in the lower gut should be preserved. If malabsorption of solid dosage forms, such as tablets and capsules, is suspected, a trial of a liquid dosage form should be attempted. If absorption is improved, as assessed by therapeutic drug monitoring (e.g., drug levels) when available or improvement in clinical symptoms, the malabsorption is likely associated with poor disintegration and dissolution. GI side effects and adherence should be closely monitored.

Although most drugs are absorbed within the proximal jejunum, drug malabsorption appears more likely to occur in patients with extensive resection of the distal jejunum and ileum, most likely because of the development of rapid intestinal transit with this bowel anatomy [36,48]. There is no specific laboratory or diagnostic test to predict the likelihood and extent of drug malabsorption in these patients. The most effective assessment is to longitudinally monitor clinical response and symptoms and perform therapeutic drug monitoring when applicable. When possible, drug levels should be monitored at baseline (i.e., before intestinal resection), immediately after surgery when oral therapy is resumed, and then weekly until the patient is clinically stable. Longitudinal monitoring is especially important for SBS patients with extensive jejunoileal resection or if they receive a growth factor such as teduglutide, since intestinal adaptation may alter the presystemic metabolism and bioavailability of drugs.

If the desired clinical responses cannot be achieved by orally administered medications, use of an alternate route of drug administration such as transdermal patches or parenteral (i.e., SC, IM, IV) administration should be considered. If a nonoral formulation is not available for a particular drug, switching to an alternate agent may be necessary.

In general, in patients with extensive resection of the distal small intestine, sustained-release or extended-release products should not be used, as the extent of drug absorption can be erratic or significantly decreased. Additionally, patients with jejunostomy and extensive ileal resection may experience reduced enterohepatic recycling of bile acids, which may also negatively affect the absorption and bioavailability of drugs that also undergo enterohepatic recirculation, such as loperamide, digoxin, and cyclosporine.

CONCLUSION

Optimizing drug therapy in patients with SBS is an important but challenging task. There is no "magic rule" with regard to drug selection and dose adjustment that can be universally applied to all patients and all drugs. Therapeutic regimens must be carefully monitored and individualized based on clinical response. Oral bioavailability of drugs can be affected by different factors ranging from dosage form, drug formulation, the length and the health of the remaining GI tract, and the magnitude of intestinal adaptation. In most patients, oral drug administration is effective in achieving treatment goals and is well tolerated. In patients who are unable to adequately absorb drugs by the oral route, alternate routes of drug administration such as rectal, parenteral, and transdermal should be explored depending on feasibility, availability of drug formulations, safety and efficacy, and long-term affordability by the patient. A close collaboration between the patient and members of the healthcare team is crucial in developing a safe, effective, successful, and sustainable therapeutic plan to improve the patient's outcome.

REFERENCES

1. Titus R et al. Consequences of gastrointestinal surgery on drug absorption. *Nutr Clin Pract.* 2013; 28(4):429–36.
2. Severijnen R et al. Enteral drug absorption in patients with short small bowel: A review. *Clin Pharmacokinet.* 2004;43(14):951–62.
3. Sabbatini M et al. Efficacy of a reduced pill burden on therapeutic adherence to calcineurin inhibitors in renal transplant recipients: An observational study. *Patient Prefer Adherence.* 2014;8:73–81.
4. Chan L-N et al. Part IV-A: A guide to front line drugs used in the treatment of short bowel syndrome. *Pract Gastroenterol.* 2015;39(3):28.
5. Jambhekar SS et al. Drug dissolution: Significance of physicochemical properties and physiological conditions. *Drug Discov Today.* 2013;18(23–24):1173–84.
6. Paine MF et al. Characterization of interintestinal and intraintestinal variations in human CYP3A-dependent metabolism. *J Pharmacol Exp Ther* 1997;283(3):1552–62.
7. Antonio L et al. Glucuronidation of catechols by human hepatic, gastric, and intestinal microsomal UDP-glucuronosyltransferases (UGT) and recombinant UGT1A6, UGT1A9, and UGT2B7. *Arch Biochem Biophys.* 2003;411(2):251–61.
8. Murakami T et al. Intestinal efflux transporters and drug absorption. *Expert Opin Drug Metab Toxicol.* 2008;4(7):923–39.
9. Nowack R. Review article: Cytochrome P450 enzyme, and transport protein mediated herb-drug interactions in renal transplant patients: Grapefruit juice, St John's Wort—and beyond! *Nephrology (Carlton).* 2008;13(4):337–47.
10. Haas CE et al. Cytochrome P450 3A4 activity after surgical stress. *Crit Care Med.* 2003;31(5):1338–46.
11. Harris RZ et al. Dietary effects on drug metabolism and transport. *Clin Pharmacokinet.* 2003; 42(13):1071–88.
12. Mouly S et al. P-glycoprotein increases from proximal to distal regions of human small intestine. *Pharmaceut Res.* 2003;20(10):1595–9.
13. Tang H et al. Protein expression pattern of P-glycoprotein along the gastrointestinal tract of the Yucatan micropig. *J Biochem Molec Toxicol.* 2004;18(1):18–22.
14. Dekaney CM et al. Expansion of intestinal stem cells associated with long-term adaptation following ileocecal resection in mice. *Am J Physiol Gastrointest Liver Physiol.* 2007;293(5):G1013–22.
15. Jiang HP et al. Differential protein expression during colonic adaptation in ultra-short bowel rats. *World J Gastroenterol.* 2011;17(20):2572–9.
16. Gillingham MB et al. Differential jejunal and colonic adaptation due to resection and IGF-I in parenterally fed rats. *Am J Physiol Gastrointest Liver Physiol.* 2000;278(5):G700–9.
17. Becker D et al. Novel orally swallowable IntelliCap(®) device to quantify regional drug absorption in human GI tract using diltiazem as model drug. *AAPS PharmSciTech.* 2014;15(6):1490–7.
18. Bansal V et al. Novel prospective in colon specific drug delivery system. *Polim Med.* 2014;44(2):109–18.
19. Vemula SK et al. Pharmacokinetics of colon-specific pH and time-dependent flurbiprofen tablets. *Eur J Drug Metab Pharmacokinet.* 2015;40(3):301–11.
20. Nishi K et al. The colon displays an absorptive capacity of tacrolimus. *Transplant Proc.* 2004;36(2):364–6.
21. Carter-Templeton H et al. Are we on the same page?: A comparison of intramuscular injection explanations in nursing fundamental texts. *Medsurg Nurs.* 2008;17(4):237–40.
22. Chung JW et al. An experimental study on the use of manual pressure to reduce pain in intramuscular injections. *J Clin Nurs.* 2002;11(4):457–61.
23. Kuzu N et al. The effect of cold on the occurrence of bruising, haematoma and pain at the injection site in subcutaneous low molecular weight heparin. *Int J Nurs Stud.* 2001;38(1):51–9.
24. Barnhill BJ et al. Using pressure to decrease the pain of intramuscular injections. *J Pain Symptom Manage.* 1996;12(1):52–8.
25. Davis MP et al. Palliative care per rectum, fast fact #257 for providers from the Center to Advance Palliative Care. www.capc.org/fast-facts/257-palliative-care-rectum/ (accessed April 10, 2015).
26. van Hoogdalem E et al. Pharmacokinetics of rectal drug administration, Part I. General considerations and clinical applications of centrally acting drugs. *Clin Pharmacokinet.* 1991;21(1):11–26.

27. David MP et al. Symptom control in cancer patients: The clinical pharmacology and therapeutic role of suppositories and rectal suspensions. *Support Care Cancer.* 2002;10:117–38.
28. Patel V et al. Rectal carbamazepine as effective long-acting treatment after cluster seizures and status epilepticus. *Epilepsy Behav.* 2014;31:31–3.
29. Cheymol G. Drug administration through the rectum: Reliability, tolerance. *Ann Gastroenterol Hepatol.* 1987;23:195–200.
30. Warren DE. Practical use of rectal medications in palliative care. *J Pain Symptom Manage.* 1996;11: 378–87.
31. Margetts L. Transdermal drug delivery: Principles and opioid therapy. *Contin Educ Anaesth Crit Care Pain.* 2007;7(5):171–6.
32. Pastore MN. Transdermal patches: History, development and pharmacology. *Br J Pharmacol.* 2015; 172(9):2179–209.
33. Prausnitz MR et al. Transdermal drug delivery. *Nat Biotechnol.* 2008;26(11):1261–8.
34. Durand C et al. Practical considerations for optimal transdermal drug delivery. *Am J Health Syst Pharm.* 2012;69(2):116–24.
35. Grissinger M et al. Transdermal Patches and Burns. *US Pharm.* 2009;34(4):43.
36. Severijnen R et al. Enteral drug absorption in patients with short small bowel: A review. *Clin Pharmacokinet.* 2004;43(14):951–62.
37. Beumer JH et al. Disposition of imatinib and its metabolite CGP74588 in a patient with chronic myelogenous leukemia and short-bowel syndrome. *Pharmacotherapy.* 2006;26(7):903–7.
38. Ueno T et al. Serum drug concentrations after oral administration of paracetamol to patients with surgical resection of the gastrointestinal tract. *Br J Clin Pharmacol.* 1995;39:330–2.
39. Broyles JE et al. Nortriptyline absorption in short bowel syndrome. *JPEN J Parenter Enteral Nutr.* 1990;14(3):326–7.
40. Mudie DM et al. Physiological parameters for oral delivery and in vitro testing. *Mol Pharm.* 2010;7(5):1388–405.
41. Ummadi S et al. Overview on controlled release dosage form. *Int J Pharma Sci.* 2013;3(4):258–69.
42. Tran PH et al. Controlled release systems containing solid dispersions: Strategies and mechanisms. *Pharm Res.* 2011;28(10):2353–78.
43. Motwani JG et al. Clinical pharmacokinetics of drugs administered buccally and sublingually. *Clin Pharmacokinet.* 1991;21(2):83–94.
44. Patel VF et al. Advances in oral transmucosal drug delivery. *J Control Release.* 2011;153(2):106–16.
45. Badgujar BP et al. The technologies used for developing orally disintegrating tablets: A review. *Acta Pharm.* 2011;61:117–39.
46. Food and Drug Administration guidance for industry: Orally disintegrating tablets. http://www.fda.gov /downloads/Drugs/GuidanceComplianceRegulatoryInformation/Guidances/ucm070578.pdf.
47. Barrett JS et al. Dietary poorly absorbed, short-chain carbohydrates increase delivery of water and fermentable substrates to the proximal colon. *Aliment Pharmacol.* 2010;31:874–82.
48. Ward N. The impact of intestinal failure on oral drug absorption: A review. *J Gastrointest Surg.* 2010;14(6):1045–51.

17 The Role of Antimotility and Antisecretory Agents in the Management of Short Bowel Syndrome

Mandy L. Corrigan and Donald F. Kirby

CONTENTS

KEY POINTS

- Understanding the surgical history, remaining bowel anatomy, and nutritional intake will guide the initiation and advancement of medications used in the treatment of Short Bowel Syndrome (SBS).
- It is important to assess a patient's past response to a medication and to consider retrialing agents over the course of time as the response may change in relation to the time from development of SBS, in part, due to the effects of intestinal adaptation.
- For patients with very short bowel, clinicians may also have to consider dosing medications in excess of manufacturer package insert recommendations due to anticipated malabsorption, but a thorough knowledge of the particular medication is needed.
- The cornerstone of medical management in SBS involves treatment with antimotility and antisecretory agents to reduce gastrointestinal secretions and slow intestinal transit to increase nutrient, fluid, and electrolyte absorption.

INTRODUCTION

Intestinal failure from short bowel syndrome (SBS) is a unique condition that may occur gradually with repeated smaller resections that slowly reduce intestinal length over time or with one massive resection from a variety of etiologies that have been discussed elsewhere in this book. The potential for intestinal rehabilitation is highly dependent on the amount, location, and quality of the remaining small bowel and the presence or absence of at least part of the colon. Understanding the surgical history, remaining bowel anatomy, and nutritional intake will guide the initiation and advancement of medications used in the treatment of SBS. It is important to assess a patient's past response to a medication and to even consider retrialing agents over the course of time as the response may change in relation to the time from development of SBS, in part, due to the effects of intestinal adaptation.

SBS is not only rare but also includes a diverse patient population that makes performance of randomized controlled trials with an adequate study population extremely difficult to measure the effectiveness of most medications, as responses can vary widely. Thus, it is unlikely that large randomized trials to produce evidence in support of the utility of older commonly used, and often generic and relatively inexpensive, medications will ever be performed. As such, the knowledge base for using these medications is often derived from use in other disease states, small uncontrolled trials, expert opinion, and anecdotal personal experience, titrating the dose to clinical response, which varies according to the SBS patient's remaining bowel anatomy. Frequently, the use of certain medications in SBS varies based on the experiences and preferences of specific institutions. For patients with very short bowel, clinicians may also have to consider dosing medications in excess of manufacturer package insert recommendations due to anticipated malabsorption, but a thorough knowledge of the particular medication is needed.

After dietary and fluid modifications, the cornerstone of medical management in SBS generally involves treatment with antimotility and antisecretory agents to reduce gastric secretions and slow intestinal transit to increase nutrient, fluid, and electrolyte absorption (Figure 17.1). Due to the absence of high-quality evidence in support of their use in SBS, the practices and dosing discussed herein are frequently based on best clinical practices.

ANTIMOTILITY AGENTS

Agents such as loperamide (Imodium), diphenoxylate-atropine (Lomotil), codeine, and tincture of opium have been used for many years to prolong transit throughout the gastrointestinal (GI) tract by reducing intestinal smooth muscle activity. Although a single agent is often initially used, occasionally in SBS, these medications are used in combination (e.g., loperamide and diphenoxylate-atropine) to increase bowel transit time to allow for more digestion and absorption (Table 17.1). If insufficiently helpful, then this may be followed by adding agents with more systemic narcotic effects such as codeine and, finally, tincture of opium, if needed. Alternatively, some clinicians may initiate loperamide and codeine together as first-line therapy based on the description of a synergistic effect of these medications [1]. However, fears of opioid use or abuse may be lessened by starting with diphenoxylate-atropine rather than codeine.

Antimotility agents are generally dosed four times daily and clinical experience suggests that it is beneficial to administer them 30–60 minutes prior to meals and at bedtime [2]. The goal of premeal dosing is to decrease the gastrocolic response, slow peristalsis, and decrease competition for absorption between medications and food [3]. Judging a response to these agents includes an evaluation of changes in stool frequency, consistency, and volume and possible medication adverse effects. Monitoring patients with Intake & Output logs can be a powerful tool in guiding therapy, and actively engaging patients in this type of data collection can be very useful to the managing clinicians and patients alike.

Whenever possible, liquid medications should be avoided in SBS patients. Sorbitol and other sugar alcohols are not absorbed by the small intestine and are often used to sweeten liquid medications. Sugar alcohols can cause significant symptoms such as nausea, vomiting, abdominal cramping, and dry mouth and increase fluid and electrolyte losses with even small amounts [4]; tablets (crushed if possible) will minimize the negative impact of sugar alcohols. Transdermal patches and subcutaneous medications (e.g., octreotide) may be preferred in select SBS patients since they bypass the GI tract for absorption.

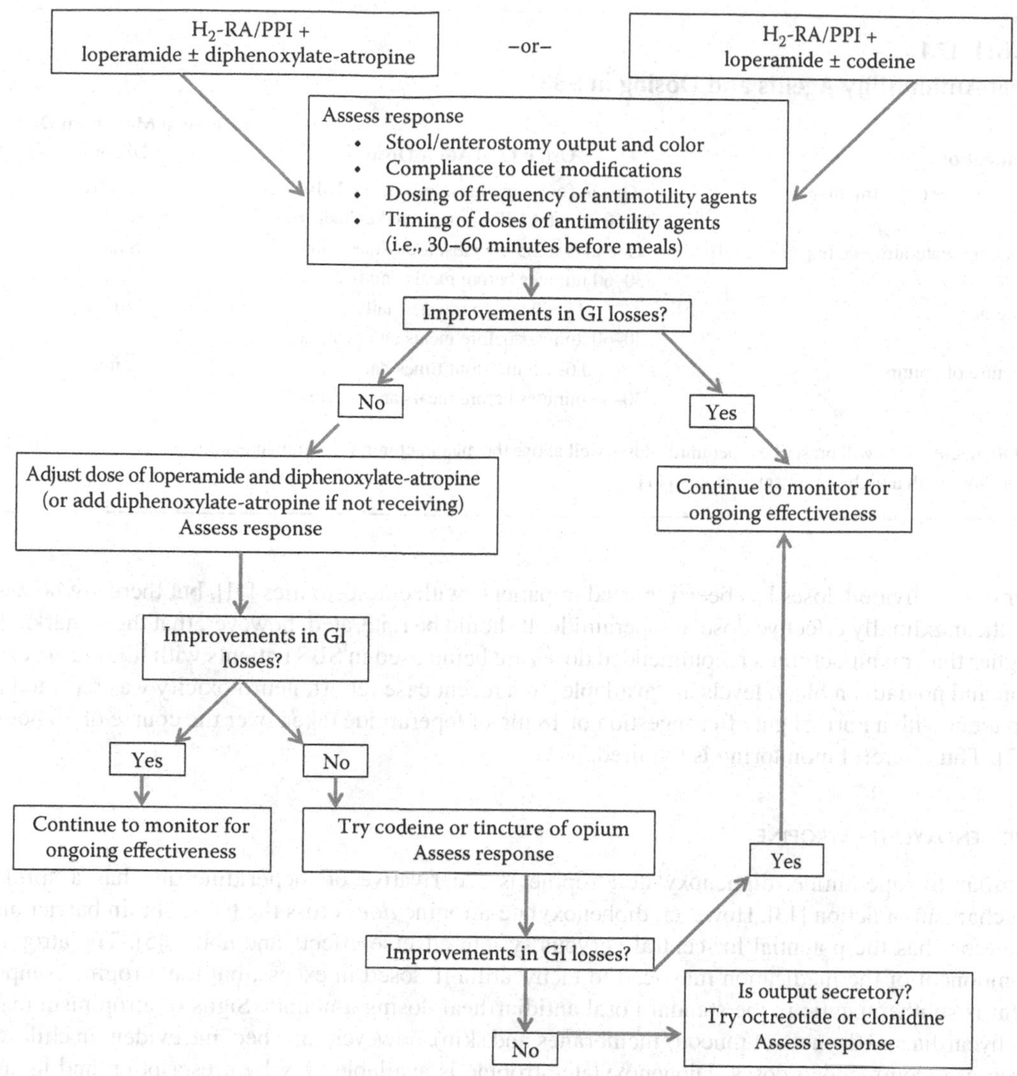

FIGURE 17.1 Algorithm for recommended use of antidiarrheal and antimotility agents.

Loperamide

The efficacy of loperamide has been well established in the treatment of diarrhea in a variety of disease states, is available over-the-counter at low cost, and is considered a first-line therapy in the management of SBS. Loperamide is a derivative of meperidine (pethidine), which targets opioid receptors on intestinal muscles to decrease peristalsis [5–7]. It increases intestinal transit time without significantly impacting gastric emptying and increases stool viscosity bulk. Loperamide also appears to reduce gastric acid secretion to some extent [8]. Additionally, loperamide increases anal sphincter tone, which may reduce the fecal urgency and stool incontinence that some patients with SBS experience [9,10]. Since loperamide has low potential to cross the blood–brain barrier, it lessens any potential for abuse. Therefore, providers may prescribe amounts in excess of the manufacturers' recommended maximum doses when treating patients with SBS [11]. Doses beyond those listed on the package insert (i.e., more than eight tablets daily) are often needed in SBS patients with extensive loss of the ileum as enterohepatic circulation of the drug is disrupted. Dosing up to 96 mg

TABLE 17.1
Oral Antimotility Agents and Dosing in SBS

Medication	Usual Oral Adult Dose	Typical Maximum Daily Dosing
Loperamide[a] (e.g., Imodium)	One to four 2 mg tabs, four times daily 30–60 minutes before meals and at bedtime	16 tabs
Diphenoxylate-atropine (e.g., Lomotil)	One to two 2.5 mg tabs, four times daily 30–60 minutes before meals and bedtime	8 tabs
Codeine	15–60 mg, four times daily 30–60 minutes before meals and bedtime	240 mg
Tincture of opium	0.6–1.5 mL, four times daily 30–60 minutes before meals and bedtime	6 mL

[a] Often, clinicians will prescribe loperamide doses well above the manufacturer's recommended dosing to patients with SBS or those with a high-output enterostomy [11].

per day in divided doses has been reported in patients with enterostomies [11], but there are no data on the maximally effective dose of loperamide. It should be reiterated, however, that these markedly higher than manufacturer's recommended doses are being used in SBS patients with limited absorption and no data on blood levels are available. In a recent case report, neurotoxicity was reported in a patient with a normal gut after ingestion of 18 mg of loperamide taken over the course of 30 hours [12]. Thus, careful monitoring is required.

Diphenoxylate-Atropine

Similar to loperamide, diphenoxylate-atropine is a derivative of meperidine and has a similar mechanism of action [13]. However, diphenoxylate-atropine *does* cross the blood–brain barrier and therefore has the potential for central nervous system adverse effects and abuse [5]. The atropine component of the medication may lead to tachycardia if dosed in excess, but the atropine component is subtherapeutic in the standard oral antidiarrheal dosing amounts. Signs of atropinism (e.g., tachycardia and dryness of mucous membranes and skin), however, may become evident in children even at recommended doses. Diphenoxylate-atropine is available only by prescription and its use should be closely monitored.

Codeine, Tincture of Opium, Paregoric, and Morphine Sulfate

Codeine is a weak–moderate opioid. Its indication for controlling diarrhea is not approved by the Food and Drug Administration (FDA); however, it is frequently used off label for this purpose in patients with SBS. Codeine dosing should be reduced by 25% with glomerular filtration rates (GFRs) in the range of 10–50 mL/min and reduced by 50% when the GFR is below 10 mL/min [14].

King and colleagues [15] compared the effectiveness of codeine and loperamide on ileostomy output. While both treatment groups experienced a significant decrease in ileostomy output, the group receiving loperamide had fewer side effects and electrolyte losses compared with the codeine group. Nightingale et al. [16] reported a synergistic effect when using loperamide and codeine in an SBS patient with Crohn's disease and an end-jejunostomy that led to the eventual discontinuation of parenteral nutrition (PN) after dependence on PN for 14 years. Using detailed balance studies, they showed that the combination of loperamide 4 mg with codeine 60 mg four times daily and 1000 mL of an oral rehydration solution daily achieved positive fluid and sodium balance.

Newton [17] compared the efficacy of codeine with that of diphenoxylate-atropine and Isogel (made from nonabsorbable fibers) in 18 patients with the presence of an ileostomy. Codeine administered at 60 mg three times daily significantly decreased ileostomy output and electrolyte and water losses [17]. In the diphenoxylate-atropine group, dosed two tablets three times daily, a nonsignificant decrease in ileostomy output was observed. Isogel was ineffective and actually increased ileostomy fluid and electrolyte losses. Of note, the codeine group showed an increase in fecal fat, and two patients in the codeine group developed obstruction and were withdrawn from the study. The study concluded that codeine was most effective, diphenoxylate-atropine lesser so.

Palmer and colleagues [18] completed a double-blind, crossover study in a cohort of 30 patients with chronic diarrhea to evaluate 4-week treatment with loperamide, diphenoxylate-atropine, and codeine. Loperamide and codeine were better at reducing rectal urgency and stool incontinence compared with diphenoxylate-atropine. Diphenoxylate-atropine was also the least effective of the agents with respect to improving stool consistency and had more CNS side effects; loperamide had the least. The study concluded that loperamide and codeine were preferred for the treatment of chronic diarrhea.

Tincture of opium is one of the most potent antimotility agents available, but there is a high potential for medication errors with prescribing and dispensing. Importantly, it should be prescribed in milliliter dosing rather than in drops. Tincture of opium is often held in reserve after patients have failed the previously discussed medications or where an allergy exists.

From a historical perspective, morphine sulfate has been utilized for its antidiarrheal side effects, but use in the SBS population has diminished over time due to the potential for abuse and other available options. The use of paregoric has also faded due to potential for medication dosing errors; however, clinicians should remain aware of the problematic nature with its use. Contemporary use of codeine, tincture of opium, and morphine sulfate may also be problematic from the payor perspective; their use often requires an appeal for insurance coverage.

ANTISECRETORY AGENTS

Gastric Hypersecretion

Early in the course of SBS, more commonly after the initial massive small bowel resection, hypersecretion of gastric acid occurs and may last for about the first 6 months [19]. The location and length of any small bowel resection are important factors in understanding the pathophysiology of gastric acid hypersecretion. Jejunal resections play a significant role in gastric acid hypersecretion due to loss of enterohormonal control (such as cholecystokinin and secretin), the mechanism for regulating gastrin secretion [2,19]. This loss leads to the continued signaling of gastrin and continued acid production. During this period, there may be a higher incidence of gastric erosions, ulcerations, strictures, and GI bleeding. Additionally, the irritant effect of excess acid can be detrimental to motility, digestion, and absorption. This increase in acid secretion can have two effects on the upper small bowel. First, it can overcome the normal physiological neutralizing effects of pancreatic bicarbonate secretion and decrease the activation of secreted exocrine pancreatic enzymes. Second, the irritation from the additional acid load may cause hypermotility of the upper small bowel, leading to less mixing of ingested food and naturally secreted pancreatic enzymes, thus resulting in further maldigestion and malabsorption.

There are two classes of antisecretory agents to target gastric acid secretion. Histamine$_2$-receptor antagonists (H_2RAs) and proton pump inhibitors (PPIs) both decrease the production of gastric acid. PPIs are typically first-line therapy and have increased effectiveness compared to H_2RAs along with the convenience of once daily dosing. The effects of H_2RAs are seen more quickly, whereas maximal response to a PPI may not be evident until after a week of treatment. For this reason, these agents may be used in combination early in the treatment course after intestinal resection. If H_2RAs and PPIs are used concurrently, they should be dosed at separate times to prevent any loss of effectiveness of the

PPI [7]. Because these drugs are absorbed in the small bowel, oral dosing above standard initial doses may be needed in SBS. Alternatively, there are orally dissolving tablets or intravenous options, which can be beneficial in treating SBS patients (Table 17.2). Intravenous H_2RAs, such as famotidine and ranitidine, are compatible with PN infusions (Table 17.2). In contrast, PPIs are not compatible with PN solutions but can be delivered as a separate intravenous solution if deemed necessary.

All patients should be treated with H_2RAs and/or PPIs after a major intestinal resection; however, not all SBS patients require acid suppression long-term. After the first 6 months after surgical resection, clinicians can either try reducing or omitting the H_2RAs or PPIs on a trial basis and observe the response by monitoring GI fluid losses and symptoms. If the GI output remains at baseline and the patient is without dyspeptic complaints, the agent can be safely discontinued. If there is an increase in GI losses or a return of persistent dyspeptic symptoms occurs and there is no other etiology or changes to other medication regimens/patient compliance responsible, then acid suppression should be resumed.

Long-term risks with chronic use of gastric antisecretory agents include decreased magnesium levels, bone fragility, and potential for small intestinal bacterial overgrowth (SIBO) and vitamin B_{12} deficiency [20–27]. Hypomagnesemia can be very problematic and difficult to correct in some SBS patients but is likely multifactorial. Nevertheless, PPIs should be considered as potential contributors and discontinued if not necessary in the patient's management. Serum magnesium levels and physical symptoms of deficiency are monitored closely in SBS patients receiving PN, which likely differs from such monitoring in the general population of patients on PPIs in the reported case studies. As described elsewhere in this book, SBS patients are at risk of SIBO; however, controversy exists in the literature as to the role of PPIs on its development [25,26]. No trials to date have specifically evaluated the role of PPIs and SIBO in SBS patients.

TABLE 17.2
Gastric Antisecretory Medications and Dosing in SBS

Medication	Medication Type	Adult Daily Dose	Intravenous Form Compatible with Parenteral Nutrition
Famotidine (Pepcid)[a]	H_2-receptor antagonist	Intravenous, 20–40 mg Oral, 20 mg twice daily	Yes
Ranitidine (Zantac)[a]	H_2-receptor antagonist	Intravenous, 150 mg Oral, 20 mg twice daily	Yes
Cimetidine (Tagament)	H_2-receptor antagonist	Oral 400 mg	n/a
Nizatidine (Axid)	H_2-receptor antagonist	Oral 150 mg twice daily	n/a
Esomeprazole (Nexium)[a,b]	Proton pump inhibitor	Intravenous, 20–40 mg	No
Pantoprazole (Protonix)[a,b]	Proton pump inhibitor	Intravenous, 80 mg q 12 hours Oral, 40 mg twice daily	No
Lansoprazole (Prevacid)[a]	Proton pump inhibitor	Oral, 15–30 mg	n/a
Omeprazole (Prilosec)[a]	Proton pump inhibitor	Oral, 20–40 mg	n/a
Dexlansoprazole (Dexilant)	Proton pump inhibitor	Oral 30–60 mg	n/a
Rabeprazole (Aciphex)	Proton pump inhibitor	Oral, 20–60 mg	n/a
Omeprazole/sodium bicarbonate (Zegerid)	Proton pump inhibitor	Oral, 20–40 mg	n/a

Note: n/a, not applicable, no intravenous form.

[a] Commonly used agents.

[b] Intravenous proton pump inhibitor may be used as an intravenous push by itself or in addition to an H_2RA that is added to parenteral nutrition.

Secretory Diarrhea

Octreotide

Octreotide is a somatostatin analog that inhibits secretions at multiple sites along the GI tract. Octreotide inhibits the release of hormones (including growth hormone, glucagon, and insulin), reduces gastric acid by suppressing gastrin, decreases gallbladder contractions, decreases both exocrine and endocrine pancreatic function, reduces bile flow, decreases gut motility, and promotes water and electrolyte absorption [28].

Octreotide is occasionally used in the SBS patient population for the net secretors—those whose stool output consistently exceeds their oral fluid intake—when conventional dietary modifications, oral rehydration solutions, and antimotility agents have not been successful in controlling GI fluid losses. Its use is not without risk of side effects that may be of particular importance in SBS. SBS patients are often prone to gallstones, and the use of octreotide may contribute to gallstone formation by decreasing gallbladder contractions and bile flow. For this reason, liver function tests should be monitored closely (consider at least monthly) during its use. Blood glucose should also be monitored closely when initiating octreotide and with dose adjustments as it inhibits both insulin and glucagon release. Since octreotide can inhibit the release of growth hormone, some prescribers will avoid its use during the period of maximal intestinal adaptation so that intestinal adaptation is not delayed or blunted. This is a plausible consideration and has been evaluated in animal studies [3,27,29,30].

Octreotide can be delivered intravenously, subcutaneously, or as long acting release (LAR) intramuscular injection. Subcutaneous injections are often prescribed every 8 hours. The use of subcutaneous octreotide 100 μg three times daily was evaluated in 10 SBS patients dependent on home PN with end-jejunosotomies. Beneficial effects observed included a significant reduction in ostomy output, decreased electrolyte losses, reduced delivery of intravenous fluid volumes, and decreased gastric acid secretions [31].

Due to patient discomfort and the frequency of injections, subcutaneous octreotide may not be the ideal route of delivery for long-term use in SBS. Octreotide may be added directly to PN solutions, a potential advantage in the SBS population. This is done as a patient additive to the PN bag immediately before administration. Octreotide can be safely added to PN solutions, although there may be a small decrease in bioavailability [32,33]. The LAR form is typically reserved for use after a patient has established the usefulness of octreotide and a stable dose has been established. The LAR form may be clinically useful for SBS patients who are transitioning off of PN or intravenous fluid support; however, cost may limit its use (Table 17.3).

TABLE 17.3
Dosing of Antisecretory Agents and Dosing in SBS

Medication	Medication Type	Typical Adult Dose	Compatible with PN	Comments
Octreotide (Sandostatin)	Somatostatin analogue	300–1200 μg/day in divided doses Subcutaneous Intravenous 10, 20, or 30 mg long-acting release (LAR) (every 28 days intragluteally)	Yes (short-acting form)	Monitor liver function tests Monitor for alterations in blood glucose
Clonidine	Alpha-adrenergic receptor agonist	Oral: 0.1–0.3 mg BID Transdermal: 0.1–0.3 mg (weekly)	n/a	Monitor blood pressure with initiation, dose changes, and discontinuation

Like other antisecretory and antimotility drugs, few trials investigating octreotide LAR exist within the SBS population. Nehra and colleagues [34] evaluated the use of octreotide LAR in eight SBS PN-dependent patients. The cohort consisted of both patients with colon-in-continuity and enterostomies [34]. Study participants were given 20 mg of octreotide LAR at study weeks 0, 3, 7, and 11. Gastric and intestinal transit was measured along with stool content for water, electrolytes, and fat at the beginning and end of the treatment period. The only statistically significant change seen was prolonged intestinal transit [34]. The potential usefulness of octreotide LAR with SBS patients needs further evaluation with a larger sized cohort before strong conclusions on its effectiveness can be made. Gomez-Herrera and colleagues [35] also evaluated the use of 20 mg octreotide LAR in six patients with SBS for over 8 months and compared them with four controls. The treatment group had a statistically significant reduction in GI output, fluid and electrolyte requirements, and PN dependence. On the basis of this scant evidence, we suggest that use of octreotide should be reserved for those SBS patients with diarrhea refractory to treatment with other antisecretory and antimotility agents and dietary modifications. As with any intervention, it is important to evaluate treatment effects, and if no change in stool output is appreciated after 2–4 weeks, the dose should be adjusted or the medication stopped.

Clonidine

Clonidine is an α-adrenergic receptor agonist that is FDA approved to treat hypertension. Clonidine has also been shown to have favorable effects in patients with SBS due to its ability to decrease motility and gastric secretions and to increase intestinal sodium and water absorption [36–39]. Clonidine has been used with some success in a variety of GI populations with chronic diarrhea, including SBS. Clonidine is available in both oral and transdermal preparations (Table 17.3). The transdermal patch offers a convenience for SBS patients that may increase compliance; it also bypasses the GI tract, thereby obviating concerns about adequate absorption and bioavailability when administered orally in patients with SBS.

McDoniel and colleagues [39] reported on two SBS patients utilizing clonidine at 0.1 or 0.2 mg twice daily by mouth. Both patients were under 30 years of age, had a small portion of colon-in-continuity (case 1: 175 cm small bowel with 8 cm colon ending in a colostomy; and case 2: 30 cm jejunum with 30 cm colon and rectum), and had excessive GI losses despite use of antimotility/antisecretory agents. Both were successfully weaned from PN solutions after treatment with clonidine [39]. Buchman et al. [40] evaluated clonidine administered via transdermal patch in eight PN-dependent SBS patients with end-jejunostomies. The patients were admitted to a General Clinical Research Center where intake was tightly controlled and output collected. A statistically significant decrease was seen in fecal weight and fecal sodium losses with a 0.3-mg clonidine patch [40]. None of the 10 patients within the Buchman and McDoniel case studies developed hypotension with the use of clonidine.

Clonidine should be reserved for secretory diarrhea refractory to treatment with antisecretory agents, antimotility agents, and dietary modifications. Existing doses of antimotility agents can be continued when clonidine is introduced but should be titrated accordingly once the goal stool volume and consistency are achieved [39,40]. As clonidine is an antihypertensive agent, caution should be taken when using this drug in patients with SBS as they are prone to difficulties with volume depletion and hypotension that often accompany states of dehydration. Clonidine has the potential to worsen hypotensive episodes, particularly in the setting of dehydration. For this reason, initiating clonidine in a monitored setting and at a low dose is prudent. Dose adjustments, including discontinuation, should be cautiously undertaken with close monitoring of blood pressure especially in a nonacute care setting.

CONCLUSION

The management of SBS encompasses both the art and science of medicine. Patients are often devastated with the lifestyle changes that are necessary due to their altered anatomy and physiology, including modifications of their diet and fluids and the need to take a large number of medications to slow their intestinal transit and improve absorption. Chief among the first-line medications used in SBS are antimotility and antisecretory agents. In this chapter, we have described the available options and provided suggestions on how to optimize their use in this setting. Although patient compliance can be a major obstacle, when the treatment plan is successful, a very significant improvement in the quality of life of SBS patients is achievable.

REFERENCES

1. Nightingale J et al. Guidelines for management of patients with short bowel. *Gut.* 2006;55:iv1–iv12.
2. Parrish CR. The clinician's guide to short bowel syndrome. *Pract Gastroenterol.* 2005;31:67–106.
3. Matarese LE. Nutrition and fluid optimization for patients with short bowel syndrome. *JPEN J Parent Enteral Nutr.* 2013;37(2);161–170.
4. Bauditz J et al. Severe weight loss caused by chewing gum. *Brit Med J.* 2008;336:96–97.
5. Bechtold ML et al. The pharmacologic treatment of short bowel syndrome: New tricks and novel agents. *Curr Gastroenterol Rep.* 2014;16:392.
6. Chan L. Medications for the management of intestinal failure. *Support Line.* 2006;28(3):8–18.
7. Chan L et al. Short bowel syndrome in adults—Part 4B. A guide to front line drugs used for the treatment of short bowel syndrome. *Pract Gastroenterol.* 2015;32–38.
8. Caldara R et al. Effect of loperamide and naloxone on gastric acid secretion in healthy man. *Gut.* 1981;22:720–723.
9. Emblem R et al. The effect of loperamide on bowel habits and anal sphincter function in patients with ileoanal anastomosis. *Scand J Gastroenterol.* 1989;24:1019–1024.
10. Sun WM et al. Effects of loperamide oxide on gastrointestinal transit time and anorectal function in patients with chronic diarrhea and faecal incontinence. *Scand J Gastroenterol.* 1997;32:34–38.
11. UK Medicines Institute. Can high dose loperamide be used to reduce stoma output? Medicines Q&A 185.3. 2013. Available at http://www.evidence.nhs.uk/search?q=%22Can+high+dose+loperamide+be+used+to+reduce+stoma+output%22. Accessed April 30, 2015.
12. Di Rosa E et al. Loperamide overdose-induced catatonia: Potential role of brain opioid system and P-glycoprotein. *Acta Neuropsychiatr.* 2014;26(1):58–60.
13. Micromedex Solutions (A). Diphenoxylate atropine. Truven Health Analytics, Inc., Greenwood Village, CO. Available at http://www.micromedexsolutions.com/micromedex2/librarian/. Accessed February 27, 2015.
14. Micromedex Solutions (B). Codeine. Truven Health Analytics, Inc., Greenwood Village, CO. Available at http://www.micromedexsolutions.com/micromedex2/librarian/. Accessed February 27, 2015.
15. King RF et al. A double blind cross over study of the effect of loperamide hydrochloride and codeine phosphate on ileostomy output. *Aust N Z J Surg.* 1982;52:121–124.
16. Nightingale JMD et al. A patient with jejunostomy liberated from home intravenous therapy after 14 years: Contribution of balance studies. *Clin Nutr.* 1992;11:101–105.
17. Newton CR. Effect of codeine phosphate, lomotil, and isogel on ileostomy function. *Gut.* 1978;19(5):377–383.
18. Palmer KR et al. Double blind cross over study comparing loperamide, codeine, and diphenoxylate in the treatment of chronic diarrhea. *Gastroenterology.* 1980;79(6):1272–1275.
19. Frantz D et al. Gastrointestinal disease. In: *The A.S.P.E.N. Adult Nutrition Support Core Curriculum*, 2nd ed. Mueller CM, ed. Silver Spring, MD: A.S.P.E.N., 2012: pp. 426–453.
20. Lam JR et al. Proton pump inhibitor and histamine 2 receptor antagonist use and vitamin B12 deficiency. *JAMA.* 2013;310:2435–2442.
21. Thomson AB et al. Safety of the long-term use of proton pump inhibitors. *World J Gastroenterol.* 2010;16:2323–2330.
22. Cundy T et al. Proton pump inhibitors and severe hypomagnesaemia. *Curr Opin Gastroenterol.* 2011;27(2).180–185.
23. Hess MW et al. Systematic review: Hypomagnesaemia induced by proton pump inhibition. *Aliment Pharmacol Ther.* 2012;36(5):405–413.
24. Kuipers MT et al. Hypomagnesaemia due to use of proton pump inhibitors—A review. *Neth J Med.* 2009;67(5):169–172.
25. Lombardo LL et al. Increased incidence of small intestinal bacterial overgrowth during proton pump inhibitor use. *Clin Gasroenterol Hepatol.* 2010;8(6):504–508.

26. Ratuapli SK et al. Proton pump inhibitor therapy does not predispose to small bowel intestinal bacterial overgrowth. *Am J Gastroenterol.* 2012;107(5):730–735.
27. Kumpf VJ. Pharmacologic management of diarrhea in patients with short bowel syndrome. *JPEN J Parent Enteral Nutr.* 2014;38:38S–44S.
28. Lamberts SW et al. Octerotide. *N Engl J Med.* 1996;334(4):246–254.
29. Bass BL et al. Somatostatin analogue treatment inhibits post-resectional adaptation of the small bowel in rats. *Am J Surg.* 1991;161:107–111.
30. Seydel AS et al. Octreotide diminishes luminal nutrient transport activity, which is reversed by epidermal growth factor. *Am J Surg.* 1996;172:267–271.
31. O'Keefe SJ et al. Octreotide as an adjunct to home parenteral nutrition in the management of permanent end-jejunostomy syndrome. *JPEN J Parenter Enteral Nutr.* 1994;18(1):26–34.
32. Seidner DL et al. Can octreotide be added to parenteral nutrition solutions? Point–Counterpoint. *Nutr Clin Pract.* 1998;13(2):84–88.
33. Ritchie DJ et al. Activity of octreotide acetate in a total nutrient admixture. *Am J Health Syst Pharm.* 1991;48:2172–2175.
34. Nehra V et al. An open trial of octreotide long-acting release in the management of short bowel syndrome. *Am J Gastroenterol.* 2001;96(5):1494–1498.
35. Gomez-Herrera E et al. The role of long acting release (LAR) depot octreotide as adjunctive management of short bowel disease. *Cir Cir.* 2004;72(5):379–386.
36. Sundaram U. Mechanism of intestinal absorption: Effect of clonidine on rabbit ileal villus and crypt cells. *J Clin Invest.* 1995;95:2187–2194.
37. DePonti F et al. Adrenergic mechanisms in the control of gastrointestinal motility: From basic science to clinical applications. *Pharmacol Ther.* 1996;69:59–78.
38. Schiller LR et al. Studies of the antidiarrheal action of clonidine. Effects on motility and intestinal absorption. *Gastroenterology.* 1985;89(5):982–988.
39. McDoniel K et al. Use of clonidine to decrease intestinal fluid losses in patients with high-output short bowel syndrome. *JPEN J Parenter Enteral Nutr.* 2004;28(4):265–268.
40. Buchman AL et al. Clonidine reduces diarrhea and sodium loss in patients with proximal jejunostomy: A controlled study. *JPEN J Parenter Enteral Nutr.* 2006;30:487–491.

18 Luminally Active Therapies

Pancreatic Enzymes, Bile Acids, Bile Acid Binders, Antimicrobials, Probiotics, and Prebiotics in Short Bowel Syndrome

Eamonn M.M. Quigley

CONTENTS

KEY POINTS

- Although potentially useful in principle, there are no data to support the use of pancreatic enzymes in the short bowel syndrome (SBS) patient, unless pancreatic insufficiency has been demonstrated.
- Although they may help to reduce diarrhea in some patients, bile acid chelators (binders) should be used with caution in SBS as they may exacerbate steatorrhea/diarrhea.
- Bile salt replacement therapy should be of value in SBS but is not widely used because of limited availability of appropriate preparations.
- The gut microbiota is disturbed in short bowel patients, with small intestinal bacterial overgrowth (SIBO) being the principal clinical manifestation.
- Antibiotics effectively manage SIBO, although their usage owes more to empiricism than to an extensive evidence base.
- In theory, probiotics and prebiotics may benefit patients with SBS, but there have been few high-quality clinical trials supporting their use.
- Based on individual case reports, some concern has been raised regarding the translocation of probiotic organisms in this patient population.

INTRODUCTION

Maldigestion and malabsorption are fundamental problems in the patient afflicted by short bowel syndrome (SBS), and several factors may contribute, including pancreatic insufficiency, depletion of the bile salt pool, and small intestinal bacterial overgrowth (SIBO); all are potential targets for therapeutic intervention. Quite apart from symptoms that may result from malabsorption, changes in luminal contents may contribute to symptomatology in other ways in this clinical context. These include spillage of unabsorbed bile acids into the colon leading to cholereic diarrhea and qualitative and quantitative changes in the microbiome of the small intestine and colon such as are now being revealed by high-throughput sequencing and metabolomics studies. This chapter will review the current status of our understanding of these issues and will attempt to provide guidance for therapy.

PANCREATIC FUNCTION AND SBS

Despite the frequent occurrence of steatorrhea in patients who suffer from SBS, and while a moderate restriction of fat has been recommended in the SBS patient with colon-in-continuity [1], exclusion of fat from the diet should be discouraged given the high caloric content of fat relative to other nutrients [2]. Furthermore, a high-fat diet has been shown experimentally to promote adaptation, enhance villus growth, and result in superior metabolic outcomes such as enhanced lean body mass [3,4]. The question then arises: could fat digestion and, thus, assimilation be augmented in the SBS patient? To answer this, an understanding of factors that may contribute to fat maldigestion and malabsorption is needed. Potential contributors include loss of intestinal surface area, presence of SIBO, accelerated intestinal transit, depleted bile salt pool (see next section), gastric hyperacidity leading to inactivation of pancreatic enzymes [5], a mismatch in nutrient and pancreatic enzyme mixing due to altered upper gut anatomy (e.g., Roux-en-Y gastroenterostomy), and perhaps, pancreatic insufficiency *per se* [6]. While the prevalence of the latter has not been estimated in this patient population, its occurrence is plausible given the well-known association between pancreatic atrophy and conditions that result in rapid and marked weight loss and/or critical illness [7–10]. Pancreatic function is reduced in patients receiving only parenteral nutrition (PN) and no enteral stimulation [11], but few SBS patients subsist on PN alone. Furthermore, although patients with extensive proximal small bowel resections may lose sites of secretin and cholecystokinin-pancreozymin synthesis and develop decreased pancreatic and biliary secretions, most SBS patients have had extensive distal small bowel resections and demonstrate normal pancreatic enzyme and bilirubin secretion [12].

Other factors may also influence pancreatic exocrine function in SBS. First, the direct instillation of carbohydrate, lipid, and mixed meals (but not protein) into the jejunum, as may occur with nasojejunal feeding or in the aftermath of certain surgical modifications of upper gastrointestinal anatomy (e.g., gastrojejunostomy), inhibits pancreatic secretion through a mechanism that has been referred to as the jejunal brake [13]. Second, loperamide, used extensively to reduce the frequency and severity of diarrhea in SBS, inhibits pancreatic and biliary secretion [12]. The clinical relevance of this finding, however, remains to be shown.

It is far from clear whether the provision of supplemental pancreatic enzymes to patients with SBS, in general, will aid fat digestion and assimilation and improve nutritional status. Acid suppression could, in theory at least, optimize pancreatic enzyme activity during the 6- to 12-month period of gastric hypersecretion after massive intestinal resection [6]; however, evidence of clinical efficacy in terms of fat assimilation is lacking [14]. The bottom line is that there, as yet, is no evidence supporting the usefulness of pancreatic enzyme supplementation in SBS, and it is rarely needed in this patient population.

BILE ACIDS AND SBS

Relevance of Bile Acid Physiology in SBS

The primary factor influencing the physiology of bile acids in SBS is loss of the terminal ileum, the primary site of bile acid absorption. It has been demonstrated that loss of segments of distal ileum of <100 cm will result in choleretic/cholereic diarrhea. Unabsorbed bile acids progress to the colon (if it is present) and are deconjugated by the colonic microbiota. In the colon, deconjugated bile acids enhance secretion, increase colonic motility, accelerate transit, impair barrier function (and, thus, increase permeability), and promote visceral sensation, the net effect being diarrhea and abdominal cramps [15]. In this circumstance, bile acid chelating agents may be of benefit.

With more extensive (>100 cm) distal ileal resections, the bile salt pool eventually becomes depleted with resultant steatorrhea. Here, bile acid chelators will exacerbate diarrhea, and bile acid replacement therapy (see "Bile Acid Replacement Therapy" section), where available, may be considered.

Changes in the absorption and enterohepatic circulation of bile acids have other implications for the SBS patient. Bile acid absorption by the ileal enterocyte is closely linked to the synthesis of bile acids in the liver (Figure 18.1). Enhanced bile acid absorption, mediated by the ileal bile acid transporter (IBAT) on the luminal surface of the enterocyte, activates the farnesoid X receptor (FXR) in ileal enterocytes to induce the expression of fibroblast growth factor (FGF) 15/19. Then, FGF 15/19 is secreted into the portal circulation and, acting as a hormone, reaches the liver, where it binds to the hepatocyte cell surface receptor complex, FGF receptor 4, to repress bile acid synthesis through

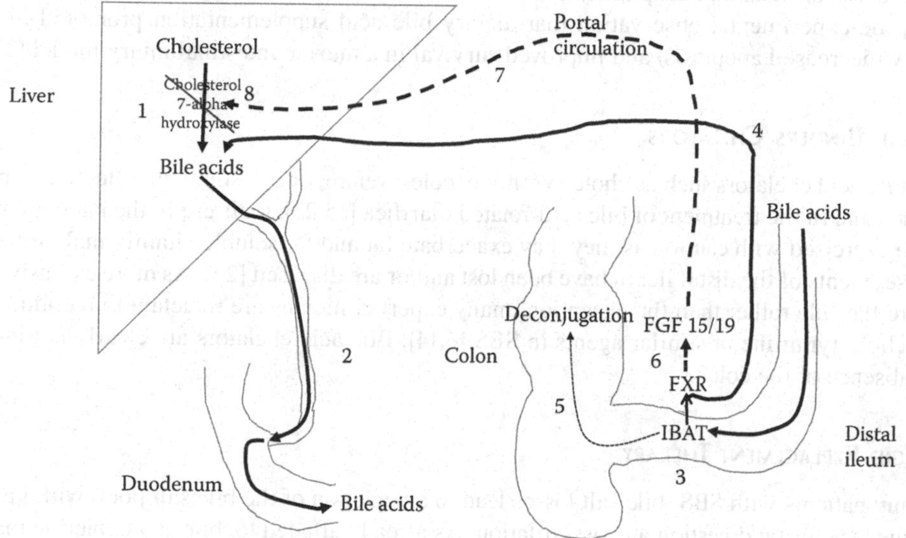

FIGURE 18.1 The enterohepatic circulation of bile acids and regulation of bile acid synthesis. (1) Bile acids are synthesized in the liver from cholesterol through a process that involves the enzyme cholesterol 7-alpha hydroxylase. Bile acids are secreted into bile and stored in the gall bladder between meals. (2) On eating, bile is secreted into the duodenum to facilitate fat digestion and assimilation. (3) On reaching the distal ileum, bile acids are reabsorbed using the ileal bile acid transporter on the ileal enterocyte. (4) Absorbed bile acids enter the portal circulation, return to the liver, and recirculate (solid line) (the enterohepatic circulation). (5) In health, minimal amounts of bile acids are lost to the colon, where they are deconjugated by colonic bacteria (6) Enhanced bile salt uptake by the enterocyte activates the farnesoid X receptor (FXR) in ileal enterocytes to induce the expression of fibroblast growth factor (FGF) 15/19. (7) FGF 15/19 is secreted into the portal circulation and, acting as a hormone, reaches the liver (dashed line) where (8) it inhibits bile acid synthesis through down-regulation of cholesterol 7 alpha-hydroxylase.

down-regulation of cholesterol 7 alpha-hydroxylase [16]. FXR is also highly expressed in the liver, kidney, and adrenal glands and regulates the activation of genes involved in the synthesis, uptake, and export of bile acids, thus conferring on it a central role in bile acid homeostasis. FGF 15/19, in turn, has metabolic effects through its promotion of gluconeogenesis, as well as glycogen and protein synthesis [17,18].

FGF15/19 also stimulates gallbladder filling, and FXR activation has been shown to protect against cholestasis-induced liver injury; these effects are of great relevance to SBS given the occurrence of cholestasis as a component of intestinal failure-associated liver disease (IFALD). Indeed, altered FXR signaling has been demonstrated in a pig model of IFALD [19], and in a much earlier study, Al-Ansari and colleagues [20] found that the IBAT was paradoxically down-regulated after massive intestinal resection.

The implications of recent research identifying diverse and far-reaching roles for bile acids as signaling molecules for the pathophysiology and management of SBS are yet to be delineated. In addition to the signaling pathways described previously related to bile acid homeostasis, it is now abundantly evident that bile acids exert diverse endocrine and metabolic actions by activating G protein-coupled bile acid receptor 1 (also referred to as TGR5), a membrane G protein-coupled receptor that is expressed in enteroendocrine cells. Activation of TGR5 on enteroendocrine cells stimulates secretion of glucagon-like peptides-1 and -2 (GLP-1 and GLP-2). GLP-1 operates as the major incretin hormone involved in glucose homeostasis [16]. These effects have led to the clinical investigation of FXR agonists, such as obeticholic acid, in nonalcoholic fatty liver disease [21] and may have relevance to steatosis in IFALD. Meanwhile, GLP-2 is a key trophic hormone in relation to the process of intestinal adaptation and growth in response to food ingestion; these effects may explain the experimental observation that dietary bile acid supplementation promoted intestinal integrity (decreased apoptosis) and improved survival in a murine intestinal injury model [22].

Bile Acid Binders/Chelators

While bile acid chelators such as cholestyramine, colesevelam, or colestipol are effective in binding bile acids and in the treatment of bile acid-related diarrhea [15,23], their use in the patient with SBS must be exercised with caution as they may exacerbate fat and fat-soluble vitamin malabsorption if longer segments of the distal ileum have been lost and/or are diseased [24]. As more extensive resections are the rule rather than the exception, many expert clinicians are reluctant to recommend the use of cholestyramine or similar agents in SBS [6,14]. Bile acid chelators are clearly not indicated in the absence of the colon.

Bile Acid Replacement Therapy

For many patients with SBS, bile salt losses lead to a depletion of the bile salt pool, with inevitable consequences for fat digestion and assimilation. As already alluded to, bile salt depletion may have other consequences for the short bowel patient, including cholestasis and cholelithiasis [25]. Other factors, including lack of oral or enteral feeding [26] and taurine deficiency [27], also play a role in the development of cholestasis.

While bile acid replacement seems logical in this context, it has not been widely studied. In an early report, ox bile was shown to reduce steatorrhea but not diarrhea in a patient who had undergone ileal and right colon resection for Crohn's disease [28]. The synthetic conjugated bile acid, cholylsarcosine, has been shown to enhance fat absorption and nutritional status and to be well tolerated in small series of patients [29–32]. However, the aforementioned studies involved a total of just 11 patients. Bile acid replacement therapy has also been shown to reduce urinary oxalate excretion in a patient with SBS [31]. Given that the induction of diarrhea is a possible adverse effect of bile acids (and probably accounted for the lack of impact of ox bile on diarrhea) [28], it is important to note that cholylsarcosine is resistant to bacterial metabolism and should therefore have no cathartic activity. Unfortunately, cholylsarcosine is not commercially available, nor are other bile acids available that do not cause diarrhea.

Bile acid therapy has also been studied in relation to IFALD. In reviewing the literature, Barclay and colleagues [33] found conflicting results from the use of either tauroursodeoxycholic acid or ursodeoxycholic acid in the prevention and treatment of IFALD in children. Although the level of evidence was low, there appeared to be a trend toward benefit from ursodeoxycholic acid [33]. For example, in one case series, ursodeoxycholic acid in a dose of 30 mg/kg/day either improved or normalized cholestasis in 11 of 12 children over a 6-month treatment period [34].

MODULATION OF MICROBIOTA IN SBS

Gut Microbiota in SBS and SIBO

The normal microbiota influences a variety of intestinal functions and plays a key role in nutrition and metabolism, as well as in maintaining the integrity of the epithelial barrier and in promoting the development of mucosal immunity. The development of SIBO in the intact intestine is normally prevented by the bacteriostatic actions of gastric acid, pancreatic and intestinal enzymes, bile salts, and secretory IgA, as well as the propulsive effects of small intestinal motility, including peristalsis and the migrating motor complex, and (maybe) the antireflux properties of the ileocecal valve (see list below). One or more of these mechanisms are often compromised in patients with intestinal failure, including SBS [35,36]. Although motor adaptation does occur in the shortened intestine, motility remains abnormal [37] and may contribute to SIBO. While the ileocecal valve forms a physical barrier to reflux of colonic material into the small bowel, results from both experimental animal models [38,39] and human studies [40] have failed to identify a major effect on either bacterial translocation or SIBO after resection of the valve. These findings would lend support to the hypothesis that specialized motor patterns in the distal ileum, and not the valve itself, are the critical elements in sustaining the propulsive functions of this region [41,42]. Many of the disorders that may result in intestinal failure, such as Crohn's disease, whether active or in remission [43,44], and radiation enteritis [45] are, in of themselves, associated with the development of SIBO. Many affected patients have undergone prior surgical procedures, such as gastrectomy, that predispose to SIBO. In both clinical and experimental surgical series, the prevalence of SIBO in the SBS has varied considerably [38,39,46–48], depending on whether or not the colon remained in continuity [46] or the terminal ileum [38] or ileocecal valve had been resected [39]. In one of the largest series, Gutierrez and colleagues [48] performed duodenal aspirates in 57 children with SBS; 70% fulfilled their criteria for SIBO. Of the multiple factors that they assessed, PN dependence alone was predictive of the presence of SIBO.

Factors that prevent small intestinal bacterial overgrowth (SIBO) in the intact intestine but may be compromised in short bowel syndrome

- Intact gastric, intestinal, and colonic anatomy
- Presence of a normal microbiome
- Bacteriostatic actions of
  - Gastric acid
  - Pancreatic secretions
  - Intestinal enzymes
  - Bile salts
  - Secretory IgA
- Propulsive effects of small intestinal motility
  - Peristalsis
  - Migrating motor complex
- Antireflux properties of the ileocecal valve

In making a diagnosis of SIBO in the patient with SBS, the limitations of the various tests (i.e., small bowel aspirate, hydrogen breath test) must be remembered [36,47]. For example, the interpretation of breath tests may be complicated in patients with SBS, not only by rapid transit but also by carbohydrate malabsorption and resultant premature delivery of unabsorbed carbohydrate to the colon, where it will undergo fermentation, potentially resulting in a false-positive result [46,49]. Indeed, colonic fermentation has been correlated with breath hydrogen concentration [46]. It must also be borne in mind that false-negative or "flat" responses to lactulose administration may be found among those whose bacterial flora has been altered by antibiotic therapy or diarrhea or in whom motility disorders coexist, situations that are commonly present in patients with intestinal failure. Although much criticized on the basis of its invasive nature, availability in the community, risk of contamination of the sample, and inability to detect overgrowth in the more distal small intestine, culture of jejunal aspirate remains the much tarnished "gold standard" for the diagnosis of SIBO [36]. This may be particularly so in the setting of SBS, where breath testing is problematic. While a variety of other serum and urinary markers have been proposed as screening tests for SIBO, none has proven sufficiently reliable for clinical use [36]. SIBO, in reality, is devoid of a true gold standard test that may ultimately be provided by the application of modern molecular analytical techniques to samples from various parts of the small intestine [50].

The clinical and nutritional consequences of SIBO in SBS depend on the clinical context; in the patient with a remnant bowel that is marginal for independent existence or in whom adaptation has been compromised, the superimposition of SIBO may prove nutritionally devastating [49,51]. SIBO, for example, has been shown to delay weaning from PN [49,52]. Apart from the usual clinical features of SIBO (see list below), some additional features may be especially prominent in the SBS patient. Bacteria may compete with the host for protein and lead to the production of ammonia [53]. In the context of an impaired mucosal barrier, encephalopathy may result, as suggested by a case of recurrent encephalopathy in an intestinal transplant recipient, which resolved after resection of an intestinal stricture [54], which presumably led to the eradication of SIBO. Moreover, SBS patients, especially those with an intact colon, may suffer D-lactic acidemia and encephalopathy as a result of the production of D-lactic acid by Gram-positive anaerobes [55,56]. The development of neurological symptoms, such as somnolence, ataxia, or altered behavior, in a patient with SBS and an unexplained anion gap metabolic acidosis should lead one to suspect D-lactic acidosis caused by SIBO [57].

Clinical features of small intestinal bacterial overgrowth

- Diarrhea
- Steatorrhea
- Fat-soluble vitamin deficiency
- Weight loss
- Bloating, distension, flatulence
- Abdominal discomfort
- Vitamin B_{12} deficiency
- Elevated serum folate levels
- D-Lactic acidosis
- Protein-losing enteropathy leading to edema
- Hepatic steatosis, abnormal liver enzymes
- Elevated vitamin K levels; may interfere with anticoagulant effects

More recently, studies of the gut bacterial populations in SBS have moved toward the application of molecular methods to define the composition of the gut microbiota. In animal models, intestinal resection resulted in a reduction in the diversity of the colonic microbiota and the development of colonic inflammation [58]. Data in human short bowel subjects remain limited but seem to contradict culture-based studies, which suggest that bacterial populations in SBS were no different from normal [59]. Lilja and colleagues [60] noted dramatic changes in the composition of the microbiota in four of five children who were PN dependent, manifest by an abundance of *Enterobacteriacae*, whereas Davidovics and colleagues [61], while also describing an abnormal fecal microbiota, reported a greater abundance of *Gammaproteobacteria* and *Bacilli* [61]. Specific microbial signatures (*Proteobacteria, Lactobacilli*) have also been linked to the development of IFALD [62]. Mayeur and colleagues [63] documented a predominance of the *Lactobacillus/Leuconostoc* group and an underrepresentation of *Clostridium* and *Bacteroides* in the fecal microbiota of 16 patients with SBS and intact colon [63]. Given the heterogeneous nature of SBS populations as well as multiple confounding factors, these limited studies are difficult to interpret. Clearly, more complete studies of the gut microbiota and its function are indicated. Whether such studies will provide new guidelines for therapeutic interventions such as antibiotics, prebiotics, and probiotics remains to be defined.

ANTIMICROBIALS

The primary goal of therapy of SIBO in intestinal failure should be the treatment or correction of any underlying disease or defect when possible. Unfortunately, for many patients with SBS, reversibility is simply not possible. For most patients with SIBO, management rests on the correction of any nutritional deficiencies and antibiotic therapy. The objective of antibiotic therapy in SIBO is not so much to eradicate the bacterial flora but rather to modify it in a manner that results in symptomatic improvement. Although, ideally, the choice of antimicrobial agent should reflect *in vitro* susceptibility testing, this is usually impractical as many different bacterial species, with different antibiotic sensitivities, typically coexist. Antibiotic treatment remains, therefore, primarily empirical. The polymicrobial nature of the contaminating flora usually requires the administration of broad-spectrum antibiotics, which cover both aerobic and anaerobic enteric bacteria [64–66]. Examples of antibiotic regimens that are frequently employed in SIBO are listed below.

Antibiotic regimens frequently employed in SIBO*

- Amoxicillin-clavulanic acid 500 mg t.i.d.
- Chloramphenicol 250 mg q.i.d.
- Ciprofloxacin 500 mg b.i.d.
- Metronidazole 250 mg t.i.d.
- Neomycin 500 mg b.i.d.
- Norfloxacin 800 mg o.d.
- Rifaximin 800–1200 mg per day
- Tetracycline 250 mg b.i.d.
- Tinidazole 500 mg o.d.
- Trimethoprim-sulfamethoxazole 1 double strength capsule b.i.d.

For regimes that have been specifically tested in short bowel syndrome patients, see text.

Bouhnik and colleagues [67] showed that amoxicillin-clavulanic acid and cefoxitin were effective against over 90% of isolated species in SIBO, indicating that they were suitable candidates for first-line therapy. Overall, a single, short (7- to 10-day) course of an antibiotic has been shown to improve symptoms for up to several months in 46–90% and render breath tests negative in 20–75% of all patients with SIBO. However, those in whom SIBO complicates intestinal failure may prove more refractory to antibiotic therapy and may require either repeated (e.g., the first 5 to 10 days out of every months) or continuous courses of antibiotic therapy [36]. Malik and colleagues [47], for example, proposed three different approaches to rotating antibiotic therapy for SIBO in children with intestinal failure based on risk stratification. For those considered moderate risk (no radiological or clinical evidence of dysmotility), they recommend rotating gentamicin 6 mg/kg/dose given

* Very few of these have been subjected to high quality-clinical trials.

twice daily for 7 days with metronidazole 10 mg/kg/dose given twice daily for 7 days with a 7-day antibiotic-free interval. For high-risk patients (radiological or clinical evidence of dysmotility), the gentamicin and metronidazole regimens are alternated every 7 days, and for individuals who are high risk and have experienced recurrent sepsis, amoxicillin-clavulanic acid in a dose of 15 mg/kg/dose given twice daily is rotated with metronidazole and gentamicin every 7 days [47].

Decisions on management should be individualized and consider the risks of long-term antibiotic therapy, such as diarrhea, *Clostridium difficile* infection, intolerance and bacterial resistance, as well as cost. For these reasons, norfloxacin, amoxicillin-clavulanic acid, and metronidazole are excellent options. Decisions regarding antibiotic therapy must also be mindful of the potential benefits of bacterial fermentation in terms of caloric salvage, especially of undigested carbohydrates [68]. In one of only a few randomized studies of antibiotic therapy for SIBO in short bowel patients, Attar and colleagues [69] found both norfloxacin and amoxicillin-clavulanic acid to be effective in improving diarrhea and reducing breath-hydrogen excretion. It was interesting to note, however, that despite excellent symptomatic response, not all patients normalized breath hydrogen excretion [69]. The more widespread availability of rifaximin, a broad-spectrum, poorly absorbed antibiotic, has presented a safe and effective alternative to the treatment of SIBO with a low risk of causing microbial resistance [70].

Among patients with SBS, antibiotic therapy may fail completely, indicating a need for alternative strategies in this clinical context and a reassessment of the role of SIBO in symptomatology. Antibiotic therapy may also prove effective in the prevention or therapy of complications of SIBO, such as liver disease [71] and D-lactic acidosis [72,73]. Although antibiotic therapy has been shown to prevent bacterial translocation in an animal model of SBS [74], it has proven more challenging to demonstrate this effect in man. Bowel segment reversal has been shown to stimulate jejunal hyperplasia and, thus, adaptation after massive resection but may promote SIBO; in an animal model, oral antibiotics have been shown to attenuate the systemic inflammatory response and weight loss associated with this procedure [75,76].

Prebiotics, Probiotics, and Synbiotics

While probiotics are defined as live microorganisms that, when ingested in adequate amount, confer a health benefit on the host [77], prebiotics are selectively fermented ingredients (typically carbohydrates) that result in specific changes in the composition and/or activity of the gastrointestinal microbiota (such as lactobacilli and bifidobacteria), thus conferring benefit(s) upon host health [78]. A synbiotic is simply a combination of a prebiotic (or prebiotics) and a probiotic (or probiotics).

Evidence for the clinical efficacy of prebiotics, whether administered alone or in conjunction with a probiotic, in human disease is scanty, and few large randomized controlled trials are extant in the literature. While some of the effects of prebiotics, such as enhanced calcium absorption and reduction in inflammation [79], might be of benefit in SBS, others, including increased gas production and increased stool frequency, might not. There is a scarcity of data on their use in SBS, intestinal failure, or SIBO [80]. Kanamori and colleagues [81] administered a synbiotic consisting of a galacto-oligosaccharide together with *Bifidobacterium breve* and *Lactobacillus casei* to seven children with SBS and refractory enterocolitis; synbiotic use resulted in a suppression of pathogenic species and increased short-chain fatty acids and promoted weight gain [81]. Similar results were reported in another small uncontrolled study [82]. In a case report, the same synbiotic combination was shown to reduce D-lactic acid levels and reverse the clinical features of D-lactic acidosis as well as prevent their recurrence in a 28-year-old with SBS who had failed to respond to antibiotics [83]. In a group of adults with SIBO unrelated to SBS, the combination of *Bacillus coagulans* and fructo-oligosaccharides rotating with antibiotics was shown to be more effective than antibiotics alone in terms of both symptom response and normalization of breath tests [84,85].

Probiotics, given their antibacterial, anti-inflammatory, and metabolic effects as well as their ability to support intestinal barrier function, should theoretically be of benefit to the SBS patient with SIBO [80]. More direct evidence of benefit comes from studies of probiotics in experimental models of translocation. In experimental models of the SBS, *Bifidobacterium lactis* reduced the rate of translocation [86–89]; others have shown that competition between probiotics and *Escherichia coli* reduced the adhesion and, thus, the translocation of the pathogen [90,91]. In another study, *Saccharmomyces boulardii* had no effect on either SIBO or translocation [92]. Animal studies suggest that probiotics may also promote adaptation [88,93].

Data on probiotic use from human studies is scanty. Sentonga and colleagues [94] failed to show any benefit of *Lactobacillus rhamnosus* on intestinal permeability in a double-blind, placebo-controlled, crossover study in 21 children with SBS. Based on their study in children with SIBO associated with SBS, Young and Vanderhoof [95] suggested that *Lactobacillus plantarum* 299v may either prevent or delay symptom recurrence after antibiotic therapy. In one randomized, double-blind trial among 12 patients with SIBO-related chronic diarrhea (but who did not have SBS), both *L. casei* and *Lactobacillus acidophilus* strains cerela proved effective [96]; in other studies, *Lactobacillus fermentum* [97] and *S. boulardii* [69] proved ineffective. In their recent systematic review, Reddy and colleagues [98] failed to retrieve any randomized controlled trial of probiotics in children or infants with SBS. In their analysis of the available data, they concluded that there was "insufficient evidence on the effects of probiotics in children with short bowel syndrome" [98].

Probiotics could be beneficial for those with complications related to SIBO in intestinal failure: the combination of a probiotic and kanamycin proved effective in a case of recurrent encephalopathy due to D-lactic acidosis [99], and experimental models have suggested a role for probiotics in non-alcoholic fatty liver disease (NAFLD) [100].

Concerns have been raised with regard to the safety of probiotics in SBS based on case reports of *Lactobacillus* sepsis [101,102] and D-lactic acidosis [103] related to probiotic therapy. With regard to the latter, it should be noted that lactobacilli are already abundant in the small intestine among children with SBS and D-lactic acidosis [63,104].

CONCLUSION

A variety of strategies employing agents that act primarily within the lumen of the small intestine or colon (if present) have been proposed to promote nutrient digestion and assimilation in the SBS. Supplemental pancreatic enzymes, bile salt binders (chelators), and supplementary bile acids each have a pathophysiological basis for their use in this context. Of these, bile acid supplementation has the best evidence base but has not been widely employed because of limited availability of appropriate preparations. Bile acid chelators, in contrast, should be used with caution, if at all, in this setting. SIBO is a well-documented and clinically important consequence of intestinal loss and/or disease. Its precise definition, however, remains problematic, and treatment strategies, although undoubtedly helpful, are largely empiric.

REFERENCES

1. Nordgaard I et al. Colon as a digestive organ in patients with short bowel. *Lancet* 1994;343:373–6.
2. Jeejeebhoy KN. Short bowel syndrome: A nutritional and medical approach. *CMAJ* 2002;166:1297–302.
3. Choi PM et al. High-fat diet enhances villus growth during the adaptation response to massive proximal small bowel resection. *J Gastrointest Surg* 2014;18:286–94.
4. Choi PM et al. The role of enteral fat as a modulator of body composition after small bowel resection. *Surgery* 2014;156:412–18.
5. Mossner J et al. Pancreatic enzyme therapy. *Dtsch Arztebl Int* 2011;108:578–82.
6. Kumpf VJ. Pharmacologic management of diarrhea in patients with short bowel syndrome. *JPEN J Parenter Enteral Nutr* 2014;38(Suppl 1):38S–44S.
7. Sauniere JF et al. Exocrine pancreatic function and protein-calorie malnutrition in Dakar and Abidjan (West Africa): Silent pancreatic insufficiency. *Am J Clin Nutr* 1988;48:1233–8.

8. Cleghorn GJ et al. Exocrine pancreatic dysfunction in malnourished Australian aboriginal children. *Med J Aust* 1991;154:45–8.
9. Huddy JR et al. Exocrine pancreatic insufficiency following esophagectomy. *Dis Esophagus* 2013;26:594–7.
10. Wang S et al. Screening and risk factors of exocrine pancreatic insufficiency in critically ill adult patients receiving enteral nutrition. *Crit Care* 2013;17:R171.
11. Kotler DP et al. Reversible gastric and pancreatic hyposecretion after long-term total parenteral nutrition. *N Engl J Med* 1979;300:241–2.
12. Remington M et al. Inhibition of postprandial pancreatic and biliary secretion by loperamide in patients with short bowel syndrome. *Gut* 1982;23:98–101.
13. Vidon N et al. Inhibitory effect of high caloric load of carbohydrates or lipids on human pancreatic secretions: A jejunal brake. *Am J Clin Nutr* 1989;50:231–6.
14. Matarese LE et al. Dietary and medical management of short bowel syndrome in adult patients. *J Clin Gastroenterol* 2006;40(Suppl 2):S85–93.
15. Camilleri M. Bile acid diarrhea: Prevalence, pathogenesis and therapy. *Gut Liver* 2015;9:332–9.
16. Burrin D et al. Digestive physiology of the pig symposium: Intestinal bile acid sensing is linked to key endocrine and metabolic signaling pathways. *J Anim Sci* 2013;91:1991–2000.
17. Li T et al. Bile acids as metabolic regulators. *Curr Opin Gastroenterol* 2015;31:159–65.
18. Kliewer SA et al. Bile acids as hormones: The FXR-FGF15/19 Pathway. *Dig Dis* 2015;33:327–31.
19. Pereira-Fantini PM et al. Altered FXR signaling is associated with bile acid dysmetabolism in short bowel syndrome–associated liver disease. *J Hepatol* 2014;61:1115–25.
20. Al-Ansari N et al. Analysis of the effect of intestinal resection on rat ileal bile acid transporter expression and on bile acid and cholesterol homeostasis. *Pediatr Res* 2003;52:286–91.
21. Ali AH et al. Recent advances in the development of farnesoid X receptor agonists. *Ann Transl Med* 2015;3:5.
22. Perrone EE et al. Dietary bile acid supplementation improves intestinal integrity and survival in a murine model. *J Pediatr Surg* 2010;45:1256–65.
23. Hofmann AF et al. Cholestyramine treatment of diarrhea associated with ileal resection. *N Engl J Med* 1969;281:397–402.
24. Hofmann AF et al. Role of bile acid malabsorption in pathogenesis of diarrhea and steatorrhea in patients with ileal resection. 1. Response to cholestyramine or replacement of dietary long chain triglyceride by medium chain triglyceride. *Gastroenterology* 1972;62:918–34.
25. Pichler J et al. Prevalence of gallstones compared in children with different intravenous lipids. *J Pediatr Gastroenterol Nutr* 2015;61:253–59.
26. Quigley EM et al. Hepatobiliary complications of total parenteral nutrition. *Gastroenterology* 1993;104:286–301.
27. Schneider SM et al. Taurine status and response to intravenous taurine supplementation in adults with short-bowel syndrome undergoing long-term parenteral nutrition: A pilot study. *Br J Nutr* 2006;96:365–70.
28. Little KH et al. Treatment of severe steatorrhea with ox bile in an ileectomy patient with residual colon. *Dig Dis Sci* 1992;37:929–33.
29. Gruy-Kapral C et al. Conjugated bile acid replacement therapy for short-bowel syndrome. *Gastroenterology* 1999;116:15–21.
30. Heydorn S et al. Bile acid replacement therapy with cholylsarcosine for short-bowel syndrome. *Scand J Gastreonterol* 1999;34:818–23.
31. Emmett M et al. Conjugated bile acid replacement therapy reduces urinary oxalate excretion in short bowel syndrome. *Am J Kidney Dis* 2003;41:230–7.
32. Kapral C et al. Conjugated bile acid replacement therapy in short bowel syndrome patients with a residual colon. *Z Gastroenterol* 2004;42:583–9.
33. Barclay AR et al. Systematic review: Medical and nutritional interventions for the management of intestinal failure and its resultant complications in children. *Aliment Pharmacol Ther* 2011;33:175–84.
34. De Marco G et al. Early treatment with ursodeoxycholic acid for cholestasis in children on parenteral nutrition because of primary intestinal failure. *Aliment Pharmacol Ther* 2006;24:387–94.
35. Vanderhoof JA et al. Short-bowel syndrome in children and adults. *Gastroenterology* 1997;113:1767–78.
36. Quigley EMM. Small intestinal bacterial overgrowth. In: Feldman M, Friedman LS, Brandt LJ, eds. *Sleisenger and Fordtran's Gastrointestinal and Liver Disease, 10th Edition*. 2016. New York, Elsevier. 1824–31.

37. Quigley EMM et al. The intestinal motor response to resection. *Gastroenterology* 1993;105:791–8.
38. Schimpl G et al. Bacterial translocation in short–bowel syndrome in rats. *Eur J Pediatr Surg* 1999;9:224–7.
39. Maestri L et al. Small bowel overgrowth: A frequent complication after abdominal surgery in newborns. *Pediatr Med Chir* 2002;24:374–6.
40. Asensio AB et al. Incidence of bacterial translocation in four different models of experimental short bowel syndrome. *Cir Pediatr* 2003;16:20–5.
41. Quigley EMM et al. Distinctive patterns of interdigestive motility at the canine ileocolonic junction. *Gastroenterology* 1984;87:836–44.
42. Quigley EMM et al. Motility of the terminal ileum and ileocecal sphincter in healthy man. *Gastroenterology* 1984;87:857–66.
43. Sanchez-Montes C et al. Small intestinal bacterial overgrowth in inactive Crohn's disease: Influence of thiopurine and biological treatment. *World J Gastroenterol* 2014;20:13999–4003.
44. Greco A et al. Glucose breath test and Crohn's disease: Diagnosis of small intestinal bacterial overgrowth and evaluation of therapeutic response. *Scand J Gastroenterol* 2015;50:1376–81.
45. Husebye E et al. Abnormal intestinal motor patterns explain enteric colonization with gram-negative bacilli in late radiation enteropathy. *Gastroenterology* 1995;109:1078–89.
46. Justino SR et al. Fasting breath hydrogen concentration in short bowel syndrome patients with colon in continuity before and after antibiotic therapy. *Nutrition* 2004;20:187–91.
47. Malik BA et al. Diagnosis and pharmacological management of small intestinal bacterial overgrowth in children with intestinal failure. *Can J Gastroenterol* 2011;25:41–5.
48. Gutierrez IM et al. Risk factors for small bowel bacterial overgrowth and diagnostic yield of duodenal aspirates in children with intestinal failure: A retrospective review. *J Pediatr Surg* 2012;47:1150–4.
49. Goulet O et al. Intestinal microbiota in short bowel syndrome. *Gastroenterol Clin Biol* 2010;34(Suppl 1):S37–43.
50. Ghoshal UC. How to interpret hydrogen breath tests. *J Neurogastroenterol Motil* 2011;17:312–17.
51. Carbonnel F et al. The role of anatomic factors in nutritional autonomy after extensive small bowel resection. *JPEN J Parenter Enteral Nutr* 1996;20:275–80.
52. Kaufman SS et al. Influence of bacterial overgrowth and intestinal inflammation on duration of parenteral nutrition in children with short bowel syndrome. *J Pediatr* 1997;131:356–61.
53. Varcoe R et al. Utilization of urea nitrogen for albumin synthesis in the stagnant loop syndrome. *Gut* 1974;15:898–902.
54. Shah SM et al. Relapsing encephalopathy following small bowel transplantation. *Transplant Proc* 2003;35:1565–6.
55. Gurevitch J et al. D-Lactic acidosis: A treatable encephalopathy in pediatric patients. *Acta Paediatr* 1993;82:119–21.
56. Angelet P et al. Recurrent episodes of acidosis with encephalophaty in a hemodialysis program patient with short bowel syndrome. *Nefrologia* 2002;22:196–8.
57. Soler Palacin P et al. D-Lactic acidosis in an 11-year-old patient with short bowel syndrome. *Ann Pediatr (Barc)* 2006;64:385–7.
58. Lapthorne S et al. Gut microbial diversity is reduced and is associated with colonic inflammation in a piglet model of short bowel syndrome. *Gut Microbes* 2013;4:212–21.
59. De Castro Furtado E et al. Cyclic parenteral nutrition does not change the intestinal microbiota in patients with short bowel syndrome. *Acta Cir Bras* 2013;28(Suppl 1):26–32.
60. Lilja HE et al. Intestinal dysbiosis in children with short bowel syndrome is associated with impaired outcome. *Microbiome* 2015;3:18.
61. Davidovics ZH et al. The fecal microbiome in pediatric patients with short bowel syndrome. *JPEN J Parenter Enteral Nutr* 2015 [epub ahead of print].
62. Korpela K et al. Intestinal microbiota signatures associated with histological liver steatosis in pediatric-onset intestinal failure. *JPEN J Parenter Enteral Nutr* 2015 [epub ahead of print].
63. Mayeur C et al. Faecal D/L lactate ratio is a metabolic signature of microbiota imbalance in patients with short bowel syndrome. *PLoS One* 2013;8:e54335.
64. Di Stefano M et al. Rifaximin versus chlortetracycline in the short-term treatment of small intestinal bacterial overgrowth. *Aliment Pharmacol Ther* 2000;14:551–6.
65. Castiglione F et al. Antibiotic treatment of small bowel bacterial overgrowth in patients with Crohn's disease. *Aliment Pharmacol Ther* 2003;18:1107–12.
66. Di Stefano M et al. Treatment of small intestine bacterial overgrowth. *Eur Rev Med Pharmacol Sci* 2005;9:217–22.

67. Bouhnik Y et al. Bacterial populations contaminating the upper gut in patients with small intestinal overgrowth syndrome. *Am J Gastroenterol* 1999;94:1327–31.
68. Royall D et al. Evidence for colonic conservation of unabsorbed carbohydrate in short bowel syndrome. *Am J Gastroenterol* 1992;87:751–6.
69. Attar A et al. Antibiotic efficacy in small intestinal bacterial overgrowth-related chronic diarrhea: A crossover randomized trial. *Gastroenterology* 1999;117:794–7.
70. Cuoco L et al. Small intestine bacterial overgrowth in irritable bowel syndrome: Retrospective study with rifaximin. *Minerva Gastroenterol Dietol* 2006;52:89–95.
71. Kubota A et al. The effect of metronidazole on TPN-associated liver dysfunction in neonates. *J Pediatr Surg* 1990;25:618–21.
72. Halperin ML et al. D-lactic acidosis: Turning sugar into acids in the gastrointestinal tract. *Kidney Int* 1996;49:1–8.
73. Bongaerts GP et al. Role of bacteria in the pathogenesis of short bowel syndrome-associated D-lactic academia. *Microb Pathog* 1997;22:285–93.
74. Tian J et al. Dietary glutamine and oral antibiotics each improve indexes of gut barrier function in rat short bowel syndrome. *Am J Physiol* 2009;296:G348–555.
75. Lee CH et al. Oral antibiotics attenuate bowel segment reversal-induced alterations in subpopulation and function of peripheral blood leukocytes, thymocytes, and splenocytes in massive bowel-resected rats. *JPEN J Parenter Enteral Nutr* 2009;33:90–101.
76. Lee CH et al. Oral antibiotics attenuate bowel segment reversal-induced systemic inflammatory response and body weight loss in massively bowel-resected rats. *JPEN J Parenter Enteral Nutr* 2007;31:397–405.
77. Hill C et al. The International Scientific Association for Probiotics and Prebiotics consensus statement on the scope and appropriate use of the term probiotic. *Nat Rev Gastroenterol Hepatol* 2014;11:506–14.
78. Gibson GR et al. Dietary prebiotics: Current status and new definition. *Food Sci Tech Bull Funct Foods* 2010;7:1–19.
79. Macfarlane S et al. Review article: Prebiotics in the gastrointestinal tract. *Aliment Pharmacol Ther* 2006;24:701–14.
80. Stoidis CN et al. Potential benefits of pro-and prebiotics on intestinal immunity and intestinal barrier in short bowel syndrome. *Nutr Res Rev* 2011;24:21–30.
81. Kanamori Y et al. Experience of long-term symbiotic therapy in seven short bowel patients with refractory enterocolitis. *J Pediatr Surg* 2004;39:1686–92.
82. Uchida K et al. Immunonutritional effects during synbiotics therapy in pediatric patients with short bowel syndrome. *Pediatr Surg Int* 2007;23:243–8.
83. Takahashi K et al. A stand-alone symbiotic treatment or the prevention of D-lactic acidosis in short bowel syndrome. *Int Surg* 2013;98:110–13.
84. Khalighi AR et al. Evaluating the efficacy of probiotic on treatment in patients with small intestinal bacterial overgrowth (SIBO)—A pilot study. *Indian J Med Res* 2014;140:604–8.
85. Chen WC et al. Probiotics, prebiotics & synbiotics in small intestinal bacterial overgrowth: Opening up a new therapeutic horizon! *Indian J Med Res* 2014;140:582–4.
86. Eizaguirre I et al. Probiotic supplementation reduces the risk of bacterial translocation in experimental short bowel syndrome. *J Pediatr Surg* 2002;37:669–702.
87. Garcia-Urkia N et al. Beneficial effects of *Bifidobacterium lactis* in the prevention of bacterial translocation in experimental short bowel syndrome. *Cir Pediatr* 2002;15:162–5.
88. Mogilner JG et al. Effect of probiotics on intestinal regrowth and bacterial translocation after massive small bowel resection in a rat. *J Pediatr Surg* 2007;42:1365–71.
89. Eizaguirre I et al. Escherichia coli translocation in experimental short bowel syndrome: Probiotic supplementation and detection by polymerase chain reaction. *Pediatr Surg Int* 2011;27:1301–5.
90. Molennar D et al. Exploring *Lactobacillus plantarum* genome diversity by using microarrays. *J Bacteriol* 2005;187:6119–27.
91. Pretzer G et al. Biodiversity-based identification and functional characterization of the mannose-specific adhesion of *Lactobacillus plantarum*. *J Bacteriol* 2005;187:6128–36.
92. Zaouche A et al. Effects of oral *Saccharomyces boulardii* on bacterial overgrowth, translocation, and intestinal adaptation after small bowel resection in rats. *Scand J Gastroenterol* 2000;35:160–5.
93. Tolga Muftuoglu MA et al. Effects of probiotics on experimental short-bowel syndrome. *Am J Surg* 2011;202:461–8.
94. Sentonga TA et al. Intestinal permeability and effects of *Lactobacillus rhamnosus* therapy in children with short bowel syndrome. *J Pediatr Gastroenterol Nutr* 2008;46:41–7.

95. Young RJ et al. Probiotic therapy in children with short bowel syndrome and bacterial overgrowth. *Gastroenterology* 1997;112:A916.
96. Gaon D et al. Effect of *Lactobacillus* strains (*L. casei* and *L. acidophilus* strains cerela) on bacterial overgrowth-related chronic diarrhea. *Medicina (B Aires)* 2002;62:159–63.
97. Stotzer PO et al. Probiotic treatment of small intestinal bacterial overgrowth by *Lactobacillus fermentum* KLD. *Scand J Infect Dis* 1996;28:615–19.
98. Reddy VS et al. Role of probiotics in short bowel syndrome in infants and children—A systematic review. *Nutrients* 2013;5:679–99.
99. Uchida H et al. D-Lactic acidosis in short bowel syndrome managed with antibiotics and probiotics. *J Pediatr Surg* 2004;39:634–6.
100. Quigley EM et al. The gut microbiota and the liver. Pathophysiological and clinical implications. *J Hepatol* 2013;58:1020–7.
101. Kunz AN et al. Two cases of *Lactobacillus bacteremia* during probiotic treatment of the short gut syndrome. *J Pediatr Gastroenterol Nutr* 2004;38:457–8.
102. de Groote MA et al. *Lactobacillus rhamnosus* GG bacteremia associated with probiotic use in a child with short gut syndrome. *Pediatr Infect Dis J* 2005;24:278–80.
103. Munakata S et al. A case of D-lactic acid encephalopathy associated with use of probiotics. *Brain Dev* 2017;32:691–4.
104. Bongaerts G, Bakkeren J, Severijnen R et al. 200. Lactobacilli and acidosis in children with short bowel. *J Pediatr Gastroenterol Nutr* 2000;30:288–93.

19 Glucagon-Like Peptide-2 in Short Bowel Syndrome

James S. Scolapio and Matt Clark

CONTENTS

KEY POINTS

- Teduglutide, a dipeptidylpeptidase degradation-resistant glucagon-like peptide-2 analog, has been shown to enhance structural and functional intestinal adaptation in humans and increase fluid absorption in patients with short bowel syndrome (SBS).
- SBS patients treated with teduglutide for 52 weeks who have >50 cm of small intestine and a segment of colon-in-continuity appear to have the highest likelihood of a favorable response in terms of weaning of parenteral support.
- Clinical trials have reported that some SBS patients have been weaned and remain off parenteral support for up to 2 years after treatment with teduglutide.
- Common side effects of teduglutide include injection site reactions, nausea and vomiting, headache, and stomal enlargement. Active gastrointestinal cancer is a contraindication to teduglutide use.

INTRODUCTION

Glucagon-like peptide (GLP)-2 is a 33-amino-acid member of the glucagon family, which includes both GLP-1 and GLP-2. Unlike GLP-1, GLP-2 has proven trophic effects on the intestinal mucosa, thereby augmenting enterocyte mass, as evidenced by an increase in villus height and crypt depth [1]. Intestinal adaptation is a natural compensatory process after intestinal resection; GLP-2 has been shown to enhance this adaptation process [1]. GLP-2 is released by enteroendocrine L cells present in the distal ileum and proximal colon in response to nutrient stimulation. The gastrointestinal physiological effects of GLP-2 in humans include an increase in intestinal and portal blood flow, a decrease in gastrointestinal secretions, epithelial proliferation and villus growth, and a slowing of gastric emptying [2].

The effects of a glucagon-like hormone on the human intestine were first reported in 1971 in a patient with an enteroglucagon-producing renal tumor and an enlarged, thickened small intestine [3]. Subsequent research in a rat model reported the trophic effects of GLP-2 on the rat intestine [4]. It was shown that the intestinotrophic effects of GLP-2 were mediated by the GLP-2 receptor in the small intestine; however, the trophic effects of GLP-2 on the intestine were limited by its rapid metabolism via circulating dipeptidylpeptidase IV (DPP-IV) enzymes. An analog of GLP-2, now known as teduglutide, was experimentally developed by substitution of the amino acid glycine for alanine in the N-terminal position of GLP-2. It was found that the glycine substitution prevents GLP-2 degradation by DPP-IV enzymes, thus prolonging its half-life and trophic effects from 7 minutes to 2 hours and making this analog potentially therapeutically useful in a clinical setting [5]. Indeed, over the past 10 years, clinical studies in humans have found that teduglutide not only has trophic effects on the human small intestine but also has positive clinical effects, including the reduction of the need for parenteral nutrition (PN) in patients with short bowel syndrome (SBS) [6–13]. In 2012, teduglutide was approved by the U.S. Food and Drug Administration (FDA) as an aid in the weaning of parenteral support (i.e., PN or intravenous fluids) in patients with SBS. In this chapter, we review the published clinical trials as well as the clinical application of teduglutide in adult patients with SBS.

CLINICAL TRIALS

In a phase I trial, subcutaneous teduglutide injection at doses ranging from 2.5 to 10 mg were shown to be safe and well tolerated in healthy volunteers [6]. Peak plasma concentrations were achieved 3 hours after injection. In 2001, an open-label study with native GLP-2 was completed in eight SBS patients without a colon [7]. These included four patients receiving PN (mean length of residual jejunum, 83 cm) and four patients not receiving PN (mean length of residual jejunum, 106 cm) [7]. All had SBS for more than 1 year (range, 4–17 years) and were considered to be in a stable phase. The mean small intestine length was 83 cm (range, 65–170 cm). None of the six patients with Crohn's disease had signs of active disease. Four hundred micrograms of subcutaneous GLP-2 was administered twice daily for a total of 35 days. A significant increase in fluid absorption was reported; however, significant increases in total energy, electrolyte, carbohydrate, protein, and fat absorption were not observed. Subject body weight increased by a mean of 1.2 kg. A significant increase in intestinal villus height and crypt depth was observed, supporting a trophic effect of GLP-2 in humans. Furthermore, GLP-2 was well tolerated by all the subjects and side effects were minimal, including erythema and tenderness at the injection site. This study concluded that GLP-2 exhibits its clinical benefit primarily by increasing fluid absorption.

In a subsequent phase II pilot study involving the longer-active GLP-2 analog, teduglutide, 16 adult patients with SBS were included [8]. All patients had undergone extensive resection of the small intestine (<150 cm of small bowel remaining) at least 1 year prior to study entry. None of the patients had signs of active Crohn's disease. Ten patients had an end-jejunostomy, 1 patient had <50% of his or her colon-in-continuity, while 5 others had their entire colon-in-continuity. Twelve of the 16 patients required PN. Patients were treated with subcutaneous teduglutide for 21 days at doses of 0.03, 0.10, or 0.15 mg/kg/day [8]. The doses used were chosen to examine dose response over a range that was expected to provide clinical benefit. A significant increase in absolute wet weight absorption and urine output, in addition to reduced fecal weight excretion, was found with teduglutide use—effects that were not dose related. Also reported in this study was an increase in small bowel villus height, crypt depth, and mitotic index, all of which supported the known trophic effects of native GLP-2 seen in the rodent model. Crypt depth and mitotic index did not change in colonic biopsies from those patients with colon-in-continuity. Effects on gastrointestinal transit were not measured in this study. This study provides further evidence that the main benefit of GLP-2 appears to be enhanced fluid absorption. Teduglutide was well tolerated in the majority of patients studied. In addition, there were no antibodies to teduglutide detected. Three patients did report minor injection site reactions and one patient reported minor lower extremity edema. Enlargement of the jejunostomy stoma was also reported by several patients, supporting the proliferation effects of teduglutide on the small intestine.

On the basis of the evidence previously described supporting an intestinotrophic role of teduglutide, thereby improving intestinal absorption, a multicenter pivotal study (32 centers) of 83 patients with SBS was conducted [9]. The mean age of patients was 48.8 years (range, 19–79 years), with an approximately equal gender distribution. Intestinal resection in the setting of Crohn's disease and acute mesenteric ischemia was the cause of SBS in 66% of the patients. Sixty-eight percent of patients had part of their colon-in-continuity, with a median remnant small intestine length of 50 cm (range, 6–125 cm). In those patients without a colon, the median small intestine length was 75 cm (range, 30–200 cm). Patients had been on PN for a mean of 7 years (range, 1–24 years). The primary end point was the ability to wean off PN. SBS patients were randomized to receive once daily subcutaneous teduglutide 0.10 mg/kg/day (n = 32) or 0.05 mg/kg/day (n = 35) or placebo (n = 16) for 24 weeks after first undergoing a period of PN optimization and stabilization [9]. These patients had been dependent on PN for at least 12 months and required parenteral support for a minimum of three times per week. Antimotility and antidiarrheal agents remained constant during the 24-week study in all patients; approximately half of the patients were taking these medications. Patients were also asked to keep diet and oral rehydration solutions as constant as possible during the study. In the standardized parenteral fluid weaning algorithm, 48-hour urine output was used to determine if a patient's parenteral fluids could be reduced. Weaning of parenteral support was allowed when 48-hour urinary volume increased by at least 10% from baseline urinary volume. Although oral intake was not strictly controlled, study subjects were asked to keep the quantity and type of oral intake as constant or as habitual as possible during the 48-hour urine collection period. A 20% reduction of infused parenteral volume at week 20 ("responder") was considered clinically significant and was the primary endpoint.

The responder rate (20% reduction in parenteral volume) at the end of the treatment period was significantly higher in the 0.05 mg/kg/day dosed group compared with the placebo group; however, there was no statistically significant difference between the 0.10 mg/kg/day dosed group and the placebo group. In the 0.05 mg/kg/day group, parenteral volume was reduced by an average of 350 mL/day (Table 19.1). The reduction in parenteral energy was not significantly different between

TABLE 19.1
Summary of Published Phase III Clinical Trials and Extension Studies of Teduglutide in SBS

	Teduglutide [9]			Teduglutide [11]	
Study Group	**(a) PBO**	**(b) TED 0.05**	**(c) TED 0.10**	**(a) PBO**	**(b) TED 0.05**
Diet	Habitual	Habitual	Habitual	Habitual	Habitual
No. of subjects	16	35	32	43	43
Remnant short bowel length (cm)	77 ± 23	58 ± 44	68 ± 43	69 ± 64	84 ± 65
Colon present	11	26	19	23	26
Study drug	None	TED 0.05 mg/kg/d	TED 0.1 mg/kg/d	None	TED 0.05 mg/kg/d
Duration	24 wks	24 wks	24 wks	24 wks	24 wks
Δ PN volume, L/wk	−0.9	−2.5	−2.5	−2.3	−4.4*** (a vs. b)
Δ PN energy, kcal/wk	−406	−1526	−749	NR	NR
>20% decrease in PN	6%	46%* (a vs. b)	25%	30%	63%** (a vs. b)
Δ body weight, kg	0.2	1.2	1.4	−0.6	1.0
Duration	–	52 wks (treatment) (N = 19/25)	52 wks (treatment) (N = 23/27)	–	–
Δ PN volume, L/wk	–	−4.9	−3.3	–	–
Δ PN energy, kcal/wk	–	−3511	−1556	–	–
>20% decrease in PN	–	68%	52%	–	–
Δ body weight, kg	–	NR	NR	–	–

Note: NR, not reported; PBO, placebo; TED, teduglutide.
* $P = 0.005$.
** $P = 0.002$.
*** $P < 0.001$.

the two active treatment doses and placebo. Neither active treatment dose resulted in a significant reduction in the number of days on parenteral support; however, three of the patients treated with the lower teduglutide dose were completely weaned from parenteral support. A significant increase in small intestine villus height was reported compared with baseline in both treatment doses. Likewise, plasma citrulline concentration and lean body mass were significantly increased in the teduglutide groups compared with the placebo group [10]. Both doses of teduglutide were well tolerated throughout the 24-week study. The most common side effects reported included abdominal pain (24%), headache (24%), and nausea (22%).

Despite the significant benefit in the lower-dose teduglutide group, this study was regarded as negative because there was no significant difference in response between the higher dose (0.10 mg/kg/day) and placebo, which was the primary endpoint [9]. As a consequence, a second trial comparing the lower teduglutide dose (0.05 mg/kg/day) and placebo was completed. Jeppesen et al. [11] performed a multicenter, randomized, double-blind, placebo-controlled phase 3 study. In this 24-week study, 86 adult SBS patients received subcutaneous teduglutide 0.05 mg/kg/day (n = 43) or placebo (n = 43) once daily. The mean age of patients studied was 50.3 years (range, 18–82 years). Patients had been receiving parenteral support for an average of 6.3 years (range, 1–25.8 years) and required parenteral support for at least three times per week. The average length of remnant small intestine in patients without a colon was 130.8 cm and 48.1 cm in those with part of their colon remaining. The intestine length was similar in both the teduglutide- and placebo-treated groups. Patients were requested to maintain a habitual diet and fluids, and no medications were started or changed during the stabilization period and throughout the 24-week treatment period. The primary efficacy endpoint was the number of responders with a >20% reduction in parenteral support volume from baseline compared with weeks 20 and 24. Parenteral support was reduced if 48-hour urine volumes exceeded baseline values by >10%. Secondary efficacy endpoints included the percentage and absolute change in parenteral support and the number of patients who stopped parenteral support at the discontinuation of treatment. Notably, the weaning plan was more aggressive in this study than in the prior teduglutide trial.

There were 27/43 (63%) responders in the teduglutide group and 13/43 (30%) in the placebo group (P = 0.002) (Table 19.1). At week 24, the mean reduction in parenteral support volume in the teduglutide group was 4.4 L/week compared with 2.3 L/week in the placebo group (P < 0.001). The percentage of patients with a 1-day or more reduction in parenteral support at week 24 was higher in the teduglutide group (54%) compared with the placebo group (23%) (P = 0.005). The most frequently reported adverse events in the teduglutide group included abdominal pain, nausea, stoma complications, and abdominal distension. No major alterations in laboratory tests (chemistry or hematology) were noted.

In an effort to determine the lasting effect of teduglutide treatment, Compher et al. [12] subsequently conducted an observational study in which 53 patients who had been treated with 24 weeks of teduglutide in the first multicenter study [9] were included to describe the change in PN use and body mass index (BMI) after stopping teduglutide. Data were collected prospectively during clinic visits at 0, 3, 6, and 12 months relative to discontinuing teduglutide treatment. Thirty-seven patients were included in the final analysis. The median age was 51 years (range, 21–68 years) and included 20 men and 17 women. Mean small intestine length was 50 cm (range, 0–213 cm) and colon length was 80 cm (range, 0–200 cm). The patients were classified according to whether their PN volume was increased, unchanged, or decreased at 12 months after stopping teduglutide. Fifteen (40.5%) had their PN volume increased during the 12 months after stopping the teduglutide, 15 (40.5%) maintained the same PN volume, and 7 (19%) had further PN volume reduction. Those who required increased PN had a shorter amount of residual colon. There was not a significant difference in PN requirements based on residual small bowel length, time since surgical resection, or patient age and gender. The median BMI did not change significantly over the 12-month study period and was not statistically different in those patients requiring increased PN versus those who remained unchanged or had decreased PN requirements. Based on the previous primary endpoint of >20% reduction from preteduglutide PN volume at the end of teduglutide treatment, there were 25 responders (i.e., those patients in whom the PN was unchanged or decreased). In the unchanged group, the three patients who had come off PN while on teduglutide remained off PN 12 months later. There was no difference in drug dose or time since last surgical resection in the responders compared with the nonresponders. The median length of small intestine was greater in responders (50 cm) than in the nonresponders (35 cm). The responders also had a longer length of colon-in-continuity compared with the nonresponders. A lower BMI at baseline and a lower PN volume reduction (i.e., receiving a lower PN volume at baseline) while on teduglutide were also predictors of a positive response. Patients with the characteristics described in the following list, once weaned using teduglutide, might be considered for a period off teduglutide under close clinical observation.

Predictors of long-term successful PN weaning in SBS patients previously treated with teduglutide [12]:

- Colon-in-continuity
- Small intestine remnant greater than 50 cm
- Lower amount of infused parenteral volume prior to treatment
- Lower amount of parenteral volume reduced during treatment

To determine the safety, tolerability, and clinical efficacy of longer use of teduglutide (beyond 24 weeks), O'Keefe and colleagues [13] subsequently completed a 28-week double-blind extension study that included patients who had received either 0.05 or 0.1 mg/kg/day dose of teduglutide and completed the first 24-week multicenter randomized controlled study [9] for a total treatment period of 52 weeks. A clinically significant response was defined as a reduction of 20% or more in weekly PN volume. Of the 56 patients who successfully completed the initial 24-week study, 52 (25 patients on 0.05 mg/kg/day and 27 patients on the 0.10 mg/kg/day dose) agreed to participate; 42 completed efficacy analyses at the end of 52 weeks. The mean age of patients in this extension study was 48.1 years, with an approximately equal gender distribution. The median length of small intestine was 60 cm (range, 10–200 cm), with 37% of patents having part of their colon-in-continuity. The median PN volume per week was 10.6 L (range, 4–33 L). Patients had been on PN for an average of 7 years (range, 1–24 years). The most common adverse events reported included headache (35%), nausea (31%), and abdominal pain (25%). No adenomatous polyps or colon cancers were found on colonoscopy at the end of the study. Seven patients did not tolerate the medication and withdrew from the study; most ($n = 4$) were the result of gastrointestinal symptoms. A greater than 20% reduction in PN was found in 68% of the 0.05 mg/kg/day and 37% of the 0.10 mg/kg/day treated groups at week 52, with four patients being completely weaned from PN. Four weeks after stopping the teduglutide, there was a need to increase the PN volume in the 0.05 mg/kg/day group, but not the 0.10 mg/kg/day group. Eleven of the 19 nonresponders at 24 weeks became responders by the end of the of this 28-week extension study. These results suggest a benefit in administering the medication for up to 52 weeks.

CLINICAL APPLICATION OF TEDUGLUTIDE

Teduglutide (Gattex, Shire Pharmaceuticals, Inc., North Reading, Massachusetts) was approved by the FDA in December 2012 for use in adult patients with SBS dependent on parenteral support [14]. Teduglutide has also been approved by the European Medicines Agency for SBS patients as a long-term aid to PN weaning (Revestive). The recommended dose is 0.05 mg/kg/day administered by subcutaneous injection. A 50% dosage reduction is recommended in patients with renal impairment (creatinine clearance less than 50 mL/min). Teduglutide is supplied in a sterile, single-use glass vial containing 5.0 mg of teduglutide as a white, lyophilized powder to be reconstituted with 0.5 mL of sterile water for subcutaneous injection. The average annual cost for teduglutide administration is $295,000. The cost for the patient is generally much lower as a result of insurance coverage and patient support programs. Insurance coverage for continued use of teduglutide once a patient is weaned from PN may prove to be a barrier with use beyond 1 year.

A practical approach to weaning PN from patients who are treated with teduglutide is important for the clinician. First, it is important to select suitable patients for its use (see list below). Suitable patients would include adults with short bowel for more than 1 year without gastrointestinal obstruction or a history of gastrointestinal cancer. Prior to beginning the weaning process, the patient's fluid and nutrition status needs to be optimized and the weight should be stable. Furthermore, the diet, hydration status, and antidiarrheal and antisecretory medications should also be optimized prior to treatment with teduglutide and PN weaning. One approach to the parenteral support (PN or intravenous fluids) weaning algorithm is based on an increase in urine output of greater than 10% from a patient's baseline urinary output. Monitoring daily urine and stool output is helpful in determining when and how much PN volume to wean. In the clinical trials previously described, 48-hour urine output collection was recommended to guide adjustments in weaning parenteral fluids. Ideally, patients should maintain a urine output of >1000 mL/day throughout this process. Reductions in parenteral support are typically recommended at 2- to 4-week intervals. Once PN infusions are <3 days per week, a trial of PN discontinuation can be considered. See Chapter 25 for further details on PN weaning.

When to consider using teduglutide:

- Require PN/IV fluids three or more times per week for ≥1 year
- <1 year on PN/IV fluids, with one or more septic episodes or liver injury present
- Clinically stable and well nourished
- Optimized short bowel diet and hydration therapy
- Maximized conventional short bowel pharmacotherapy
- Motivated with a desire to reduce or discontinue the parenteral support
- Demonstrated compliance/reliability with other therapies
- Partnership exists between treatment team and patient
- Absent GI structural defects (e.g., obstruction) precluding adequate oral intake
- Absent contraindications for use
  - Active GI neoplasia
  - Active non-GI malignancy—assess risk vs. benefit

The clinician needs to be aware of the side effects and contraindications associated with teduglutide therapy (see Risk Evaluation and Mitigation Strategy [REMS] at http://www.gattexrems.com). The most common adverse effects are abdominal pain, injection site reactions, nausea and vomiting, and headaches. Stomal enlargement, in those with an ostomy, also occurs commonly and can be a source of frustration due to leakage and require revision of the ostomy appliance. As might be expected, fluid overload has been reported, and caution is advised in those with congestive heart failure or severe kidney disease. Although no data regarding enhanced medication absorption have been reported, caution should be given with oral medications with a narrow therapeutic index and those absorbed predominantly from the small intestine. Laboratory testing (bilirubin, alkaline phosphatase, lipase, and amylase) is recommended every 6 months while on therapy given the occurrence of gallbladder disease and pancreatitis observed in the clinical trials. Adequate studies with teduglutide have not been conducted in pregnant and nursing women or pediatric patients.

Listed on the teduglutide warning label is the potential for neoplastic growth. Teduglutide use is not recommended in patients with active or a history of a gastrointestinal malignancy. The clinical decision to continue teduglutide in patients with nongastrointestinal malignancy should be made based on risk–benefit considerations. It is recommended that patients being treated with teduglutide undergo a screening colonoscopy within 6 months of starting therapy, 1 year after, and at 5-year intervals thereafter while on treatment.

CONCLUSION

The collective evidence from both preclinical studies on intestinal adaptation and randomized controlled clinical trials supports the benefit of teduglutide in the treatment of adult patients with SBS requiring parenteral support. The clinical benefit appears to be modulated primarily by enhanced intestinal fluid absorption. Many SBS patients treated with teduglutide have been able to reduce parenteral support by at least 1 day and several patients have been able to completely discontinue all parenteral support. Some patients who did not experience a significant reduction in parenteral support after 24 weeks of treatment did experience a reduction in parenteral support after 52 weeks of treatment. These observations underscore the importance of individualizing treatment in this heterogeneous population. Overall, teduglutide use appears safe and well tolerated; however, a REMS program is in place and is required for all providers of this therapy. Additional clinical follow-up and reporting will be helpful as more SBS patients are treated. Finally, the cost of teduglutide and insurance coverage may prove to be a limiting factor for use. Cost analyses are needed comparing teduglutide to more traditional therapies.

REFERENCES

1. Tappenden KA. Intestinal adaptation following resection. *JPEN J Parenter Enteral Nutr* 2014;38:23S–31S.
2. Estall JL et al. Glucagon-like peptide-2. *Annu Rev Nutr* 2006;26:391–411.
3. Gleeson MH et al. Endocrine tumor in the kidney affecting small bowel structure, motility, and absorptive function. *Gut* 1971;12:773–782.
4. Drucker DJ et al. Induction of intestinal epithelial proliferation by glucagon-like peptide 2. *Proc Natl Acad Sci USA* 1996;93:7911–7916.
5. Drucker DJ et al. Regulation of the biological activity of glucagon-like peptide 2 in vivo by dipeptidyl peptidase IV. *Nat Biotechnol* 1997;15:673–677.
6. Metcalfe AJ et al. An evaluation of single dose administration of ALX-0600, a GLP-2 analog, in healthy male subjects. *Gastroenterology* 2000;118;Abstract 1072.
7. Jeppesen PB et al. Glucagon-like peptide 2 improves nutrient absorption and nutritional status in short bowel patient with no colon. *Gastroenterology* 2001;120:806–815.
8. Jeppesen PB et al. Teduglutide (ALX-0600), a dipeptidyl peptidase IV resistant glucagon-like peptide 2 analogue, improves intestinal function in short bowel syndrome patients. *Gut* 2005;54:1224–1231.
9. Jeppesen PB et al. Randomized placebo-controlled trial of teduglutide in reducing parenteral nutrition and/or intravenous fluid requirements in patients with short bowel syndrome. *Gut* 2011;1136:1–13.
10. Tappenden KA et al. Teduglutide enhances structural adaptation of the small intestine mucosa in patients with short bowel syndrome. *J Clin Gastroenterol* 2013;47:602–607.
11. Jeppesen PB et al. Teduglutide reduces need for parenteral support among patients with short bowel syndrome with intestinal failure. *Gastroeneterology* 2012;143:1473–1481.
12. Compher C et al. Maintenance of parenteral nutrition volume reduction, without weight loss, after stopping teduglutide in a subset of patients with short bowel syndrome. *JPEN J Parenter Enteral Nutr* 2011;35:603–609.
13. O'Keefe SJ et al. Safety and efficacy of teduglutide after 52 weeks of treatment in patients with short bowl intestinal failure. *Clin Gastroenterol Hepatol* 2013;11:815–823.
14. Shire Pharmaceuticals, Inc., North Reading, Massachusetts (http://www.GATTEX.com and http://www.Shire.com).

20 Utility of Growth Hormone and Other Potential Agents to Restore Enteral Autonomy in Short Bowel Syndrome

John K. DiBaise

CONTENTS

KEY POINTS

- Despite advances in the provision of parenteral nutrition (PN), this mode of nutritional support carries with it significant risks to the patient, impairs quality of life, and is costly.
- Intestinal adaptation plays a key role in the successful management of patients with short bowel syndrome (SBS). Recent investigations have focused on the use of trophic substances to increase the absorptive function of the remaining gut.
- In patients with PN-dependent SBS, treatment with somatropin (i.e., recombinant human growth hormone) has shown conflicting results in terms of effects on intestinal absorption but impressive reductions in PN requirements, leading to controversy and lack of certainty on the clinical utility of this treatment approach.
- Somatropin appears to be well tolerated, with manageable side effects including fluid retention, gastrointestinal symptoms, and injection site reactions occurring commonly and serious adverse effects being uncommon.
- Somatropin should be used under the guidance of clinicians experienced in the management of SBS, with an expectation that these patients need to be monitored closely, both during and after its use.

INTRODUCTION

After the 1- to 2-year period of greatest intestinal adaptation following massive resection, a homeostatic/maintenance stage begins where no further spontaneous intestinal adaptation is thought to occur. Intestinal failure is frequently considered permanent when parenteral nutrition (PN) is required beyond this stage. This is exemplified by the <6% probability of eliminating PN use if not successfully accomplished in the first 2 years after the individual's last bowel resection [1]. Fortunately, >50% of adults with SBS are able to be weaned completely from PN within 5 years of diagnosis [1,2]. Despite the life-saving nature of PN and advances in its provision, it is associated with significant risks to the patient, such as catheter-related sepsis, venous thrombosis, and liver disease; notably, it also impairs quality of life and is very costly. Therefore, an important goal when treating the SBS patient who requires PN is to reduce dependency on it and, whenever possible, eliminate its use altogether. As such, there has been intense investigation to identify treatments that maximize intestinal adaptation and absorption.

The current understanding of the adaptation process (see Chapter 4) has led to the study of hormones, nutrients, and growth factors in experimental models and in humans with SBS. A number of pharmacological agents have been demonstrated to induce trophic properties on the intestinal epithelium in animal models of SBS. These reports have been followed by conflicting information regarding efficacy in humans with respect to the adaptive changes to the gut, enhancement of intestinal absorption, and usefulness to restore enteral autonomy. In this chapter, pharmacologic agents other than glucagon-like peptide-2 (GLP-2) (see Chapter 19) that are available for use or in development to aid in weaning PN will be discussed, including recombinant human growth hormone (rhGH), GLP-1, glutamine, epidermal growth factor (EGF), and peptide YY.

GROWTH HORMONE

Effect on Intestinal Adaptation and Absorption

In animal models of SBS, the exogenous administration of growth hormone (GH) has been shown to enhance intestinal epithelial hyperplasia, resulting in an increase in body weight, small bowel length, colonic mass, and biomechanical strength [3–7]. While enhanced intestinal absorption has been consistently demonstrated in animal models of SBS [8–13], there have been conflicting reports on GH use in humans (Table 20.1) [14–20]. GH has also been shown to favorably affect bone mineral density and markers of bone turnover [21]. It is likely that the mixed results in humans are, at least partly, attributable to methodological differences, including study design and patient characteristics, and thereby prevent definitive conclusions regarding the benefit (or lack thereof) of this therapy on intestinal absorption.

Effect on PN Weaning

On the basis of the results on intestinal absorption, Byrne et al. [22] conducted an open-label study involving 47 SBS patients who received rhGH (mean dose, 0.11 mg/kg/day; range, 0.03–0.14) together with oral glutamine (30 g/day) and a high-complex-carbohydrate, low-fat diet for 4 weeks while admitted to a clinical research facility. After this 4-week treatment with rhGH, patients continued at home with oral glutamine and the modified diet. Follow-up data were reported after 1 year. Patients were allowed to continue use of other standard treatments used in SBS such as antimotility and antisecretory medications and oral rehydration solutions (ORSs). Most patients ($n = 39$) were dependent on PN, while several ($n = 8$) were referred with progressive malnutrition to prevent the need to initiate PN. The primary endpoint was PN weaning rather than intestinal absorption or body composition. After 4 weeks of treatment, 27 patients (57%) had eliminated PN use, 14 (30%) were able to reduce their PN requirements, and 6 (13%) experienced no change in PN requirements. Only

TABLE 20.1
Efficacy of rhGH on Intestinal Absorption and PN Weaning in SBS Patients

Author	*N*	Study Design	Remnant Small Bowel Length, Mean (Range)	Colon Present (*N*)	Mean Time on PN (Years)	Treatment (Duration)	Results
Byrne et al. [15]	10	Open	37 (8–90) cm	10	6	rhGH (0.14 mg/kg/day), glutamine, HCLF diet (3–4 weeks)	Improved nutrient and water absorption; decreased stool output
Ellegard et al. [18]	10	RCCT	130 (90–170) cm	4	Only 1 patient on PN	rhGH (0.024 mg/kg/day) (8 weeks)	Increased body weight, lean body mass, total body potassium, bone mineral content; no change in energy or fluid absorption
Scolapio et al. [19]	8	RCCT	71 (55–120) cm	2	12.9	rhGH (0.14 mg/kg/day), glutamine (3 weeks)	Transient increase in body weight and lean body mass; increased sodium and potassium absorption
Skudlarek et al. [20]	8	RCCT	104 (30–150) cm	4	7	rhGH (0.14 mg/kg/day), glutamine (4 weeks)	No improvement in intestinal absorption; increased body weight
Byrne et al. [23]	61 (49 on PN)	Open	61 (0–183) cm	37	4	rhGH (0.09 mg/kg/day), glutamine, individualized diet (4 weeks)	41% off PN, 51% on reduced amount of PN, 8% no change in PN after 1 year
Seguy et al. [14]	12	RCCT	48 (0–120) cm	9	7.5	rhGH (0.05 mg/kg/day), hyperphagic diet (3 weeks)	Improved nitrogen, energy, and carbohydrate absorption; increased body weight and lean body mass; no change in plasma citrulline

(*Continued*)

TABLE 20.1 (CONTINUED)
Efficacy of rhGH on Intestinal Absorption and PN Weaning in SBS Patients

Author	*N*	Study Design	Remnant Small Bowel Length, Mean (Range)	Colon Present (*N*)	Mean Time on PN (Years)	Treatment (Duration)	Results
Zhu et al. [24]	27	Open	47 (15–80) cm	14	NR	rhGH (0.05 mg/kg/day), glutamine, modified diet (3 weeks)	Treated during period of adaptation; 77% off PN at 1 year; 50% off PN at 2 years
Weiming et al. [25]	37	Open	45 (15–100) cm	20	NR	rhGH (0.05 mg/kg/day), glutamine, HCLF diet, EN (3 weeks)	All but 3 treated ≤2 years from resection; 21 of 23 patients followed for >2 years weaned completely from PN (18 maintained on HCLF diet + EN)
Guo et al. [26]	12	Open	59 (10–100) cm	11	NR	rhGH (0.05 mg/kg/day), glutamine, HCLF diet, EN (4 weeks)	All but one treated during period of adaptation; reduced PN requirements (6 off PN); increased nitrogen absorption
Byrne et al. [27]	41	RCPGT	73 (NR) cm	36	4	rhGH (0.1 mg/kg/day), glutamine, individualized diet (4 weeks)	Reduced PN requirements (9 off PN); stable body weight

Note: EN, enteral nutrition; HCLF, high carbohydrate, low fat; NR, not reported; PN, parenteral nutrition; RCCT, randomized, controlled, crossover trial; RCPGT, randomized, controlled, parallel group trial; rhGH, recombinant human growth hormone; SBS, short bowel syndrome.

the end-jejunostomy patients were unable to make any reductions in PN requirements. One year later, 19 patients (40%) remained off PN, while 19 (40%) others were on reduced PN and 9 (19%) were receiving PN at levels similar to their initial pretreatment requirements. This report ushered in the concept of "intestinal rehabilitation."

In a follow-up to this study, these investigators conducted a larger open-label study involving 61 SBS patients who were treated with a mean rhGH dose of 0.09 mg/kg/day plus 30 g/day of oral glutamine in combination with an individualized diet based upon their remaining bowel anatomy [23]. Forty-nine were PN dependent and 12 were treated to prevent initiation or resumption of PN. Treatment continued for 4–6 weeks, once again while admitted to a clinical facility for intense monitoring and education, and then patients continued the glutamine and the modified diet after discharge. PN status after 1 year of follow-up was the primary endpoint. Of the 49 patients infusing PN at study entry, 20 (41%) were completely weaned from PN and remained off PN at 1 year, 25 (51%) had a reduction in PN requirements, and 4 (8%) had no change in PN requirements. In patients without a colon, elimination of PN occurred only in those patients who had >100 cm of remaining small bowel. Of the 12 patients not on PN at study entry, 75% remained PN-free at 1 year.

In another open-label case series, Zhu et al. [24] treated 27 SBS patients with rhGH, glutamine, and modified diet. Interestingly, these patients were treated much earlier in relation to the onset of SBS compared with the other studies (mean, 86 ± 105 days post resection). Of 13 patients followed for more than 1 year, 10 (77%) were weaned completely from PN, prompting the investigators to conclude that early initiation of this therapy may enhance intestinal adaptation and increase a patient's ability to wean from PN. Weiming and colleagues [25] treated 37 SBS patients with rhGH and oral glutamine for 4 weeks in addition to a high-complex-carbohydrate, low-fat diet and supplemental enteral nutrition (EN) support via a feeding tube. Most were treated within 2 years of the onset of SBS. Of the 23 patients followed for >2 years, 21 were weaned completely from PN; 18 of these were maintained on an oral diet supplemented with EN, while the other 3 were received an oral diet alone. Most recently, Guo et al. [26] treated 12 SBS patients (including 2 children) with a 4-week course of rhGH, oral glutamine, and supplemental EN followed by continued use of glutamine, EN, and a high-complex-carbohydrate, low-fat oral diet. Most were treated <1 year from their last intestinal resection. Of the 11 PN-dependent patients followed over a period ranging from 3 months to 1 year, 1 patient was weaned from both PN and EN, 5 were weaned from PN and lived on EN and an oral diet, while 4 others experienced a reduction in PN frequency and/or volume. The single patient treated >2 years after resection did not experience a significant PN reduction, suggesting that the interval from resection to treatment may be an important factor in its success. Alternatively, it may be that the treatment success during the adaptive period as found in these studies [24–26] simply reflects the effects of spontaneous adaptation rather than a hyperadaptive response due to the treatment regimen used. Clearly, further controlled trials during the period of intestinal adaptation are needed.

The studies described are limited by their uncontrolled design, making it difficult to determine the relative importance of the individual components of this bowel rehabilitation regimen (i.e., diet/education, ORS, glutamine, or rhGH) in helping to wean patients from PN. To address some of these concerns, Byrne et al. [27] completed a randomized, double-blind, controlled trial of rhGH combined with an individualized specialized oral diet (SOD) and oral glutamine in 41 patients with PN-dependent SBS requiring >3000 calories/week [27]. These patients were admitted to a clinical facility at two centers and were stabilized for 2 weeks on a SOD, antimotility and antisecretory medications, ORS, and the PN formula they were receiving at home. After the optimization and stabilization period, they randomly received one of three treatments: oral glutamine (30 g/day) plus rhGH placebo (control group) ($n = 9$), glutamine placebo plus rhGH (0.1 mg/kg/day) ($n = 16$), or glutamine plus rhGH ($n = 16$). Treatment continued "in-house" for 4 more weeks together with intensive diet education. After 4 weeks of treatment, the patients were discharged to home with instructions to continue on the SOD and glutamine or glutamine placebo for 12 additional weeks. The primary endpoint was the change from baseline in the weekly total PN volume (defined as the combined volumes of PN + lipids + supplemental intravenous fluids). Secondary endpoints included the reduction from baseline in weekly PN calories and frequency of PN administration (i.e., number of days infusing PN). Intestinal absorption studies were not performed in this study, nor were morphological or transit assessments of the small intestine.

After 4 weeks of treatment, patients receiving rhGH and SOD, with or without glutamine, showed significantly greater reductions in total PN volume, calories, and frequency compared with patients receiving glutamine and SOD (i.e., the control group) (Figure 20.1). Importantly, the patients receiving all three interventions (i.e., rhGH, glutamine, and SOD) achieved the greatest reductions in these parameters, with a mean reduction in PN volume, PN calories, and PN infusions compared with baseline. PN reduction remained significant during the 12-week observation period in the group treated with both rhGH and glutamine only (Figure 20.1). Nine patients were weaned completely from PN. Although generally well tolerated, peripheral edema and musculoskeletal complaints were common in the rhGH-treated groups. Importantly, a weight loss of about 5 kg was also observed in both groups that had received rhGH.

The modest benefits of the intestinal absorption studies are hard to reconcile with the dramatic findings from the PN weaning studies contributing to the lack of certainty on the clinical utility of this treatment approach. This has led to a considerable amount of skepticism surrounding the long-term benefits of this treatment modality, and its clinical use remains controversial. Indeed, a recent Cochrane review that included five randomized controlled trials of GH in SBS patients concluded that while GH, with or without glutamine, appeared to provide benefit in terms of increased weight, lean body mass, energy, and nitrogen absorption, the effects were generally short-lived after cessation of therapy, questioning the long-term clinical utility of the treatment [28]. Of the studies reviewed, only a single randomized controlled trial that focused on PN weaning as the primary endpoint was included [27]. They concluded that the evidence to date was inconclusive and that the temporary benefit based on the nutrient absorption studies questioned the clinical utility with respect to PN weaning. A similar conclusion was reached by Guo and colleagues [29] in their systematic review and meta-analysis of four randomized controlled trials.

Despite these conclusions, the limitations of the studies included should be considered, as the differences may be related to one or more of a number of factors:

- Small number of patients studied;
- Numerous differences in study methods, including the dose of rhGH used (from 0.024 mg/kg/day to 0.14 mg/kg/day);
- Length of treatment (from 3 to 8 weeks);
- Variable oral diet (none, hyperphagic, high carbohydrate–low fat, individualized based on bowel anatomy);
- Patient characteristics (presence of colon, etiology of SBS);
- Variable length of time on PN;
- Addition of glutamine; and
- Use of conventional pharmacotherapies, including dose, frequency, timing, and form.

Finally, the difficulty of performing high-quality, reliable nutrient balance studies may also have contributed.

Appropriate Patient Selection: "Skepticism > Enthusiasm"

Appropriate patient selection appears to be important for the successful use of rhGH as an adjunct to PN weaning in SBS patients [30]. The gain of about 300–550 mL/day in fluid and about 250–450 kcal/day in energy versus the control group in the Byrne et al. study [27] is consistent with the gain (427 kcal/day) observed in the study by Seguy and colleagues [14] in which balance studies were

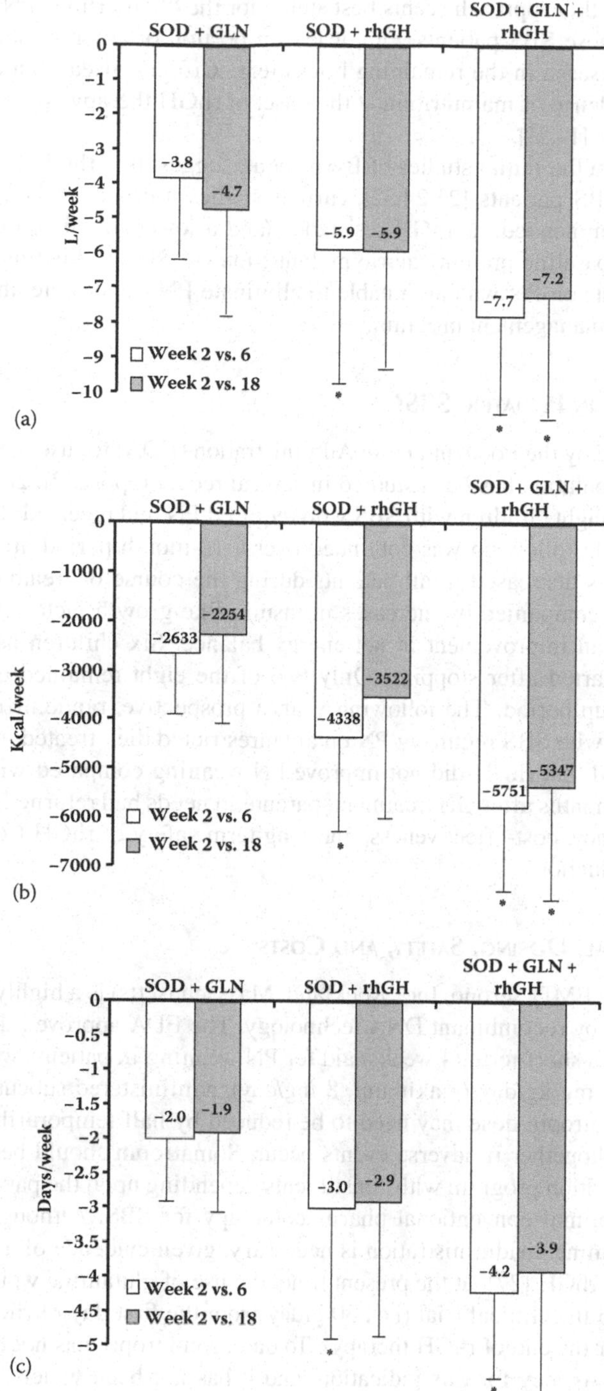

FIGURE 20.1 Changes from baseline in parenteral nutrition (PN) requirements after 4 weeks of treatment with SOD + rhGH, SOD + glutamine (GLN), or SOD + GLN + rhGH (week 6) and after a 12-week follow-up, during which patients continued to receive glutamine only or the glutamine placebo along with the specialized oral diet (week 18). (a) Reduction in PN volume per week, (b) reduction in PN calories per week, and (c) reduction in PN frequency per week. *$P < 0.05$ vs. SOD + GLN control.

performed. Therefore, this approach seems best suited for the "borderline" PN-dependent patients. While not absolute, those SBS patients with at least a portion of colon remaining, those without underlying mucosal disease in the remaining bowel (e.g., Crohn's disease and radiation enteritis), and those without evidence of malnutrition at the onset of rhGH therapy appear to be the best candidates for this therapy [14,31].

While findings from the initial studies of Byrne et al. suggest that rhGH can be used to prevent the need for PN in SBS patients [23,24,32], further studies are needed before this preventative approach can be recommended, as rhGH resistance (and a lower likelihood of response) may be seen in patients with baseline protein calorie malnutrition [14,31]. At this time, rhGH should only be used in SBS patients on PN who are unable to eliminate PN use despite an optimized diet and conventional medical management program.

What about Its Use in Pediatric SBS?

Although not approved by the Food and Drug Administration (FDA) for use in the pediatric population, its use in this population has been studied in several recent reports. In 2010, Goulet et al. [33] prospectively studied eight children with SBS who required PN and received rhGH 0.13 mg/kg/day over a 12-week period. Follow-up was continued over a 12-month period after rhGH discontinuation. PN requirements decreased in all patients during the course of treatment, which was well tolerated. This was accompanied by increases in insulin-like growth factor 1 (IGF-1) and plasma citrulline, as well as an improvement in net energy balance. Six children had to be maintained on PN or have it restarted after stopping. Only two of the eight remained off PN at the end of the 12-month follow-up period. The following year, a prospective, randomized, open-label study involving 14 children with SBS requiring PN on an unrestricted diet, treated with or without rhGH for 4 months, reported that rhGH did not improve PN weaning compared with the control group [34]. Furthermore, 6 months after GH treatment, parenteral needs had returned to their basal values. The indications, efficacy, cost-effectiveness, and long-term safety of rhGH treatment for pediatric SBS need further evaluation.

Somatropin Approval, Dosing, Safety, and Costs

Somatropin (Zorbtive; EMD Serono, Inc., Rockland, Massachusetts) is a highly purified human GH preparation produced by recombinant DNA technology. The FDA approved the use of somatropin in December 2003 as a short-term (4 weeks) aid for PN weaning in patients with SBS. The recommended dosage is 0.1 mg/kg/day (maximum, 8 mg/day), administered subcutaneously once daily for 4 weeks. The somatropin dose may need to be reduced by half temporarily, stopped temporarily, or discontinued altogether if adverse events occur. Somatropin should be used in conjunction with a specialized nutrition program with constituents depending upon the patient's bowel anatomy, caloric needs, and optimal conventional pharmacotherapy for SBS. Although it remains controversial whether glutamine coadministration is necessary, given evidence of a potential synergistic role of glutamine and rhGH [27], at the present time, the use of glutamine would be prudent in this setting as was used in the clinical trial (i.e., 30 g/day from the first day of rhGH administration to at least 12 weeks after the end of rhGH therapy). To date, somatropin has not been approved by the European Medicines Agency for this indication, and it has not been widely adopted into clinical practice more than a decade after its approval in the United States.

A factor that may have played an important role in the successful outcomes of the studies focusing on PN weaning as the primary endpoint [22–27,32] is their conduct in a controlled inpatient-like setting that allowed close monitoring of the patient status and intensive dietary, educational, and behavioral modification. This likely required a very motivated patient with adequate financial resources and enhanced compliance with the program both during and after completion of the rhGH administration period. How the use of this agent would translate into the ambulatory setting where visits and supervision would not be as intensive is unknown. Clearly, admitting a patient for 4 weeks to optimize diet, hydration, and medical therapy and administer somatropin would be rather challenging in the present healthcare environment.

Adverse events are common with the relatively high dose of somatropin used for SBS, further limiting its adoption into clinical practice. Fluid retention, gastrointestinal symptoms, and injection site reactions occur commonly; however, serious adverse effects appear to be uncommon. GH use has also been associated with acute pancreatitis, impaired glucose tolerance, type 2 diabetes mellitus, carpal tunnel syndrome, and arthralgias.

Somatropin is contraindicated in patients with active neoplasia. Although FDA approval of somatropin is based on a 4-week administration period, the balance studies indicate that the duration of effect is limited to the treatment period and the safety of long-term continuous or intermittent 4-week treatments with GH needs to be considered. In particular, the potential for promoting the development of colon cancer with long-term rhGH has been raised as a concern [35,36]. In this regard, it should be noted that patients receiving rhGH (in which the IGF-1 levels are maintained in the normal range) have not been shown to have an increased rate of colon cancer [37]. Moreover, mice with transgenic overexpression of GH do not develop colon cancer [38]. This may be related to GH-dependent up-regulation of suppressor of cytokine signaling-2, with subsequent inhibition of the proliferative effects of IGF-1 [39].

In the United States, the cost of a 4-week course of somatropin is approximately $20,000 [40]. An economic analysis of healthcare costs associated with GH use estimated a 2-year savings of $85,474 assuming that 34% of GH-treated patients eliminated PN use within 6 weeks of treatment and 31% remained PN-free after 2 years [41]. However, patients in the clinical trial were studied in an inpatient setting (albeit not hospital) for 4 weeks and received daily visits and education/counseling, costs not factored into the dollar amount mentioned above.

OTHER AGENTS UNDER INVESTIGATION TO AID PN WEANING

GLUCAGON-LIKE PEPTIDE-1

The GLP-1 receptor agonist exenatide (Byetta; Amylin Pharmaceuticals, San Diego, California), an FDA-approved treatment of type 2 diabetes mellitus, was recently reported in a retrospective, open-label study to reduce PN requirements in five adult SBS patients (four with at least part of colon remaining in continuity), presumably through the slowing of gut transit by pharmacologically mimicking the "ileal brake" given its lack of intestinotrophic properties [42]. A subsequent placebo-controlled multiple crossover study evaluating the acute effects of continuous infusions of GLP-1, GLP-2, and a combination of both GLP-1 and GLP-2 in nine adults with SBS (seven with end-jejunostomies) found that all treatment regimens significantly reduced fecal wet weight, energy, nitrogen, sodium, and potassium losses compared with placebo [43]. Only GLP-2-containing treatments increased absolute absorption of wet weight and sodium, while only the combination of GLP-1 and -2 improved hydration status. The effects of GLP-1 were less potent than those of GLP-2, while the combination of the two showed additive effects. Although a tendency toward nausea and reduced appetite was seen with GLP-1, this was ameliorated by the coadministration of GLP-2. The authors concluded that larger, long-term randomized controlled studies are warranted to further assess the potential role of the GLPs or analogs, alone or in combination, in the treatment of SBS. Most recently, the preliminary results of an open-label "proof-of-concept" pilot study were published in abstract form, demonstrating a reduction in jejunostomy output and improvement in intestinal absorption in eight SBS patients with a jejunostomy who received daily subcutaneous injection of liraglutide (titrated up to 1.8 mg/day), a GLP-1 agonist, for 8 weeks [44]. No changes in gastric emptying or intestinal epithelial growth were noted. Further studies of GLP-1 agonists in humans, with or without concomitant GLP-2 agonist use, seem warranted to evaluate the clinical potential of these agents.

Glutamine

Glutamine, a highly abundant amino acid in intact proteins and the primary energy source of enterocytes, becomes "conditionally essential" in states of severe physiological stress [45,46]. It has been shown to prevent mucosal atrophy and deterioration of gut permeability in patients receiving PN [47]. Nevertheless, when glutamine was added to an ORS provided to adult SBS patients with an end-jejunostomy, no benefit was seen in terms of fluid or sodium absorption [48]. Furthermore, in a randomized, controlled, crossover study involving eight adult SBS patients, no difference in small bowel morphology, transit time, D-xylose absorption, or stool output was seen [49].

Despite these negative studies of glutamine use by itself, there is evidence that glutamine may have a synergistic effect with GH with regard to intestinal adaptation and PN weaning in SBS [10,27,50], suggesting a role for combined GH and glutamine in enhancing intestinal adaptation. Indeed, the combination of GH and glutamine has been shown to synergistically increase IGF-1 plasma levels, intestinal DNA and villus growth in rodent models of SBS [10,51–53]. However, not all studies have demonstrated positive effects of this combination on intestinal adaptation [54]. Furthermore, a recent randomized controlled study involving a small number of severe SBS patients on PN found that rhGH improved de novo synthesis and intestinal absorption, thereby increasing the availability of glutamine over the physiologic range, suggesting that the beneficial effects of rhGH might be achieved without concomitant glutamine use [55].

Epidermal Growth Factor

Following demonstration of proabsorptive and proadaptive effects in experimental models of SBS [56], recombinant EGF was investigated in a study involving five children with SBS [57]. EGF (100 µg/kg/day mixed with enteral formula for 6 weeks) was well tolerated and resulted in an increase in the amount of enteral feeding consumed (enteral energy as percentage of total energy, 25% ± 28% pretreatment vs. 36% ± 24% posttreatment) and a transient improvement in carbohydrate absorption. EGF treatment was not associated with significant changes in intestinal permeability, the rate of weight gain, or liver function tests. Further study of EGF seems warranted.

Peptide YY

Peptide YY, also produced by L-cells in the distal small bowel and proximal colon, is an important motility-modulating hormone that, because of its effects to slow gastrointestinal transit (mediator of the ileal and colonic brakes), might play a role in facilitating fluid and nutrient absorption. As might be expected, its levels are diminished in patients without ileum or colon, but levels are markedly elevated in SBS patients with a colon remaining [58]. Furthermore, despite earlier reports not identifying intestinotrophic properties of peptide YY, a recent report found that peptide YY induces intestinal proliferation in peptide YY knockout mice also receiving total EN after massive small bowel resection [59]. Although a peptide YY analog is available, to our knowledge, it has yet to be studied in humans with SBS.

CONCLUSION

An important goal in the treatment of SBS is to reduce and, whenever possible, eliminate the need for parenteral support. Following optimization of diet, hydration, and conventional pharmacological strategies (and occasionally surgical reconstructive procedures), the use of trophic factors has the potential to bring about further reductions. Somatropin was the first agent approved for this purpose in PN-dependent SBS patients. While conflicting data and skepticism regarding its long-term benefit exist, it has been shown to enhance intestinal absorption of nutrients in SBS patients and seems to play a role in allowing many of these patients to be weaned from PN completely or to reduce their PN requirements. Whether these results can be reproduced when patients are not treated in an inpatient-like facility and by less experienced practitioners remains to be seen. At this time, somatropin is only approved for adults with SBS who require PN support. It should be used under the guidance of a multidisciplinary team of clinicians experienced in the management of SBS, with an expectation that these patients need to be monitored closely during and after its use. Long-term safety and efficacy, timing of administration in relation to the onset of SBS, cost effectiveness, and use in the pediatric and geriatric populations will require further study.

REFERENCES

1. Messing B et al. Long-term survival and parenteral nutrition dependence in adult patients with the short bowel syndrome. *Gastroenterology* 1999;117:1043–1050.
2. Amiot A et al. Determinants of home parenteral nutrition dependency and survival of 268 patients with non-malignant short bowel syndrome. *Clin Nutr* 2013;32:368–374.
3. Shulman DI et al. Effects of short-term growth hormone therapy in rats undergoing 75% small intestinal resection. *J Pediatr Gastroenterol Nutr* 1992;14:3–11.
4. Hart MH et al. Augmentation of post-resection mucosal hyperplasia by pleceroid growth factor (PGF)—Analog of human growth hormone. *Dig Dis Sci* 1987;32:1275–1280.
5. Christensen H et al. Growth hormone increases the mass, the collagenous proteins and the strength of rat colon. *Scand J Gastroenterol* 1990;25:1137–1143.
6. Verhage AH et al. Effects of growth hormone in rats with 80% small bowel resection fed totally by parenteral nutrition. *Nutr Res* 1998;18:823–832.
7. Benhamou PH et al. Human recombinant growth hormone increases small bowel lengthening after massive small bowel resection in piglets. *J Pediatr Surg* 1997;32:1332–1336.
8. Mainoya JR. Effects of bovine growth hormone, human placental lactogen and ovine prolactin on intestinal fluid and ion transport in the rat. *Endocrinology* 1975;96:1165–1170.
9. Mainoya JR. Influence of bovine growth hormone on water and NaCl absorption by the rat proximal jejunum and distal ileum. *Comp Biochem Physiol* 1982;71:477–479.
10. Zhou X et al. Glutamine enhances the gut trophic effect of growth hormone in rat after massive small bowel resection. *J Surg Res* 2001;99:47–52.
11. Park JH et al. Growth hormone did not enhance mucosal hyperplasia after small-bowel resection. *Scand J Gastroenterol* 1996;31:349–355.
12. Iannoli P et al. Epidermal growth factor and human growth hormone accelerate adaptation after massive enterectomy in an additive nutrient-dependent and site-specific fashion. *Surgery* 1997;112:721–729.
13. Ljungmann K et al. GH decreases hepatic amino acid degradation after small bowel resection in rats without enhancing bowel adaptation. *Am J Physiol Gastrointest Liver Physiol* 2000;279:G700–G706.
14. Seguy D et al. Low-dose growth hormone in adult home parenteral nutrition-dependent short bowel syndrome patients: A positive study. *Gastroenterology* 2003;124:293–302.
15. Byrne TA et al. Growth hormone, glutamine and a modified diet enhance nutrient absorption in patients with severe short bowel syndrome. *JPEN J Parenter Enteral Nutr* 1995;222:296–302.
16. Zhu W et al. Rehabilitation therapy for short bowel syndrome: Experimental study and clinical trial. *Chin Med J (Engl)* 2002;115:776–778.
17. Wu GH et al. Effects of bowel rehabilitation and combined trophic therapy on intestinal adaptation in short bowel patients. *World J Gastroenterol* 2003;9:2601–2604.
18. Ellegard L et al. Low-dose recombinant growth hormone increases body weight and lean body mass in patients with short bowel syndrome. *Ann Surg* 1997;22:88–96.
19. Scolapio JS et al. Effect of growth hormone, glutamine, and diet on adaptation in short bowel syndrome: A randomized, controlled study. *Gastroenterology* 1997;113:1074–1081.
20. Skudlarek J et al. Effect of high dose growth hormone with glutamine and no change in diet on intestinal absorption in short bowel patients: A randomized, double-blind, crossover, placebo-controlled study. *Gut* 2000;47:199–205.
21. Tangpricha V et al. Growth hormone favorably affects bone turnover and bone mineral density in patients with short bowel syndrome undergoing intestinal rehabilitation. *JPEN J Parenter Enteral Nutr* 2006;30:480–486.
22. Byrne TA et al. A new treatment for patients with short-bowel syndrome: Growth hormone, glutamine, and a modified diet. *Ann Surg* 1995;222:243–254.

23. Byrne TA et al. Bowel rehabilitation: An alternative to long-term parenteral nutrition and intestinal transplantation for some patients with short bowel syndrome. *Transplant Proc* 2002;34:887–890.
24. Zhu W et al. Rehabilitation therapy for short bowel syndrome. *Chin Med J (Engl)* 2002;115:776–778.
25. Weiming Z et al. Effect of recombinant human growth hormone and enteral nutrition on short bowel syndrome. *JPEN J Parenter Enter Nutr* 2004;28:377–381.
26. Guo M et al. Effect of growth hormone, glutamine, and enteral nutrition on intestinal adaptation in patients with short bowel syndrome. *Turk J Gastroenterol* 2013;24:463–468.
27. Byrne TA et al. Growth hormone, glutamine and an optimal diet reduces parenteral nutrition in patients with short bowel syndrome. A prospective, randomized, placebo-controlled, double-blind clinical trial. *Ann Surg* 2005;242:655–661.
28. Wales PW et al. Human growth hormone and glutamine for patients with short bowel syndrome. *Cochrane Database Syst Rev* 2010;6:CD006321.
29. Guo MX et al. Growth hormone for intestinal adaptation in patients with short bowel syndrome: Systematic review and meta-analysis of randomized controlled trials. *Curr Ther Res Clin Exp* 2011;72:109–119.
30. Byrne T et al. Does growth hormone and glutamine enhance bowel absorption? *Gastroenterology* 1998;114:1110–1112.
31. Thissen JP et al. Nutritional regulation of the insulin-like growth factors. *Endocr Rev* 1994;15:80–101.
32. Wilmore DW et al. Factors predicting a successful outcome after pharmacologic bowel compensation. *Ann Surg* 1997;226:288–293.
33. Goulet O et al. Effect of recombinant human growth hormone on intestinal absorption in children with short bowel syndrome. *JPEN J Parenter Enteral Nutr* 2010;34:513–520.
34. Peretti N et al. Growth hormone to improve short bowel syndrome intestinal autonomy: A pediatric randomized open-label trial. *JPEN J Parenter Enteral Nutr* 2011;35:723–731.
35. Giovannucci E. Insulin, insulin-like growth factors and colon cancer: A review of the evidence. *J Nutr* 2001;131:3109S–3120S.
36. Giovanucci E et al. Risk of cancer after growth-hormone treatment. *Lancet* 2002;360:268–269.
37. Beentjes JA et al. One year growth hormone replacement therapy does not alter colonic epithelial proliferation in growth hormone deficient adults. *Clin Endocrinol (Oxf)* 2000;52:457–462.
38. Williams KL et al. Enhanced survival and mucosal repair after dextran sodium sulfate-induced colitis in transgenic mice that overexpress growth hormone. *Gastroenterology* 2001;120:925–937.
39. Theiss AL et al. Growth factors in inflammatory bowel disease: The actions and interactions of growth hormone and insulin-like growth factor-1. *Inflamm Bowel Dis* 2004;10:871–880.
40. Parekh NR et al. Criteria for the use of recombinant human growth hormone in short bowel syndrome. *Nutr Clin Pract* 2005;20:503–508.
41. Migliaccio-Walle K et al. Economic implications of growth hormone use in patients with short bowel syndrome. *Curr Med Res Opin* 2006;22:2055–2063.
42. Kunkel D et al. Efficacy of the glucagon-like peptide-1 agonist exenatide in the treatment of short bowel syndrome. *Neurogastroenterol Motil* 2011;23:739–745.
43. Madsen KB et al. Acute effects of continuous infusions of glucagon-like peptide (GLP)-1, GLP-2 and the combination (GLP-1 + GLP-2) on intestinal absorption in short bowel syndrome (SBS) patients. A placebo-controlled study. *Regul Pept* 2013;184:30–39.
44. Hvistendahl M et al. The glucagon-like peptide 1 agonist liraglutide reduces jejunostomy output and improves intestinal absorption in short bowel syndrome patients with intestinal failure: A pilot study. *Gastroenterology* 2015;148(Suppl 1):S188–S189 (abstract).
45. Kovacevic Z et al. Mitochondrial metabolism of glutamine and glutamate and its physiological significance. *Physiol Rev* 1983;63:547–605.
46. Askanazi J et al. Muscle and plasma amino acids following injury. Influence of intercurrent infection. *Ann Surg* 1980;192:78–85.
47. van der Hulst RR et al. Glutamine and the preservation of gut integrity. *Lancet* 1993;341:1363–1365.
48. Beaugererie L et al. Effects of an isotonic oral rehydration solution, enriched with glutamine, on fluid and sodium absorption in patients with a short bowel. *Aliment Pharmacol Ther* 1997;11:741–747.
49. Scolapio JS et al. Effect of glutamine in short-bowel syndrome. *Clin Nutr* 2001;20:319–323.
50. Biolo G et al. Growth hormone decreases muscle glutamine production and stimulates protein syntheses in hypercatabolic patients. *Am J Physiol* 2000;279:E323–E332.
51. Ziegler TR et al. Gut adaptation and the insulin-like growth factor system: Regulation by glutamine and IGF-1 administration. *Am J Physiol* 1996;271:G866–G875.

52. Gu Y et al. Effects of growth hormone and glutamine supplemented parenteral nutrition on intestinal adaptation in short bowel rats. *Clin Nutr* 2001;20:159–166.
53. Waitzberg DL et al. Small bowel adaptation with growth hormone and glutamine after massive resection of rat's small bowel. *Nutr Hosp* 1999;14:81–90.
54. Vanderhoof JA et al. Growth hormone and glutamine do not stimulate intestinal adaptation following massive small bowel resection in the rat. *J Pediatr Gastroenterol Nutr* 1997;25:327–331.
55. Seguy D et al. Growth hormone enhances fat-free mass and glutamine availability in patients with short-bowel syndrome: An ancillary double-blind, randomized crossover study. *Am J Clin Nutr* 2014;100:850–858.
56. Sham J et al. Epidermal growth factor improves nutritional outcome in a rat model of short bowel syndrome. *J Pediatr Surg* 2002;37:765–769.
57. Sigalet DL et al. A pilot study of the use of epidermal growth factor in pediatric short bowel syndrome. *J Pediatr Surg* 2005;40:763–768.
58. Andrews NJ et al. Human gut hormone profiles in patients with short-bowel syndrome. *Dig Dis Sci* 1992;37:729–732.
59. Zhu W et al. Peptide YY induces intestinal proliferation in peptide YY knockout mice with total enteral nutrition after massive small bowel resection. *J Pediatr Gastroenterol Nutr* 2009;48(5):517–525.

21 Surgical Considerations in the Short Bowel Syndrome

Jon S. Thompson

CONTENTS

KEY POINTS

- Surgical management of the short bowel syndrome begins in the perioperative period.
- Primary goals are to minimize complications, improve quality of life, and enhance survival.
- Preserving and optimizing the intestinal remnant are the priority.
- Surgical rehabilitation procedures are useful in selected groups of patients.

INTRODUCTION

The surgical management of patients with short bowel syndrome (SBS) should aim to minimize the development of predictable complications, improve quality of life, and enhance patient survival. In some cases, these efforts begin in the preoperative period prior to SBS. Prevention of SBS would be ideal given the morbidity and mortality associated with long-term treatment. There are intraoperative strategies to be employed at the initial operation and any subsequent reoperation. Postoperative management of SBS and surgical rehabilitation, procedures intended to improve intestinal function, also have a profound effect on overall outcome. In this chapter, we review the preoperative, intraoperative, and postoperative strategies that can be utilized to optimize the chance for the best outcome. Additionally, surgical aspects of selected gastrointestinal (GI) complications occurring in SBS patients are discussed.

SURGICAL MANAGEMENT OF SBS

Prevention

Preoperative strategies to prevent SBS are determined primarily by the patient's underlying disease. The incidence of postoperative SBS can be minimized by avoiding technical errors, preventing adhesions, diagnosing intestinal ischemia in a timely fashion, and approaching the frozen abdomen cautiously [1]. Intestinal ischemia due to hypoperfusion or vascular injury is increasingly recognized as a complication of laparoscopic procedures [2]. Patients undergoing bariatric procedures are at risk for internal hernias, and this diagnosis should always be suspected when these patients experience abdominal pain [3]. Intestinal ischemia from mesenteric vascular disease and hypercoagulability needs expeditious diagnosis to permit attempts at revascularization. Intestinal viability should be carefully assessed intraoperatively and second-look procedures should be used judiciously to prevent unnecessary resection [4]. Radiation enteritis can be reduced by minimizing bowel exposed to radiation [5]. Patients with Crohn's disease may develop SBS due to errors in diagnosis, aggressive resectional therapy, and postoperative complications [6,7]. SBS can be minimized in trauma patients by early diagnosis of vascular injuries, appropriate resuscitation, and damage control laparotomy [8]. Bowel-preserving strategies are now being used in the treatment of infants with necrotizing enterocolitis and may decrease the incidence of SBS due to this condition [9].

Preoperative Management

Discussion with the patient and family about the potential consequences of SBS, including the need for prolonged parenteral nutrition (PN) support, should be undertaken before operative decision making whenever possible. There are some patients, such as the elderly patient with extensive comorbidity or advanced malignancy, in whom it might be appropriate to avoid surgical intervention that would result in SBS. Obviously, this can be a very difficult decision. For patients who have had previous resections and might predictably require further resection leading to SBS, there should be greater discussion and consideration of management issues.

The surgeon should try to gain as much information as possible about preexisting bowel anatomy and intestinal disease when considering further operative procedures in patients who have had previous intestinal resection. Contrast-enhanced radiographic studies of the intestinal tract are helpful in estimating the residual intestinal length and in assessing the presence of dilation, potential points of obstruction and mucosal disease. Ultrasonography of the gallbladder should be obtained because patients who have had previous intestinal resection are at increased risk for cholelithiasis. Nutritional status should be assessed so that appropriate nutritional support can be provided during the perioperative period.

In patients with acute intestinal conditions likely to require massive resection, management consists of stabilizing the patient hemodynamically and correcting fluid and electrolyte deficits. Preoperative antibiotics should cover colonic bacterial organisms. Nasogastric decompression may be appropriate in some cases for anticipated ileus. If need for an ostomy is predicted, consultation with a stomal therapist and marking the optimal site for the ostomy should be done preoperatively if time permits. These stomas often become difficult-to-manage, high-output stomas, and proper construction and positioning are paramount.

Intraoperative Management

An important intraoperative strategy is to avoid extensive resection when it is not clearly necessary. Decisions about resection margins and management of intestinal lesions should not be carried out until the entire situation has been fully assessed. Salvaging even a few inches of small intestine in the setting of a severely shortened remnant may be appropriate, despite the potential morbidity of additional anastomoses. Strategies such as stricturoplasty, intestinal tapering, and serosal patching may be helpful in managing specific lesions that would otherwise require resection [10]. Avoiding extensive enterolysis and using resection cautiously can prevent SBS in patients with extensive adhesions from conditions such as radiation enteritis [5].

Management of the intestinal ischemia is an important and common intraoperative issue [4]. Any obstruction or constriction of the mesentery should be relieved, and the bowel should be covered with warm, moist packs to allow the bowel to recover. Signs of viability include improved color, visible mesenteric pulsations, and peristalsis. Palpation of pulses in the main mesenteric arteries should be done to assess the etiology of the ischemia. Other useful modalities include intravenous injection of a fluorescent probe with visualization of fluorescent staining using a Wood's lamp to assess diffuse changes and the use of a Doppler ultrasonic flow probe to evaluate blood flow at the margins of the bowel. Newer quantitative techniques to assess intestinal perfusion such as indocyanine green fluorescein angiography are also now available. Revascularization should be performed, if feasible, to salvage reversible ischemic bowel. Bowel which is obviously nonviable requires resection. When recovery of viability is a possibility, a second-look procedure should be considered after resuscitation to reevaluate questionable bowel.

Intestinal obstruction should be excluded intraoperatively if this possibility has not been adequately assessed preoperatively. Passing a balloon-tipped catheter (e.g., Baker's tube or Foley catheter) through the intestinal tract to identify possible stenoses may be necessary. Intestinal bypass, rather than resection, is appropriate in certain situations such as dense adhesions. In patients who already have a short bowel, there may be opportunities to reconstruct the bowel (e.g., to eliminate blind loops causing stasis and small intestinal bacterial overgrowth [SIBO], or recruit bypassed segments).

Formation of an ostomy should be considered when the patient is unstable, intestinal viability is questionable, and the patient will be left with a very shortened intestinal remnant, for example, less than 60 cm. When a second-look procedure is planned, leaving the stapled ends of the bowel in discontinuity at the initial procedure may be appropriate. Duodenal and high jejunal ostomies may create difficult management problems because of their high stoma output. They need to be properly constructed. Occasionally, the intestine will not reach the abdominal wall, and tube decompression is required. In general, restoring intestinal continuity should be considered strongly whenever distal viable bowel is present.

Because patients with SBS are at increased risk for development of cholelithiasis and acute biliary complications, a prophylactic cholecystectomy should be considered [11]. This decision needs careful evaluation in the patient undergoing a massive resection in an emergent situation. Cholecystectomy would be more reasonable in stable patients who are undergoing elective procedures or who require subsequent reoperation.

Postoperative Management

The key issues in the management of SBS in the early postoperative period are control of sepsis, maintenance of fluid and electrolyte balance, and initiation of nutritional support. As the patient recovers, important priorities become maintaining adequate nutritional status, maximizing the absorptive capacity of the remaining intestine, and preventing the development of complications related to SBS and its management. The clinical manifestation of SBS varies greatly among patients depending on intestinal remnant length, location, and function. The status of the remaining digestive organs and the adaptive capacity of the intestinal remnant are also important (see the following list). Recently, other patient-related factors have also been recognized, including age, diagnosis, and body mass index [12–15]. Thus, while intestinal length is important, the outcome of SBS is not entirely dependent on a given length of remaining intestine. Consideration of these factors allows assessment of the patient's nutritional prognosis and guides nutritional management.

Factors affecting the outcome of short bowel syndrome
- Intestinal anatomy
  - Remnant function
  - Remnant length
  - Remnant location
- Status of digestive organs
  - Colon
  - Liver
  - Pancreas
  - Stomach
- Intestinal adaptation
- Patient factors
  - Age
  - Bocy mass index
  - Intestinal disease
  - Medical commorbidity

The length of the small intestine from the ligament of Treitz to the ileocecal junction is generally about 16 ft (480 cm). Approximately the proximal two-fifths is jejunum and the distal three-fifths is ileum [16–18]. Adult patients with less than 180 cm of small intestine, about one-third the normal length, may develop SBS. Permanent PN support, however, is more likely to be needed in patients with less than 120 cm of intestine remaining without colon-in-continuity and less than 60 cm remaining with colonic continuity [14,19,20]. In infants, the intestinal length is 125 cm at the start of the third trimester and 250 cm at term. The length then doubles again as the child reaches adulthood [21]. While children with less than 75 cm small intestine may develop SBS, they are further classified as short small bowel (>38 cm), very short small bowel (15–38 cm) and ultrashort small bowel (<15 cm). These categories predict PN independence and survival.

Site of resection, jejunum versus ileum, is another important factor. Patients with an ileal remnant generally fare better because the ileum has specialized absorptive properties for bile salts and vitamin B_{12}, unique motor properties that prolong transit time, a hormone profile different from the jejunum, and a greater capacity for intestinal adaptation [22,23]. The presence of the terminal ileum and ileocecal junction improves the functional capacity of the intestinal remnant [23]. However, most patients with SBS have undergone ileal resection.

The status of the other digestive organs is an important determinant of outcome. The stomach influences oral intake, mixing of nutrients, transit time, pancreatic secretion, and protein absorption. Since SBS patients typically develop hyperphagia, which aids in intestinal adaptation, loss of the stomach, which is fortunately uncommon in the setting of SBS, would be a limiting factor [24,25]. Therefore, patients with a history of a Roux-en-Y gastric bypass for obesity, for example, may benefit from reconstruction of the stomach. Pancreatic enzymes are important in the digestive process and particularly influence fat absorption. The colon absorbs fluid and electrolytes, slows transit, and participates in the absorption of energy from malabsorbed carbohydrates [26–28]. Compared with an end-jejunostomy (type 1 anatomy), a jejunoileal anastomosis with an intact colon (type 3 anatomy) is equivalent to 60 cm of additional small intestine, and a jejunocolic anastomosis (type 2 anatomy) is equivalent to about 30 cm of additional small intestine [19] (Figure 21.1). The presence of the colon is also important in children with very short and ultrashort small bowel [29].

The underlying disease leading to resection is an important patient-related outcome factor. Patients with an active inflammatory disease (e.g., Crohn's disease and radiation injury) in the intestinal remnant may have compromised intestinal function. The incidence of hepatobiliary disease is increased in these patients [30]. The cause of resection will also influence outcome because of the effect on other digestive organs. For example, patients with SBS due to malignancy and trauma often have involvement of other digestive organs, such as the stomach and pancreas [8].

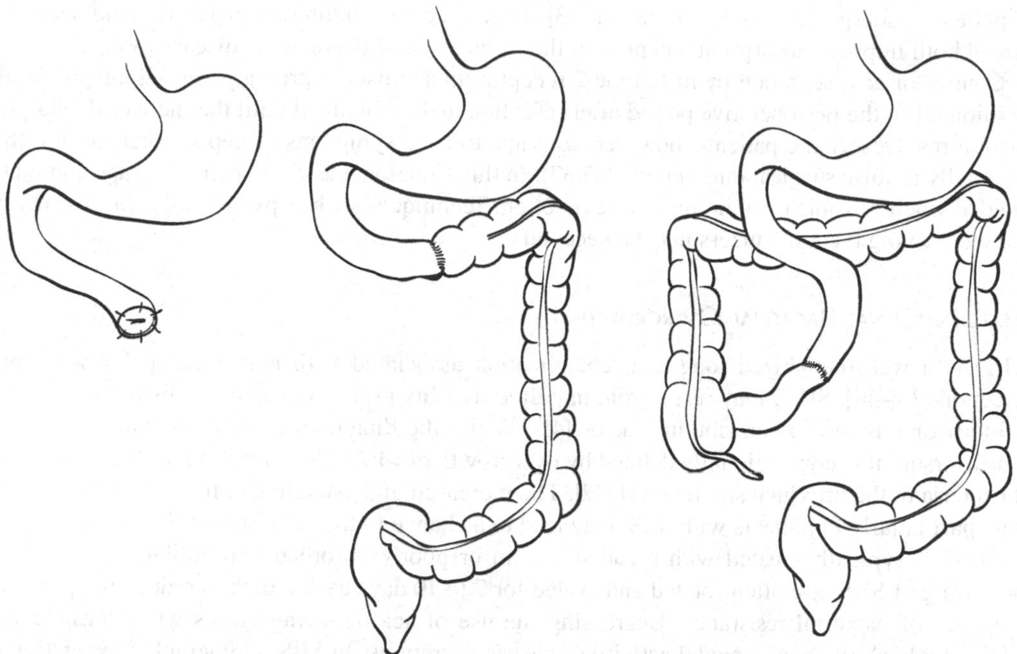

FIGURE 21.1 Intestinal anatomy in SBS type 1 anatomy (left) is a proximal jejunostomy. Type 2 anatomy (center) is a jejunocolonic anastomosis. Type 3 anatomy (right) is a jejuno-ileo-colonic anastomosis. (Reprinted from Thompson JS et al. *Current Problems in Surgery*, Elsevier, New York, 2012, p. 57. With permission.)

SURGICAL ASPECTS OF GI COMPLICATIONS

Cholelithiasis

Cholelithiasis occurs in 30–40% of adult patients and 20% of pediatric patients with SBS [11,31,32]. Altered hepatic bile metabolism and secretion, gallbladder stasis, and malabsorption of bile acids are important contributing factors. Long-term PN itself is associated with gallbladder stasis and alters hepatic bile metabolism. Since patients receiving PN develop both cholelithiasis and hepatocellular dysfunction, they require careful clinical evaluation to distinguish between the two [11,31]. Intestinal mucosal disease and resection, particularly of the ileum, cause bile acid malabsorption leading to lithogenic bile and increased formation of cholesterol stones. Having colon-in-continuity does not affect the incidence of cholelithiasis [28]. In general, the risk for cholelithiasis is significantly increased if less than 120 cm of intestine remains, the terminal ileum has been resected, and PN is required.

Cholelithiasis leads to complications such as acute cholecystitis and choledocholithiasis more frequently in SBS patients compared with the general population. These conditions require more complex surgical treatment. Thus, prophylactic cholecystectomy has been recommended when laparotomy is being undertaken for other reasons in SBS patients [11,31]. However, cholecystectomy is performed in only 10% of SBS patients [32].

Gastric Hypersecretion

Gastric hypersecretion is a common problem in both adult and pediatric patients with SBS [33–35]. Massive intestinal resection can cause gastric hypersecretion as a result of parietal cell hyperplasia and hypergastrinemia. This is a transient phenomenon, usually lasting several months, possibly from loss of an inhibitor of acid secretion from the resected intestine. The hyperacidity exacerbates malabsorption and diarrhea and can lead to development of peptic ulcer disease in up to one-fourth of patients undergoing massive resection [33]. Pharmacologic inhibition of gastric acid secretion should both improve absorption and prevent the occurrence of peptic ulcer disease [36].

Control of acid secretion by histamine-2 receptor antagonists or proton pump inhibitors should be initiated in the perioperative period after resection and maintained until the increased acid production resolves. Some patients, however, continue to have symptoms of peptic ulcer disease that eventually require surgical intervention [33,37]. In this situation, gastric resective therapy should be avoided when possible to maintain gastric function. Techniques such as pyloroplasty for obstruction and oversewing bleeding ulcers may be necessary.

Small Intestinal Bacterial Overgrowth

SIBO is a well-recognized long-term complication associated with both intestinal disease and resection [38–40]. SIBO may result from impaired motility or stasis caused by obstructive lesions. Achlorhydria is also a contributing factor [41]. While the diagnosis of SIBO remains somewhat controversial, it is conventionally defined by overgrowth of $>10^5$ colony forming units per milliliter of bacteria in the proximal small bowel [42]. The increased understanding of the intestinal microbiome, particularly in patients with SBS, may lead to a change in the definition of this disorder [43].

SIBO is typically treated with broad-spectrum or poorly absorbed oral antibiotics, which, in the setting of SBS, are often rotated and cycled for 7 to 10 days each month to reduce the potential induction of bacterial resistance. Decreasing the use of acid-reducing agents when feasible will help bring back the bacteriocidal activity of gastric secretions. In SBS, radiographic evaluation of the GI tract is recommended because SIBO may result from a mechanical obstruction or a blind loop, which can be relieved by operation. SIBO often occurs related to a primary intestinal motor abnormality, particularly in children. Surgical options in this setting include resection of dysfunctional bowel, stricturoplasty for obstruction, or intestinal tapering to correct dysmotile dilated bowel segments.

SURGICAL REHABILITATION

Surgical rehabilitation for patients with SBS primarily aims to increase the intestinal absorptive capacity of the existing intestine. This can be achieved by procedures designed to improve intestinal function or by increasing the area of absorption (see list below). Strategies to improve absorption include recruiting additional intestine into continuity, relieving mechanical obstruction, or slowing intestinal transit. Intestinal lengthening procedures to expand the area of absorption and improve function are feasible in selected patients. Patients developing life-threatening complications of SBS therapy may ultimately benefit from intestinal transplantation. The latter two procedures are covered in Chapters 23 and 24, respectively. The choice of surgical therapy for the patient with SBS is influenced by intestinal remnant length and caliber and the clinical condition of the patient (Table 21.1).

Surgical approach to short bowel syndrome

- Preserve the intestinal remnant
    - Minimal resection
    - Nonresection procedures
    - Recruitment of additional intestine
- Improve intestinal motility
    - Procedure to relieve obstruction
    - Tapering enteroplasty
    - Reversed intestinal segments
- Increase absorptive area
    - Intestinal lengthening
    - Intestinal transplantation

TABLE 21.1
Surgical Therapy for Short Bowel Syndrome

Intestinal Length	Intestinal Caliber	Clinical Status	Surgical Therapy
Adequate (>120 cm)	Normal diameter	Enteral nutrition only	Optimize intestinal function Recruit additional length
	Dilated bowel	Bacterial overgrowth	Treat obstruction Intestinal tapering
Marginal (60–120 cm)	Normal diameter	Need for PN Rapid transit	Recruit additional length Procedures to slow transit
	Dilated bowel	Bacterial overgrowth Need for PN	Intestinal lengthening
Short (<60 cm)	Normal diameter	Need for PN	Optimize intestinal function Recruit additional length
	Dilated bowel	Bacterial overgrowth Need for PN	Intestinal lengthening
	Normal or dilated	Complications of PN	Intestinal transplantation

Preserving the Intestinal Remnant

About one-half of adult patients with SBS will undergo further abdominal procedures after their initial discharge from the hospital [32]. Usually, this is necessitated by intestinal problems caused by complications such as adhesions, anastomotic strictures, or underlying disease. At any reoperation in patients with established SBS, an important goal is to preserve the intestinal remnant length. The length, location, and characteristics of the remnant should be carefully documented at the time of any operation to help guide subsequent management. Several strategies can be employed to achieve remnant preservation when subsequent intestinal disease requires operation. For instance, further resection can often be avoided by employing stricturoplasty for benign strictures and utilizing serosal patching for certain strictures and chronic perforations (Figure 21.2). Tube enterostomy is another useful approach to controlling output from acute perforations and chronic enterocutaneous fistulas. Intestinal tapering can be used to improve the function of dilated segments. Intestinal resection should be limited in extent when it cannot be avoided. End-to-end anastomosis is favored both to prevent blind loops and to maximize functional length of the intestine. Depending on the previous operations performed, SBS patients occasionally have intestinal segments that can be recruited into continuity. However, there are also conditions, such as radiation injury or intestinal pseudo-obstruction, where resection of often lengthy intestinal segments will result in overall improvement of function.

The majority of stricturoplasties can be performed in the fashion of a Heineke-Mikulicz pyloroplasty. With this technique, the stricture is incised longitudinally and then closed transversely. The incision should be large enough to achieve a satisfactory luminal orifice, usually extending at least 1 cm proximal and distal to the stricture. The enterotomy can be repaired with either a single-layer or a two-layer anastomosis. Longer or multiple closely associated strictures can be resolved with a side-to-side stapled anastomosis. Blind loops should be minimized because of risk of stasis and SIBO.

Serosal patch repair is a useful technique for dealing with a nonhealing fistula, stricture, or other focal defect. It is particularly useful in intestinal segments that are difficult to mobilize. This type of repair involves apposition of an adjacent serosal surface, usually either small intestine or colon, to the intestine around the lesion. A single-layer seromuscular-to-seromuscular anastomosis is created in either an interrupted or continuous fashion. The serosal patch eventually becomes covered by the normal mucosa of the patched intestine by lateral in-growth from the adjacent tissue [44]. This

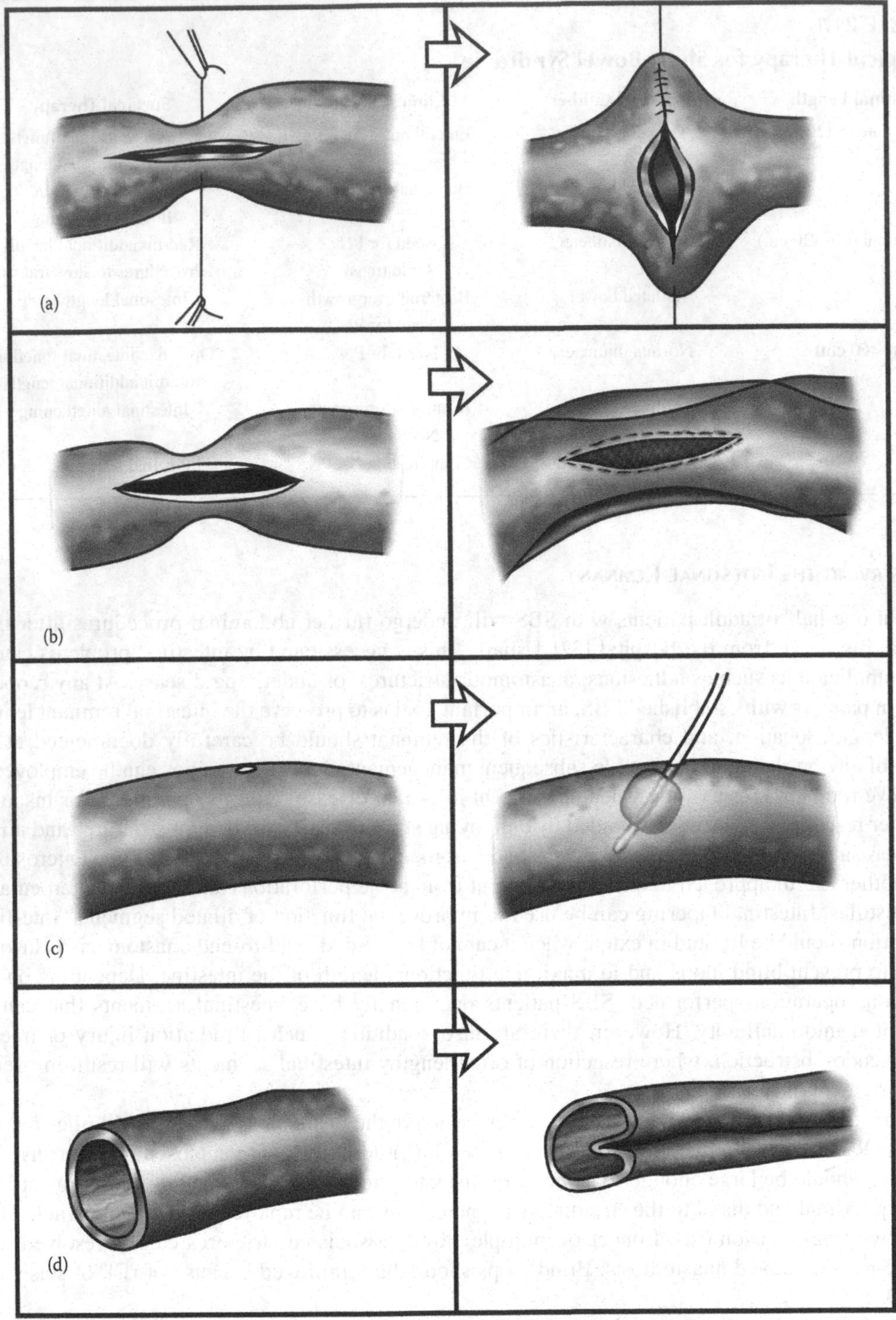

FIGURE 21.2 Techniques for preserving intestinal length include stricturoplasty for strictures (a), serosal patches for strictures and perforation (b), tube enterostomy for fistula (c), and tapering of dilated segments rather than resection (d).

technique is most applicable to smaller defects because the patched defects contract, potentially leading to a stenotic segment.

Restoring Intestinal Continuity

Whether and when to restore intestinal continuity in patients who have a distal intestinal or colonic remnant are important management issues [45,46]. More than 50% of patients will have ostomies performed at the time of resection leading to SBS due to the often emergent nature of their initial resection, questionable blood supply to the intestinal remnant, presence of colonic disease, and/or anticipated poor functional outcome.

There are several advantages to restoring intestinal continuity, which are provided in the list below. Recruited small intestine will improve absorption. The colon may augment intestinal absorption by increasing the absorptive surface area, deriving energy from short-chain fatty acids, and prolonging transit time, particularly if the ileocecal valve is intact [47]. The colon can serve as a "brake" to gastric emptying in SBS patients, perhaps mediated by peptide YY and other hormones secreted from the terminal ileum and colon. Eliminating a stoma may improve the quality of life and reduce complications, including the risk of central venous catheter infection.

Restoration of intestinal continuity

- Advantages
  - Intestinal stoma eliminated
  - Decreased central line infections
  - Energy absorbed from short-chain fatty acids
  - Increased absorptive capacity
  - Prolonged transit time
- Disadvantages
  - Bile acid diarrhea
  - Dietary restrictions
  - Perianal complications
  - Risk of nephrolithiasis

Unfortunately, the response of the colon and other recruited intestine to exposure to luminal contents is somewhat unpredictable. Bile acids may cause a secretory diarrhea. Perianal problems can be quite severe, leading to disability and a decrease in the patient's oral intake. Because oxalate is absorbed primarily in the colon, restoring continuity with the colon places the patient at increased risk for the formation of calcium oxalate stones [28]. Thus, these issues need consideration in the decision-making process.

In our experience, only about 25% of SBS patients with an initial stoma eventually underwent ostomy closure [45,46]. In some patients, the stoma may be the end of the GI tract. Prohibitive surgical risk is another factor. Anticipated poor functional outcome is a further deterrent to ostomy closure. Ultimately, the decision should be considered on an individual basis, depending on the length of the intestinal remnant, the status of the ileocecal valve and the colon, and the patient's overall condition. In our experience, 60–90 cm of small intestine is required to prevent severe diarrhea and perianal complications. Restoring continuity, however, should always be given strong consideration because of possible improvements in absorption, which may obviate the need for PN. We are generally aggressive in this regard. In some patients, opting to exchange a proximal stoma for a more distal one is appropriate as this may improve nutrition while preventing issues with disabling diarrhea [48].

Improving Motility

Patients with SBS may develop dilated intestine secondary to chronic mechanical obstruction or as a consequence of intestinal adaptation. Adaptive dilation occurs more frequently in children. Intestinal dilatation may lead to stasis and SIBO, which can further aggravate the malabsorption associated with the shortened intestinal remnant. Mechanical obstruction from anastomotic stenosis, adhesions, or strictures related to the underlying disease process should always be sought in these patients and corrected using the nonresective techniques mentioned previously. If dilated segments are not associated with distal obstruction, then tapering the dilated segments may improve motility. Restoring more normal luminal size permits closure of the lumen during contraction of the bowel wall, which improves peristalsis. Tapering enteroplasty has been demonstrated to improve intestinal function in SBS patients [13]. Both simple imbrication of the redundant bowel and longitudinal transection with excision of intestine along the antimesenteric border have been employed. A continuous nonabsorbable suture line is usually most expeditious for imbrication. Excisional techniques are more easily performed with the various stapling devices. As blind loops may be associated with SIBO, they should be sought and corrected, preferably by revising the anastomosis rather than resection.

Prolonging Intestinal Transit

Operations designed to prolong intestinal transit time to improve absorption have been performed clinically for a variety of motility disorders for several decades, but both their short-term and long-term efficacy remains unclear [49–53] (Figure 21.3). These adjunctive procedures are often performed during the adaptive phase of SBS, and it is difficult to determine whether further improvement in intestinal absorption and nutritional status are due to the surgical procedure or of the normal adaptive process. They are also frequently performed at the time of ostomy closure or other surgical interventions, which might independently improve intestinal function [53]. Three procedures (reversed intestinal segments, colon interposition, and intestinal valves) have been attempted in sufficient numbers to be considered further.

Reversing segments of intestine to slow intestinal transit is the procedure that has been reported most extensively for SBS [49–53]. The antiperistaltic segment functions by inducing retrograde peristalsis distally and disrupting the motility of the proximal intestine. In addition, the disruption of the intrinsic nerve plexus slows myoelectrical activity in the distal remnant. Reversed segments also alter the hormonal milieu normally found after resection [54]. Most experimental studies of antiperistaltic segments demonstrate slowed intestinal transit, improved absorption, reduced weight loss, and prolonged survival after intestinal resection, but this has not been uniformly reported [54,55].

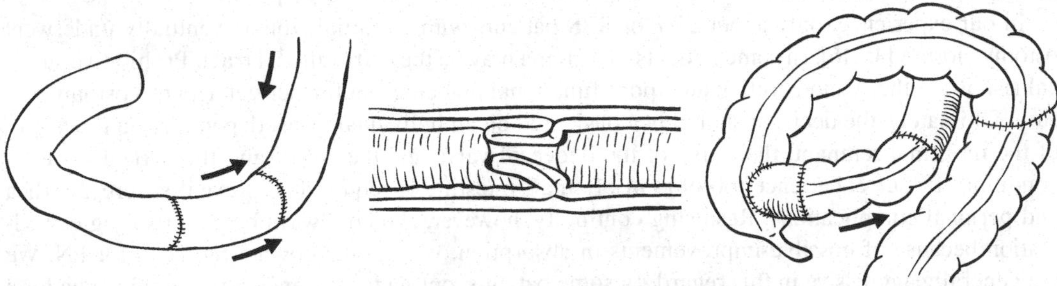

FIGURE 21.3 Techniques for slowing intestinal transit: antiperistaltic segment (left), intestinal valve (center), colon interposition (right). (Reprinted from Thompson JS et al. *Current Problems in Surgery*, Elsevier, New York, 2012, p. 85. With permission.)

The antiperistaltic segment ideally slows intestinal transit without causing complete functional obstruction. To achieve this, several technical details are important. The optimal length of the reversed segment would appear to be about 10 cm in adults [49–53]. The reversed segment should be created as distal in the small intestinal remnant as feasible to get the benefit of proximal absorptive surface. This may be proximal to an ostomy or a colonic anastomosis. A satisfactory vascular arcade to the segment must be identified and complete rotation of the mesentery avoided during reversal to prevent intestinal ischemia.

Antiperistaltic segments have been reported clinically in more than 80 SBS patients; 90% were adults [49–53]. The length of the segment has varied from 5 to 15 cm in adults in these reports. Clinical improvement has been reported in 80% of SBS patients in these anecdotal reports with slowed intestinal transit and increased absorption demonstrated. While long-term function of antiperistaltic segments has been demonstrated, our experience and that of others suggest only 50% derive long-term clinical benefit [50–53]. Transient obstructive symptoms, intestinal ischemia, and anastomotic leak are potential early problems that have been described. Loss of function of the reversed segment and SIBO are long-term concerns. This procedure has been reported in patients with Crohn's disease, with acceptable outcomes, and does not appear to influence recurrence rates [51,53,56]. Obviously, caution has to be exercised in patients with mesenteric scarring or residual intestinal disease in which case reversed intestinal segments may not be feasible.

There are several potential mechanisms for the effect of surgically constructed valves on intestinal motility. They create a partial mechanical obstruction, disrupt the normal motor pattern of the small intestine, and prevent retrograde reflux of colonic contents [49,57]. In experimental studies, intestinal valves and sphincters have been shown to prolong intestinal transit time, increase absorptive capacity, and improve survival after intestinal resection, although the results have been inconsistent. Effective valves usually result in some dilation of the proximal intestine and may cause, at least transiently, obstructive symptoms. Necrosis of the valve, complete obstruction, and intussusception are potential complications. Durability of the sphincter function of valves is a concern.

Techniques for creating intestinal valves include external constriction of the intestine, segmental denervation, and intussuscepting intestinal segments to increase intraluminal pressure, with the latter being employed most frequently. Intussuscepted or nipple valves should be 2 cm in length if created retrograde and 4 cm if the valve is prolapsed antegrade. We have generally created a retrograde sphincter similar to that employed in the continent ileostomy procedure but only 2 cm in length [57]. There is little experience, however, to recommend one technique over another.

Intussuscepted valves have been reported in clinical studies as primary treatment of SBS in 25 adults and one infant [45,49,58,59]. The primary endpoints were improved diarrhea and maintenance of body weight. Twenty-four patients improved markedly, one had questionable benefit and the other required takedown of the valve. Importantly, nipple valves were lost in one-third of patients followed for more than 5 years in one study, again raising the issue of durability. Nipple valves have also been employed successfully in six infants as the initial step of a staged approach to cause initial dilation of the intestine with the intent to permit subsequent intestinal lengthening [59].

Interposing a colonic segment within the small intestinal remnant in either an isoperistaltic or antiperistaltic fashion has been attempted to retard intestinal transit. Isoperistaltic interposition is performed proximally and functions by slowing the rate at which nutrients are delivered to the distal small intestine [49]. The antiperistaltic colon interposition is placed distally, similar to the reversed small intestinal segment. Interposed colonic segments absorb water, electrolytes, and nutrients in addition to their effect on intestinal transit. It has been suggested that interposed colon might develop structural and functional similarities to the small intestine, but this has not been substantiated [60]. In experimental studies, isoperistaltic colon interposition has generally resulted in slower transit time, less weight loss, and improved survival after resection, but results with antiperistaltic colon interposition have been less consistent. The length of colon interposed seems to be less critical for efficacy than with reversed segments of small intestine.

The use of colon interposition has been reported in a dozen SBS patients, of which 11 were isoperistaltic interposition [49,60]. The interposed colon segment varied between 8 and 24 cm in length. Eleven of these patients were infants younger than 1 year of age and all were PN dependent preoperatively. Half of the patients demonstrated sustained clinical improvement. The other half, including one with an antiperistaltic colon, did not improve and subsequently died of sepsis or hepatic failure. Colonic stasis with bacterial overgrowth may have contributed. Overall, this experience suggests that isoperistaltic colon interposition may have some merit, but long-term results are uncertain.

Final Considerations

Procedures designed to slow intestinal transit should be applied cautiously in SBS patients with demonstrated rapid transit. While we generally use an 80–90 cm remnant as the minimum cutoff, the group from France, which has the greatest experience, will consider the procedure in patients with as little as 40 cm intestine remaining [53]. These procedures are best considered only after maximal intestinal adaptation has occurred, but the opportunity to perform them may come earlier. Antiperistaltic segments should be used in patients with longer remnants so that the 10-cm segment utilized still leaves sufficient intestinal remnant for absorption. Valves should be considered in patients with shorter remnants because less bowel is used. Colon interposition has largely been restricted to children where the small intestinal remnant is much shorter. Overall, despite their potential benefit, these procedures are applicable to only a small proportion of patients with SBS (<5% in our experience) and their long-term efficacy remains uncertain.

CONCLUSION

The surgical management of SBS should aim to minimize complications, improve quality of life, and enhance survival. This begins in the preoperative period with consideration of ways to prevent SBS. Intraoperative strategies to minimize resection are imperative. Other surgical considerations in SBS include the management of cholelithiasis, gastric hypersecretion, and SIBO. Surgical rehabilitation aims to preserve the intestinal remnant, restore intestinal continuity when feasible, and improve intestinal motility. Procedures to prolong intestinal transit should be applied cautiously to selected patients.

REFERENCES

1. Thompson JS et al. Postoperative short bowel syndrome. *J Am Coll Surg* 2005; 201:85–9.
2. McBride CL et al. Short bowel syndrome after laparoscopic procedures. *Am Surg* 2014; 80:382–5.
3. McBride CL et al. Short bowel syndrome following bariatric surgical procedures. *Am J Surg* 2006; 192:828–32.
4. Thompson JS et al. Mesenteric ischemia: Acute mesenteric arterial ischemia. In: Schein M, Wise L, eds. *Critical Controversies in Surgery*. New York: Springer, 2001:167–74.
5. Boland E et al. A 25-year experience with postresection short bowel syndrome secondary to radiation therapy. *Am J Surg* 2010; 200:690–3.
6. Thompson JS et al. Short bowel syndrome and Crohn's disease. *J Gastrointest Surg* 2003; 7:1069–72.
7. Thompson JS et al. Short bowel syndrome after continence-preserving procedures. *J Gastrointest Surg* 2008; 12:73–6.
8. Dabney A et al. Short bowel syndrome after trauma. *Am J Surg* 2004; 188:792–5.
9. Petty JK et al. Operative strategies for necrotizing enterocolitis: The prevention and treatment of short-bowel syndrome. *Semin Pediatr Surg* 2005; 14:191–8.
10. Thompson JS. Strategies for preserving intestinal length in the short-bowel syndrome. *Dis Colon Rectum* 1987; 30:208–13.
11. Thompson JS. The role of prophylactic cholecystectomy in the short-bowel syndrome. *Arch Surg* 1996; 131:556–9.

12. Thompson JS et al. Pre resection BMI influences post resection BMI in short bowel syndrome. *Medimond Int Proc* 2009; 103–9.
13. Thompson JS et al. Surgical approach to short-bowel syndrome. Experience in a population of 160 patients. *Ann Surg* 1995; 222:600–5.
14. Messing B et al. Long-term survival and parenteral nutrition dependence in adult patients with the short bowel syndrome. *Gastroenterology* 1999; 117:1043–50.
15. Vantini I et al. Survival rate and prognostic factors in patients with intestinal failure. *Dig Liver Dis* 2004; 36:46–55.
16. Underhill BM. Intestinal length in man. *Br Med J* 1955; 2:1243–6.
17. Fanucci A et al. Small bowel length measured by radiography. *Gastrointest Radiol* 1984; 9:349–51.
18. Nightingale JM et al. Length of residual small bowel after partial resection: Correlation between radiographic and surgical measurements. *Gastrointest Radiol* 1991; 16:305–6.
19. Carbonnel F et al. The role of anatomic factors in nutritional autonomy after extensive small bowel resection. *JPEN J Parenter Enteral Nutr* 1996; 20:275–80.
20. O'Keefe SJ et al. Short bowel syndrome and intestinal failure: Consensus definitions and overview. *Clin Gastroenterol Hepatol* 2006; 4:6–10.
21. Touloukian RJ et al. Normal intestinal length in preterm infants. *J Pediatr Surg* 1983; 18:720–3.
22. Thompson JS et al. Factors affecting outcome following proximal and distal intestinal resection in the dog: An examination of the relative roles of mucosal adaptation, motility, luminal factors, and enteric peptides. *Dig Dis Sci* 1999; 44:63–74.
23. Cosnes J et al. Role of the ileocecal valve and site of intestinal resection in malabsorption after extensive small bowel resection. *Digestion* 1978; 18:329–36.
24. Crenn P et al. Net digestive absorption and adaptive hyperphagia in adult short bowel patients. *Gut* 2004; 53:1279–86.
25. Cosnes J et al. Adaptive hyperphagia in patients with postsurgical malabsorption. *Gastroenterology* 1990; 99:1814–19.
26. Nordgaard I et al. Colon as a digestive organ in patients with short bowel. *Lancet* 1994; 343:373–6.
27. Jeppesen PB et al. Significance of a preserved colon for parenteral energy requirements in patients receiving home parenteral nutrition. *Scand J Gastroenterol* 1998; 33:1175–9.
28. Nightingale JM et al. Colonic preservation reduces need for parenteral therapy, increases incidence of renal stones, but does not change high prevalence of gall stones in patients with a short bowel. *Gut* 1992; 33:1493–7.
29. Diamond IR et al. Does the colon play a role in intestinal adaptation in infants with short bowel syndrome? A multiple variable analysis. *J Pediatr Surg* 2010; 45:975–9.
30. Thompson JS et al. Radiation therapy increases the risk of hepatobiliary complications in short bowel syndrome. *Nutr Clin Pract* 2011; 26:474–8.
31. Dray X et al. Incidence, risk factors, and complications of cholelithiasis in patients with home parenteral nutrition. *J Am Coll Surg* 2007; 204:13–21.
32. Lawiński M et al. Cholelithiasis in home parenteral nutrition (Hpn)patients—Complications of the clinical nutrition: Diagnosis, treatment, prevention. *Pol Przegl Chir* 2014; 86:111–15.
33. Thompson JS. Reoperation in patients with the short bowel syndrome. *Am J Surg* 1992; 164:453–6.
34. Hyman PE et al. Gastric acid hypersecretion in short bowel syndrome in infants: Association with the extent of resection and enteral feeding. *J Pediatr Gastroenterol Nutr* 1986; 5:191–7.
35. Frederick PL et al. Relation of massive bowel resection to gastric secretion. *N Engl J Med* 1965; 272:509–14.
36. Jeppesen PB et al. Effect of intravenous ranitidine and omeprazole on intestinal absorption of water, sodium, and macronutrients in patients with intestinal resection. *Gut* 1998; 43:763–9.
37. Safioleas M et al. Short bowel syndrome: Amelioration of diarrhea after vagotomy and pyloroplasty for peptic hemorrhage. *Tohoku J Exp Med* 2008; 214:7–10.
38. Quigley EM et al. Small intestinal bacterial overgrowth. *Infect Dis Clin North Am* 2010; 24:943–59, viii–ix.
39. Stoidis CN et al. Potential benefits of pro- and prebiotics on intestinal mucosal immunity and intestinal barrier in short bowel syndrome. *Nutr Res Rev* 2011; 24:21–30.
40. DiBaise JK et al. Enteric microbial flora, bacterial overgrowth, and short bowel syndrome. *Clin Gastroenterol Hepatol* 2006; 4:11–20.
41. Compare D et al. Effects of long-term PPI treatment in producing bowel symptoms and SIBO. *Eur J Clinic Invest* 2011; 41:380–6.
42. Singh VV et al. Small bowel bacterial overgrowth: Presentation, diagnosis, and treatment. *Curr Treat Options Gastroenterol* 2004; 7:19–28.

43. Joly F et al. Drastic changes in fecal and mucosa-associated microbiota in adult patients with short bowel syndrome. *Biochimie* 2010; 92:753–61.
44. Thompson JS et al. Morphologic and nutritional responses to intestinal patching following intestinal resection. *Surgery* 1988; 103:79–86.
45. Thompson JS et al. Surgical approaches to improving intestinal function in the short bowel syndrome. *Arch Surg* 1999; 134:706–9.
46. Nguyen BT et al. Should intestinal continuity be restored after massive intestinal resection? *Am J Surg* 1989; 158:577–9.
47. Jeppesen PB et al. The influence of a preserved colon on the absorption of medium chain fat in patients with small bowel resection. *Gut* 1998; 43:478–83.
48. Diamond IR et al. Advantages of the distal sigmoid colostomy in the management of infants with short bowel syndrome. *J Pediatr Surg* 2008; 43:1464–7.
49. Thompson JS. Surgical approach to the short-bowel syndrome: Procedures to slow intestinal transit. *Eur J Pediatr Surg* 1999; 9:263–6.
50. Panis Y et al. Segmental reversal of the small bowel as an alternative to intestinal transplantation in patients with short bowel syndrome. *Ann Surg* 1997; 225:401–7.
51. Thompson JS et al. Predicting outcome of procedures to slow intestinal transit. *Transplant Proc* 2006; 38:1838–9.
52. Layec S et al. Increased intestinal absorption by segmental reversal of the small bowel in adult patients with short-bowel syndrome: A case-control study. *Am J Clin Nutr* 2013; 97:100–8.
53. Beyer-Berjot L et al. Segmental reversal of the small bowel can end permanent parenteral nutrition dependency: An experience of 38 adults with short bowel syndrome. *Ann Surg* 2012; 256:739–44.
54. Thompson JS et al. Effect of reversed intestinal segments on intestinal structure and function. *J Surg Res* 1995; 58:19–27.
55. Digalakis M et al. Interposition of a reversed jejunal segment enhances intestinal adaptation in short bowel syndrome: An experimental study on pigs. *J Surg Res* 2011; 171:551–7.
56. Kozlowski D et al. Surgically reversed segment of small bowel segment in Crohn's disease. *Gastroenterology* 1999; 116:A688.
57. Quigley EM et al. Disruption of canine jejunal interdigestive myoelectrical activity by artificial ileocolonic sphincter. Studies of intestinal motor response to surgically fashioned sphincter substitute. *Dig Dis Sci* 1989; 34:1434–42.
58. Zurita M et al. A new neovalve type in short bowel syndrome surgery. *Rev Esp Enferm Dig* 2004; 96:110–18.
59. Georgeson K et al. Sequential intestinal lengthening procedures for refractory short bowel syndrome. *J Pediatr Surg* 1994; 29:316–20.
60. Kono K et al. Interposed colon between remnants of the small intestine exhibits small bowel features in a patient with short bowel syndrome. *Dig Surg* 2001; 18:237–41.

22 Ostomy, Fistula, and Skin Management

Christine T. Berke and Cathi Brown

CONTENTS

KEY POINTS

- High-output ostomy, enterocutaneous fistula, slow healing wounds, enteral feeding tubes, and/or fecal incontinence with related skin problems are relatively common in short bowel syndrome (SBS) and greatly affect quality of life.
- Wound, ostomy, continence (WOC) nurses play a critical role in the care of patients with SBS who experience ostomy, wound, and/or skin complications.
- Treatments for patients with SBS and wound, ostomy, and/or skin issues are unique for each person, but there are guiding principles that allow for successful management of these complex problems.

INTRODUCTION

The presence of a diverting bowel ostomy and/or open surgical wound healing by secondary intention is encountered commonly in patients with short bowel syndrome (SBS). These conditions can lead to complications such as high-output ostomies contributing to painful peristomal skin damage with poor ostomy adaptation and enterocutaneous fistula (EF) formation resulting in complex painful delayed wound healing [1,2]. These complications often contribute to a significant decrease in quality of life for the SBS patient [3], as the patient often feels "tethered" to his or her bathroom or home.

In SBS patients with an ostomy, chronic wounds, EFs, and/or fecal incontinence, the wound, ostomy, continence (WOC) nurse plays a particularly important role. The care related to skin, wound, and ostomy management present challenges and treatments as unique as the individual bodies they belong to. Ideally, each patient with a complex ostomy and/or wounds will have access to a board-certified WOC nurse to assist the team in meeting the patient's physical and psychological needs. In this chapter, the general principles of care for each of these specialty nursing-focused areas are presented.

OSTOMY CARE OF THE HIGH-OUTPUT STOMA

Many patients with SBS will have an intestinal stoma. Knowledge of the amount and type of bowel remaining is important, as this will impact the "treatment plan" and the expected consistency and volume of effluent discharging from the stoma [1]. In general, ostomy output will be relatively liquid and caustic to the skin because of the presence of digestive enzymes and the alkaline nature of the effluent. Effluent consistency and causticity will depend on the bowel response and adaptation to the "treatment plan" and the patient's adherence to this plan [4].

The general principles of ostomy management are unchanged in patients with SBS. The care focus includes finding a pouch system that provides predictable, reliable wear-time while maintaining the integrity of the peristomal skin [5]. The majority of the patients with SBS will initially have a high-output stoma (i.e., >2 L/day) [2,4,6]. Oftentimes, this will lessen as adaptation occurs. Colwell [7] defined a high-output stoma in more simple terms as the degree of output occurring in "patients with reduced small bowel … who are symptomatic," *symptomatic* being the key term. The primary immediate postoperative symptoms in SBS are dehydration, electrolyte imbalances, and weight loss; malnutrition is a later manifestation [1,2,4,7].

The average wear-time of an ostomy appliance is 3 or 4 days for a standard colostomy and ileostomy, respectively [8]. The anticipated wear-time of an ostomy system for a patient with a high-output stoma has not been established. The wear-time is determined by the erosion of the barrier seal next to the stoma secondary to the amount of liquid output [7], the presentation of the stoma above the skin surface, the location of the lumen/os on the stoma and the topography of the abdominal plane surrounding the stoma [5,7].

The barrier seal needs to be carefully evaluated with each pouch change (planned or not). Upon removal of the old wafer from the patient's skin (gently remove to avoid stripping of the epidermis), the patient should be taught to look at the back of the barrier wafer for evidence of washing of the barrier edge next to the stoma, excess moisture absorption on the back of the barrier, and/or evidence of leaks (Figure 22.1). This exam will offer clues to reinforce the barrier wafer in specific locations with additional caulking materials [5,7,9].

The stoma location on the abdomen and the stoma height or protrusion above the surrounding skin surface is very important to determine the success of managing an ostomy appliance, especially for high-volume and/or very liquid output. Even though these properties of the stoma cannot readily be changed, it is important to understand how they affect the success or failure of a pouching system. Ideally, the stoma should have a profile above the skin of about 2 cm, with the os/lumen located at the apex/top of the stoma. Situated this way, effluent is directed out and down into the pouch system. Stomas located in skin folds (Figure 22.2), near scars or incisions (Figure 22.3), with low profiles (Figure 22.4), and/or the lumen off-center or at skin level (Figure 22.5) contribute to leaks and erosion of the barriers [9].

Many patients with SBS have experienced significant weight loss and/or multiple abdominal surgeries that contribute to loose skin, wrinkles, and scarring. The abdomen may be soft and doughy (from weight loss), firm and fibrotic (from scarring), or a combination of the two. It is important to evaluate the patient in different positions, including when lying supine and lateral decubitus, sitting, standing, and bending (Figures 22.6 through 22.8). Observing the changes in the skin surrounding the stoma (about four inches in all directions) during these activities will provide valuable information about the mechanical stresses that the adhesive barrier is placed under with patient activity/mobility [9,10].

BARRIER PRODUCTS AND WAFERS

Barrier products are used to protect the peristomal skin from effluent and to even the peristomal skin plane. Skin rashes, erosions, and ulcers are *not* an expected outcome of having an ostomy [5]. Reasons for readmission to the hospital for patients with SBS are often related to peristomal skin breakdown secondary to inability to maintain a pouch seal [2,4,6]. Because the effluent from the SBS ostomy is typically more caustic, the skin is at higher risk for breakdown (moisture-associated dermatitis) [11]

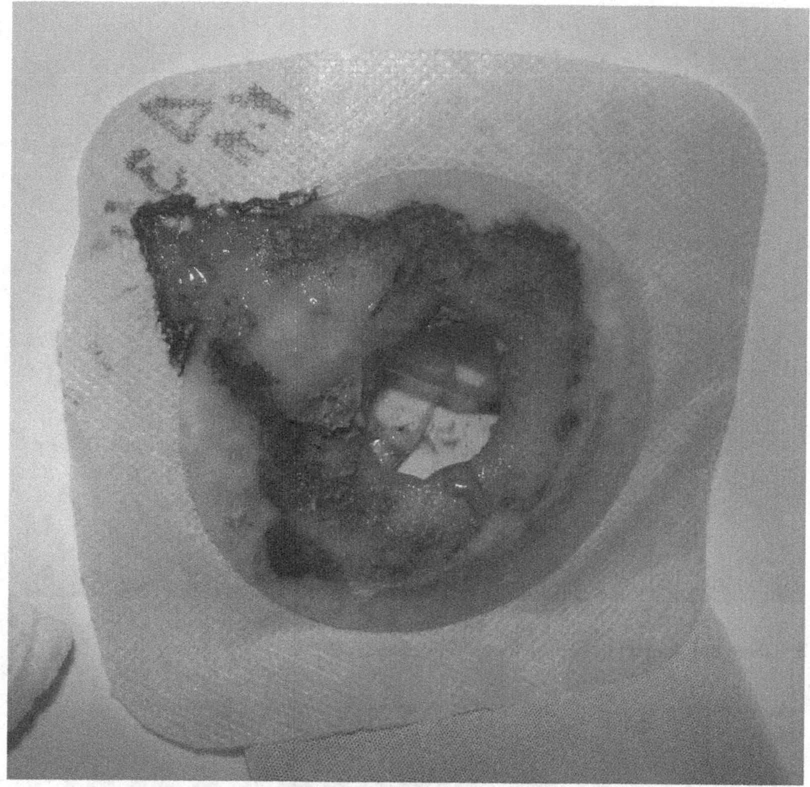

FIGURE 22.1 **(See color insert.)** Evaluating leaking on the back of worn ostomy wafer.

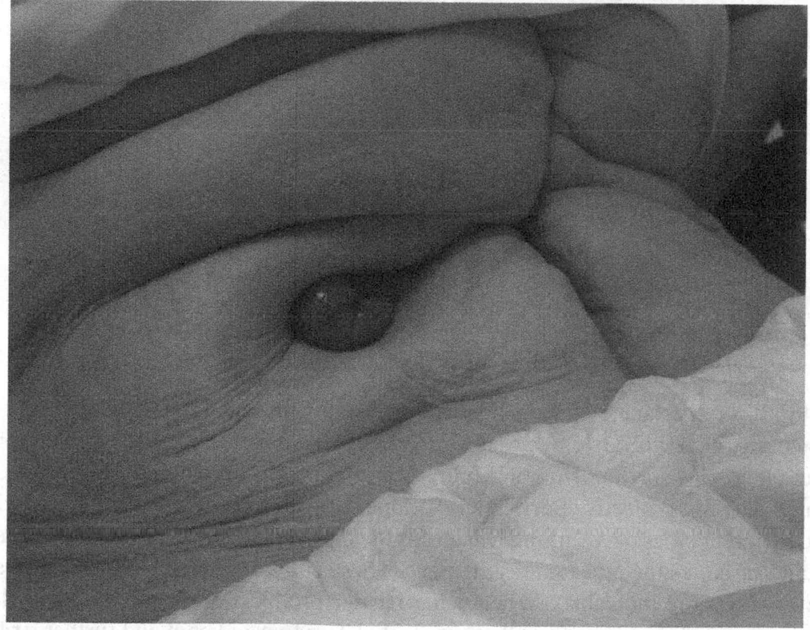

FIGURE 22.2 **(See color insert.)** Stoma with deep peristomal skin creases.

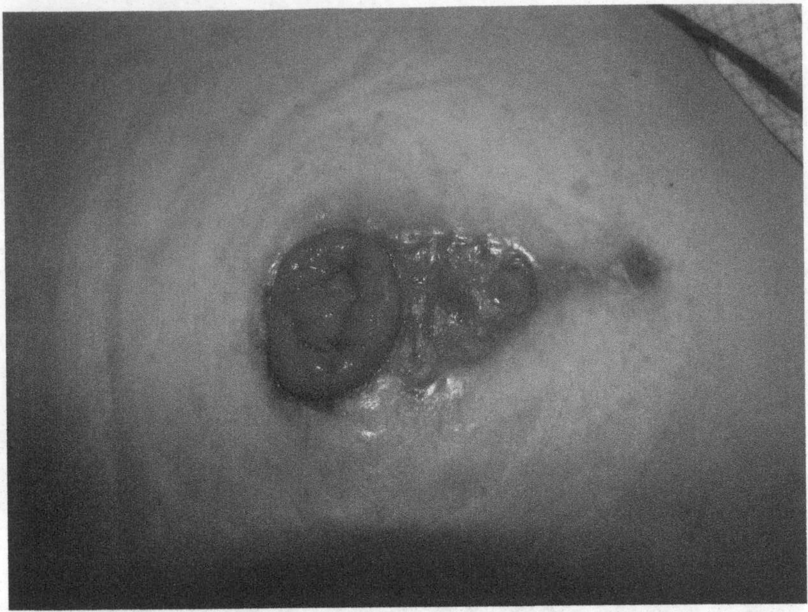

FIGURE 22.3 **(See color insert.)** Stoma located near a scar.

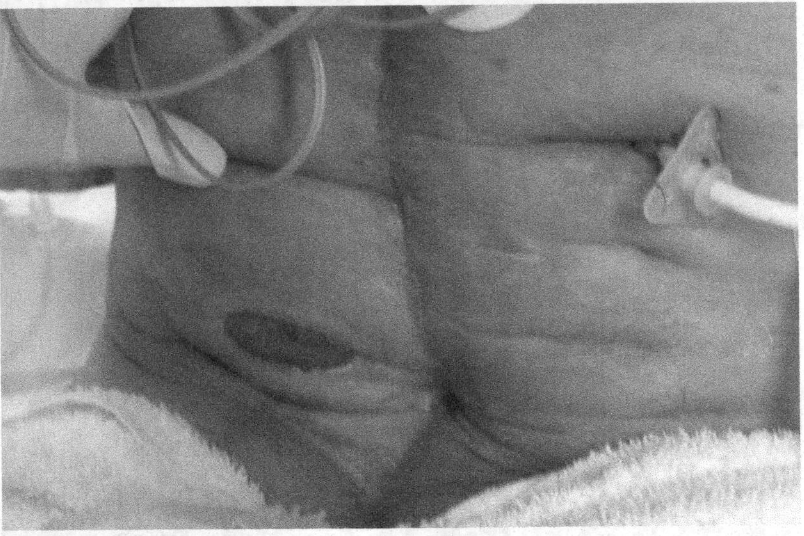

FIGURE 22.4 **(See color insert.)** Stoma with low profile, crease, near fistula (distal midline); gastrostomy site with hypergranulation tissue.

and trauma [8]. It is important to understand different ostomy products and their correct/intended uses to protect the peristomal skin. Ostomy products are divided into barriers and pouches. Barriers include liquid barriers (e.g., 3M Cavilon No-sting Film, Marathon Skin Protectant, Smith & Nephew Skin Prep, Convatec AllKare Protective Barrier, and Coloplast Brava Skin Barrier), the wafer with adhesive backing, and different types of "caulking" materials to help seal the inner wafer edge next to the stoma and to even and/or flatten the peristomal skin plane. These caulking barriers include pastes, strips and rings (some products are moldable). When using barrier products on irritated, denuded peristomal skin, it is recommended to use products that are alcohol-free to avoid pain and further irritation of the skin. Pectin-based (ostomy) powder can be used to absorb moisture from denuded skin. It is dusted

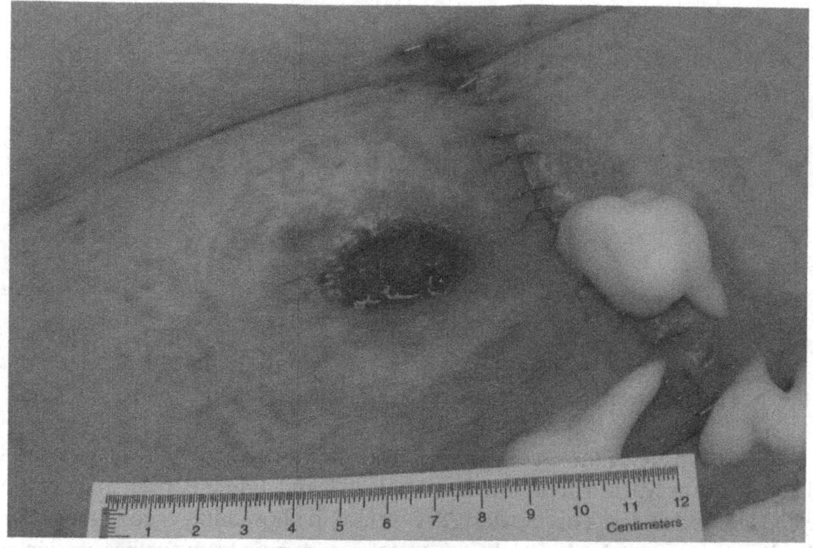

FIGURE 22.5 **(See color insert.)** Stoma with low profile and skin level lumen.

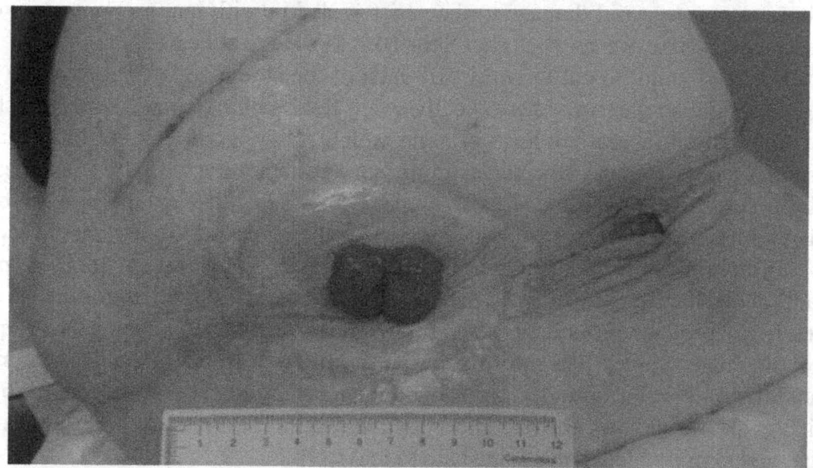

FIGURE 22.6 **(See color insert.)** Stoma presentation with patient lying supine.

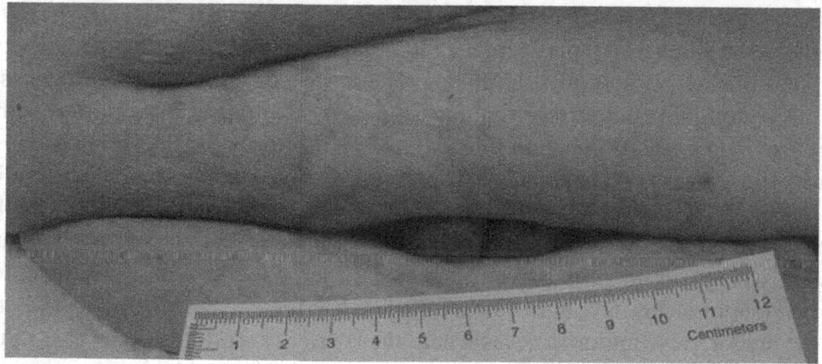

FIGURE 22.7 **(See color insert.)** Stoma presentation with patient sitting upright.

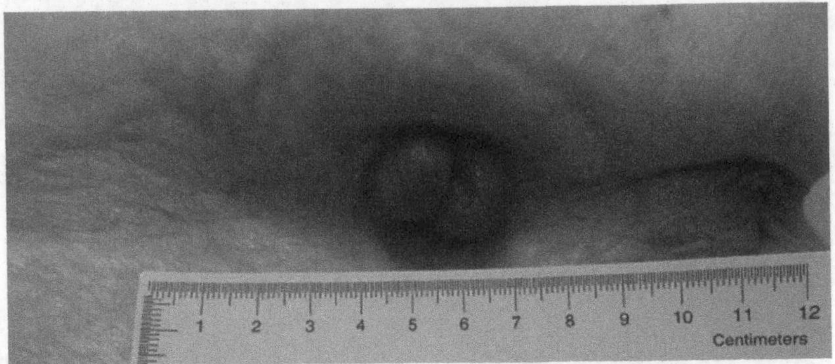

FIGURE 22.8 **(See color insert.)** Stoma presentation with patient standing.

lightly over weeping skin areas; the excess powder is brushed away, leaving the powder to stick only to the denuded areas. The powdered areas are then "sealed" with a liquid barrier spray or blotting with a barrier wipe and allowed to dry. This creates a dry "crust" to allow adherence of the wafer to denuded skin. Liquid skin barriers can also be used to protect the epidermis from further erosion and irritation [5,9]. None of these barrier products add more adhesion to the wafer system even though they may feel "tacky" before they are dry. There are actual adhesive products (spray, wipe, or brush-on) that should be used with great care to avoid damage to the peristomal skin with inappropriate or excessive use (e.g., Hollister medical adhesive spray, Torbot Skin TAC, Nu-Hope adhesive).

The barrier wafer should be cut to within 1/8 inch of the stoma edge to protect the peristomal skin. The stoma should be measured periodically, every few weeks, to make sure the cut is still the correct size, especially if the patient loses or gains weight. New-onset leaks or immediate peristomal skin irritation could be clues to changes in the stoma shape or size [5,9]. The adhesive wafers are available in standard and extended-wear preparations. Typically, extended wear barriers are recommended with high-output, very liquid ostomies as they have additional chemicals in them to resist erosion. Each brand of product has a little different terminology or name for these products, so it is important to familiarize yourself with the products before ordering them for the patient [5]. All of the major ostomy product manufacturers (e.g., Coloplast, Hollister, Convatec, Nu-Hope, Marlen, Torbot) have telephone support and information on the Internet to help educate on correct use of their products. It is important to understand how the barrier products are intended to be used correctly to gain the most benefit for the patient's peristomal skin. Incorrect use of products can lead to further peristomal skin problems and contribute to leaks [9].

Barrier wafers can be flat or convex. Convexity means the back of the wafer "bumps out" on the side that adheres to the skin around the stoma. Convexity is used to stabilize flexible peristomal skin, smooth wrinkles/creases, or "mirror/match" peristomal skin indentations to improve the protrusion of the stoma. Convexity can be soft and more flexible or rigid and firm. Soft convexity is usually indicated for more firm peristomal abdominal planes, and rigid/firm convexity is usually best for soft and pliable peristomal skin planes. These are not hard and fast rules, as each individual patient's abdominal contours are unique. Convexity is often best supported with the use of an ostomy belt as long as the stoma is in line with the natural waist. If the stoma is above or below the natural waistline, an ostomy belt may be displaced (roll) into the waistline with bending or other movements pulling the wafer loose. This will need to be monitored as the belt may not be effective or a different style of belt (similar to an abdominal binder) may need to be obtained/created [5,9,10].

Anecdotally, when working with barriers and ostomies in patients with SBS, the more moldable and soft the barrier product is, the more quickly the soft barrier tends to erode/wash when the output is high volume and/or very liquid. In cases where the barrier is eroding and/or absorbing moisture quickly, it may be better to use solid barrier products (sheets, nonmoldable rings, barrier adhesive strips) [7]. Lastly, we encourage seeking assistance from outside sources when multiple attempts and/or plans for pouching have not been successful. The Wound, Ostomy, Continence Nurse Society (WOCN) maintains a database (www.wocn.org) of board-certified ostomy nurses. You can search by city or state. Most of the facilities that treat patients with SBS have one or more WOC nurses on staff that can be an excellent resource for pouching suggestions in complex situations.

POUCHES

Ostomy pouches are designed to be odor proof and water resistant. They are typically changed along with the wafer two to three times a week, depending upon whether it is a one- or two-piece system. One-piece pouches come with an adhesive barrier wafer fused to the pouch. Two-piece pouch systems can be detached from the wafer using either a plastic flange or an adhesive coupling. Pouch tail closures are either integrated into the tail or require a separate clip. Some pouches have built-in filter systems with charcoal inserts to assist with odor and gas management; these filters are often ineffective if they become wet with liquid output. Pouches come in various sizes based on volume. Most of the features on pouches are used based on patient preferences [5,9].

For ostomies in SBS patients, a high-output pouch may be beneficial for increased liquid volumes. The tail closure for these pouches is a spout outlet with a cap or plug [7]. Liquid effluent is heavy and can disturb/pull on the wafer-skin seal if the pouch is allowed to overfill. Patients should be taught to empty their pouch when it is one-third to one-half full. If the patient has very high volume output, it may be helpful to connect the system to a larger dependent drainage bag positioned at the side of the patient's bed or chair when he or she is at home. These can be placed in reusable grocery bags for carrying and concealment when leaving the house. Most high-output pouches come with a device to connect the system to dependent drainage. Dependent drainage systems are usually replaced one to two times per month and can be rinsed with a 10% solution of bleach and water and allowed to air dry when not in use [7,9].

GENERAL OSTOMY CARE PRINCIPLES

Peristomal skin care should include gentle cleansing with plain water or a pH-balanced soap, tap water rinse, and patted dry. Do not scrub the skin or use alcohol, betadine, hydrogen peroxide, or other harsh chemicals. If there is build-up of adhesive or caulking materials on the peristomal skin, an adhesive remover wipe or spray can be used to gently remove this residue. Some adhesive removers are oil based and will need to be washed off with soap [12]. The patient should be taught to avoid scrubbing or picking off excess barrier from the skin to limit skin damage. If the stoma is very active during the wafer/pouch change, a bedside suction machine with a Yankauer tip can be used to suction the effluent; however, be careful not to apply the suction directly to the stoma tissue to avoid damage to the mucosa.

Ostomy supplies are usually covered by a predetermined percentage (copay may or may not apply) under Durable Medical Equipment in the patient's insurance plan. The patient or his or her family/caregiver can contact the insurance plan for specifics. If a home health agency is involved, the supplies are usually provided by the agency while they are contracted to provide care to the patient (check with the agency). It is often best to locate and work with an agency that is familiar with SBS and/or complex ostomy/wound patients. Ostomy supplies can quickly become expensive when leaks and peristomal skin breakdown are present and/or allowed to persist. If the current pouch system has been determined to be the most effective for the patient and excess supplies (more than the standard allowed 20 wafers and pouches per month) are required, a letter of medical necessity may need to be sent to the insurance company explaining the situation and requesting coverage of the excess supplies. It is essential to understand the challenges of managing a complicated ostomy and the importance of a consistent methodical process to find the most effective pouch system for the patient's situation. Eliciting help from ostomy experts is often beneficial in challenging situations and before allowing the peristomal skin condition to deteriorate to the point of requiring hospitalization. Some situations are so complex or challenging that referral to a surgeon for evaluation of possible surgical intervention to aid with ostomy management is highly recommended.

PREOPERATIVE MARKING OF A PLANNED STOMA SITE

In 2007, the American Society of Colon and Rectal Surgeons and the WOCN prepared a joint position statement instructing on the importance of preoperative marking of patients prior to a planned bowel diversion surgery. This paper provides the rationale/purpose, recommendations, and step-by-step procedure for stoma site marking [13]. The paper does not specifically address preoperative marking of a patient with an existing ostomy and/or EF(s), but the same principles still apply, taking into consideration these existing sites [14]. Studies consistently support that those patients who have preoperative marking by a trained ostomy clinician experience fewer postoperative complications related to the ostomy [13]. General principles include placement of the stoma within the rectus abdominis muscle, use of multiple patient positions to identify appropriate stoma sites, avoidance of folds and scars, and consideration of the clothing/beltline [13].

As previously mentioned, ostomy location may significantly affect the predictable wear-time of pouches and the self-management skill adaptation required by the patient with a new ostomy. It is understood that certified ostomy nurses and/or colorectal surgeons are not available in every surgical situation. Surgeons ultimately have the final determination in the placement of the ostomy during the intraoperative period and should familiarize themselves with the general principles of ostomy site selection for promotion of best patient outcomes.

MANAGEMENT OF ENTEROCUTANEOUS FISTULAS AND WOUNDS

EFs may result from a multitude of conditions and circumstances. Ninety percent of fistulas develop as a result of abdominal surgeries. Classification is determined by output volume, site of origin, etiology, and/or the number of fistula tracts. Managing the patient with a fistula can be challenging to the physician(s), WOC nurse, nursing staff, and the nutritionist involved in the patient's care [15]. Fistulas, unlike the creation of a stoma, where the site is selected and surgically created, are not predetermined and often occur in areas where management/pouching is challenging (e.g., skin fold, a wound or wound edge, and a scar) (Figure 22.4).

Many of the principles of ostomy management can be applied to fistula management. The goals of management are ultimately the same: protecting and maintaining the integrity of the perifistular skin, managing effluent, controlling odor, and finding a pouching system, whenever possible, to provide adequate wear-time.

Fistulas with drainage of less than 100 mL in 24 hours can often be managed with wound dressings such as gauze, absorptive foam, or alginate/hydrofiber. Dressings should be replaced when saturated and care taken to protect the perifistular skin with a protective barrier ointment, zinc paste, or a combination [15]. Fistulas that drain more than 100 mL per 24 hours generally require pouching. The pouching system should be selected based on the amount of drainage and the size, location, and the number and presentation (e.g., stomatized or not) of the fistula. The patient should be evaluated in multiple body positions to determine skin changes and how the pouch system will contour with patient movement [16]. Prior to application of a pouch system, it is important to create a level pouching surface around the EF. Caulking barriers (as previously discussed in the ostomy section) are effective in filling creases and defects around the perifistular skin. Another option that creates a pliable, moldable filler is the combination of ostomy paste and powder mixed to the consistency of clay/putty (ingredient amounts are dependent on the humidity and moisture content of the ostomy paste). This filler is soft and conforming and provides flexibility with patient movement (Figure 22.9).

Pouching options include standard ostomy appliances, commercially designed fistula management systems that come in a variety of shapes and sizes to conform to abdominal planes and accommodate the size of the wound/fistula, or a custom-made system [16]. Two to three inches of intact

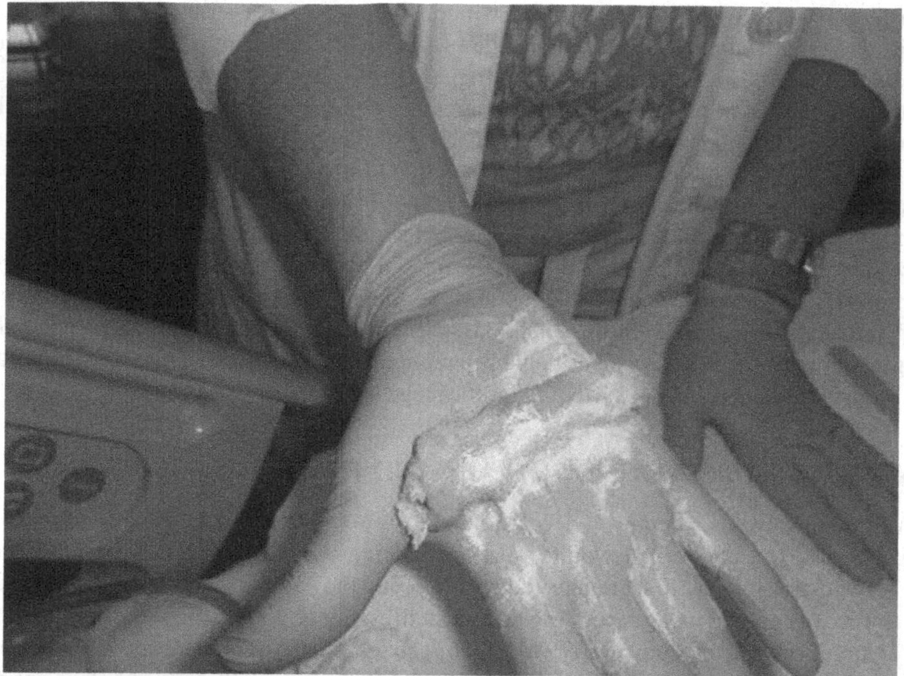

FIGURE 22.9 (See color insert.) Combination of stoma paste and powder to create putty.

skin is needed around the wound perimeter for best adherence of the appliance. Using a piece of clear plastic, a template/pattern of the wound/fistula area is created, allowing one-quarter to one-half inch of intact skin exposure around the area. The edge of the wound manager should not be cut directly at the edge of the wound/fistula. The pattern is traced onto the back of the appliance, cut out, and adhered onto the periwound/perifistular skin. Filling agents may be used along the cut edge of the appliance to fill in creases and/or provide additional protection to the exposed skin (Figure 22.10).

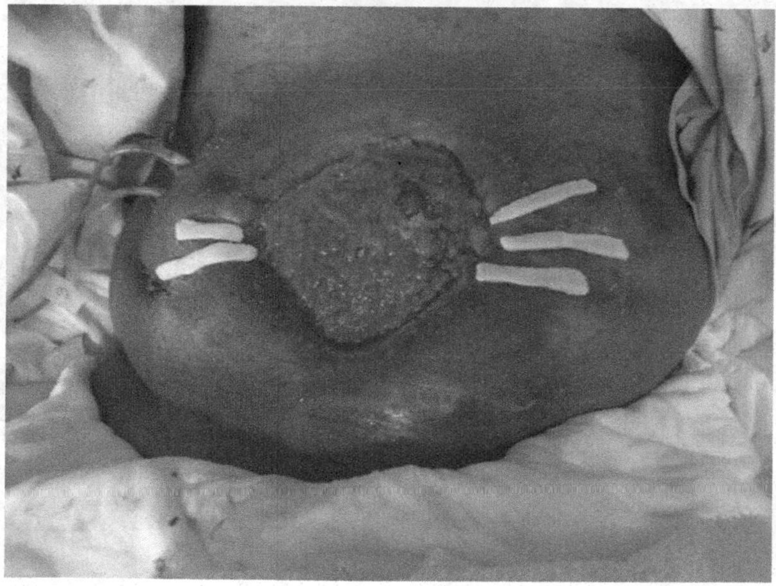

FIGURE 22.10 (See color insert.) Filling in periwound creases with barrier product to even the plane for pouching.

Many commercial systems have a built-in window/lid on the front of the pouch allowing access to the fistula(s) and wound bed. This feature allows dressings to be changed within the wound manager to extend the life of the appliance. The frequency of dressing changes is determined by the amount of effluent. In our experience, internal dressing changes vary between 2 and 6 hours. The time varies with each manufacturer. Fistula pouching systems have odor-proof components. Many systems feature a spigot/port to drain effluent from the system. A Foley bag may be connected to the system for dependent drainage. A tube (e.g., red robin catheter, chest tube, JP drain) can be run through the drainage port in the wound manager and connected to low continuous suction. A tube stabilizer placed on/in the manager will keep the tube in place. The stabilizer should be applied to the section of the manager where effluent drains. Effluent must be liquid in consistency to drain through a tube. If the patient is eating solid foods, particulates will clog the tubing. If not connected to straight drainage, the pouch system should be emptied when one-third to one-half full as effluent can add weight and contribute to system failure/leakage [16,17].

NEGATIVE PRESSURE WOUND THERAPY AND FISTULA MANAGEMENT

Negative pressure wound therapy (NPWT) and an ostomy pouch can be used to manage fistula drainage in an open abdominal wound while promoting wound healing. Barrier products are placed around the fistula to segregate the fistula from the wound bed. NPWT foam/gauze is placed in the wound bed using layers of wide mesh dressing (e.g., Adaptic) to cover any exposed bowel or organ before placing the NPWT foam/gauze. A transparent drape covers the entire wound bed/fistula and negative pressure is initiated. Once a seal is obtained, a hole is cut directly over the segregated fistula and an ostomy appliance is placed to capture effluent from the fistula, allowing the wound bed to heal and drainage from the fistula to be controlled. This technique is most effective when the fistula is stomatized, easily visualized, and segregated. It is important to note that NPWT should never be applied to manage the effluent from the fistula(s) as the drainage is too thick for the wound dressings and will clog the suction system (Figure 22.11). For complete instructions on NPWT, refer to KCI Clinical Guidelines (http://www.kci1.com/KCI1/vactherapyformsandbrochures).

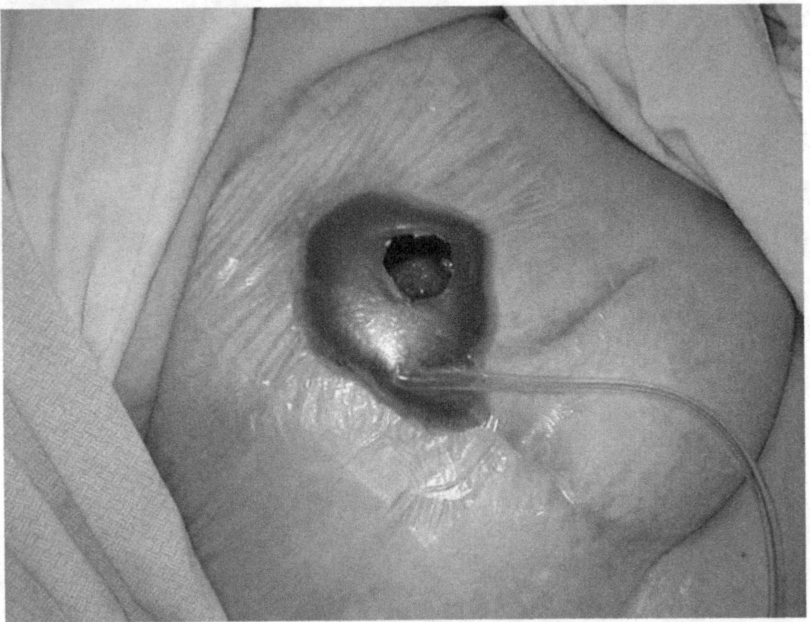

FIGURE 22.11 **(See color insert.)** Negative pressure wound therapy for wound treatment with a fistula.

CUSTOM-MADE SYSTEM FOR FISTULA MANAGEMENT

Conventional wound management systems are not always effective in molding to abdominal contours or achieving adequate wear time. Skin protection remains a top priority. With a custom-made system, a protective layer is applied onto the periwound skin (e.g., sheets of hydrocolloid or adherent foam dressings). A soft pliable catheter is wrapped in slightly moistened gauze and laid in the wound bed (e.g., a 28-Fr red radiopaque catheter). The tubing is flexible and connects easily to low continuous suction. A transparent drape is placed over the entire dressing, and strip paste and/or moldable caulking rings/seals are used around the tubing to achieve/maintain a seal (Figure 22.12).

GENERAL FISTULA MANAGEMENT GUIDELINES

When suction is required for containment of high-output effluent, it is a limiting factor for patient mobility. If portable suction is not readily available, the patient will be limited to the length of tubing connected to wall suction during his or her inpatient stay. In the home setting, portable units can be noisy and difficult to obtain. Working with a Durable Medical Equipment provider in the patient's community is often the best resource for procuring a device for home use.

There may be multiple attempts at management of a fistula or heavily draining wound before an effective plan is established. The plan will need to be modified if skin contours change, patient activity levels increase, or the amount of effluent changes. Importantly, treatment modalities that are effective in the inpatient setting may need to be modified when the patient is discharged home. The patient and caregiver skill level must be assessed during the development of a fistula management plan. If the dressing application or general maintenance is not easily completed, then the plan will need to be modified to meet the skill level of those involved with the care.

When every effort to maintain a pouch system has been exhausted, the fistula drainage, regardless of amount of output, may need to be managed with dressings. Barrier ointments/pastes are used to protect and maintain the periwound/perifistular skin integrity. Barrier ointments/pastes may consist of zinc oxide, petrolatum, dimethicone, or a mixture of these. It is important to apply the barrier to the surrounding skin in a thick layer for protection with each dressing change. Manufacturer's guidelines should be followed for application and removal of all barrier products. A surfactant-based

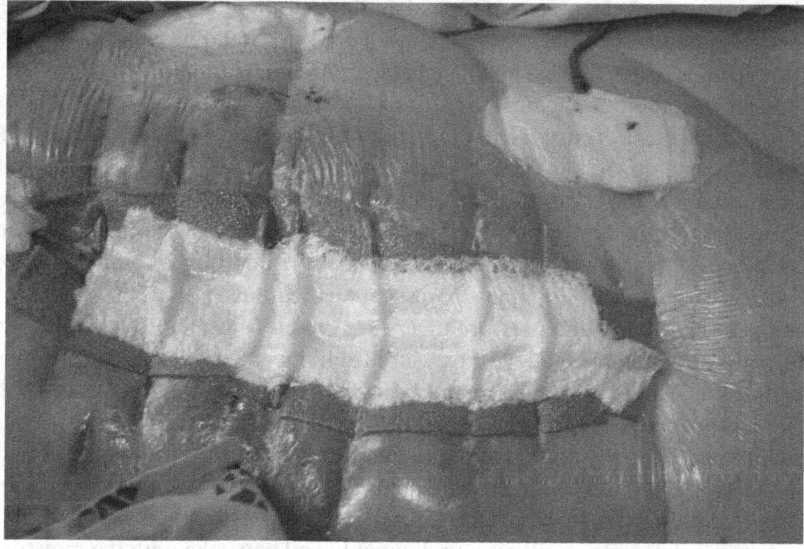

FIGURE 22.12 **(See color insert.)** Custom-made fistula/wound management system connected to low intermittent suction.

cleanser or mineral oil will ease the removal of most ointments/pastes. Avoid scrubbing and use of harsh chemical as the skin often becomes denuded to the point that barrier ointments/pastes will not adhere to the weeping moist skin. Ostomy powder can be lightly dusted over the wet/weepy areas, allowing the barrier ointment/paste to adhere on top [18]. Product choices for absorption of the effluent may include alginates, gauze, ABD pads, infant or feminine products, or, when finances are limited, absorptive soft towels/linens that can be laundered and reused. Dressings may be secured with an abdominal binder or snug-fitting undergarments or taped at the edges of the outer dressing. The patient and/or caregiver must be vigilant, changing dressings as often as required to manage effluent and keep the periwound/perifistular skin intact. This is a very labor-intensive plan and should be used only as a last resort.

While pouching systems offer the best odor control, there are products made for ostomy pouches to reduce and/or eliminate bowel odors (e.g., M9 Odor eliminating drops, Adapt or Brava lubricating deodorant, and Safe-n-Simple ostomy pouch deodorant). These can be expensive as they usually require more than the typical amount used in a standard ostomy pouch. Other options include oral body deodorants such as Devrom or Derifil. Charcoal dressings and filters neutralize odor; however, when they become wet, the charcoal is deactivated, making the dressing or filter ineffective at managing odor [9].

Fistula management can be expensive. Consideration must be made for the cost of dressings, the management systems, and the labor incurred with application and management. Fistula pouches can cost upward of $150.00 per system. Medicare may cover up to 80% of the cost of some of the supplies, with the patients paying 20% if they do not have coinsurance [16,17]. In our experience, full and sometimes partial coverage for fistula supplies and portable suction is difficult to obtain, especially for long-term use.

MANAGEMENT OF PERCUTANEOUS ENTERAL TUBE SITES

Minor complications are reported in 13–40% of patients with a percutaneous gastrostomy tube [19]. The most common complications of the stoma site include peristomal skin irritation/breakdown, leaking, bleeding, hypergranulation tissue growth, and infection at the stoma site. General care of the tube site includes daily assessment for skin problems and gentle washing under the retention bumper with mild soap and water using cotton-tipped applicators. Hydrogen peroxide, rubbing alcohol, and/or routine/prophylactic use of topical antibiotic ointments/creams is not recommended as these can contribute to peristomal skin problems. The skin should be examined for excess moisture, denudation from leakage, rashes, nonblanchable erythema from too much pressure applied by the external bolster (i.e., too tight against the skin), skin stripping from adhesives and/or increased warmth, redness, or purulent drainage from infection. The retention bumper and flange should not be moved or "slid up and down" the tube during care as this can contribute to bumper failure over time. During examination, the edges of the retention bumper should be gently lifted on all sides to access and assess the tube insertion site. The site will be at increased risk for complications if it is located in a skin crease, fold, or scar and when the patient is obese or immunocompromised (e.g., diabetes mellitus, posttransplant, immunosuppressant medications) [19–21].

Skin irritation, denudement, and pressure ulcers are typically related to leakage, drainage from hypergranulation tissue, and/or infection or pressure from the external retention bumper positioned too tightly on the skin. The first step is to identify and eliminate or treat the cause of the problem. Irritated skin that is not open or weeping can best be treated with an alcohol-free topical skin barrier wipe applied daily under the retention bumper; make sure the skin is dry before laying the bumper back down on the skin. Oil-based ointments are appropriate for minimal leakage, minor skin irritation, or medication delivery. Water-based creams will wash quickly if the site is leaking and are not generally recommended. Powders will also wash quickly and can cake with the moisture at the site, contributing to skin irritation; powders can be used with a barrier wipe/spray to create a "crust," as described earlier in this chapter on ostomy management. Only visibly soiled ointment, powder, and/or paste should be gently removed when the dressing is changed. Reapply fresh barrier on top; do not remove the entire barrier every time, as this will irritate the skin more. Frequency of dressing changes will depend upon the amount of leakage. Old paste/barrier can be easily removed with mineral oil to avoid damaging the skin; this needs to be done only one to two times a week. Only use one layer of fenestrated gauze under the retention bumper (additional layers can be added on top of the retention bumper as needed). If the site is leaking actively/frequently, it is critical that the dressings be changed quickly and frequently to avoid caustic stomach effluent from sitting on and digesting the peristomal skin. Gauze absorbs but does NOT wick the drainage *away from the skin*. The retention bumper should generally be positioned about 0.5 to 1 cm from the skin surface, so it is sitting lightly but not tightly on the skin. The tube can be marked so the caregiver knows where the bumper should always be located. Some tubes have external markings, and this can easily be noted for the caregiver to check. The position of the bumper should be checked daily and with major changes in body position if the patient/caregiver notices that the retention bumper "seems to move on its own." This can happen over time (age of tube) or with frequent manipulation of the bumper manually (loosens the grip of the bumper against the tube). Thin foam or alginate wound dressings can be used around the tube site for treatment of pressure ulcers. The cause of the pressure ulcer (e.g., sutures, retention bumper too tight, and "button" length too short for abdominal wall) must be addressed. While systemic antibiotics are generally used to treat peristomal infections, depending upon the signs and symptoms present, a topical antifungal powder or antibacterial dressings two to three times a day may also be utilized either alone or together [19–21].

Correct anchoring of the tube with an external retention bumper or device to prevent mobility of the tube in the stoma site is critical to eliminate leaks and hypergranulation tissue formation. If the tube is allowed to move around or in/out of the site, the stoma will enlarge, contributing to leaking (Figures 22.4 and 22.13). Simply placing a larger-diameter tube will only temporarily "fix the problem," especially if the tube is not anchored and is still mobile in the stoma, and is not the recommended first step when dealing with tube site leakage. Feeding tubes that do not have "built-in" external retention bumpers can be immobilized by using commercially available retention devices (e.g., Hollister tube attachment device, Bard StatLock device, Dale Hold-n-Place adhesive patch, Convatec FlexiTrac anchoring device) or a custom-made anchoring device using a baby bottle nipple and a solid ostomy skin barrier wafer. The skin barrier opening is enlarged to accommodate the tube diameter size from the top and fit around the tube site, adhering it to the clean dry skin. The baby bottle nipple is slit along the side through the end of the nipple, which can be enlarged slightly to accommodate the diameter of the tube and placed around the tube (the bottom of the nipple sits inside the flange of the wafer) and is anchored to the flange with waterproof tape [20].

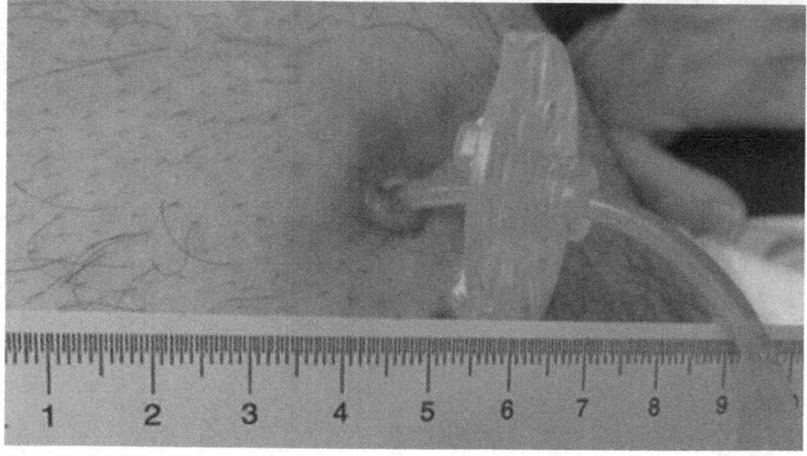

FIGURE 22.13 **(See color insert.)** Gastrostomy tube mobility allowing hypergranulation tissue growth.

Hypergranulation tissue can cause pain and bleed with tube movement and contributes to drainage and moisture at the site. Hypergranulation tissue can be treated with silver nitrate cautery, a topical high-potency steroid cream (e.g., triamcinolone), foam wound dressings placed snugly around the tube site (to manage moisture better), or with excision and cautery of excess tissue (after infiltration with lidocaine) [19–21].

MANAGEMENT OF FECAL INCONTINENCE-ASSOCIATED DERMATITIS

SBS patients with chronic diarrhea who do not have a stoma are at high risk for fecal incontinence-associated dermatitis (IAD) (Figure 22.14), even if they are continent. The anal sphincters function most effectively with solid or semiformed stool. With frequent or large-volume loose or liquid stool, there is a high likelihood of fecal incontinence and/or periodic seepage of stool from the anus. The fecal material will contain digestive enzymes that can compromise the skin if allowed to remain on the skin for even a short time. The prevalence of IAD in SBS is unknown, although, anecdotally, it is commonly reported. As such, reviews on prevention and treatment of IAD in the wound/continence literature are based mostly on expert opinion with a paucity of data from small research studies [22–24]. The literature consistently promotes using a systematic skin care regimen that includes gentle cleansing, moisturizing, and applying a skin barrier with each incontinence/leakage episode [22–25]. It is important to note that these types of products (cleansers, moisturizers and barriers) are rarely covered by insurance. It is essential to use the products in the manner and amount according to the manufacturers' recommendations to avoid waste.

Cleansers should be used with each incontinence episode to gently remove irritants from the skin. Stool should not be allowed to dry on the skin. Cleansers should be free of strong perfumes and alcohol. Ideally, the cleanser should be pH balanced to closely match the acid mantle of normal human skin (5–6.5 pH range). Bar soaps should be avoided as they are typically alkaline (pH greater than 7) and will contribute to skin irritation. Scrubbing or rubbing of the affected skin should also be avoided, especially if redness, irritation, and/or denudement are present as this will contribute to further skin breakdown and pain [22–24]. Dove Body wash and Johnson's Baby Wash have been cited as being closer in pH to normal skin [26]. For SBS patients residing in a care facility, pH-balanced perineal skin cleansers and/or disposable cleaning cloths are appropriate to use.

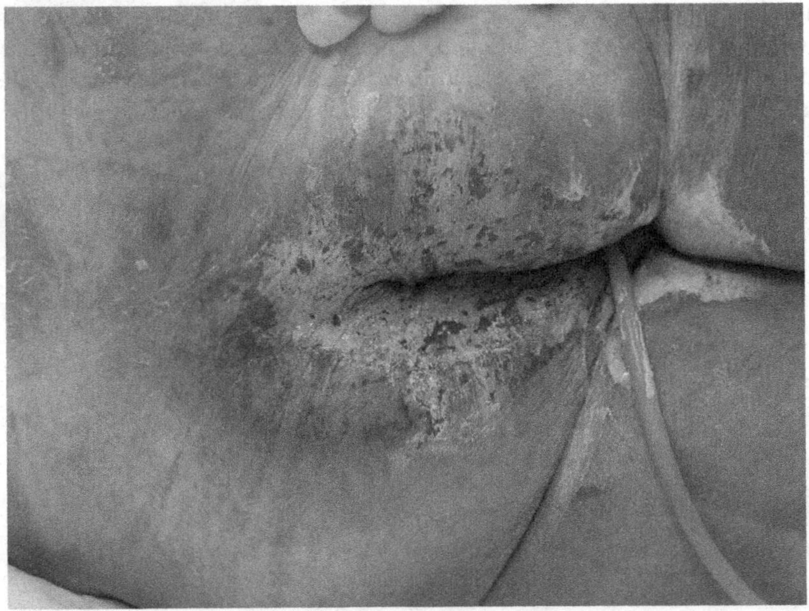

FIGURE 22.14 **(See color insert.)** Severe fecal incontinence association dermatitis.

One of the primary functions of the human skin is to act as a barrier to external contaminants. The layers of the skin have a lipid component that is depleted/stripped with frequent washing, especially with standard soaps and antimicrobial cleansers. It is critical, therefore, that the affected skin be replenished with a moisturizer after each cleansing/rinsing episode to repair and maintain skin integrity. Lotions are water-based preparations and should not be used for fecal incontinence skin care. Effective moisturizers will be creams (50% oil:50% water) or ointments (greater than 50% oil content) [26]. Many of the disposable cleansing cloths in licensed healthcare settings will be a combination of a gentle cleansing agent and moisturizer (i.e., all-in-one product). These products can be expensive to use in the home setting as they are not covered by insurance. These disposable products should *not* be flushed into city or septic plumbing systems as they may contribute to clogs requiring costly repairs.

Protective barrier products consist of ointments and pastes. Ointments are the most occlusive and prevent skin breakdown by creating a barrier between the offending agent (e.g., feces) and the skin. The most frequently used barrier product is petrolatum, but others include dimethicone, calamine, allantoin, lanolin, or zinc oxide. Pastes are ointment preparations with an absorptive powder (zinc, carboxymethylcellulose) mixed in [22–24,26]. Another category of barriers is liquid film-forming acrylates, as previously discussed in the ostomy section. These should be applied after cleansing and moisturizing and allowed to dry before letting skin folds rest together. Follow the manufacturers' directions for frequency and method of application. It is important to use non-alcohol-based (no-sting) liquid barriers if the skin is denuded.

In general, pastes tend to "wash"/erode more quickly with frequent liquid fecal incontinence. In our experience, a combination of an ointment and paste is usually more durable but still needs to be applied with each incontinence episode regardless of the amount of leakage (after gentle cleansing and moisturizing). There is no "perfect" barrier for caustic liquid stool. The most important concept is to follow the regimen of gentle cleansing, moisturizing, and barrier protection as soon as leakage/incontinence occurs. There are multiple combination (often compounded by pharmacies) "butt pastes" listed on the Internet. It is important to evaluate each ingredient and see if it is appropriate for the patient's skin you are treating. For example, many contain antifungal powders or creams, but the patient may not have a fungal skin infection, while some have a steroid cream to control inflammation but should not be used for longer than several weeks. We recommend that these types of compounds be used only when indicated and for the appropriate length of time. Our final recommendation is to use a product for a reasonable period (5–7 days) before discarding as ineffective as many SBS patients will have numerous butt pastes, creams, and ointments in their possession but are using them inappropriately, inconsistently, or not in conjunction with correct cleansing and moisturizing routines.

FINAL THOUGHTS: THE ROLE OF NURSING IN THE MANAGEMENT OF THE PATIENT WITH SBS

The WOC nurse plays an essential role in communicating, reinforcing, and evaluating the treatment plan (e.g., skin, wound and ostomy care, dietary intake, fluid prescriptions—oral and parenteral—and medication administration) prescribed by the multidisciplinary SBS team. Nurses are expected to reinforce, educate, and support the patient and caregiver in adhering to the plan. Written care instructions, step-by-step photographic directions, and treatment observation with return demonstration are beneficial for most patients and their caregivers to learn and master the prescribed clinical treatments. Accurate documentation is important in monitoring successes and failures so ineffective treatments and/or management plans are not carelessly repeated. The nurse is involved in identifying and evaluating the patient and/or caregiver's learning styles, ability to cope/adapt with stress and significant lifestyle changes, and the support systems available to promote success for the patient. Lastly, communication with team members regarding identified areas of concern that impact the patient's response/adherence to the treatment plan is vital for successful follow-up and outcomes [1–3,5,27].

REFERENCES

1. DiBaise JK et al. Short bowel syndrome in adults—Part 1: Physiological alterations and clinical consequences. *Pract Gastroenterol* 2014;132:30–39.
2. Sica J et al. Management of intestinal failure and high-output stomas. *Br J Nurs* 2007;16(13):772–777.
3. Carlsson E et al. Living with an ostomy and short bowel syndrome: Practical aspects and impact on daily life. *J Wound Ostomy Continence Nurs* 2001;28(2):96–105.
4. McDonald A. Orchestrating the management of patients with high-output stomas. *Br J Nurs* 2014;23(12):645–649.
5. Wound Ostomy and Continence Nurse Society. *Management of the Patient with a Fecal Ostomy: Best Practice Guideline for Clinicians.* Mount Laurel, NJ: Author, 2010, pp. i–44.
6. Baker ML et al. Causes and management of a high-output stoma. *Colorect Dis* 2010;13:191–197.
7. Colwell J. Managing the patient with a high output stoma. Presented at the WOCN Society's 46th Annual Conference, Nashville, Tennessee, June 21–25, 2014.
8. Richbourg L et al. Ostomy pouch wear time in the United States. *J Wound Ostomy Continence Nurs* 2008;35(5):504–508.
9. Colwell J. Principles of stoma management. In: *Fecal & Urinary Diversions: Management Principles.* Eds, Colwell JC, Goldberg MT, Carmel JE. St. Louis: Mosby, 2004, pp. 240–262.
10. Hoeflok J et al. Use of convexity in pouching. *J Wound Ostomy Continence Nurs* 2013;40(5):506–512.
11. Gray M et al. Peristomal moisture-associated skin damage in adults with fecal ostomies. *J Wound Ostomy Continence Nurs* 2013;40(4):389–399.
12. Rolstad BS et al. Relating knowledge of anatomy and physiology of the skin to peristomal skin care. *WCET* 2011;32(1):4–10.
13. Wound Ostomy and Continence Nurses Society. *WOCN Society and ASCRS Position Statement on Preoperative Stoma Site Marking for Patients Undergoing Colostomy or Ileostomy Surgery.* Mt. Laurel: NJ. Author, 2014, pp. 1–9. http://c.ymcdn.com/sites/www.wocn.org/resource/resmgr/Publications/ASCRS_Stoma_Site_Marking_PS_.pdf.
14. Colwell JC. Stoma site selection in a patient with multiple enterocutaneous fistulae. *J Wound Ostomy Continence Nurs* 2001;28:113–115.
15. Hoedema RE et al. Enterostomal therapy and wound care of the enterocutaneous fistula patient. *Clin Colon Rectal Surg* 2010;23(3):161–168.
16. Bryant BA et al. Management of draining wounds and fistulas. In: *Acute & Chronic Wounds: Current Management Concepts*, 4th ed. Eds, Bryant RA, Nix DP. St. Louis: Mosby, 2012, pp. 514–533.
17. Willcutts K et al. Ostomies and fistulas: A collaborative approach. *Pract Gastroenterol* 2005;33:63–79.
18. Lekan-Rugledge D. Management of urinary incontinence: Skin care, containment devices, catheters, absorptive products. In: *Urinary and Fecal Incontinence: Current Management Concepts*, 3rd ed. Ed, Doughty DB. St. Louis: Mosby, 2006, pp. 310–324.
19. Blumenstein I et al. Gastroenteric tube feeding: Techniques, problems and solutions. *World J Gastroenterol* 2014;20(26):8505–8524.
20. Carmel JE et al. Tube management. In: *Fecal & Urinary Diversions: Management Principles.* Eds, Colwell JC, Goldberg MT, Carmel JE. St. Louis: Mosby, 2004, pp. 351–380.
21. Wound Ostomy and Continence Nurse Society. *Management of Gastrostomy Tube Complications for the Pediatric and Adult Patient.* Mount Laurel, NJ: Author, 2008, pp. 1–10.
22. Wound Ostomy and Continence Nurse Society. *Incontinence Associated Dermatitis (IAD): Best Practice for Clinicians.* Mount Laurel, NJ: Author, 2011, pp. 2–15.
23. Gray M et al. Incontinence-associated dermatitis: A comprehensive review and update. *J Wound Ostomy Continence Nurs* 2012;39(1):61–74.
24. Haugen V et al. Prevention and management of incontinence-associated dermatitis. *Safe Pract Patient Care* 2012;6(1):1, 7–11. http://www.safe-practices.org/pdf/SafePractices16.pdf.
25. Gray M et al. Incontinence-associated dermatitis: A consensus. *J Wound Ostomy Continence Nurs* 2007;34(1):45–54.
26. Dixon M. When what comes out is way more than what goes in: Perineal skin care. *Pract Gastroenterol* 2009;76:11–23.
27. Parrish CR et al. Short bowel syndrome in adults—Part 2: Nutrition therapy for short bowel syndrome in the adult patient. *Pract Gastroenterol* 2014;134:40–51.

23 Autologous Gastrointestinal Reconstruction

David F. Mercer

CONTENTS

KEY POINTS

- Autologous gastrointestinal reconstruction refers to the surgical modification of a short bowel patient's existing small or large intestine and typically involves surgical techniques developed to manage intestinal dilation, thereby optimizing the exposure of the mucosal absorptive surface to the enteric stream.
- A short bowel patient should have failed conventional medical management and have dilation of the small intestine >3.5 cm to be considered for autologous reconstruction.
- There are a variety of surgical reconstruction techniques that can be used to modify dilated intestine with the goal of improving overall function. The short- and longer-term outcomes with these techniques are essentially equal.

INTRODUCTION

Autologous reconstruction of the gastrointestinal (GI) tract refers to the surgical modification of a patient's own existing small or large intestine to improve overall enteral absorption. In its simplest form, this represents basic general surgical principles that include restoration of intestinal continuity, repair of enteroenteral or enterocutaneous fistulas, resection of extensively diseased bowel segments, and repair or removal of fixed intestinal strictures. With these procedures, the surgeon seeks to optimize exposure of the mucosal absorptive surface to the nutrient-laden enteric stream. Within the field of intestinal failure management, however, autologous reconstruction has, in large part, come to be defined as surgical techniques developed to deal primarily with intestinal dilation. In this chapter, we outline the theoretical goals of autologous reconstruction, the indications and process of evaluation for considering surgical options, and the various surgical options which have been described in this regard.

GOAL OF AUTOLOGOUS GI RECONSTRUCTION

One consequence of shortened intestinal length can be the development of progressive dilation of the residual small bowel. The mechanism underlying this dilation is not clear at the present time. In many cases, this dilation occurs in the absence of any discernible obstruction to forward flow and seems to be a development that is inherent to the condition of short bowel syndrome (SBS) itself, possibly because, at least in part, of the process of intestinal adaptation. There are instances where dilation occurs as a sequela of some form of mechanical obstruction of the intestine; this would typically be dealt with by relieving the obstructing process, allowing the intestine to recover a normal luminal diameter. The deliberate creation of a complete or near-complete small bowel obstruction has been proposed, however, with the goal of creating intestinal dilation to then allow the performance of an autologous reconstruction procedure [1].

Autologous reconstruction procedures of the intestine are often referred to as "lengthening" procedures, as the overall length of the intestine is generally increased as a result of the procedure. It is not necessarily the case, however, that it is the absolute increase in length that leads to improvement in function, but rather it is the reduction in dilation and creation of a uniform luminal diameter that lead to successful advancement in enteral feeding. Dilated segments of the intestine display poor antegrade peristalsis, with frequent remixing of the enteric stream, and have a propensity for developing clinically significant bacterial overgrowth. These features often lead to the inability to advance calories provided enterally due to noxious symptoms experienced by the patient. By performing an enteroplasty, the surgeon seeks to reduce the overall luminal diameter down to a more appropriate size, thus improving the volume-to-surface area ratio of the intestine and hopefully also improving antegrade motility and eliminating small intestinal bacterial overgrowth. These improvements may combine to lead to successful weaning of parenteral nutrition support. In this view then, the increase in length is not the primary goal of the surgery, but rather a consequence of the reduction in luminal diameter. In effect, it becomes an easy surrogate to describe the change in intestinal shape.

It is necessary to point out that a contrary view is that dilation is actually a desirable future and that it can be manipulated to increase the total absorptive surface area of the intestine to lead to better overall long-term outcomes. Proponents of this view support the deliberate creation of obstructing or near obstructing anatomies, with the ultimate intention of effecting dilation and then performing a subsequent enteroplasty. This same view would also suggest merit to performing an early enteroplasty on congenitally obstructed intestine, rather than simply relieving the obstruction and allowing the intestine to return to normal luminal diameter, if possible. At the present time, it is not certain which of these views is most correct.

PREOPERATIVE EVALUATION

For most autologous reconstruction procedures of the intestine, there is a prerequisite for intestinal dilation; however, there are different thresholds for what dilation is deemed the minimum for surgical intervention. In general, it is accepted that the intestine needs to be dilated to >3.5 cm in diameter; ideally, somewhat more. This minimum diameter is required simply to ensure that the diameter of the loops after enteroplasty is still sufficient to permit forward progression of the enteric stream. The determination of the degree of intestinal dilatation may be done with a number of different radiographic methods. Most commonly, a barium-contrast small bowel series is used. This imaging technique has the advantage of providing not only structural/anatomic information but also dynamic information about the function of the intestine, including the evidence of propulsive contractions versus insufficient or retrograde contractions, which can be seen in isolated dilated segments. Because the presence of overlapping small bowel loops can make interpretation of studies difficult, especially where there have been prior autologous reconstruction interventions, the availability of a radiologist skilled in the evaluation of patients with SBS and reconstructive procedures is beneficial, as is a close relationship between the examining radiologist and treatment team in discussing study findings. A computed tomography scan with or without enteral contrast may also be used and can have the advantage of eliminating the confounder of overlapping bowel loops, but at the expense of losing the ability to dynamically examine the intestine. Any assessment of the degree of dilation performed at the time of endoscopy is imprecise at best. There is no practical way to be quantitatively accurate in assessing dilation during endoscopy; however, it can be used to indicate whether some degree of dilation is present, although even this can be misleading at times.

Although the presence of intestinal dilation is required for autologous reconstruction, it is generally not sufficient on its own to be an indication for surgical intervention. Intervention to address intestinal dilation may be best reserved for instances where a patient is showing failure of advancement of enteral feeds and/or failure to wean parenteral nutrition, treatment of bacterial overgrowth, endoscopic management of intestinal strictures where present, and use of pharmacologic promotility agents. Possible indications for autologous reconstruction procedures include

- Intestinal dilation >3.5 cm in diameter
- Patient is showing failure of advancement of enteral feeds and/or failure to wean parenteral nutrition, after attempts have been made to:
  - Optimize and maximize medical management
    - Including alternative formulas and method of delivery
  - Treat bacterial overgrowth if present
  - Manage mucosal inflammation
  - Manage intestinal strictures (e.g., endoscopically or surgically) where present
  - Use pharmacologic promotility or antimotility agents as required

A possible exception to this guideline would be instances where autologous reconstruction is considered as a primary procedure in cases of neonatal bowel obstruction or in defined experimental programs, where an obstruction is created deliberately as a precursor to reconstruction. It should be noted that there is very little evidence to support the deliberate creation of dilation for the purpose of subsequent autologous reconstruction over simply relieving any obstructions in the intestine, optimizing medical management, and then intervening with autologous reconstruction to address dilation only when it occurs naturally. The management outcomes in the latter approach are at least equivalent to the former.

THE LONGITUDINAL INTESTINAL LENGTHENING AND TAPERING PROCEDURE

The longitudinal intestinal lengthening and tapering (LILT) procedure, commonly referred to as the "Bianchi procedure," is a technique for reducing luminal diameter and increasing intestinal length that was developed and popularized in the early 1980s [2]. It takes advantage of the fact that the vascular supply to a loop of the intestine comes up through the mesentery and then decussates around the bowel on either side. It may be used on any primarily dilated segment of the intestine, with the exceptions of short segments of dilated bowel (generally <10 cm) and dilation of the duodenum. It also cannot be used on a segment of the bowel that has undergone a prior enteroplasty, with the exception of an excisional tapering enteroplasty (see below), where it would still be technically possible.

After marking off the selected segment of dilation, the antimesenteric side of the intestine is divided longitudinally along its midline, thus opening up the entire lumen of the bowel and exposing the mucosa on the mesenteric side. The plane between the two leaves of mesentery is then developed, and stay sutures are placed on the edge of the bowel wall on either side of the midline. With gentle upward traction on the sutures, a space opens up between the two separate vascular pedicles, and then the surgeon can carefully come along the longitudinal midline of the bowel wall, dividing it into equal portions, each supplied by a separate leaf of mesentery. These open segments can then be sewn into parallel tubes, with the distal end of one tube being gently turned back and sewn to the proximal end of the other tube, creating a "lazy S" conformation of the bowel and rendering the segment isoperistaltic. In the original description by Bianchi, division of the intestine was done using bipolar electrocautery, and all sewing was done by hand. In a variation of the procedure, the plane between the leaves of the mesentery was developed bluntly, and then a longitudinal stapler was used to divide the bowel into two separate tubes prior to reanastomosis as described previously. This has the advantage of being a much quicker technique but may be fraught with a higher rate of complications, as described further in the chapter.

In skilled hands, the LILT procedure can be done with relatively minimal operative morbidity [3,4]. The major risks in the short term are those of any complex GI surgery, including anastomotic or staple line leaks, bleeding, and wound complications. One early complication specific to the procedure and typically considered a technical performance issue, however, is segmental necrosis related to interruption of blood supply to one of the intestinal loops. Longer term complications from the procedure include late stricturing and the formation of intraloop fistulas between the new tapered loops of bowel. The latter complication is found more commonly after a LILT procedure that is performed with surgical staplers. When the procedure is performed entirely by hand, this risk is distinctly minimized.

It is difficult to accurately describe the positive long-term outcomes because of variability in center experience and differing management strategies used to wean children from parenteral nutrition over the decades since this procedure was first described. Rates of reported weaning from parenteral nutrition, the preferred measurement of success, have varied from 4% to 100% of treated patients, with a mean of approximately 70% [3]. Weaning of parenteral nutrition generally occurs over the period of 1–2 years after performance of the procedure. It is obviously highly influenced by both the preoperative anatomy of the patient as well as the postoperative management strategy of the treating program.

THE SERIAL TRANSVERSE ENTEROPLASTY PROCEDURE

The serial transverse enteroplasty (STEP) procedure was first described in 2003 and has subsequently become the most commonly performed enteroplasty in most centers around the world [5–8]. In STEP, a series of alternating staple firings using a GI anastomosis-type stapler are performed in a zigzag pattern along a dilated segment of bowel, thereby reducing the luminal diameter to a degree that is better suited for the patient as judged by the operating surgeon but typically to a diameter of approximately 2 cm. The actual change in length of an affected segment of bowel is dependent upon its initial diameter. As such, an increase in bowel length exceeding 100% can be achieved with the STEP procedure. This degree of lengthening is not possible with the LILT procedure, which has a maximum increase in length of 100%. The staple firings can be performed in a transverse fashion extending from side to side along the dilated segment or can be done in a mesenteric–antimesenteric fashion. It is most critical during the performance of STEP that the orientation of the intestine be strictly maintained regardless of which technique a surgeon chooses. This is, perhaps, more easily achieved in the mesenteric to antimesenteric fashion but with experience and care can be achieved equally as easily using transverse staple firings. It is also important that the individual staple firings traverse across the longitudinal midline of the intestine, to create a true overlapping zigzag pattern. Failure to do so will ultimately result in an ineffective pattern of enteroplasty, with no meaningful change in the overall dilation of the intestinal segment. This will entail making a small opening in the mesentery just at the edge of the intestine, taking care to go between existing blood vessels, thus maximizing the blood supply to the intestine. After completion of the procedure, all staple lines are checked to ensure that they are intact and reinforced where necessary.

The STEP procedure may be repeated through an area that has previously undergone a STEP enteroplasty, on segments that have previously undergone a LILT procedure, on short dilated segments, and, to an extent, on segments of dilated duodenum. Performing the procedure in repeat fashion can be more challenging depending upon the techniques used in the previous operation. Indeed, it is during the performance of a reoperation that the surgeon truly appreciates the importance of maintaining strict orientation of the intestine at the original operation. Where the staple firings have been placed off axis, it can be extremely difficult to get effective reduction in luminal diameter with a repeat procedure. Where the staple lines have been regularly placed, it is the goal of reoperative surgery to then restore a uniform luminal diameter along the segment of the bowel; this can involve extending existing staple lines, placing new staple lines, or even performing excisional tapering on certain segments as required. An excellent result can be achieved after repeat operation, with outcomes very similar to those of a primary procedure [7,9].

A more recent variant indication for the STEP procedure is for the management of segments of dilated intestine found in children at their initial infant surgery (e.g., at the time of primary management of intestinal atresia) [1]. This is done, in part, to assist in managing the diameter of the dilated upstream segment of the intestine with the typically much smaller diameter of the patent downstream segment of the intestine. Traditionally, it has been taught that without modification, the discrepancy in size between the proximal and distal segments of the intestine will lead to a poorly functioning anastomosis, in effect acting like a functional obstruction. This has typically been dealt with by performing a proximal tapering enteroplasty; however, as surgeons have gained familiarity with the STEP procedure, it has been adapted to the circumstances. While it is possible that this may have a positive effect on the anastomosis itself, in general, these enteroplasty staple lines are quite short and typically prove ineffective in causing a persistently reduced diameter in the affected segment of the intestine. This becomes manifest when the need for reoperative surgery arises some number of months after the primary surgery and the increased challenges of performing a STEP along this already stapled segment of the intestine become evident. Intermediate- and longer-term data on this relatively new procedure are not yet available. As such, it should be used cautiously and only in experienced hands, ideally in specialized institutions where comprehensive intestinal failure care is provided.

In skilled hands, a STEP procedure can be performed with minimal operative morbidity [5,7]. The pattern of complications after the procedure is very similar to that of the LILT procedure, with the exception that there appears to be a lower rate of intraloop fistulization after the STEP procedure [3]. This may reflect technical factors of performing the LILT procedure, such as the use of stapling devices rather than hand-sewing the anastomotic lines, however, and may not be inherent to the procedure itself. After successful performance of a STEP procedure, there are reports demonstrating a progressive reduction in parenteral nutrition requirements over the course of 12 months, along with a concomitant increase in enteral calories [7]. Published series show rates of weaning from parenteral nutrition that range from 20% to 100%, with a mean around 60–70%, similar to that seen for the LILT procedure [3].

At the present time, the major long-term complications of the STEP procedure include recurrent bowel dilation, stricturing, and delayed GI bleeding. Recurrent dilation can result from ineffective technical performance of the procedure but can also be the result of an ongoing process of dilation within the intestine; thus, it may not technically be a complication of the procedure. Strictures, in contrast, are typically the result of overaggressive attempts at gaining intestinal length at the expense of reducing the luminal diameter, thus leading to areas that are too narrow to allow antegrade progression of the enteric stream. When these occur, they often prevent advancement in enteral feeding and generally require operative intervention with repair by stricturoplasty or resection. A final complication that is of uncertain etiology is the development of an inflammatory process in distal segments of the small intestine. This is generally found in areas adjacent to the large intestine. The segments do not obviously appear ischemic, and there is no propensity for a similar phenotype elsewhere in the intestine. It may be related to altered microbial populations within the affected segment of the bowel, as in some cases it has been seen to recur in a previously normal segment of the intestine after resection of a more distal affected segment. Some anecdotal success in management has been achieved using immunomodulator therapies.

THE SPIRAL INTESTINAL LENGTHENING AND TAPERING PROCEDURE

A more recently described enteroplasty procedure, coming from the same group that developed the LILT procedure, is the spiral intestinal lengthening and tapering (SILT) procedure [10]. At the present time, this procedure seems to be indicated in segments of the intestine that are also suitable for an LILT procedure. While it does not appear suitable for reoperation after a prior enteroplasty, it does appear to have potential utility in short segment dilations, which are not amenable to the LILT procedure. The SILT procedure is performed by first carefully marking the orientation of the intestine, followed by the creation of a series of 60° angled cuts on alternating sides along a dilated segment of the intestine. This creates, in effect, a helical segment of the intestine, which may then be lengthened by gentle longitudinal traction along the segment, followed by reanastomosis of the cut edges of the bowel to create a new, narrower, and longer isoperistaltic segment of the intestine. This is purported to have the advantage of maintaining the longitudinal orientation of the intestine, in contrast to a STEP procedure, which alters the wave of peristalsis in a zigzag fashion. Because this procedure is very new, there are very few published data about outcomes as of yet. Preliminary reports suggest a perioperative morbidity equivalent to other enteroplasty procedures.

TAPERING ENTEROPLASTY

A final reconstructive tool in the armamentarium of the surgeon is the use of a tapering enteroplasty. This procedure is performed along a dilated segment of the intestine with the goal of reducing the luminal diameter toward normal, without altering the longitudinal orientation of smooth muscle fibers or the myenteric plexus. It achieves the primary goal of improving the volume:surface area ratio of the intestine with some reduction in overall surface area.

The most common technique used is a longitudinal excisional tapering enteroplasty. After marking off the dilated segment of the intestine, a series of clamps are placed longitudinally along the antimesenteric midline of the intestine, with the bowel then being stretched out flat, which is elevated up. Using either cautery and suture or, more commonly, a series of firings of a stapler, a portion of "excess" tissue is excised, reducing the remaining bowel back to a diameter more appropriate for the age of the patient. In addition to maintaining the original orientation of peristalsis, this technique also permits later application of any other enteroplasty technique, including LILT, SILT, or STEP. This technique is most useful when there is a reasonable length of the intestine present already and where the creation of additional "length" is not felt to materially improve overall functioning. It is very effective along the duodenum when there is significant dilation that impacts on emptying of the gastroduodenal complex and is also very useful in short segment dilations in areas of previous STEP procedures, where the creation of new transverse staple lines is rendered impossible by the orientation of existing staple lines. The disadvantage relative to other enteroplasties is a reduction in absorptive surface; however, when applied in the correct circumstances, the advantage gained by improving volume:surface area and creating uniformity of the intestinal lumen typically outweighs the loss of absorptive surface.

There are certain rare conditions, such as intestinal myopathies with dilation or idiopathic intestinal dilation where there is still evidence of peristalsis, where this procedure may be performed over a longer segment, in some cases up to 200 cm or more at one time. This can require the use of multiple staple loads, in excess of 20–30 or more, and care must be taken to carefully maintain the orientation of the intestine along the entire segment and to avoid reducing the residual lumen too aggressively. With modern stapling devices, leaks are very rare, and staple lines typically do not have to be oversewn.

A variation in the tapering enteroplasty is a nonexcisional type, in which the antimesenteric surface of the intestine is imbricated, reducing the overall luminal diameter of the segment with invagination of the excess tissue into the lumen of the remaining intestine. This has the advantage, when properly performed, of eliminating the risk of leak. However, the result is often unsatisfying when working with a bulky segment of the intestine due to alteration of flow and peristalsis in the affected segment. Another downside of this technique is that, over time, the segment has a tendency to redilate and "outstretch" the modified segment. Nevertheless, it has found some utility in the alteration of a dilated duodenum, where there is fear of a potential duodenal leak. In general, an excisional tapering enteroplasty is preferable to the nonexcisional version.

CONCLUSIONS

The objective of autologous intestinal reconstruction is to optimize the volume:surface area of a segment of dilated intestine while at the same time improving antegrade motility to reduce stasis and bacterial overgrowth. The goal at the forefront of the surgeon's mind when undertaking these procedures should be to create uniformity of the intestine rather than extend bowel length—the creation of length is usually a by-product of an effective enteroplasty procedure rather than the primary goal. An overzealous desire to lengthen the intestine can, and will be met by, the development of strictures, which will have a greater negative impact on the advancement of enteral nutrition than any potential "benefit" gained from additional length. The bowel should be reduced down to a diameter that is age appropriate to the patient, and no further. None of the enteroplasty techniques described (Figure 23.1) offers conclusive benefit over the other and, in skilled hands, can be used

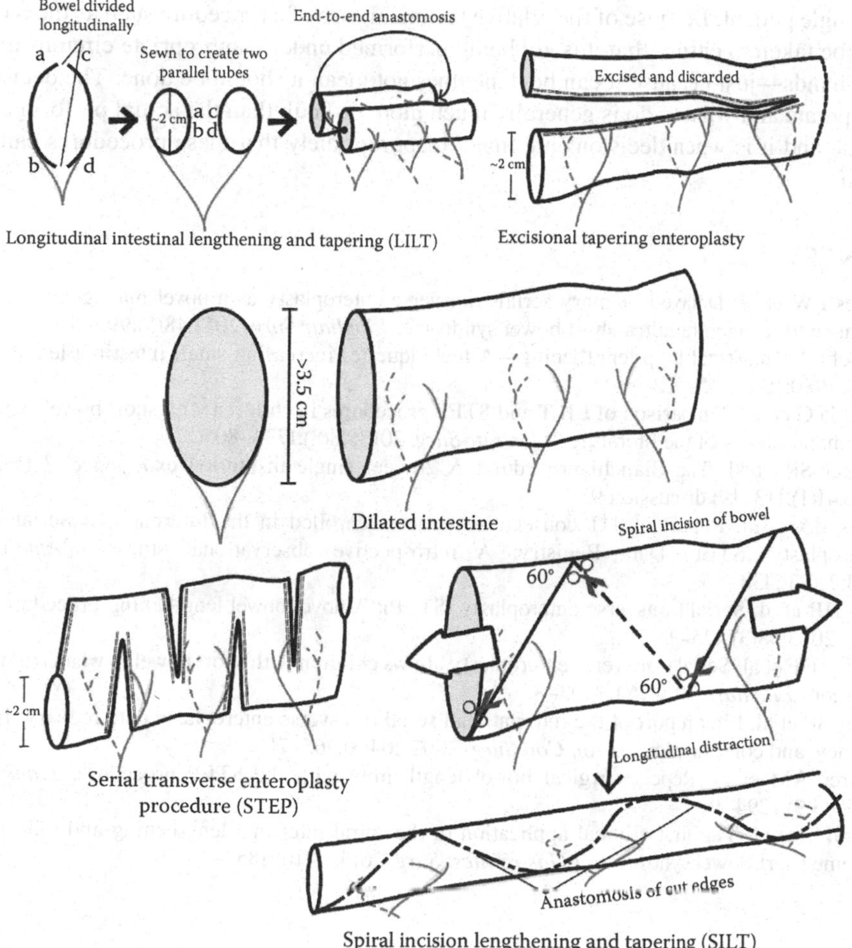

FIGURE 23.1 Schematic representation of surgical options for autologous reconstruction of a dilated small intestine. See text for descriptions of the procedures illustrated.

TABLE 23.1
Comparison of Common Techniques of Autologous Reconstruction

Procedure	Anatomic Requirements	Advantages	Disadvantages
LILT	Intestine dilated >3.5 cm, no prior enteroplasty of bowel	Bowel remains isoperistaltic, future enteroplasties can still be performed (except repeat LILT)	Maximum length increase 2×, technically more challenging with equivalent results, cannot be repeated
STEP	Intestine dilated >3.5 cm	Easy to perform, can achieve lengthening >2×, can be repeated or can follow prior LILT	Possible effect on peristalsis due to interruption of longitudinal muscle
SILT	Intestine dilated >3.5 cm	? Isoperistaltic	Inadequate data
Tapering enteroplasty	Intestine dilated >3.5 cm	Isoperistaltic, easy to perform, can be done repeatedly	Loss of absorptive surface area

interchangeably when indicated (Table 23.1). In some cases, multiple techniques can be applied within a single patient. Because of the relative technical ease of a procedure such as the STEP, great care must be taken to ensure that it is not being performed under inappropriate circumstances or in untrained hands—just because it can be done does not mean it should be done. The decision about when to operate and what to do is generally much more difficult than the actual performance of the procedures, and it is when decisions are made inappropriately that these procedures can have the most harm.

REFERENCES

1. Wales PW et al. Delayed primary serial transverse enteroplasty as a novel management strategy for infants with congenital ultra-short bowel syndrome. *J Pediatr Surg*. 2013;48(5):993–9.
2. Bianchi A. Intestinal loop lengthening—A technique for increasing small intestinal length. *J Pediatr Surg*. 1980;15(2):145–51.
3. Frongia G et al. Comparison of LILT and STEP procedures in children with short bowel syndrome—A systematic review of the literature. *J Pediatr Surg*. 2013;48(8):1794–805.
4. Walker SR et al. The Bianchi procedure: A 20-year single institution experience. *J Pediatr Surg*. 2006;41(1):113–19; discussion 9.
5. Jones BA et al. Report of 111 consecutive patients enrolled in the International Serial Transverse Enteroplasty (STEP) Data Registry: A retrospective observational study. *J Am Coll Surg*. 2013;216(3):438–46.
6. Kim HB et al. Serial transverse enteroplasty (STEP): A novel bowel lengthening procedure. *J Pediatr Surg*. 2003;38(3):425–9.
7. Mercer DF et al. Serial transverse enteroplasty allows children with short bowel to wean from parenteral nutrition. *J Pediatr*. 2014;164(1):93–8.
8. Modi BP et al. First report of the international serial transverse enteroplasty data registry: Indications, efficacy, and complications. *J Am Coll Surg*. 2007;204(3):365–71.
9. Andres AM et al. Repeat surgical bowel lengthening with the STEP procedure. *Transplantation*. 2008;85(9):1294–9.
10. Cserni T et al. The first clinical application of the spiral intestinal lengthening and tailoring (silt) in extreme short bowel syndrome. *J Gastrointest Surg*. 2014;18(10):1852–7.

24 Intestinal Transplantation

Sherilyn Gordon Burroughs and Douglas G. Farmer

CONTENTS

KEY POINTS

- The increased effectiveness of modern immunosuppression paved the way for intestinal transplantation to emerge as a viable treatment option for many patients with intestinal failure.
- Use of refined patient and graft selection and operative and postoperative prophylaxis management strategies has resulted in decreased morbidity and mortality after intestinal transplantation.
- Despite these advances, sepsis and chronic rejection remain formidable obstacles to universal long-term success after intestinal transplantation.

INTRODUCTION

Since its introduction into clinical practice over five decades ago, the field of intestinal transplantation (ITx) has undergone significant advances. Limited initial clinical attempts in the 1960s were met with a 30-day mortality of nearly 90% [1]. Overall, 1-year patient survival rates of 85% are now consistently demonstrated, while rates of ≥92% have been achieved in select ITx recipients [2]. In this chapter, we review the development of ITx and discuss its indications and surgical approaches. Outcomes and challenges associated with broadened utility and improved long-term outcomes are also reviewed.

HISTORY

In the late 1950s, the experimental era of ITx was initiated by the pioneering work of Lillehei [3] and Starzl [4], who independently established successful canine auto- (Lillehei) and allo- (Starzl) ITx models. Their orthotopic models were an advanced iteration of the heterotopic model created in 1902 by French Nobel laureate Alexis Carrel, in which vascularized intestinal segments were implanted into the necks of dogs [5]. Nine human ITx clinical attempts worldwide, spanning from 1964 to 1970, resulted [1] (Table 24.1). The outcomes of these attempts performed under immunosuppression of that era—corticosteroids, azathioprine, and antilymphocyte globulin in some combination—were suboptimal due to uncontrollable rejection or technical failure. It was readily apparent that survival after transplantation of the lymphoid-rich intestine would require more potent and specific immunosuppression and advanced surgical techniques before success could be achieved. Simultaneously, the development of parenteral nutrition (PN) by Wilmore and Dudrick in 1968 [6] and long-term central venous catheters by Broviac in 1972 [7] enabled the prolonged provision of intravenous fluids, electrolytes, and nutrients to patients with congenital or acquired absorptive, motility, anatomic, or functional gastrointestinal (GI) disorders. The collective diagnoses constituting these disorders are now referred to as causes of intestinal failure.

PN use, initially limited to short-term, in-hospital therapy, had a dramatic effect on the ability to acutely stabilize patients with intestinal failure. Subsequently, long-term PN use in the home setting has increased over time [8,9], conveying a greater survival benefit (Figure 24.1), and as a consequence, ITx was relegated purely to a research entity. In 1984, the successful use of the novel calcineurin inhibitor, cyclosporine, for other solid organ transplants led to renewed interest in human ITx.

TABLE 24.1
Early Attempts at Human Intestinal Transplantation

Year	Center	Graft	Graft Survival	Cause of Graft Loss
1964	Boston Floating Hospital	Living related isolated intestine	12 hours	Intestinal necrosis
1964	Boston Floating Hospital	Isolated intestine	2 days	Intestinal necrosis
1967	University of Minnesota	Intestine + colon	12 hours	Pt mortality, pulmonary embolism
1968	University of Sao Paulo	Isolated intestine	12 days	Rejection
1969	University of Paris	Intestine + colon	23 days	Rejection
1969	University of Mississippi	Living related isolated intestine	32 days	Rejection
1969	University of Sao Paulo	Isolated intestine	5 days	Rejection
1969	Albert Einstein Hospital	Isolated intestine	18 hours	Pt mortality, hypovolemic shock
1970	Cornell University Hospital	Living related isolated intestine	79 days	Rejection

Source: McAllister, V., Grant, D.R., in Grant, D.R., Wood, R.F.M., eds. *Small Bowel Transplantation*, Edward Arnold, London, 1994, p. 121.

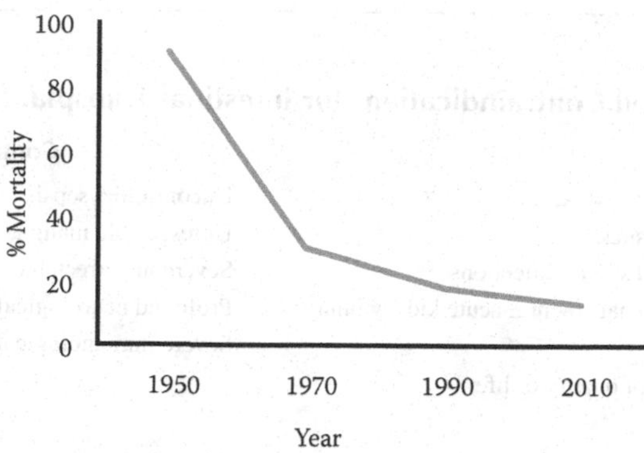

FIGURE 24.1 Five-year mortality before and after chronic PN availability.

TABLE 24.2
Outcomes of Initial Experience in Clinical Intestinal Transplantation with Cyclosporine Immunosuppression

Year	Author	Graft	Graft Survival	Cause of Graft Loss
1985	Cohen	Isolated intestine	12 days	Rejection
1987	Goulet	Isolated intestine	3 hours	Thrombosis
1987	Goulet	Isolated intestine	211 days	Rejection
1987	Deltz	Living related isolated intestine	12 days	Rejection
1987	Starzl	Multivisceral	192 days	Patient mortality, multisystem organ failure
1988	Grant	Combined liver/small bowel	5 years	Unknown

Source: Grant, D. et al. *Lancet*, 335, 181–184, 1990.

Several landmark case reports emerged, including the first successful human multivisceral transplant by Starzl and associates in 1987 [10], isolated ITx by Deltz and colleagues in 1987 [11], and combined liver–ITx by Grant and associates in 1988 [12] (Table 24.2). Unfortunately, rejection remained a major obstacle to graft survival, preventing consideration of ITx as a feasible treatment option.

The modern era of transplantation was heralded by the development and subsequent availability of tacrolimus in the 1990s. Reports of a series of patients successfully undergoing ITx with survival exceeding 1 year were published thereafter [1], and tacrolimus use, along with surgical and critical care advances, cemented the establishment of ITx as a viable treatment option for intestinal failure. This culminated in October 2000 with the decision of the Centers for Medicaid and Medicare Services in the United States to approve ITx as a definitive therapy for patients with intestinal failure and associated complications [13].

INDICATIONS

Although analysis of patients maintained on contemporary long-term home PN therapy reveals that many do well with few serious complications, not all patients tolerate PN in the intermediate or long-term. Recent reports demonstrate 85–88% 5-year survival rates on home PN, but with a 19–26% rate of serious complications [14,15]. Debilitating complications include poor glycemic regulation, severe chronic fatigue, severely impaired quality of life, and employment obstacles [16,17]. Potentially lethal complications include intestinal failure-associated liver disease (IFALD), loss of central vascular access sites, recurrent central line infections with or without septic extravascular foci, osteoporosis with spontaneous fractures, and difficult fluid and electrolyte management with recurrent episodes

TABLE 24.3
Common Indications and Contraindications for Intestinal Transplant

Indications—Absolute	Contraindications
Intestinal failure-associated liver disease	Uncontrolled sepsis
Loss of central vascular access sites	Unresectable malignancies
Recurrent catheter-related blood stream infections	Severe uncorrectable cardiopulmonary disease
Difficult fluid and electrolyte management ± acute kidney injury	Profound neurological/cognitive impairment
Indications—Relative	Severe immunologic deficiencies
Severe fatigue and impairment of quality of life	
Growth retardation	

of ischemic acute tubular necrosis and chronic kidney disease [18–20]. Once irreversible intestinal failure is present, and life-threatening PN-related complications are imminent, ITx should be considered. We describe in the following the major indications for ITx (Table 24.3).

Liver Disease

IFALD, when manifested as irreversible liver failure, is the most straightforward indication for ITx, as death from liver disease is inevitable without transplantation. IFALD occurs to some degree in 40–60% of chronic PN patients [19]. Microbiome alterations, intestinal stasis with resultant small bowel bacterial overgrowth, reduced clearance of hepatic bile acids, nutrient deficiencies, and toxic components of PN have been implicated as causative factors [21–23]. The most widely accepted hypothesis, however, is that hepatic steatosis with progression to hepatitis, fibrosis, and cirrhosis is stimulated by oxidative injury mediated by the proinflammatory arachidonic acid omega-6 fatty acids in soy-based lipid emulsions used in traditional PN [24].

The clinicopathological presentation and disease progression differ in patients depending upon multiple factors, including age, GI anatomy, PN formulation administered, use of enteral nutrition, as well as other less-defined genetic and metabolic characteristics. The progression of liver failure based on PN exposure alone is thus not always predictable. As such, patients are typically managed preemptively according to the best evidence of risk. For example, lipid management in PN formulations is critically reviewed in high-risk populations, namely, premature newborns and infants with physiologic hepatic immaturity, patients with hereditary or acquired hepatic comorbidities (e.g., cystic fibrosis-related liver disease and chronic hepatitis), and those with disorders of lipid metabolism and recurring sepsis. Analysis of wait-list mortality from the United Network for Organ Sharing (UNOS) Annual Report data reveals that liver failure experienced in IFALD patients, particularly the pediatric subset, may result in a more rapidly progressive deterioration than in patients with other forms of liver disease [25]. The ability to reverse or arrest early hepatic dysfunction with alternative lipid formulations, such as omega-3 fatty acid-based lipid emulsions (Omegaven) [21,26] or alternative lipid mixtures (SMOFlipid) [24] has been reported. Their increased use is thought to correlate with the trend of decreased need for utilization of liver-inclusive grafts in the last decade [2,24]. Validation of this association requires further study. An obstacle to widespread use in the United States is the fact that these alternatives have not been approved by the U.S. Food and Drug Administration.

Loss of Central Venous Access

The inability to establish or safely maintain central venous access is also an indication for ITx. Patients on chronic PN often develop central venous occlusion due to thrombi of hypercoagulable or septic origin, resulting in limited options for PN delivery. Limited access is appropriately defined as loss of approximately half the standard jugular, subclavian, or iliac vein access sites, and not the extreme cases in which transhepatic, intra-atrial, or intrathoracic access lines are the only available options due to superior or inferior vena cava (IVC) thrombus. Increasingly, collaboration with interventional radiologists or cardiologists who have demonstrated improved success in thrombectomy and stenting central veins has allowed for more durable patency of central access sites, preserving same-site access for longer duration in patients on chronic PN [27].

Catheter-Related Bloodstream Infections

Recurrent central venous catheter sepsis in patients with intestinal failure is also a central venous access-related indication for ITx. In general, this indication does not include patients with the occasional infection but instead refers to those with fungemia, multiple recurring bacterial infections, infections associated with metastatic foci such as endocarditis and osteomyelitis, infections associated with multiple organ failure syndromes, and infections caused by multiple antibiotic-resistant microbes. Although use of ethanol lock prophylaxis protocols has recently been demonstrated to reduce the incidence of catheter-related bloodstream infections in both high-risk pediatric [28] and adult [29] PN-dependent patients, the risk of mortality in this cohort remains high [14,26,30].

Miscellaneous

Another subset of intestinal failure patients that should be considered for early ITx referral includes those at high risk for early death or PN failure during attempts at gut rehabilitation. This group includes patients with ultrashort remnant bowel (<20 cm in adults/<10 cm in infants with absence of the colon), high proximal unreconstructable duodenostomy or gastrocolonic discontinuity, desmoid tumors, or extensive portomesenteric thrombosis. In addition, patients with congenital epithelial functional disorders with no realistic prognosis for adaptation (e.g., microvillus inclusion disease, tufting enteropathy, and congenital villus atrophy) are included. Earlier referral and transplant allows for a more straightforward perioperative and intraoperative course and decreased overall mortality.

Finally, patients with intestinal failure because of disorders associated with high morbidity and poor quality of life should be considered for ITx. This group includes patients with fluid and electrolyte challenges rendering them hospital bound or committed to continuous 24-hour infusions, patients with motility disorders such as chronic intestinal pseudo-obstruction, and patients with frozen peritoneal cavities complicated by uncontrolled enterocutaneous/enteroatmospheric fistulae. Irrespective of the diagnosis, early referral to a center capable of intestinal rehabilitation and ITx is critical for optimizing both pre-ITx care and post-ITx outcomes. While the aforementioned indications were established within the last decade, improvements in the overall management of intestinal failure have led to a new dialogue on the standard indications. Whether a real revision of these will be forthcoming remains to be seen [31].

EVALUATION/LISTING

A comprehensive evaluation of major organ systems must be undertaken before listing an individual for ITx. As with all potential transplant recipients, medical suitability and surgical suitability are critical considerations. Extraintestinal comorbidities may influence a transplant center's decision in determining ITx candidacy. Contraindications potentially unmasked at evaluation include profound cognitive or neurologic impairment, uncontrolled systemic sepsis, and uncorrectable systemic illnesses not directly related to the digestive system that cannot be treated by transplantation. Examples of the latter include fixed, severe cardiopulmonary disease, severe immunologic deficiencies, and the presence of unresectable malignancies.

The University of California at Los Angeles evaluation protocol is described in Table 24.4. Studies were designed to assist with operative planning, including the type of transplant to be performed, target vascular access sites, and inflow and outflow vessels for the graft. Diseased organs to

TABLE 24.4
Prelisting Evaluation of Intestinal Transplant Recipients at the University of California, Los Angeles, Intestinal Transplant Program

Laboratory Tests	Other Diagnostic Tests
Type and screen	Upper/lower GI contrast
HLA typing	MR venography
Cytotoxic antibody screen	MRI central veins
Flow class I and II PRA	Nuclear medicine glomerular filtration
Reflex single antigen testing	Nuclear medicine gastric emptying study
Micronutrients/serum vitamins	Cardiac echo
Complete blood count/platelets	Pulmonary function testing
Fibrinogen, PT/INR, PTT	
Urinalysis	
Viral serologies	
• Epstein-Barr Virus IgM, IgG	
• Cytomegalovirus IgM, IgG	
• Human immunodeficiency virus	
• Hepatitis B, C	

Note: HLA, human leukocyte antigen; IgG, immunoglobulin G; IgM, immunoglobulin M; INR, international normalized ratio; MR, magnetic resonance; MRI, magnetic resonance imaging; PT, prothrombin time; PTT, partial thromboplastin time.

be resected and the potential sites of GI reconstruction are included. Risk of immune complications is determined via measurement of panel of reactive antibodies (PRA) and human leukocyte antigen (HLA) typing. Highly sensitized candidates (e.g., multiparous women, retransplant candidates, or recipients of multiple blood products) may require desensitization prior to acceptance. Once deemed a suitable ITx candidate, patients are listed with UNOS as a function of urgency: status 1, urgent; status 2, nonurgent; or status 7, temporarily inactive. Separate listing according to the Model for End Stage Liver Disease (MELD, adult) or Pediatric End Stage Liver Disease (PELD, pediatric) system is required if concomitant liver transplantation is necessary [32]. If pancreatic transplantation is also required, a third separate listing is initiated.

A comment regarding listing and waiting for liver-inclusive grafts is warranted at this point. Pediatric ITx recipients are allocated according to the liver portion of their grafts based on PELD score. Because the progression of IFALD differs significantly from that of other forms of pediatric liver disease, however, mortality in candidates with IFALD has historically been high relative to non-ITx recipients with equivalent PELD scores [25]. In 2004, a major UNOS allocation policy change occurred allowing multiorgan recipients with IFALD to become more competitive for liver-inclusive grafts. As a result, pediatric ITx candidate wait-list mortality was reduced by 50% in the 4 years after the change [2]. A modification in allocation for adult liver-inclusive grafts was approved in 2013 and has the potential to favorably impact adult wait-list times.

GRAFT SELECTION

Five general graft options are available to ITx candidates. Selection depends upon the integrity of the remnant GI tract and the status of the other viscera. Nomenclature consensus among all centers worldwide has been a challenge; the most common classification system [33] is listed in the following and depicted in Figure 24.2:

1. Isolated intestine graft consisting of all or part of the jejunoileum (Figure 24.2A)
2. Combined liver and intestine graft (Figure 24.2B)

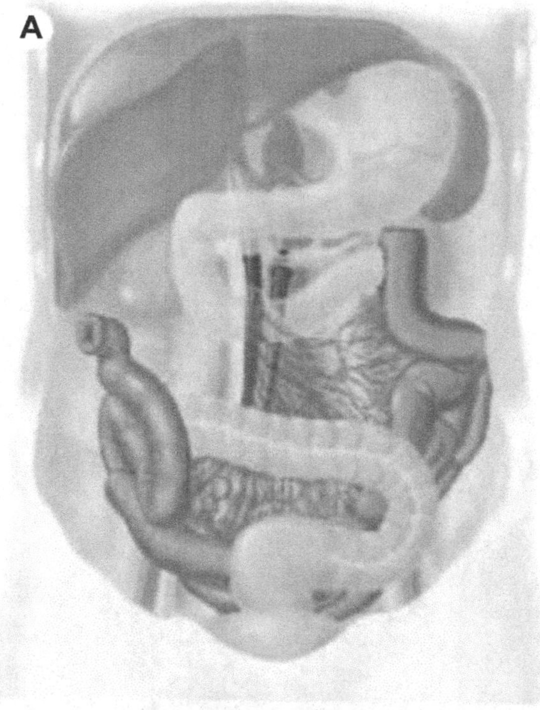

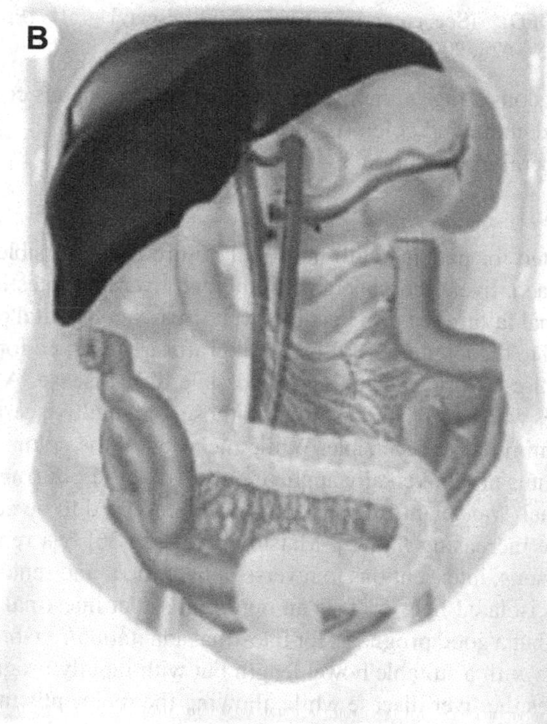

FIGURE 24.2 **(See color insert.)** (A) Isolated intestinal graft. (B) Combined liver–intestinal graft.

(*Continued*)

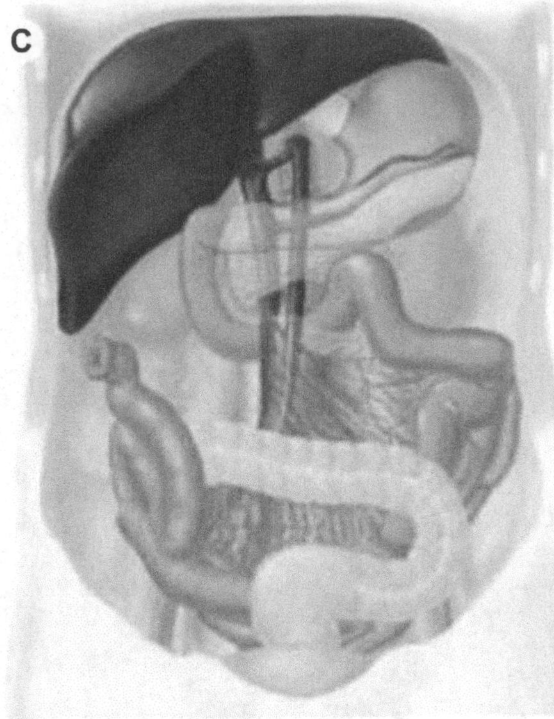

FIGURE 24.2 (CONTINUED) **(See color insert.)** (C) Multivisceral graft. (From Fishbein, T.M. et al. *Gastroenterology*, 124, 1615–1628, 2003. With permission.)

3. Multivisceral graft consisting of the liver, jejunoileum, and various combinations of stomach, pancreas, duodenum, and colon (Figure 24.2C)
4. Modified multivisceral graft (option 3 without the liver)
5. Isolated liver graft

Isolated ITx is indicated for patients with intestinal failure and reversible or no disease in other viscera such as the stomach, liver, and pancreas. Combined liver and intestine grafts are offered to patients who have intestinal failure with irreversible liver disease (congenital or acquired) and without GI tract disease proximal to the jejunum. Multivisceral grafts are reserved for patients with extensive disease involving the entire GI tract, including irreversible liver disease. A modified multivisceral graft is used in candidates who have criteria similar to those for a multivisceral graft except that their liver disease is deemed minimal or reversible. While inclusion of the colon may improve posttransplant fluid management, it is not universally applied; only 20% of ITx during the most recent reporting period of the Intestinal Transplant Registry (ITR) were reported to be colon-inclusive, although this number seems to be increasing [34,35]. Matsumoto et al. [36] has reported that this strategy results in fewer readmissions, interventions to reverse dehydration, and renal complications.

Finally, the use of an isolated liver graft is an option in select intestinal failure candidates with irreversible liver disease but a good prognosis for intestinal adaptation/rehabilitation. This scenario is most common in patients with a suitable bowel length but with rapidly progressive IFALD. Isolated liver transplantation cures the liver disease while allowing the recipient's intestine time to enhance adaptation and wean from PN support. Appropriate candidate selection is critical; isolated liver transplantation in a patient with intestinal failure in whom adaptation does not occur and the need for PN persists carries a poor prognosis [14]. A list of causes of intestinal failure currently leading to ITx in children and adults, together with the frequency of graft types employed, is shown in Figure 24.3.

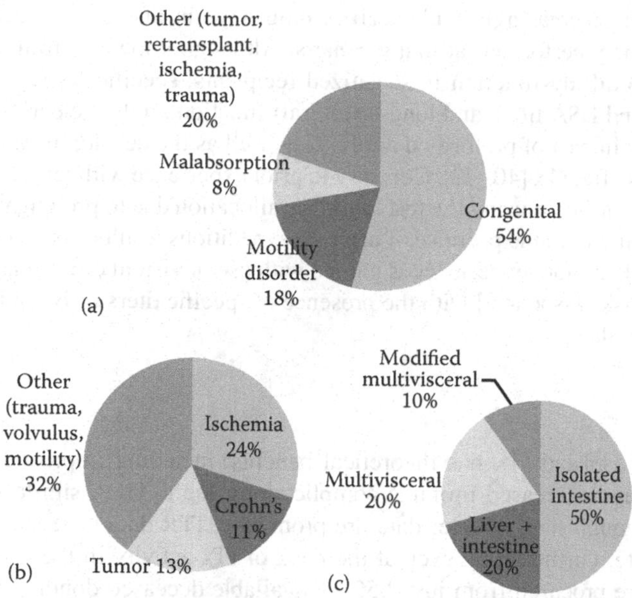

FIGURE 24.3 (a) Indications for pediatric intestinal transplant reported to the Intestinal Transplant Registry (2013). (b) Indications for adult intestinal transplant reported to the Intestinal Transplant Registry (2013). (c) Frequency of type of intestinal graft used worldwide as reported to the Intestinal Transplant Registry (2010). (From Intestinal Transplant Registry, available at http://www.intestinaltransplants.org. With permission.)

DONOR SELECTION

Deceased Donors

The standard selection criteria for deceased donor solid organ grafts, including the absence of recent systemic viral, bacterial, or fungal infection or malignancy, also apply to the ITx donor. Additional considerations are size, circumstances surrounding donor death, and cytomegalovirus (CMV) status. The majority of ITx candidates have had multiple abdominal and pelvic surgeries, loss of bowel length, and adhesive disease resulting in loss of abdominal domain needed to accommodate organs from a donor of similar age and size. To circumvent this, targeting a donor:recipient weight ratio of 0.70 or 0.75:1 is optimal. Furthermore, because of the sensitivity of allograft mucosa to ischemia, donor mechanism of death, including periods of asystole with prolonged resuscitative efforts and the use of high-dose vasopressors that shunt blood from the bowel, should be critically evaluated. For this reason, the rate of ITx has not benefitted from the increased utilization of non-heart-beating donors seen with other solid organ transplants [37]. Similarly, geographic location of the donor can be a limiting factor due to increased cold ischemia time (CIT). Prolonging the CIT beyond the optimal window of 8–12 hours generally results in graft mucosal permanent storage and ischemia-reperfusion injury with initial villous blunting, crypt loss, epithelial detachment, and graft nonfunction [38]. Some ITx clinicians discourage the use of CMV-positive donors due to a higher risk of CMV reactivation and resistant viremia with graft loss [39]. Historically, this may have been a result of powerful immune-depleting induction therapies and is likely less relevant with contemporary immunosuppression. Furthermore, donor availability can be significantly impaired with this policy, particularly for infants who are likely to be seronegative.

Regarding immune risks, the donor and recipient should be blood group identical/compatible to avoid hyperacute (a type of antibody-mediated) rejection. The significance of HLA-preformed antibodies is becoming increasingly evident. HLA antigen typing and donor-specific antibody (DSA) testing is now routinely performed at many centers. Although known to translate to an increased likelihood of early graft dysfunction in sensitized recipients, specifics regarding the interplay of elevated non-DSA and DSA titers and long-term graft function are less clear. Several studies demonstrate the negative impact of preformed antibody as well as the development of *de novo* antibody on clinical outcomes after ITx [40–42]. Contrary to prior experience with lengthy cross-match times (precluding practical utility in using the test for donor allocation due to prolongation of CIT), virtual cross-match techniques have the promise of offering expeditious results. As shown in a small cohort of ITx recipients [43], as more experience is gained with use of virtual cross-match for organ allocation, the long-term risks associated with the presence of specific titers of B- and T-cell alloantibodies can be better elucidated.

Live Donors

Living donation for isolated ITx has theoretical benefits, including improved graft function due to minimized CIT and decreased immune complications due to HLA similarity of living related donors [44,45]. Although single-center data are promising, ITR data have shown no difference in graft survival to date. Furthermore, even at the peak of ITx activity in the United States in 2007, intestinal grafts were procured from just 2.5% of available deceased donors [2]. Thus, there is no shortage of high-quality intestinal donors compelling use of live-donor intestinal grafts. Living intestinal donation does not fill an unmet gap seen with other organ shortages.

While reports from a single-center practice of donor follow-up do not suggest life-threatening donor morbidity [45], there remain concerns of increased risk of perioperative medical sequelae and significant complications, including wound infection, hernia, adhesive small bowel obstruction, and the potential impairment of long-term GI function that must be considered in the risk–benefit analysis of living intestinal donation.

OPERATIVE PROCEDURES

All multivisceral procurement techniques represent modifications of original descriptions by Starzl and colleagues [46]. Subsequent modifications have been published by Grant [12], Starzl [47], Bueno [48], and Abu-Elmagd [49] and their colleagues. Common to all techniques is that procurement of thoracic and renal organs is not precluded and that minor modifications enable procurement of all visceral grafts described herein. The general principles as outlined in a previous report [50] include use of a midline incision, obtaining vascular control of the donor supraceliac and infrarenal aorta, mobilization of the target graft organ or organs, and coordinated donor perfusion (Figure 24.4).

Isolated Intestine

For the isolated intestine graft, either the superior mesenteric artery or the infrarenal aorta supplies recipient arterial inflow, while the IVC, superior mesenteric vein, and portal vein are options for venous outflow of the graft. GI continuity is reestablished proximally by anastomosis of native (recipient) to donor jejunum, while distally, the donor bowel is brought out as an ileostomy, with or without a distal anastomosis to the native colon. The ostomy creation allows for precise measurement of stool volume and ease of endoscopic graft surveillance.

Liver–Intestine

For the recipient of a liver–intestinal allograft, neither hilar dissection nor biliary reconstruction is required, and native portocaval shunting has been utilized for foregut decompression, with good results. Importantly, dissection and removal of diseased remnant gut occur after graft reperfusion.

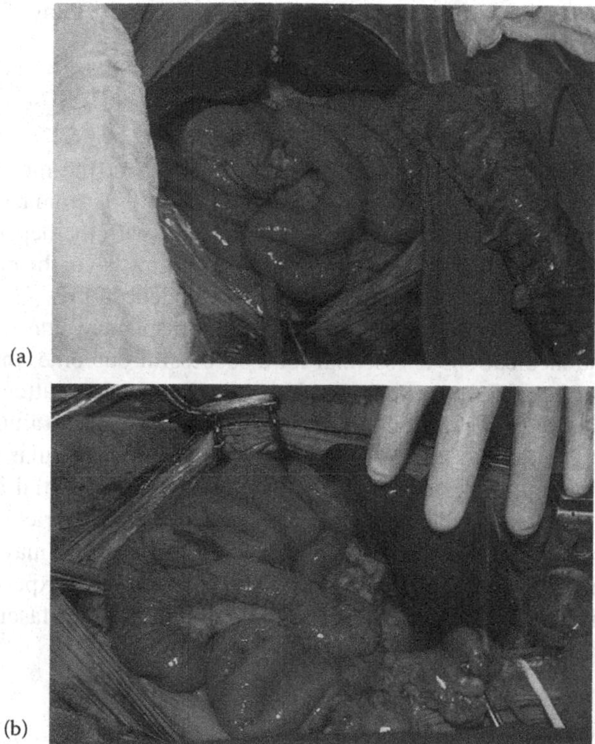

FIGURE 24.4 Operative approach to a multivisceral donor. (a) The round and falciform ligaments were divided and the liver was completely mobilized. In addition, the left colon has been mobilized to the splenic flexure, the terminal ileum has been stapled (lower left corner), and the aortic cannula has been positioned. (b) The aortic cannula is in position with the supraceliac aorta encircled with umbilical tape (lower right). The donor is prepared for systemic heparinization, cross-clamping, and organ perfusion. (From Yersiz, H. et al. *Liver Transpl.*, 9, 881, 2003. With permission.)

We use this technique to avoid extensive dissection before native hepatectomy in the presence of portal hypertension and coagulopathy and have been able to successfully stage the liver–intestine operation in challenging cases. The abdomen is packed and closed after graft implantation, completion of vascular anastomoses, and drainage of the distal bowel. The patient is then resuscitated in the intensive care unit, returning for completion native enterectomy and graft-to-native intestinal anastomosis after stabilization [51]. Regardless of the graft used, ITx recipients require dissection of diseased bowel with restoration of intestinal continuity as described above.

Multivisceral

For recipients of a multivisceral graft, the entire native viscera, including the liver, requires resection prior to implantation. Usually, the stomach and left colon are divided to leave a viable perfused remnant. The entire small and large bowel as well as the pancreatico-duodeno-splenic complex is mobilized off the retroperitoneum. The liver is then mobilized off the retroperitoneum and IVC. Then, the superior mesenteric artery (SMA), celiac trunk, infrahepatic IVC, and suprahepatic IVC are clamped. The native viscera are removed. The donor *en bloc* allograft consisting of the stomach (optional), duodenum, pancreas, liver, jejunoileum, and colon (optional) is then implanted. Arterial inflow is established directly off the aorta, while venous outflow is via the suprahepatic IVC. Proximal GI continuity is restored with either a gastrogastrostomy or a Roux-en-Y gastrojejunostomy. Distal continuity is restored when possible with a colocolostomy or ileocolostomy. The routine use of stomas is applied for graft monitoring in most centers.

Modified Multivisceral

The modified multivisceral graft proceeds exactly as described for the multivisceral graft except that the native liver is retained and the allograft consists of an *en bloc* stomach (optional), pancreas, duodenum, jejunoileum, and colon (optional). The celiac trunk with the hepatic artery is spared to maintain blood supply to the native liver. Allograft venous outflow is via the portal vein, and biliary reconstruction is usually accomplished with a choledochoduodenostomy.

In all types of ITx operations described, access to the transplanted intestine for administration of enteral nutrition and medications is essential for a successful outcome; thus, the final phase of the operation consists of establishment of enteral access. Furthermore, attention to the closure of the abdominal cavity is necessary as compression due to spatial constraints resulting from loss of abdominal domain can lead to ischemic allograft necrosis and vascular thrombosis and is to be avoided. Splenectomy, split-liver donor grafts, liver resection, or partial allograft enterectomy are strategies that have been advocated, particularly in small pediatric patients. Synthetic or bioprosthetic-assisted or skin-only closures with delayed reconstruction may also need to be considered. The Miami and Indiana transplant groups have reported their experience with a series of patients with transplantation of same-donor abdominal wall [52] or rectus fascia with intestinal graft in combination with ITx [53], respectively, with excellent results.

POSTOPERATIVE MANAGEMENT

Early Medical and Nutritional Care

ITx recipients are monitored in the intensive care unit, where serial assessment of volume status, GI losses, renal function, and indicators of graft perfusion, including serial serum lactate, chemistry panels, liver function studies, and arterial blood gas analysis, can be performed via invasive lines for the first several days postoperatively. Recipient hemodynamic assessment can be complicated by the unpredictable timing of volume shifts resulting from resolution of graft edema. Anticoagulation is a critical component of early postoperative care as predisposition to thrombosis is compounded by hemoconcentration with volume shifts. Agents such as prostaglandin, dopamine, dextran, and low-dose heparin are used at our center to promote splanchnic perfusion and prevent thrombosis. It is anticipated that the patient will require PN until the absorptive capacity of the intestinal graft is demonstrated; enteral feedings are usually held for the first several days to weeks after transplantation depending on the type of allograft, technical issues, and the graft condition. Our center defaults to an intraoperative surgical approach to enteral access. This is particularly important in children with oral aversions as the administration of adequate enteral nutrients can be a challenge. Standard gastrostomy tubes can be used in patients with normal gastric motility pretransplant; however, in those with short bowel syndrome and poor gastric emptying, jejunal enteral access is required. In these cases, we place a combination gastrojejunostomy tube. An optimal enteral formula for use after ITx has not been determined; the formula used tends to be center specific.

Immunosuppression

Graft and patient survival rates have improved as immunosuppression has become more potent and specific. Although maintenance protocols vary, >70% of recipients as recently as 2012 received an induction agent for the purpose of T-lymphocyte depletion to encourage microchimerism and tolerance [34]. Drugs/strategies used to achieve induction have included antithymocyte globulin [54], altemtuzumab (off-label) [55] infusion of donor bone marrow-derived cells [56], and interleukin-2 receptor blockade [57,58]. Tacrolimus is the most common agent used as maintenance therapy. Our protocol consists of induction with an interleukin-2 receptor antagonist such as daclizumab (Zenepax, Roche Laboratories, Nutley, New Jersey; off-label use; no longer commercially available) or basiliximab (Simulect, Novartis Pharmaceuticals, East Hanover, New Jersey; off-label use) administered both preoperatively and postoperatively, followed by initiation of enterally administered maintenance tacrolimus within 24 hours of ITx. We also introduce secondary and tertiary immunosuppression consisting of an intravenous steroid pulse and taper and mycophenolic acid (CellCept, Roche Laboratories; off-label use). Enteric conversion is started after allograft absorptive capacity has been demonstrated. With this regimen, we have observed a marked increase in patient and graft survival along with a decrease in rejection and infection when compared with a T-cell depleting induction regimen [58]. In cases of tacrolimus intolerance and/or increased risk of rejection, we have demonstrated graft salvage in a subset of both adults and children who have converted to mammalian target of rapamycin inhibitors (mTORi) (Rapamune, Wyeth or Zortress, Novartis; both off-label use) rescue therapy [59].

Intermediate and long-term immunosuppressive goals include steroid weaning and a reduction in trough serum levels of tacrolimus to avoid cumulative morbidity. In addition to the universal risk for infection with immunosuppression, the well-known adverse effects of prolonged steroid use such as osteoporosis, adrenal insufficiency, peptic ulcer disease, psychosis, cataracts, growth failure in children, and glucose intolerance are augmented by the toxicities associated with other immunosuppressants used in ITx. For tacrolimus, neurotoxicity, nephrotoxicity, glucose intolerance, and hypertension predominate. With mycophenolic acid, bone marrow depression, mucosal ulcerations, and GI disturbances are problematic. The use of mTORi can result in bone marrow depression, nephrotic syndrome, stomatitis, pneumonitis, and dyslipidemia. Weaning of immunosuppression to avoid these complications must be tempered by the long-term risk for acute and chronic rejection, both significant problems after ITx.

COMPLICATIONS

Rejection

After sepsis, acute cellular rejection is the second most common cause of death after ITx. The Scientific Registry of Transplant Recipients (SRTR) reports that 40% of ITx recipients are diagnosed with acute rejection in the first year [2]; this subset has a 50% risk of mortality [60]. Rejection is also the primary reason for graft loss [34], in part because the diagnosis may be delayed when relying upon nonspecific clinical signs and symptoms. Symptoms often include fever, high-output GI losses, abdominal pain, and hematochezia; rarely, obstructive GI symptoms predominate. Serum or stool levels of intestinal fatty acid binding protein [61], citrulline [62], calprotectin [63] and granzyme B [64] have been championed as markers of rejection; however, due to a lack of specificity, none is currently considered of clinical utility. A high index of suspicion is therefore necessary to diagnose rejection early to initiate early treatment and preserve the health of the graft. Endoscopy with intestinal graft biopsy is the gold standard for the early detection of acute rejection after ITx. Endoscopic features of acute rejection include edema, hyperemia, mucosal granularity, loss of fine mucosal vascular pattern, diminished peristalsis, and mucosal ulceration. Histologic features include mononuclear infiltration, crypt injury with nuclear enlargement and hyperchromasia, decreased cell height, mucin depletion, crypt apoptosis, and distortion of villus and crypt architecture (Figure 24.5). Zoom video endoscopy has been reported to allow improved mucosal visualization [65]; however, widespread clinical application has not yet been achieved.

Given the low sensitivity of clinical indicators and the risk for graft loss with untreated rejection, surveillance endoscopy in the early post-ITx period is a common practice. The frequency with which surveillance endoscopy is performed tends to be center specific. Most initiate surveillance endoscopy within 1 to 2 weeks after ITx and continue at least weekly for the first 6 to 8 weeks. In addition, when clinical signs and symptoms suspicious for rejection are noted, diagnostic endoscopy and biopsy are immediately performed, regardless of timing.

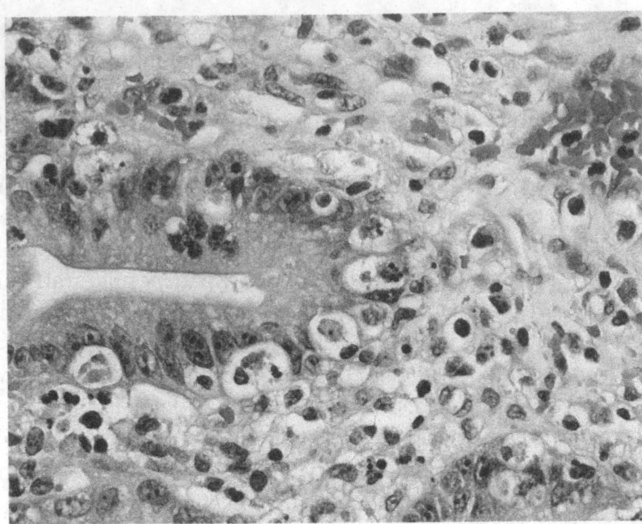

FIGURE 24.5 Histologic features of intestinal allograft acute cellular rejection, including crypt distortion with apoptosis and an extensive inflammatory infiltrate.

Although the mechanism is not well delineated, several reports have observed that recipients of liver-inclusive intestinal grafts experience fewer episodes of acute rejection and a more favorable profile of graft survival in the first 3 years [2,34]. This phenomenon is perhaps explained by the presence and persistence of passenger donor leukocytes in the host peripheral blood, also known as microchimerism [66]. It is unclear as to how the presence of the liver facilitates the favorable balance of tolerogenic to immunogenic lymphocytes. Others have proposed that, much like the kidney in the combined heart/kidney recipient with a decreased risk of rejection, the liver serves as a "sink," either for antigens or for lymphocytotoxic antibodies, mitigating the expected immunoreactivity of the lymphoid-rich intestinal graft [67]. More studies are required to clarify these observations. When rejection does occur in liver-inclusive grafts, the liver portion of the composite graft is usually late to reject, and therefore, the use of liver enzymes to signal rejection proves unreliable.

Treatment of acute rejection is based on clinical and histologic severity. Severe episodes warrant monoclonal antilymphocytic antibody therapy and carry a high risk of graft loss. Antilymphocyte therapies carry a cumulative risk for posttransplant lymphoproliferative disorder (PTLD) and CMV disease and require concomitant empiric antiviral therapy. In contrast, mild to moderate rejection episodes can be treated with increased maintenance immunosuppression and/or a steroid pulse and taper regimen. In patients refractory to increased immunotherapy, it is critical to proceed swiftly to enterectomy and cessation of immunosuppression to avoid sepsis and death. In the case of refractory rejection, a distinct disadvantage of the combined liver–intestine graft is that the entire bloc of donor organs must be resected, necessitating immediate retransplantation. For this reason, some centers advocate a technique of individual implantation of liver and bowel at the time of ITx [68].

Late or chronic graft dysfunction, likely underdetected and underreported, is thought to be immune mediated. Clinically, worsening malabsorption and GI losses are often seen, and radiologically, loss of fine mucosal patterns and mucosal thickening may be noted. Prior episodes of acute rejection are not reliable predictors of chronic graft dysfunction. If DSAs are elevated, the clinical picture is thought to be consistent with antibody-mediated rejection. Although histology often demonstrates microangiopathy, necrosis, and chronic vasculopathy, classic histologic C4d complement staining is not consistently seen. A variety of B-lymphocyte and plasma cell-targeted therapies have been utilized with some success to deplete important effector cells. These include humanized anti-CD20 monoclonal antibody (rituximab), intravenous immunoglobulin, plasmapheresis, and eculizumab [69,70]. Highly sensitized patients may receive targeted desensitization therapy before or immediately after ITx to mitigate graft damage.

Infection

ITx recipients are often the most heavily immunosuppressed solid organ transplant recipients. It is not surprising, therefore, that infection is the primary cause of mortality after ITx [34]. The necessity of a long, complex abdominal procedure renders these patients susceptible to bacterial translocation with intra-abdominal and blood-borne sepsis. Other common sources of infection are catheter related and pulmonary based. Extubation and removal of central venous catheters as early as permissible post-ITx are critical to reduce the incidence of infections. Aggressive monitoring, evaluation, and treatment must be undertaken when clinical signs of infection arise, as they may be subtle. The most critical infections unique to this population are the infectious enteritides such as adenovirus and rotavirus, *Cryptosporidium*, *Giardia lamblia*, and *Clostridium difficile*. These infections can mimic rejection and are often incorrectly treated as such [71]. They can also precipitate a subsequent rejection episode and graft loss.

CMV and Epstein-Barr virus (EBV) present unique problems after ITx. Rates of viremia have been documented to range from 11% to 40% [72], rates much higher than those seen in any other solid organ population. Both viruses can directly infect the bowel and represent a major source of morbidity and mortality. Several protocols exist to control viral replication after ITx. We utilize a standard prophylaxis protocol consisting of intravenous ganciclovir for the first 100 days post-ITx, followed by conversion to oral valganciclovir. Because of the high rate of CMV relapse and its associated increase in post-ITx mortality [73], we use a preemptive monitoring and therapeutic protocol consisting of frequent plasma polymerase chain reaction testing for EBV and CMV. CMV or EBV detection prompts preemptive therapy that includes intravenous ganciclovir or CMV immune globulin (or both). With this protocol, we have significantly reduced the incidence of CMV and EBV viremia, infection, and tissue invasion after ITx [71].

Posttransplant Lymphoproliferative Disorder

PTLD is a lymphocytic malignancy frequently caused by EBV infection that typically occurs in the setting of intensive immunosuppression. The spectrum of disease ranges from B-cell predominant lymphoid hyperplasia to aggressive, non-EBV, monotypic lymphomas; prognosis varies by histopathological type. The overall cumulative incidence at 5 years in the most recent ITx cohort reported by SRTR (2006–2010) was 9% [2]. The pediatric seronegative population is most at risk. ITR data reveal that PTLD is the cause of graft loss in 1.6% and patient death in 6.1% of pediatric ITx recipients [34]. Prompt diagnosis and treatment are imperative to improve outcomes. Once suspected, a thorough evaluation to include physical examination with attention to lymph nodes should be performed. Adenopathy on chest and abdominal cross-sectional imaging should be evaluated by biopsy. Once diagnosed, positron emission tomography–CT scan, bone marrow biopsy, and lumbar puncture are employed for staging. Treatment regimens consist of ganciclovir, CMV immune globulin, and paradoxically, a reduction in immunosuppression. Rituximab and chemotherapy are also options depending upon monomorphic or polymorphic populations on immunohistochemistry.

Renal Impairment

Although not unique to ITx, renal dysfunction in the post-ITx recipient has been shown both in single-center and registry analyses to carry a significantly greater risk of mortality when compared with ITx recipients with normal renal function [74]. The mortality associated with renal dysfunction after ITx is also higher compared with other solid organ recipients [75]. Accurate pretransplant assessment of renal function to gauge the need for including renal grafts in the bloc of transplanted organs and postoperative immunosuppressive regimens modified to spare renal injury are two strategies utilized to minimize this effect.

OUTCOMES

Several data sources are available to evaluate ITx outcomes. Large, single-center U.S. series have been reported from the Universities of Pittsburgh, Miami, Nebraska, California (Los Angeles), and Indiana, as well as the transplant programs at Georgetown and Mount Sinai. Additionally, pooled center data are available from two sources. The ITR is a worldwide, voluntary registry that is believed to contain data regarding all human ITx. From this standpoint, it is a unique data source. Additionally, mandatory data from U.S. centers through UNOS are made available in the SRTR Annual Report. Outcome data mentioned will reflect these major sources.

As previously noted, outcomes after ITx are dependent upon the era of immunosuppression. From the ITR, overall 1-year patient and graft survival rates in the most recent era now exceed 75% in select recipients (Figure 24.6) [34]. Further observations include differential prognoses based upon the type of ITx and type of induction therapy used (Figure 24.7) [34]. In addition to the usual benchmarks of graft and patient survival, it is important to note secondary post-ITx outcomes such as enteral autonomy and quality of life (QOL). Recent data demonstrate that ITx is associated with a 90% rate of enteral autonomy [61] and improved QOL in some, but not all, spheres as measured by the Child Health Questionnaire and the Pediatric QOL 4.0 (pediatric) [76,77] and short form-36 (SF-36) (adult) [78] validated survey instruments.

Long-term ITx data reveal decreased 3- and 5-year patient and graft survival for isolated intestine grafts compared with other solid organ transplants and for intestinal grafts that are transplanted in combination with a liver graft [2]. Although patient loss due to sepsis is the primary reason, this decrease in survival is also a direct result of immune-related graft loss or chronic rejection [2].

COST

Few studies have accurately enumerated the cost of ITx versus long-term home PN. While transplant-associated costs including the first year of care were reported to exceed US$1 million a decade ago, consideration of the long-term cumulative cost of PN (including that of associated

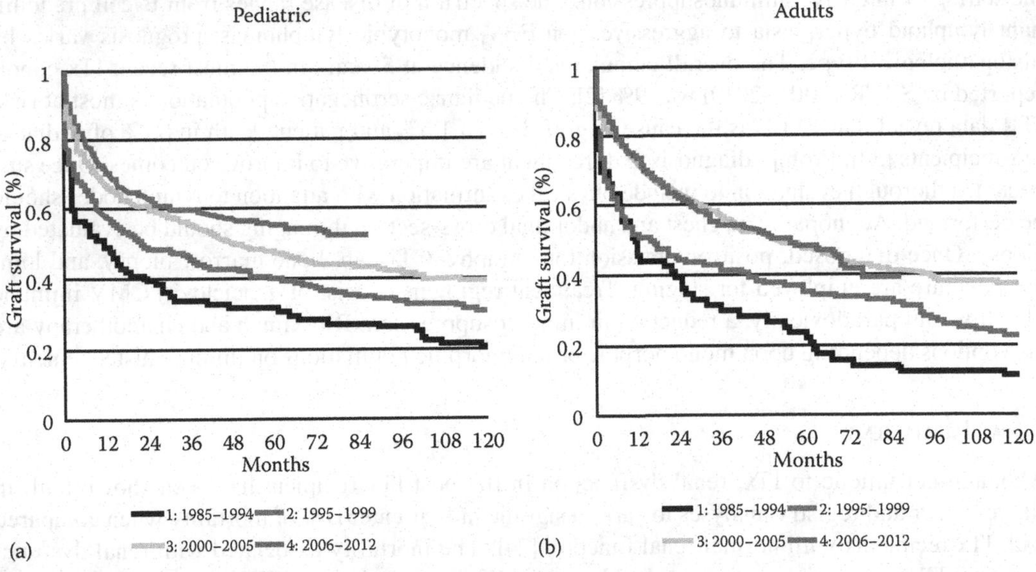

FIGURE 24.6 **(See color insert.)** (a) Pediatric and (b) adult survival after intestinal transplantation by era. (From Intestinal Transplant Registry, available at http://www.intestinaltransplants.org. With permission.)

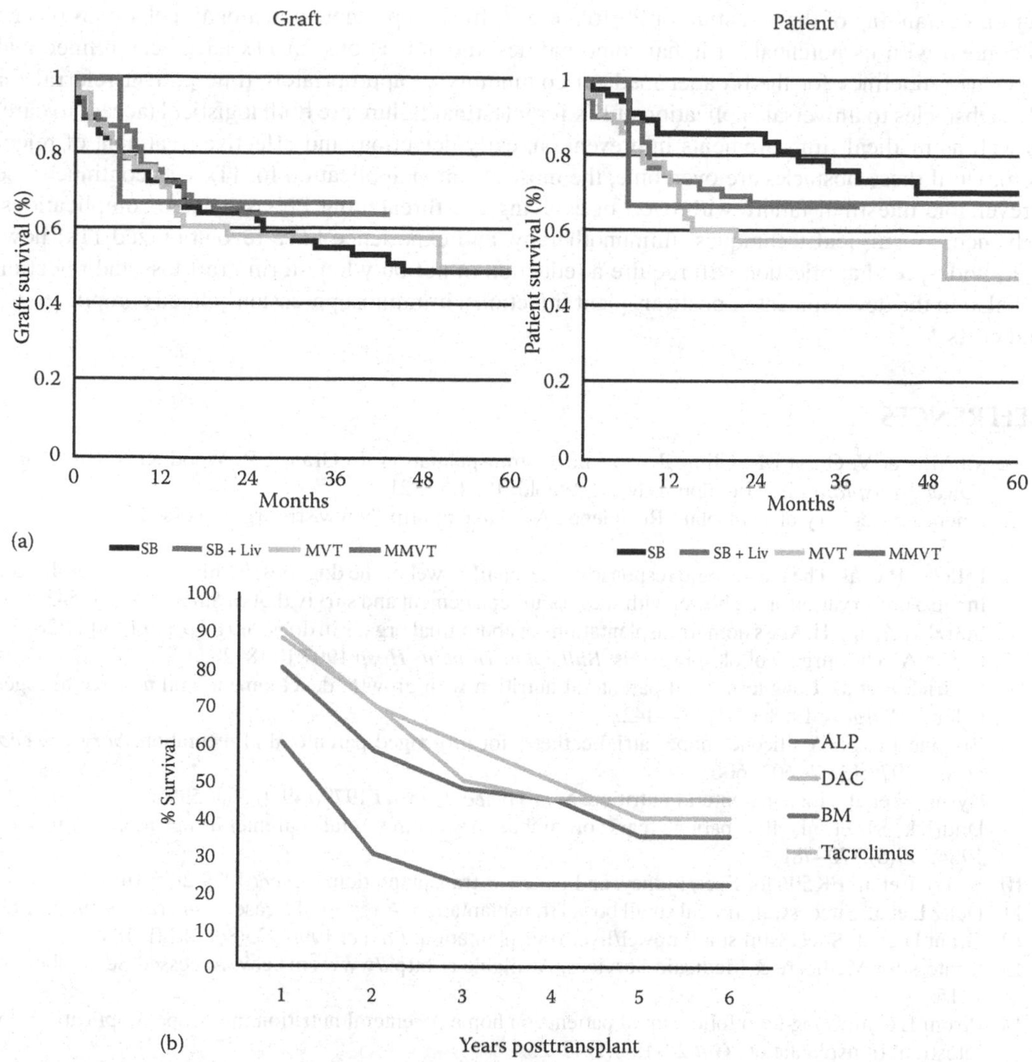

FIGURE 24.7 (See color insert.) (a) Graft survival after intestinal transplantation by graft type (2008–2012). (b) Graft survival by induction agent. ALP, antilymphocyte product; BM, bone marrow; DAC, dacluzimab. (From Intestinal Transplant Registry, available at http://www.intestinaltransplants.org. With permission.)

care and potential morbidities) suggested, at that time, that a cost breakeven point would occur well within the expected range of graft survival, making ITx the more cost-effective option [79]. The unquantifiable costs on both sides of the equation such as lost productivity, the impact of chronic infusions on quality of life, sleep quality, and socialization are impossible to include in these calculations.

CONCLUSION

The field of ITx has changed dramatically since the experimental eras of the 1950s to 1970s. At present, ITx is performed at a limited number of specialized transplant centers worldwide and ITx recipients are enjoying unprecedented successful patient and graft survival not previously seen. As our understanding of the potential for PN to preserve life and promote nutritional repletion is placed in context with its potential for lethal comorbidities, the indications for ITx have been refined and serve as guidelines for the broader medical community to appropriately time patient referral for ITx. Obstacles to universal application of ITx for intestinal failure are both logistical (access to care) as well as medical (improvements in prevention, early detection, and effective treatment of rejection). Until these obstacles are overcome, the most common application for ITx will continue to be irreversible intestinal failure with overt or evolving life-threatening PN-associated complications. Advances in surgical techniques, immunotherapy, and experience have revolutionized ITx; however, widespread application will require a reduction in not only long-term graft loss and rejection but also in the development of posttransplant infections, immunosuppression-related complications, and costs.

REFERENCES

1. McAllister V, Grant DR. Clinical small bowel transplantation. In Grant DR, Wood RFM (eds) *Small Bowel Transplantation*. London, Edward Arnold, 1994, p. 121.
2. Scientific Registry of Transplant Recipients. Available at http://www.srtr.org. Accessed September 20, 2015.
3. Lillehei R et al. The physiologic response of the small bowel of the dog to ischemia including prolonged in vitro preservation of the bowel with successful replacement and survival. *Ann Surg* 1959;150:543–559.
4. Starzl T, Kaupp H. Mass homotransplantations of abdominal organs in dogs. *Surg Forum* 1960;11:28–30.
5. Carrel A. The surgery of blood vessels. *Bull Johns Hopkins Hosp* 1907;18:18–28.
6. Dudrick S et al. Long-term total parenteral nutrition with growth, development, and positive nitrogen balance. *Surgery* 1968: 64(1):134–142.
7. Broviac J et al. A silicone rubber atrial catheter for prolonged parenteral alimentation. *Surg Gynecol Obstet* 1973;136(4):602–606.
8. Byrne W et al. Home parenteral nutrition. *Surg Gynecol Obstet* 1979;149(4):593–599.
9. Dudrick SJ et al. 100 patient-years of ambulatory home total parenteral nutrition. *Ann Surg* 1984;199(6):770–781.
10. Starzl T et al. FK506 for liver, kidney, and pancreas transplantation. *Lancet* 1989;2(8670):1000–1004.
11. Deltz E et al. Successful clinical small bowel transplantation: A report of a case. *Clin Transpl* 1989;21:89.
12. Grant D et al. Successful small bowel/liver transplantation. *Lancet* 1990;335(8683):181–184.
13. Centers for Medicare & Medicaid Services. Available at http://www.cms.gov. Accessed September 20, 2015.
14. Pironi L et al. Long-term follow up of patients on home parenteral nutrition in Europe: Implications for intestinal transplantation. *Gut* 2011;60(1):17–25.
15. Squires RH et al. Natural history of pediatric intestinal failure: Initial report from the Pediatric Intestinal Failure Consortium. *J Pediatr* 2012;161(4):723–728.
16. Huisman-deWall G et al. The impact of home parenteral nutrition on daily life—A review. *Clin Nutr* 2007;26(3):275–288.
17. Tung Y et al. Clinical improvement following home parenteral nutrition in pediatric patients with intestinal failure. *J Formos Med Assoc* 2006;105(5):399–403.
18. Kaufman SS. Prevention of parenteral nutrition-associated liver disease in children. *Pediatr Transplant* 2002;6(1):37–42.
19. Kelly D. Liver complications of pediatric parenteral nutrition—Epidemiology. *Nutrition* 1998;14(1):153–157.
20. Lauverjat M et al. Chronic dehydration may impair renal function in patients with chronic intestinal failure on long-term parenteral nutrition. *Clin Nutr* 2006;25(1):75–81.
21. Cheung HM et al. Rescue treatment of infants with intestinal nutrition-associated cholestasis (PNAC) using a parenteral fish-oil-based lipid. *Clin Nutr* 2009;28(2):209–212.
22. Greenberg GR et al. Effect of total parenteral nutrition on gut hormone release in humans. *Gastroenterology* 1981;80:988–993.
23. Kubota A et al. Total parenteral nutrition-associated intrahepatic cholestasis in infants: 25 years' experience. *J Pediatr Surg* 2000;35(7):1049–1051.
24. Chang M et al. The use of fish oil lipid emulsion in the treatment of intestinal failure associated liver disease (IFALD). *Nutrients* 2012;4(12):1828–1850.

25. Fryer J et al. Mortality in candidates waiting for combined liver-intestine transplants exceeds that for other candidates waiting for liver transplants. *Liver Transpl* 2003;9(7):748–753.
26. Willis T et al. High rates of mortality and morbidity occur in infants with parenteral nutrition-associated cholestasis. *JPEN J Parenter Enteral Nutr* 2010;34(1):32–37.
27. Bourdaud N et al. Intestinal and pancreatic transplantation: Anesthetic considerations. In Bissonette B (ed) *Considerations in Pediatric Anesthesia*. Shelton, CT: People's Medical Publishing, 2011, pp. 1850–1858.
28. Ardura M et al. Central catheter-associated bloodstream infection reduction with ethanol lock prophylaxis in pediatric intestinal failure: Broadening quality improvement initiatives from hospital to home. *JAMA Pediatr* 2015;169(4):324–331.
29. Corrigan M et al. Hospital readmissions for catheter-related bloodstream infection and use of ethanol lock therapy: Comparison of patients receiving parenteral nutrition or intravenous fluids in the home vs a skilled nursing facility. *JPEN J Parenter Enteral Nutr* 2013;37(1):81–84.
30. Bueno J et al. Factors impacting the survival of children with intestinal failure referred for intestinal transplantation. *J Pediatr Surg* 1999;34(1):27–32.
31. Burghardt K et al. Pediatric intestinal transplant listing criteria—A call for a change in the new era of intestinal failure outcomes. *Am J Transplant* 2015;15(6):1674–1681.
32. McDiarmid SV et al. Principal Investigators and Institutions of the Studies of Pediatric Liver Transplantation (SPLIT) Research Group. Development of a pediatric end-stage liver disease score to predict poor outcome in children awaiting liver transplantation. *Transplantation* 2002;74(2):173–181.
33. Fishbein TM et al. Intestinal transplantation for gut failure. *Gastroenterology* 2003;124(6):1615–1628.
34. Intestinal Transplant Registry. Available at http://www.intestinaltransplants.org. Accessed September 20, 2015.
35. Sudan D. The current state of intestine transplantation: Indications, techniques, outcomes, and challenges. *Am J Transplant* 2014;14(9):1976–1984.
36. Matsumoto CA et al. Inclusion of the colon in intestinal transplantation. *Curr Opin Organ Transplant* 2011;16(3):312–315.
37. Cobianchi L et al. Experimental small bowel transplantation from non-heart-beating donors: A large-animal study. *Transplant Proc* 2009;41(1):55–56.
38. Lopez-Garcia P et al. Histochemical evaluation of organ preservation injury and correlation with cold ischemia time in 13 intestinal grafts. *Transplant Proc* 2014;46:2096–2098.
39. Manez R et al. Incidence and risk factors associated with the development of cytomegalovirus disease after intestinal transplantation. *Transplantation* 1995;59:1010–1014.
40. Abu-Elmagd KM et al. Preformed and *de novo* donor specific antibodies in visceral transplantation: long-term outcome with special reference to the liver. *Am J Transplant* 2012;12(11):3047–3060.
41. Farmer DG et al. Pretransplant predictors of survival after intestinal transplantation: Analysis of a single-center experience of more than 100 transplants. *Transplantation* 2010;90(12):1574–1580.
42. Gerlach UA et al. Clinical relevance of the *de novo* production of anti-HLA antibodies following intestinal and multivisceral transplantation. *Transplant Int* 2014;27(3):280–289.
43. Hawksworth JS et al. Successful Isolated intestinal Transplantation in Sensitized recipients with use of virtual crossmatching. *Am J Transplant* 2012;12:S33–S42.
44. Pollard S. Intestinal transplantation: Living related. *Br Med Bull* 1997;53:868–878.
45. Tesi R et al. Living-related small bowel transplantation. Donor evaluation and outcome. *Transplant Proc* 1997;29:686–687.
46. Starzl T et al. A flexible procedure for multiple cadaveric organ procurement. *Surge Gynecol Obstet* 1984;158:223–230.
47. Starzl T et al. The many faces of multivisceral transplantation. *Surg Gynecol Obstet* 1991;172:335–344.
48. Bueno J et al. Composite liver-small bowel allografts with preservation of donor duodenum and hepatic biliary system in children. *J Pediatr Surg* 2000;35:291–295; discussion 295–296.
49. Abu-Elmagd K et al. Logistics and technique for procurement of intestinal, pancreatic, and hepatic grafts from the same donor. *Ann Surg* 2000;232:680–687.
50. Yersiz H et al. Multivisceral and isolated intestinal procurement techniques. *Liver Transpl* 2003;9:881–886.
51. Renz J et al. Application of combined liver-intestinal transplantation as a staged procedure. *Transplant Proc* 2004;36:314–315.
52. Levi D et al. Transplantation of the abdominal wall. *Lancet* 2003;361:2173–2176.
53. Mangus RS et al. Closure of the abdominal wall with aceullar allograft in intestinal transplantation. *Am J Transplant* 2012;12(Suppl 4):S55–S59.
54. Starzl T et al. Tolerogenic immunosuppression for organ transplantation. *Lancet* 2003;361:1502–1510.

55. Tzakis A et al. Alemtuzumab (Campath 1-H) combined with tacrolimus in intestinal and multivisceral transplantation. *Transplantation* 2001;75:1512–1517.
56. Mathew JM et al. Immune responses and their regulation by donor bone marrow cells in clinical organ transplantation. *Transplant Immunol* 2003;11:307–321.
57. Farmer D et al. Induction therapy with interleukin-2 receptor antagonist after intestinal transplantation is associated with reduced acute cellular rejection and improved renal function. *Transplant Proc* 2004;36:331–332.
58. Sudan D et al. Basiliximab decreases the incidence of acute rejection after intestinal transplantation. *Transplant Proc* 2002;34:940–941.
59. Gordon S et al. Rescue immunotherapy using sirolimus after small bowel transplantation. Presented at the IXth International Small Bowel Transplantation Symposium 2005.
60. Lauro A et al. Mortality after steroid-resistant acute cellular rejection and chronic rejection episodes in adult intestinal transplants: Report from a single center in induction/preconditioning era. *Transplant Proc* 2013;45:2032–2033.
61. Kaufman S et al. Lack of utility of intestinal fatty acid binding protein levels in predicting intestinal allograft rejection. *Transplantation* 2001;71:1058–1060.
62. Gondolesi G et al. Serum citrulline is a potential marker for rejection of intestinal allografts. *Transplant Proc* 2002;34:918–920.
63. Mercer DF et al. Stool calprotectin monitoring after small intestine transplantation. *Transplantation* 2011;91:1166–1171.
64. McDiarmid S et al. Perforin and granzyme B. Cytolytic proteins up-regulated during rejection of rat small intestine allografts. *Transplantation* 1995;69:762–766.
65. Kato T et al. The first case report of the use of a zoom video endoscope for the evaluation of small bowel graft mucosa in a human after intestinal transplantation. *Gastrointest Endosc* 1999;50:257–261.
66. Rana A et al. The combined organ effect: Protection against rejection? *Ann Surg* 2008248:871–879.
67. Narula J et al. Outcomes in recipients of combined heart-kidney transplantation: Multiorgan, same-donor transplant study of the international society of heart and lung transplantation/united network for organ sharing scientific registry. *Transplantation* 1997;63:861–867.
68. Sudan D et al. A new technique for combined liver-intestinal transplantation. *Transplantation* 2001;72:1846–1848.
69. Fan J et al. Eculizamab salvage therapy for antibody-mediated rejection in a desensitization-resistant intestinal retransplant patient. *Am J Transplant* 2015;15:1995–2000.
70. Gondolesi G et al. Pretransplant immunomodulation of highly sensitized small bowel transplant candidates with intravenous immune globulin. *Transplantation* 2006;81(12):1743–1746.
71. Ziring D et al. Infectious enteritis after intestinal transplantation: Incidence, timing, and outcome. *Transplantation* 2005;79:702–709.
72. Florescu DF et al. Opportunistic viral infections in intestinal transplantation. *Expert Rev Anti Infect Ther* 2014;11:367–381.
73. Beath S et al. Risk factors for death and graft loss after small bowel transplantation. *Curr Opin Organ Transplant* 2003;8:195–201.
74. Watson M et al. Renal function impacts outcomes after intestinal transplantation. *Transplantation* 2008;86:117–122.
75. Ojo A et al. Chronic renal failure after transplantation of a nonrenal organ. *N Engl J Med* 2003;349: 931–940.
76. Sudan D et al. Quality of life after pediatric intestinal transplantation: The perception of pediatric recipients and their parents. *Am J Transplant* 2004;4:407–413.
77. Ngo KD et al. Pediatric health-related quality of life after intestinal transplantation. *Pediatr Transplant* 2001;15:849–854.
78. Pironi L et al. Assessment of quality of life on home parenteral nutrition and after intestinal transplantation using treatment-specific questionnaires. *Am J Transplant* 2012;Suppl 4:S60–S66.
79. Sudan D. Cost and quality of life after intestinal transplantation. *Gastroenterology* 2006;130:S158–S162.

25 Home Parenteral Nutrition Initiation, Monitoring, and Weaning

Jithinraj Edakkanambeth Varayil, John K. DiBaise, and Ryan T. Hurt

CONTENTS

KEY POINTS

- Home parenteral nutrition (PN) can be life-saving in patients with short bowel syndrome.
- One of the most important decisions before the initiation of home PN is appropriateness of the candidate.
- Partnering with a home infusion company that provides high-quality care and has nutrition support professionals on staff is essential.
- The choice of central venous catheter depends on the anticipated duration of home PN.
- Close monitoring of patients on home PN can help prevent complications.

INTRODUCTION

Home parenteral nutrition (PN) is often the most critical life-sustaining therapy available for many patients with severe short bowel syndrome (SBS) [1–4]. There are a number of factors that must be considered when deciding who can be safely managed in the home setting, including [5,6]:

- Insurance coverage of PN and nursing support
- Availability of laboratory and other monitoring
- An acceptable home environment
- Social support systems to ensure its safe administration

Importantly, the successful delivery of home PN (HPN) requires partnering with infusion companies that provide 24-hour support, 7 days per week, along with other members of the healthcare team caring for the patient. In addition to the high cost of HPN (estimated at $250,000/year), there are a number of risks associated with it, including catheter-related blood stream infection (CRBSI), intestinal failure-associated liver disease (IFALD), and central venous thrombosis [7–12]. Providing the patient with education about these complications and instituting a plan for the monitoring and reporting if any of these complications is suspected are critical. Furthermore, it is vital to determine the anticipated duration of PN and the eventual plan for weaning of PN. In this chapter, we discuss the initiation, monitoring, and weaning of HPN.

INITIATION OF HPN

Prior to initiating HPN, a number of factors should be considered. The first decision that has to be made is whether or not PN delivery at home is appropriate for the patient. Given the high costs associated with HPN, this decision should be closely followed by a determination of insurance/Medicare coverage. After these issues have been reconciled, the type of central venous catheter (CVC) to use is determined, and proper education and training regarding PN administration and monitoring, usually while still in the hospital, are provided. A determination regarding PN weaning is typically made at a later time based on the degree of gut adaptation, nutrient absorption, and hydration status. The following sections will address these issues further.

Is HPN Appropriate?

Determining whether HPN is appropriate has to be made on an individual basis, taking into consideration the clinical indication/underlying disease, prognosis, and patient goals of care [7,10,11]. Although HPN can be a life-saving therapy, it is expensive and there are potentially life-threatening complications associated with its use. Furthermore, PN does not promote improvements in the adaptive function of the remnant bowel; thus, lifelong dependence on this form of nutrition may be required. Discussions with both the patient and their family regarding their goals and expectations of care should take place prior to central line placement and PN initiation. They should also be informed of the potential effects of HPN on their quality of life, interference with sleep, and the lifelong monitoring required. Furthermore, more than one patient and family have misunderstood that it is they who will be administering the therapy, not the home care nurse. It is important to make it clear that patients and caregivers will be taught how to administer the therapy themselves to liberate them from constant oversight.

Insurance/Medicare Coverage

HPN is a very expensive therapy, and insurance/Medicare coverage should be approved prior to initiation [13]. A high percentage of HPN consumers are Medicare recipients, either because they are older than 65 years or they have medical disability. To be approved for Medicare coverage for HPN in the setting of SBS-intestinal failure, there are number of criteria that need to be met [14] (Figure 25.1), including the need for PN for at least 3 months' duration according to the clinician's best medical judgment, intestinal resection within the prior 3 months leaving <152.4 cm (i.e., 5 ft) residual small intestine from the ligament of Treitz, and use of a PN formula that provides an average daily energy per week of 20–35 kcal/kg actual body weight, 0.8–1.5 g protein/kg actual body weight, and at least 10% dextrose content. Formulas outside these parameters must be documented in the clinical record and explained to Medicare for justification. If the amount of small bowel remaining cannot be determined, or it has been longer than 3 months, then other Medicare criteria need to be met. These include fecal fat testing on the basis of a 72-hour stool collection (patient must malabsorb 50% of fat ingested), documentation of small intestinal dysmotility, or excessive fluid losses. All require clinical documentation. The clinician needs to work closely with coverage specialists at the home infusion companies to ensure approval prior to initiation. Importantly, Medicare does not reimburse for additional parenteral fluids that are occasionally used in patients with SBS. Similarly, while there may be a benefit from a combination of both PN and enteral nutrition (EN) to meet the nutritional needs and minimize the dependence on PN in some SBS patients, Medicare will typically not reimburse for both therapies unless the patient is transitioning off of PN to EN and the "3-month permanence" criterion has been met.

Determining the Duration of HPN

It can be difficult to determine the duration that HPN will be required; however, an anticipated duration of HPN has to be made at the time of initiation of HPN. Insurance companies require HPN providers make this clinical judgment based on their best judgment. The duration of PN is not only important for determining insurance coverage but also plays a role in determining other important HPN-related issues, including the type of CVC to utilize. The estimated duration of HPN may also assist in decisions regarding the eventual weaning of HPN and transitioning to oral or enteral nutrition.

Partnering with the Home Infusion Company

Most medium- and large-size hospitals compound PN for their inpatients but do not provide PN for patients who subsequently are discharged home on PN. While some hospitals have their own infusion companies, most HPN ordering providers will need to partner with commercial/private infusion companies to provide HPN and other home services. An infusion company that provides excellent HPN management will have Medicare and insurance coverage specialists to help verify and investigate HPN coverage during the initiation process. This is an essential first step in approval because if the infusion company does not investigate benefits initially, then the patient will run the risk of incurring the full cost of the PN and associated services ($300–500/day) if the claim is rejected (often months after services are provided).

Inpatient versus Outpatient HPN Initiation and Training

Once HPN has been approved, the decision can be made by the ordering provider, in partnership with the infusion company, about where the PN initiation and training will occur—either the outpatient or inpatient setting. A key factor that should be considered when deciding on location is the risk of refeeding syndrome. In those patients who are felt to be at risk for refeeding syndrome or significant hyperglycemia, arrangements should be made for hospital admission for PN initiation and close monitoring. Although there are limited data on who is most at risk for refeeding, the National Institute for Health and Care Excellence (NICE) guidelines have been proposed [15] (Table 25.1). For those who are determined to be at risk, PN should be initiated at less than the estimated energy needs of the patient while closely monitoring laboratory values for electrolyte shifts (i.e., potassium, magnesium, and phosphorus) and physical examination for evidence of fluid overload and decline

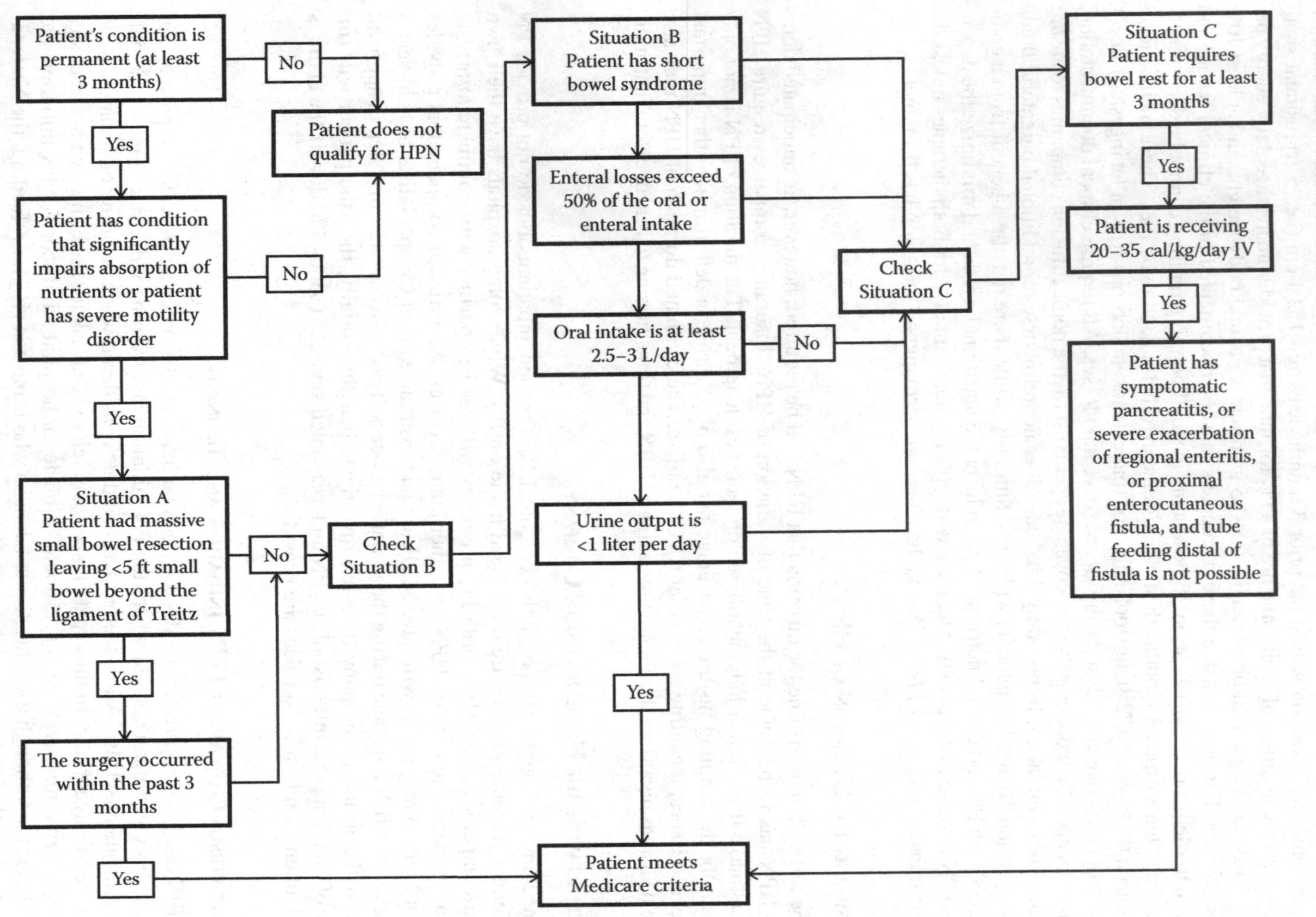

FIGURE 25.1 Medicare criteria for management of HPN in patients with short bowel syndrome (National Coverage Determination [NCD] for Enteral and Parenteral Nutrition, Medicare, http://www.cms.gov/medicare-coverage-database/details/ncd-details.aspx).

TABLE 25.1
NICE Guidelines for Determining the Risk of Refeeding Syndrome in Adult Patients on PN

Refeeding Risk Guidelines
Patient has *one or more* of the following:
• Body mass index less than 16 kg/m^2
• Unintentional weight loss >10% in the last 3–6 months
• Little or no nutritional intake for more than 5 days
• Low levels of potassium, phosphate, magnesium prior to the initiation of feeding
Or…
Patient has *two or more* of the following:
• Body mass index less than 18.5 kg/m^2
• Unintentional weight loss >10% in the last 3–6 months
• Little or no nutritional intake for more than 5 days
• A history of alcohol abuse or drugs including insulin, chemotherapy, antacids, or diuretics

in cardiorespiratory status. Vitamins (especially thiamine) and minerals need to be added when PN starts, if not before. This is particularly important if the patient receives intravenous (IV) fluids with dextrose prior to initiation of PN. The PN formula can then be advanced over the next several days to the goal based upon observed tolerance. Although most patients who receive PN at home had it initiated in the hospital setting, it has been suggested that potential candidates for initiation of PN at home instead of in the hospital include patients who have failed enteral feedings, those who have gastrointestinal diseases without excessive gastrointestinal losses, and those with an oncology diagnosis and inability to tube feed [16]. Of course, this requires close partnership and monitoring by a willing patient, the PN ordering provider, and a home infusion company willing to do a home start-up. If any of these is missing, the patient is best served by being hospitalized for initiating PN.

We prefer that the education portion of the HPN be completed in the hospital setting during the initiation of PN because our multidisciplinary team is available to participate in the education process and the patient can demonstrate the ability to safely and independently deliver/administer PN prior to discharge. In many other centers, however, while the PN is typically initiated in the hospital, the HPN education is done with the help of home care nursing agency after discharge. This is particularly important if the pump used in the hospital will be different than the one used at home. Wherever the education takes place, periodic assessment of patient and/or caregiver knowledge of important elements of HPN delivery and monitoring should be performed.

What Should Patient/Caregiver Education Entail?

The most important part of HPN initiation is the patient and caregiver education required to allow its safe delivery. Many complications of HPN, including infection, can be minimized by proper education of optimal HPN practices. As previously mentioned, at some institutions, the patients receive the training while in the hospital. At others, most of the training is performed after discharge at home. One of the primary goals of educating patients is to assess the ability to administer PN at home safely. Although formal cognitive testing is not generally employed or advocated, an assessment of the physical abilities and mental well-being of all patients and caregivers to administer PN effectively and safely at home is necessary. Patients and/or their caregivers should be required to redemonstrate proper technique and gain approval from their nurse educator(s) before they are allowed to administer PN independently at home. Typical training takes 8 hours divided over 3 or 4 days (Table 25.2 [17]). At least 2 days prior to the patient's anticipated discharge home (and never on a Friday for a weekend discharge), communication should be made with the infusion company to ensure that they are aware of the PN formula and that it will be available when the patient reaches

TABLE 25.2
Preparing the Patient for HPN

Area of Preparation	Items to Cover
Psychosocial assessment	• Physical abilities • Mental well-being
Administration training	• Provide an example of a typical day on HPN • Instructions for hand hygiene • Care of the CVC • Catheter site care—aseptic technique • Changing injection caps • Instilling antibiotic or ethanol locks • Some home infusion companies and institutions will teach patients to use chlorhexidine sponges to cover the catheter insertion site; however, there are no data to support their use with tunneled CVC catheters and we do not recommend their routine use[a] • Monitoring for possible complications • Who to contact with questions or concerns
Detailed instructions on various procedures	• Starting and stopping PN • Adding insulin to PN • Adding vitamins to PN
Obtaining supplies	• Provide education about the supplies they need at home • How to obtain these required supplies • How to contact the home infusion company and the HPN team with any questions

[a] Corrigan, M.L. et al., *JPEN J. Parenter. Enteral Nutr.*, 37, 81–84, 2013.

home. In addition, infusion company representatives, including nursing whenever possible, should meet with the patient prior to discharge to ensure a smooth transition from the hospital to the home setting. Furthermore, it is preferred that the home environment is evaluated prior to the dismissal of patients to ensure a safe environment. A number of factors should be evaluated to ensure a safe home environment, including the use of a designated space for PN initiation, use of a separate refrigerator to store PN, and maintaining adequate hygiene. It is also important to periodically evaluate and review the technique of patients during follow-up visits.

Choice of the CVC

Determining the most appropriate type of CVC to use is an important decision when initiating HPN [18]. This choice is often dependent upon the anticipated duration of HPN. In general, in patients who are anticipated to require HPN for short-term (6–12 weeks), a single-lumen peripherally inserted central catheter is often preferred [19,20]. It is worth noting, however, that this is highly variable among the experts based on the institutional policies and clinical experience. In patients with anticipated requirement of HPN for more than 12 weeks, a single-lumen tunneled catheter or subcutaneously implanted IV access device (i.e., port) is often advised [19]. Advantages of tunneled catheters are ease of self-care, protection from bacterial migration from the skin (due to the cuff), and the possibility for catheter repair. Several studies have reported the linear relation between the incidence of CRBSI and the number of lumens in the CVC [19–21]. Patients may prefer a port because there is a perception of less alteration in body image and less concern for accidental pulling or cutting of the device. The main disadvantage of implanted ports is that they have to be surgically removed if they become infected compared with the simpler procedure to remove a tunneled catheter. In addition, because ports typically need to be accessed weekly with a needle, the port diaphragm deteriorates with time and the number of punctures and will need to be changed periodically.

Cycling of PN

In the hospital setting, PN is typically infused continuously over a 24-hour period for a number of reasons. Habit is one. Another relates to the fluid volume status in hospitalized patients and a desire to avoid fluid overload. A more practical reason is the convenience for the nursing staff not having to start and stop the infusion. When patients are discharged home on PN, it is customary to transition the patient to a cycled infusion over 10–14 hours [22]. This will require an increase in the rate of PN infusion to decrease the infusion time, thus allowing the patient to have more independence from the infusion pump. It is very important at this juncture to ensure that all parenteral fluids are consolidated. For example, the patient who has been receiving 2 L of PN in the hospital with a second IV running at 100 mL/hour to maintain hydration does not want to end up at home with only the 2 L of PN and a readmission shortly after discharge from dehydration. It is also important to recognize that HPN bags hold a maximum of 4 L, so if a patient requires more volume than this, he or she will need parenteral fluid "chasers" during the period when he or she is not infusing PN. Furthermore, mimicking the actual home plan for 2 days prior to discharge to ensure all remains stable is ideal. When patients are switched to a cycled run, all the nutrients will be delivered over that 10- to 14-hour time frame. As such, concern has been raised about exceeding a glucose infusion rate of 5 mg/kg/minute (or 7.2 g/kg); however, it should be noted that this formula came into being in the critical care arena, and there are no data in noncritically ill patients that exceeding this is clinically important.

Importantly, in patients at risk of refeeding syndrome, hyperglycemia, or fluid overload, it is recommended that the PN be cycled prior to discharge home from the hospital [23]. This will allow for continued close monitoring. Cycled HPN is generally infused nocturnally as this allows patients to be disconnected and, potentially, more active during the day. Nocturnal HPN does have its drawbacks, however, including increased interruption of sleep due to increased urination and noise from the infusion pump. As such, some patients prefer to infuse PN during the day. These patients will often benefit from the use of a portable programmable infusion pump that can be carried in a backpack or tote to keep them mobile and independent while they "infuse and cruise."

MONITORING OF HPN

In our experience, most initial HPN mistakes are made within the first 48 hours of returning home. Because of this, both the HPN team and the infusion company should call the patient to ensure the safe transition from the hospital to the home. Because of the importance of detecting mistakes early, it is recommended that only infusion companies that provide 24-hour clinician support to patients should be used. In addition, it is preferred that one of the HPN team members and a physician covering the service after hours are available to help troubleshoot any problems the infusion company clinicians may have.

Laboratory Monitoring

After the patient is discharged from the hospital on a stable HPN formula, routine lab monitoring is recommended. This lab monitoring should include electrolytes, liver enzymes, and micronutrient levels at baseline and weekly, monthly, and then quarterly intervals (Table 25.3). During the first month the patient is at home, we measure electrolytes and liver enzymes weekly. If stable, we decrease the frequency of monitoring to every other week for another month or two. If still stable, monthly lab monitoring is usually appropriate. Due to the recent national shortages of trace elements and vitamins in the United States, we monitor these quarterly after the initial/baseline lab draw. A complete blood count is also typically checked at least quarterly. If the patient is having acute symptoms such as fever and chills suggestive of infection, labs including blood cultures will be drawn outside the regular schedule (Table 25.3). Additionally, if liver function tests become elevated or changes are made to the PN formula, labs will often be obtained outside the regular lab schedule.

TABLE 25.3
Example of Typical Initial Laboratory Monitoring Routine of HPN Patients

Time	Labs Monitored
Initiation	Comprehensive metabolic panel[a]; magnesium, phosphorus; complete blood count with differential; trace element panel[b]; vitamins A, D, and E (prior to PN start so not measuring what is being infused)
Week 1	Basic metabolic panel,[c] magnesium, phosphorus
Week 2	Comprehensive metabolic panel,[a] magnesium, phosphorus, complete blood count
Week 3	Basic metabolic panel,[c] magnesium, phosphorus
Week 4	Comprehensive metabolic panel,[a] magnesium, phosphorus, complete blood count
Week 6	Comprehensive metabolic panel,[a] magnesium, phosphorus, complete blood count
Week 8	Comprehensive metabolic panel,[a] magnesium, phosphorus, complete blood count, trace element panel,[b] and vitamins if previously abnormal and being supplemented

[a] Comprehensive metabolic panel includes sodium, potassium, creatinine, blood urea nitrogen (BUN), bicarbonate, chloride, aspartate aminotransferase (AST), alanine aminotransferase (ALT), total bilirubin, alkaline phosphatase, albumin, calcium, and glucose.

[b] Trace element panel includes zinc, selenium, and copper.

[c] Basic metabolic panel includes sodium, potassium, creatinine, BUN, bicarbonate, chloride and calcium.

Importantly, the time intervals of laboratory monitoring including various electrolyte panels are not based on evidence or guidelines but instead on expert recommendation/clinician experience [21].

Monitoring for CRBSI

CRBSI is one of the most common causes of morbidity and mortality in patients on HPN and is the most common reason for hospital admission in these patients [17,24–26]. A number of risk factors have been implicated in the development of CRBSI, including the catheter type, the number of catheter lumens, HPN education, and quality of follow-up [24]. Signs and symptoms of CRBSI may include fever, lethargy, chills, rigors, and elevated white blood cell count. Liver enzymes often become elevated in the setting of a CRBSI. Other types of catheter infection include an exit site infection, which may present with discharge from the skin at the catheter tunnel exit site, and a tunnel tract infection, which may present with redness and tenderness along the catheter tract. If a bloodstream infection is suspected, blood cultures should be obtained immediately from the catheter and a peripheral vein [20]. Furthermore, a large study conducted at a tertiary care academic medical center found that continuing PN after a positive blood culture was associated with increased hospital stay after adjusting for other comorbidities [27]. Therefore, it has been recommended that PN be temporarily discontinued in the setting of a newly diagnosed CRBSI; the optimal number of days of discontinuation remains uncertain. Broad-spectrum antibiotics should be started empirically if the suspicion of infection is high. The most common causes of CRBSI include coagulase-negative *Staphylococci*, *Staphylococcus aureus*, and *Staphylococcus epidermidis*. Gram-negative and fungal infections are less common; however, because of the need for catheter removal if they are present, fungal cultures should also be obtained as part of the initial cultures. Antibiotics should be adjusted depending on the organism isolated and antibiotic sensitivities. If the patient is stable, the infection can often be treated without removal of the catheter in most cases; pseudomonas and fungal infections will require catheter removal. In cases where catheter salvage is possible, antibiotics should be delivered through the CVC that is thought to be the source (Figure 25.2). If the patient is hemodynamically unstable, the catheter should be removed immediately. A 14-day course of IV antibiotic therapy is recommended in most cases. In some cases, repeat cultures to make sure the infection has been cleared are recommended. Persistently positive blood cultures may indicate an

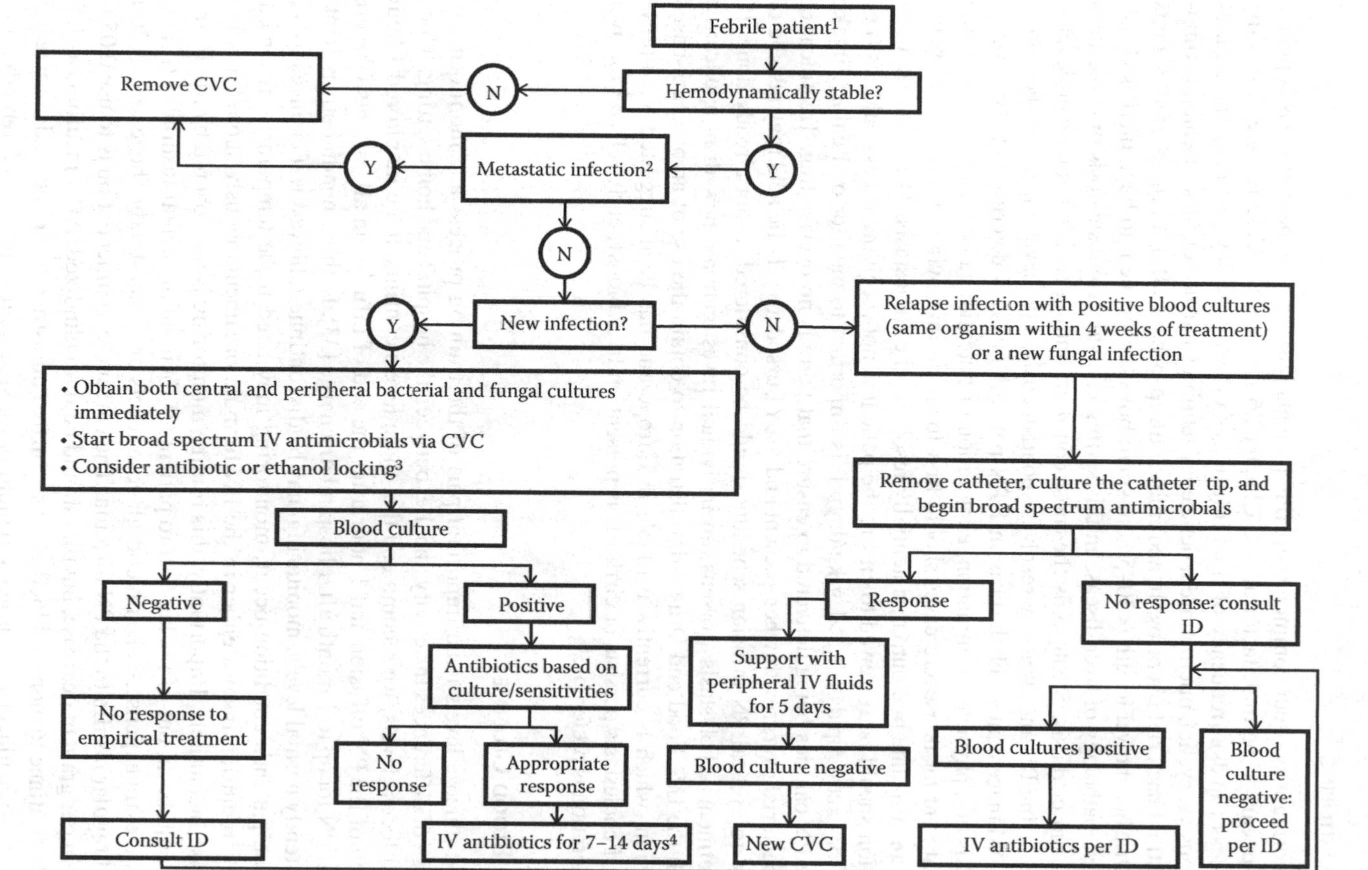

FIGURE 25.2 Catheter salvage guidelines in hemodynamically stable HPN patients. CVC indicates central venous catheter; ID, Department of Infectious Diseases; IV, intravenous; N, no; Y, yes. [1] Temperature >1.0°C or >1.5°F above baseline, shaking chills with infusion, or other symptoms of sepsis. [2] Abscess, infectious endocarditis, or bone or joint infections. [3] Administration of a small amount of antibiotic or 70% ethanol in the catheter lumen while HPN is not being infused. [4] Catheter tunnel or pocket infections generally require CVC removal and treatment with appropriate antimicrobials for full resolution of the infection. (Adapted from Edakkanambeth Varayil, J. et al., *JPEN J. Parent. Enteral Nutr.*, 2015. With permission.)

infected heart valve or thrombus and will require additional testing and consultation with Infectious Diseases specialists. See Chapter 27 for further information regarding CVCs and management of their complications.

Liver Enzyme Monitoring

Liver enzyme abnormalities occur commonly in HPN patients [28–30]. The pathogenesis is poorly understood and appears to be multifactorial (see Chapter 26 for details). Caloric excess, specific macronutrient excess (lipids), frequency of lipid infusions (3 days vs. 7 days a week), duration of infusion (continuous vs. cyclic), micronutrient deficiency (choline, carnitine), lack of enteral stimulation, small intestinal bacterial overgrowth, and infection/sepsis have all been implicated. Infants and those with ultrashort bowel length (<30–50 cm small bowel) also seem to be at increased risk [24,31,32]. The histopathology of liver disease in this setting can vary from steatosis or cholestasis to steatohepatitis and cirrhosis. Steatosis is the most common finding in adults and can develop within weeks of starting PN and typically resolves spontaneously. The development of cholestasis is more ominous. Management of cholestasis in HPN patients involves determining the severity through clinical history, physical examination, exploration of potential causes, and further testing as indicated. Treatment for nonsevere cases should first focus on improving oral or enteral nutrition intake as it can stimulate bile output, potentially resolving the cholestasis. The caloric content of the HPN solution should be reviewed to ensure the patient is not receiving excess calories (i.e., >35 kcal/kg/day) or excess lipids (i.e., >1 g/kg/day). It is important to monitor oral calorie intake in addition to the PN calories being delivered to ensure that there is no overfeeding. Treatment of small intestinal bacterial overgrowth when present and use of ursodeoxycholic acid may also be of benefit. A change to cyclical PN infusion schedule should be considered, if not already done. If, despite these treatments, cholestasis worsens, an individual investigational new drug application can be made with the U.S. Food and Drug Administration to obtain the use of an omega 3-based novel lipid emulsion, which is currently available in Europe and has been suggested to improve IFALD [28–30]. If cholestasis persists or cirrhosis is present on liver biopsy, early referral for liver transplant consideration is preferable.

Monitoring of Blood Glucose

Monitoring blood glucose levels is an important part of the training process and monitoring of HPN [31]. Because of differences in activity and diet between the hospital and home setting, which can affect blood glucose levels, we recommend that these levels continue to be monitored 1 hour after the initiation of the PN infusion and 1 hour after the end of infusion in all patients who are receiving cyclical PN for up to 1 month after hospital discharge [33]. In those nondiabetic patients who show consistently normal levels, monitoring may be discontinued; however, if changes to the PN formula or the patient's condition occur, monitoring may need to be temporarily resumed. Those individuals requiring insulin either in the PN formula or subcutaneously should monitor their blood glucose indefinitely. Importantly, this routine monitoring is not covered by Medicare. Therefore, this could be an out-of-pocket cost to patients if their supplemental insurance (if any) does not cover the extra expense. When blood glucose levels are consistently above 180 to 200, we generally add regular insulin to the PN formula. The current recommendation is to use 0.05 to 0.1 units of insulin per gram of dextrose, but this should be individualized. After insulin is added, the patient should continue to monitor blood glucose; further adjustments will be made as needed. In addition to hyperglycemia, clinicians need to monitor for signs and symptoms of hypoglycemia especially after stopping the PN infusion. An uncommon occurrence is rebound hypoglycemia, where hypoglycemia occurs following the presence of PN-related hyperglycemia shortly after the PN infusion is stopped [22]. In this case, reducing the PN rate in half for 1–2 hours then stopping it typically avoids the problem.

Metabolic Bone Disease Monitoring

Metabolic bone disease (MBD) occurs commonly in HPN patients (see also Chapter 8) [34–36]. In addition to the standard risk factors (e.g., female, thin, tobacco use), contributors to the development of MBD in HPN patients include preexisting disease, malabsorptive syndromes (including SBS), corticosteroid therapy, inactivity, hypogonadism, and hypercalciuria. Calcium, phosphorus, and magnesium deficiency are often present in SBS and may also play a role. Vitamin D deficiency as a result of malabsorption (by suppressing parathyroid hormone secretion) may also contribute to MBD. Current HPN formulations provide limited vitamin D (200 IU) due to concern that higher levels could potentially worsen bone mineral density. In our experience, SBS patients often require enhanced vitamin D supplementation (50,000 IU or more weekly) to achieve serum levels of 20–50 ng/mL. Some practitioners prefer to use daily dosing of liquid vitamin D. Therapies to minimize bone mineral density loss include calcium and vitamin D supplementation and, occasionally, the use of bisphosphonates or calcitonin. Annual or biannual bone mineral density testing should be considered in all HPN patients because of their increased risk.

Micronutrient and Trace Element Monitoring

Micronutrients including vitamins and trace elements are added to the PN formula in the form of a multiple vitamin preparation containing 12 different vitamins and a multiple trace element (MTE) preparation most commonly containing five trace elements (in adults). Even though there are a number of micronutrients that are important for various metabolic functions, we routinely monitor selenium, zinc, vitamins D and B_{12}, folate, iron, and copper in all patients on HPN at the time of initiation and every 3 to 6 months thereafter depending upon the presence of a deficiency or excess at baseline. This is particularly important in light of recent shortages in parenteral individual and MTE preparations available for use in PN. Clinicians substituting a different MTE should be made aware of differences in the amount of the individual trace elements included and the potential absence of certain trace elements in different MTEs. For example, MTE-4 does not contain selenium. Close monitoring of trace elements is therefore essential in patients with SBS receiving HPN. Chapters 12 and 13 provide details on vitamin and trace element issues in SBS and HPN [31].

Annual Monitoring

Medicare requires all HPN patients to follow up with their HPN program at least annually. During this follow-up visit, we recommend reviewing their CVC care, PN infusion technique, inspection of their catheter, and routine laboratory and other relevant monitoring. Importantly, an assessment of their readiness for weaning of PN should also occur.

WEANING OF HPN

Over 50% of adults with SBS are able to be weaned completely from PN within 5 years of diagnosis [32,37]. In contradistinction, the probability of eliminating PN use is <6% if not successfully accomplished in the first 2 years after the individual's last bowel resection. Weaning HPN is defined as the safe transition from artificial nutrition support to another form of nutrition support, which may include either enteral and/or oral nutrition. All patients who are to be considered eligible for weaning should be nutritionally optimized and maintain weight and adequate fluid balance. Furthermore, the patient should be motivated with a desire to reduce or discontinue HPN support. The presence/absence of a colon and the length of the remaining small bowel do not necessarily factor into the selection of appropriate candidates, and virtually any bowel anatomies can be considered. While successful weaning depends on the degree of adaptation of the remaining small intestine and the presence of the colon, other factors such as the presence of stricture, obstruction/

narrowing, or active Crohn's disease could potentially interfere with successful weaning and need to be considered.

It should be established early on whether the goal is to reduce PN requirements or to completely eliminate PN. An SBS patient needs to recognize that the "tradeoff" to not being on PN is the need to take several medications orally and increase the amount of food and fluid ingested daily. As such, major lifestyle changes and increased out-of-pocket expenses are often required. As a result, patient education and ongoing support are important to enhance compliance with the care plan. This is best done in the setting of a multidisciplinary practice with healthcare providers experienced in the care of SBS patients.

PN weaning involves multiple modalities, including an optimized diet and fluid regimen, use of antidiarrheal and antisecretory agents, and, in appropriate patients, use of novel trophic agents such as recombinant human growth hormone (somatropin; Zorbtive) or the glucagon-like peptide-2 analog (teduglutide; Gattex). Furthermore, it is necessary to ensure that all efforts at medication intervention have been maximized, including dose, timing, form, and frequency. It is also important to remember that oral micronutrient supplementation becomes necessary as PN is weaned and levels require periodic monitoring. Similarly, electrolyte supplementation, usually magnesium and/or potassium and sometimes bicarbonate, may be needed and require monitoring. The frequency of monitoring will depend upon the stage of PN weaning and the presence of existing or prior deficiencies. Vitamin B_{12} requires supplemental administration, most commonly by the subcutaneous or intramuscular route on a monthly basis.

Before PN weaning begins, the SBS patient's diet, fluid intake, and medications should be optimized. In addition, previously established daily calorie and fluid intake goals should be met. Frequent follow-up is necessary with subsequent PN reductions based on tolerance as determined by the development of symptoms, hydration status, electrolytes, and weight [38]. A useful approach to monitor hydration status is to maintain the urinary sodium concentration >20 mEq/L and daily urinary volume >1 L and enteral balance (oral fluid intake minus stool output) between 500 and 1000 mL/day. Although monitoring stool and urine output is cumbersome, SBS patients attempting to wean PN tend to be highly motivated. Providing the patient with a diary to record this information for review and discussion at the office and over the phone is helpful.

PN reductions can be made by either decreasing the days that PN is infused per week or by decreasing the daily PN infusion volume equally throughout the week (e.g., 10–30% reduction) [37]. Patients tend to prefer the former; however, dehydration is less of a potential concern with the latter. An optimal interval for making PN reduction decisions has not been defined. At most, once weekly would seem appropriate while acknowledging that this needs to be individualized. Once PN infusions are <3 days/week, a trial of PN discontinuation should be considered. Although the occasional patient may successfully discontinue PN without the gradual weaning strategy, this approach is not recommended for the SBS patient who has been receiving PN for an extended period of time.

CONCLUSION

HPN has evolved into a very successful, lifesaving treatment in the management of intestinal failure. Nevertheless, the provision of PN remains intrusive and expensive and continues to be associated with significant morbidity. Fortunately, most patients with intestinal failure are able to be weaned from PN within 2 years. Although HPN is associated with a number of factors that may result in a restriction of activities and deleteriously impact daily life, with time and experience, patients on HPN can modify their lifestyles to minimize the impact of this therapy. Additionally, patient support groups such as the Oley Foundation (www.oley.org) are important sources of information on practical topics (e.g., body image, travel), education, and support and may reduce the risk of complications and enhance survival and the quality of life of the patient on either EN or PN support. Finally, the management of PN by an interdisciplinary nutrition support team reduces PN-related morbidity and may reduce costs associated with its use. Because SBS is an uncommon condition and clinical expertise in its management is not widely available, the referral of these patients to experienced centers for periodic assessment is encouraged.

REFERENCES

1. Howard L et al. Four years of North American registry home parenteral nutrition outcome data and their implications for patient management. *JPEN Journal of Parenteral and Enteral Nutrition.* 1991;15(4):384–393.
2. Howard L et al. Current use and clinical outcome of home parenteral and enteral nutrition therapies in the United States. *Gastroenterology.* 1995;109(2):355–365.
3. Van Gossum A et al. Home parenteral nutrition in adults: A multicentre survey in Europe in 1993. *Clinical Nutrition.* 1996;15(2):53–59.
4. Jeong SH et al. Factors affecting postoperative dietary adaptation in short bowel syndrome. *Hepatogastroenterology.* 2009;56(93):1049–1052.
5. Barnadas G. Preparing for parenteral nutrition therapy at home. *American Journal of Health-System Pharmacy.* 1999;56(3):270–272.
6. Nightingale J et al. Guidelines for management of patients with a short bowel. *Gut.* 2006;55(Suppl 4):iv1–12.
7. Howard L. Home parenteral nutrition: Survival, cost, and quality of life. *Gastroenterology.* 2006;130(2 Suppl 1):S52–59.
8. Reddy P et al. Cost and outcome analysis of home parenteral and enteral nutrition. *JPEN Journal of Parenteral and Enteral Nutrition.* 1998;22(5):302–310.
9. Richards DM et al. Cost-utility analysis of home parenteral nutrition. *The British Journal of Surgery.* 1996;83(9):1226–1229.
10. Detsky AS et al. A cost-utility analysis of the home parenteral nutrition program at Toronto General Hospital: 1970–1982. *JPEN Journal of Parenteral and Enteral Nutrition.* 1986;10(1):49–57.
11. Wesley JR. Home parenteral nutrition: Indications, principles, and cost-effectiveness. *Comprehensive Therapy.* 1983;9(4):29–36.
12. Wateska LP et al. Cost of a home parenteral nutrition program. *JAMA.* 1980;244(20):2303–2304.
13. Naghibi M et al. A systematic review with meta-analysis of survival, quality of life and cost-effectiveness of home parenteral nutrition in patients with inoperable malignant bowel obstruction. *Clinical Nutrition.* 2014;34(4):924–930.
14. National Coverage Determination (NCD) for Enteral and Parenteral Nutrition, Medicare. Accessed on July 19, 2015, at: http://www.cms.gov/medicare-coverage-database/details/ncd-details.aspx.
15. National Institute of Health and Care Excellence. Accessed on July 19, 2015, at: https://www.nice.org.uk/guidance/cg32.
16. Newton AF et al. Home initiation of parenteral nutrition. *Nutrition in Clinical Practice.* 2007;22:57–64.
17. Corrigan ML et al. Hospital readmissions for catheter-related bloodstream infection and use of ethanol lock therapy: Comparison of patients receiving parenteral nutrition or intravenous fluids in the home vs a skilled nursing facility. *JPEN Journal of Parenteral and Enteral Nutrition.* 2013;37(1):81–84.
18. Pittiruti M et al. ESPEN Guidelines on Parenteral Nutrition: Central venous catheters (access, care, diagnosis and therapy of complications). *Clinical Nutrition.* 2009;28(4):365–377.
19. Chopra V et al. PICC-associated bloodstream infections: Prevalence, patterns, and predictors. *The American Journal of Medicine.* 2014;127(4):319–328.
20. Edakkanambeth Varayil J et al. Catheter salvage after catheter-related bloodstream infection during home parenteral nutrition. *JPEN Journal of Parenteral and Enteral Nutrition.* May 13, 2015. pii: 0148607115587018. Epub ahead of print.
21. Kirby DF et al. Home parenteral nutrition tutorial. *JPEN Journal of Parenteral and Enteral Nutrition.* 2012;36(6):632–644.
22. Stout SM et al. Metabolic effects of cyclic parenteral nutrition infusion in adults and children. *Nutrition in Clinical Practice.* 2010;25(3):277–281.
23. Kirby DF. Improving outcomes with parenteral nutrition. *Gastroenterology & Hepatology.* 2012;8(1):39–41.
24. Bech LF et al. Environmental risk factors for developing catheter-related bloodstream infection in home parenteral nutrition patients: A 6-year follow-up study. *JPEN Journal of Parenteral and Enteral Nutrition.* April 7, 2015. Epub ahead of print.
25. Muir A et al. Preventing bloodstream infection in patients receiving home parenteral nutrition. *Journal of Pediatric Gastroenterology and Nutrition.* 2014;59(2):177–181.
26. Reimund JM et al. Catheter-related infection in patients on home parenteral nutrition: Results of a prospective survey. *Clinical Nutrition.* 2002;21(1):33–38.
27. Patel V et al. Longer Hospitalization of patients with positive blood cultures receiving total parenteral nutrition. *Surgical Infections.* 2014;15(3):227–232.

28. Diamanti A et al. Long-term outcome of home parenteral nutrition in patients with ultra-short bowel syndrome. *Journal of Pediatric Gastroenterology and Nutrition*. 2014;58(4):438–442.
30. Burrin DG et al. Impact of new-generation lipid emulsions on cellular mechanisms of parenteral nutrition-associated liver disease. *Advances in Nutrition*. 2014;5(1):82–91.
31. Pogatschnik C. Trace element supplementation and monitoring in the adult patient on parenteral nutrition. *Practical Gastroenterology*. 2014;38(5):27.
32. Messing B et al. Long-term survival and parenteral nutrition dependence in adult patients with the short bowel syndrome. *Gastroenterology*. 1999;117(5):1043–1050.
33. Edakkanambeth Varayil J et al. Hyperglycemia during home parenteral nutrition administration in patients without diabetes. *Journal of Parenteral and Enteral Nutrition*. 2015. pii: 0148607115606116. Epub ahead of print.
34. Winkler MF et al. Clinical, social, and economic impacts of home parenteral nutrition dependence in short bowel syndrome. *JPEN Journal of Parenteral and Enteral Nutrition*. 2014;38(1 Suppl):32S–37S.
35. Ellegard L et al. High prevalence of vitamin D deficiency and osteoporosis in out-patients with intestinal failure. *Clinical Nutrition*. 2013;32(6):983–987.
36. Staun M et al. ESPEN guidelines on parenteral nutrition: Home parenteral nutrition (HPN) in adult patients. *Clinical Nutrition*. 2009;28(4):467–479.
37. Amiot A et al. Determinants of home parenteral nutrition dependence and survival of 268 patients with non-malignant short bowel syndrome. *Clinical Nutrition*. 2013;32(3):368–374.
38. DiBaise JK et al. Strategies for parenteral nutrition weaning in adult patients with short bowel syndrome. *Journal of Clinical Gastroenterology*. 2006;40(Suppl 2):S94–S98.

26 Intestinal Failure-Associated Liver Disease

Deirdre A. Kelly and Sue V. Beath

CONTENTS

KEY POINTS

- Intestinal failure-associated liver disease (IFALD) encompasses a spectrum of disease from mild abnormalities of liver function to extensive fibrosis and decompensated liver disease.
- Children are more likely than adults to develop severe IFALD.
- IFALD can develop insidiously and severe fibrosis can develop in the absence of jaundice and near-normal liver function tests.
- There are multiple causes for IFALD—frequently, several etiologies act in concert.
- IFALD can be reversed if steps are taken to minimize inflammatory processes and encourage enteral nutrition.
- Intestinal failure/rehabilitation teams have an important role in reducing severe (Type 2–3) IFALD.

INTRODUCTION

Intestinal failure-associated liver disease (IFALD) has been the leading indication for intestinal transplantation since the beginning of the 1990s, especially in children. Other terms for this condition are parenteral nutrition-associated cholestasis (PNAC), often applied in the context of premature neonates with intestinal immaturity, and parenteral nutrition-associated liver disease (PNALD); the term *IFALD* is preferred as it focuses attention on the whole context of intestinal failure and not just the parenteral nutrition (PN) infusions. In this chapter, the term *IFALD* will be understood to include both PNAC and PNALD.

Understanding the causes of IFALD and identifying ways to prevent or treat IFALD have been the focus of hundreds of publications [1–14], and after 25 years of endeavor, substantial progress has been made. Although the incidence of mild IFALD (defined as liver function tests [LFTs] 1.5 times above reference range, in absence of jaundice/features of portal hypertension) appears to be unchanged in the last four decades [11], the number of children and adults requiring liver and bowel transplantation appears to have decreased, possibly relating to improvements in the management of IFALD [15]. Overall, while the outlook for adults and children with IFALD is much improved, some individuals still go on to develop end-stage liver disease and need organ transplantation [16]. In the setting of short bowel syndrome (SBS), these improvements seem to result, at least in part, from the management by a nutritional care team that monitors the PN and the patient closely and makes adjustments to optimize PN, promotes enteral autonomy, ensures proper maintenance of central venous catheters, and treats infections promptly [17–19].

DEFINITION

It is important to keep in mind that IFALD is a diagnosis of exclusion, and before concluding that liver dysfunction in a patient who has intestinal failure is in fact IFALD, it is essential to screen for other etiologies such as biliary obstruction (e.g., biliary atresia in an infant or gallstones or malignancy in adult patients), viral hepatitis, autoimmune hepatitis, endocrine disorders, drug toxicity, and genetic cholestatic syndromes.

IFALD is an umbrella term encompassing a wide spectrum of pathology from minor transient abnormalities in liver function to established cirrhosis within the context of intestinal failure and PN. It is often divided into three categories: early, intermediate, and advanced [12], which approximately corresponds to the categories described in the consensus document on prevention of complications in intestinal failure [8] (Table 26.1). All definitions include a combination of biochemical, clinical, and histological criteria that mostly correlate [13]. Reliance on LFTs alone is not recommended as IFALD can develop insidiously and major histological changes can occur in the absence of jaundice and near-normal LFTs [20]. Recognizing IFALD and its subcategories is important because it allows for detection at an earlier and more reversible stage than was the case historically and helps ensure that different groups of patients are compared fairly when evaluating treatments.

CLINICAL COURSE OF IFALD

IFALD in children is usually a consequence of a systemic inflammatory response syndrome most frequently related to sepsis. Scenarios that increase the intensity of a systemic inflammatory response, such as surgery or invasive care required in neonatal units, increase the risk of IFALD, which may only become clinically apparent and more severe when a precipitant such as a bloodstream infection occurs. Other clinical factors that increase the risk and severity of IFALD include

TABLE 26.1
Severity Categories of IFALD According to Biochemistry and Clinical Features of Liver Disease Including Jaundice

IFALD Type	0 None	1 Early	2 Intermediate	3 Advanced	3+ End Stage
LFTs[a]	Normal	Raised ×1.5[a]	Raised[b]	Raised	Raised
Bilirubin	Normal	2–2.9 mg/dL	3–6 mg/dL	>6 mg/dL	>12 mg/dL
Clinical	Normal	Normal	Jaundiced	Jaundiced, portal hypertension, splenomegaly	Coagulopathy

[a] LFTs: alkaline phosphatase or γ-glutamyl transferase sustained for 6 months in adults and 6 weeks in children. (From Beath S. et al., *Transplantation*, 85, 1378–1384, 2008.)

[b] May include elevations in alanine transaminase and aspartate aminotransferase or a moderate increase in γ-glutamyl transferase >150 IU.

prolonged hospitalization, prematurity, and abdominal surgery (Tables 26.2 and 26.3). Several studies have shown that IFALD is usually a slowly progressive condition with an insidious rise in total bilirubin (conjugated fraction 50% or more) until an inflammatory event such as a catheter-related bloodstream infection occurs, which then causes the serum bilirubin to rise sharply, often >6 mg/dL [19]. After recovery from sepsis, the bilirubin concentrations fall but often remain above baseline. Recurrent septic episodes (more than three) are associated with progression in liver disease to Type 3 IFALD [21]. Early IFALD may occur within weeks or months of commencing PN, and although progression to cirrhosis is relatively uncommon, it can occur after as short a period as 5 months on PN [22].

Liver biopsy in the context of IFALD reveals a wide spectrum of pathology from steatosis to biliary cirrhosis. In adults, hepatic steatosis is relatively common and may develop without signs of inflammation, cholestasis, or hepatocyte necrosis [23]. In contrast, infants are more likely to present with centrilobular cholestasis, portal inflammation, and necrosis with or without fatty infiltration. More advanced liver disease is rare in adults but has been reported in children who are being evaluated for combined liver and small bowel transplantation and includes portal fibrosis (100%),

TABLE 26.2
Clinical Factors Associated with IFALD in Children

Risk Factor for IFALD	References	Evidence Level
Prematurity	9, 21, 24, 25	3
Need for abdominal surgery	26	3
Need for stoma	27	3
Less than 30 cm small bowel	28	2–
	27, 29	3
History of gastroschisis and dysmotility	30	3
History of severe necrotizing enterocolitis	24, 26	3
Early colonization with Pseudomonas or Enterobacter	31	3
Catheter-related bloodstream infections (CRBSI) within 28 days of birth	2, 32	3
Recurrent CRBSI	9, 21, 31	3

Note: Evidence level: below the rank of 1 is considered weak (observational or cohort studies) and a negative suffix indicates a risk of bias (page 16 at http://www.sign.ac.uk/pdf/qrg50.pdf).

TABLE 26.3
Clinical Factors Associated with IFALD in Adults

Risk Factor for IFALD	References	Evidence Level
Age >40 years	33	3
History of Crohn's disease	34	3
Repeated abdominal surgery associated with recurrent fistulization	35	4
Less than 100 cm small bowel	5, 36	3
Absence of ileocaecal valve	5	3
History of malignancy	6, 36	4, 3
Infection with hepatitis C	1	2
Duration of treatment	36	3

Note: Evidence level: below the rank of 1 is considered weak (observational or cohort studies) and a negative suffix indicates a risk of bias (page 16 at http://www.sign.ac.uk/pdf/qrg50.pdf).

pericellular fibrosis (95%), and bile ductular proliferation (90%) [22]. Pigmented Kupffer cells (81%) and portal bridging (86%) were also prominent features (see Figure 26.1).

Features of portal hypertension, including hepatosplenomegaly, may be present even when liver biopsy does not demonstrate significant fibrosis. It is important to recognize the adverse significance of gastrointestinal bleeding even in the absence of esophageal varices, as this is a sign of raised portal pressure affecting collaterals in atypical sites generated by previous intestinal surgery. Children and adults sometimes remain deceptively well, as the PN masks the malabsorption and cachexia that commonly accompanies life-threatening liver disease. Once hepatic decompensation begins (Type 3+ IFALD), as indicated by deterioration in coagulation times, falling plasma albumin, ascites, and hypoglycemia when the PN is interrupted, IFALD progresses rapidly and accounts for the extremely high mortality rate of adult and pediatric patients with IFALD awaiting transplantation [33].

EXTENT OF THE PROBLEM/EPIDEMIOLOGY

Abnormal LFTs occur in over 50% of babies and young children [3,19,33] at some point in their treatment of intestinal failure. Progression to Type 2 (intermediate) IFALD is less common, but a systematic review of 23 papers reporting on 2447 premature neonates given PN because of gastrointestinal immaturity found that 35% (range, 0–68%) developed cholestasis, defined as serum bilirubin >2 mg/dL [11]. In children with intestinal failure, four papers reporting on 283 patients found that 126 (44.5%) became jaundiced. In adults, jaundice is most uncommon, but abnormalities of LFTs occur in 30–43% of patients with short-term intestinal failure, and these generally normalize [37]. For adults receiving PN in the hospital or where there is underlying sepsis, the abnormalities of LFTs may be more extreme. Where histology is available, the findings in this setting are often characterized by hepatic steatosis, with accumulation of both macrovesicular and microvesicular fat within the hepatocytes, which may be accompanied by a degree of steatohepatitis. Gallstones are frequently detected (45% of patients) [38], and it has been recommended that prophylactic cholecystectomy be performed if abdominal surgery is needed for other reasons [13].

PATHOPHYSIOLOGY

The pathophysiology in IFALD can be divided in two: first, the effects of exogenous factors such as excessive nutrient provision in PN and, second, the endogenous patient-related risk factors. Taking the exogenous factors first, excessive nutrient provision in PN may overwhelm normal metabolic processes and endotoxin produced from the cell wall of bacteria during episodes of sepsis, including CRBSI and proinflammatory mediators that promote cytotoxic reactions, and disrupt the integrity of the biliary system and health of hepatocytes—leading to IFALD. Underprovision of micronutrients has also been proposed as a mechanism for IFALD, with reports that the amino acid taurine may be conditionally essential in neonates [39] and the relative lack of the antioxidant α-tocopherol in soya-derived lipid infusions may be an exacerbating factor in IFALD [12]. In adults, lack of choline was shown to cause reversible changes in LFTs, and hepatic computed tomography scan appearances suggested that steatosis recurred 10 weeks after choline supplements were stopped in a placebo-controlled study of 15 adult subjects [40]. Second, the endogenous patient-related factors include abdominal wall defects, ultrashort gut (<10 cm residual small bowel in a child and <100 cm in an adult), and inadequate or immature homeostatic mechanisms in neonates and older adults >40 years. But of all these factors, the inflammatory response provoked by infections and the cascade of cytotoxic reactions are the most important in causing acute deteriorations resulting in IFALD [41]. These effects are amplified in the very young [9,24,32] and malnourished because of immaturity and depletion of natural homeostatic mechanisms. In adults as well as children, the provision of PN during a septic episode or immediately after a major surgical procedure needs to be restrained and calibrated to the capacity of the liver to metabolize the nutrients, since cytokines

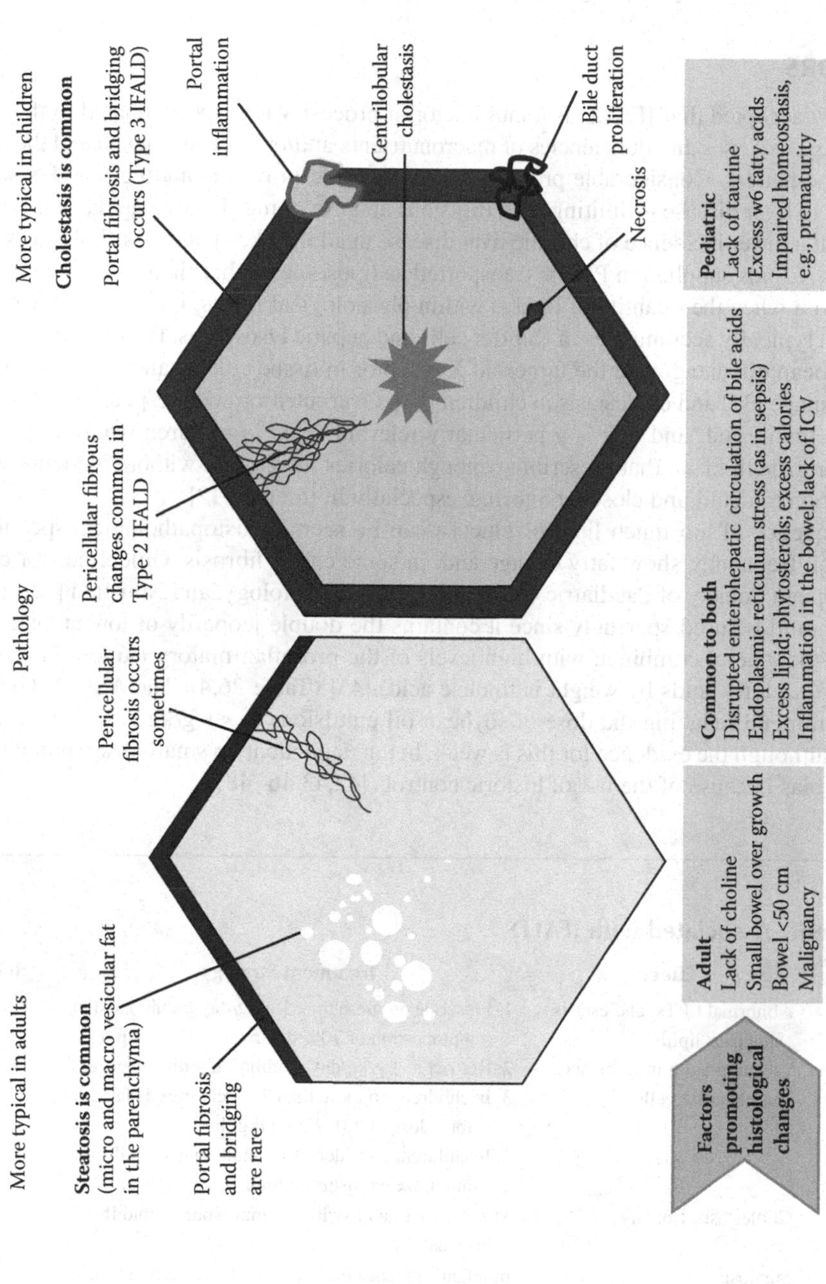
Pathology
More typical in adults
Steatosis is common
(micro and macro vesicular fat in the parenchyma)
Portal fibrosis and bridging are rare
Pericellular fibrosis occurs sometimes
Pericellular fibrous changes common in Type 2 IFALD
More typical in children
Cholestasis is common
Portal fibrosis and bridging occurs (Type 3 IFALD)
Portal inflammation
Centrilobular cholestasis
Bile duct proliferation
Necrosis
Factors promoting histological changes
Adult
Lack of choline
Small bowel over growth
Bowel <50 cm
Malignancy
Common to both
Disrupted enterohepatic circulation of bile acids
Endoplasmic reticulum stress (as in sepsis)
Excess lipid; phytosterols; excess calories
Inflammation in the bowel; lack of ICV
Pediatric
Lack of taurine
Excess w6 fatty acids
Impaired homeostasis, e.g., prematurity

FIGURE 26.1 Histopathology and underlying mechanisms of IFALD.

and stress hormones such as adrenaline tend to drive hepatocytes toward catabolism rather than anabolism. The long-term development of fibrosis with or without jaundice often results from a combination of provision of excess nutrients together with patient-related risk factors such as SBS (<100 cm in adults), lack of ileocecal valve, prematurity, necrotizing enteritis or gastroschisis, and uncontrolled sepsis [24,26,30,37]. Understanding these elements of pathophysiology is important in managing IFALD effectively (see Figure 26.1).

RISK FACTORS

It is universally accepted that IFALD is a multifactorial process with aspects related to the components of PN (e.g., excesses and deficiencies of macronutrients and/or micronutrients) and the medical condition of the patient. Considerable progress has been made in understanding how PN solutions can contribute to liver disease—limiting lipid infusions and use of multisource lipids have both been associated with a lower incidence of chronic liver disease in adults [4,37] and less cholestasis in children [14,42,43]. Lipids supplied in PN are transported as liposomes rather than chylomicrons, which implies that even when the quantity of lipid is within physiological limits, it can lead to hepatic steatosis, where it typically accumulates in Kupffer cells and hepatic lysosomes. Phytosterols, which are present in soybean oil, antagonize the farnesoid X receptor in tissue culture and are associated with hepatocyte damage [37] and cholestasis in children [44]. Overnutrition with respect to carbohydrates has also been implicated, and this is a particularly relevant issue in children whose higher metabolic needs for growth mean that prescribing enough calories for growth without inducing steatosis requires attention to detail and close monitoring, especially in infancy [12].

The consequence of too much lipid or glucose can be seen in histopathological specimens of the liver, which frequently show fatty change and, in some cases, fibrosis. Guidelines for children from the European Society of Paediatric Gastroenterology, Hepatology, and Nutrition [12] state that soybean oil should be used sparingly since it contains the double jeopardy of low amounts of the antioxidant α-tocopherol combined with high levels of the proinflammatory ω6 fatty acid linoleic acid (53% of total fatty acids by weight is linoleic acid) [45] (Table 26.4). The ASPEN Guidelines [14] also recommend reducing the dose of soybean oil emulsions to <1 g/kg/day to treat children with IFALD, although the evidence for this is weak, being dependent on small observational studies with a risk of bias because of the use of historic controls [42,43,46–48].

TABLE 26.4
PN Components Associated with IFALD

PN Component	Effect	Treatment Strategy	References
Lipids	Abnormal LFTs, cholestasis, steatosis, lipid accumulation in lysosomes and Kupffer cells	1. Prescribe no more than 1 g/kg/day (adults) and in a proportion of 70% dextrose and 30% lipid.	4, 37
		2. Restrict to 1 g/kg/day in children with cholestasis.	14
		3. In children, no more than 25% calories as fat; aim for a dose of 1.0–2.5 mg/kg/day.	13
		4. In children, consider using multisource lipids to minimize exposure to linoleic acid (18:2).	12
Soybean oil	Cholestasis, fibrosis	Monitor LFTs and switch to multisource lipid if abnormal	14
Glucose	Steatosis	In infants, glucose infusion should be no more than 1.2 g/kg/hour (20 mg/kg/minute)	49
Phytosterols	Antagonizes FXR cholestasis	Reduce exposure to soya oil	50
Amino acids (in neonates)	Cholestasis	Switch to amino acid-free PN with premature infant formula and whey protein	1

In adults, the risk factors associated with IFALD include malignancy, hepatitis C, Crohn's disease, the presence of an enterocutaneous fistula, age >40 years, and lack of enteral nutrition, which is also associated with gallstones [5,6]. Cholestasis in adults, which is less common compared with children, has been associated with the residual length of the small bowel (<50 cm). A number of adverse factors probably contribute, including difficulty in establishing stable enteral feeding, which may worsen fluid balance, poor intestinal adaptation, interruption of the enterohepatic circulation leading to abnormal bile acid metabolism, or the short or diseased gut may be more prone to bacterial translocation and systemic sepsis [5,38]. A prospective study that evaluated the prevalence of liver disease in adults on home PN for permanent intestinal failure associated the development of cholestasis to the provision of lipid infusions of >1 g/kg/day [4].

The clinical circumstances that increase the risk of IFALD occurring in a child on PN include prematurity and surgery (Tables 26.2 and 26.3). Duration of PN is also a risk factor; however, this is likely secondary to increasing the exposure to other risk factors such as CRBSI. In one of the largest systematic reviews on this subject [11], intermediate IFALD (defined as conjugated bilirubin >2 mg/dL) occurred in 15% (105/667) of children who received PN for up to 28 days, which increased to 37% (85/229) after 30–60 days of PN, and after 60 days of PN, 61% (31/51) were jaundiced. The immaturity of homeostatic mechanisms and detoxification pathways in very young children means that the impact of CRBSI is greater, making sepsis an important factor leading to cholestasis in young children. Endotoxin has a direct inhibitory effect on bile acid transporters, especially the bile salt export pump [41].

PROPOSED BIOLOGICAL MECHANISMS AND THERAPEUTIC TARGETS

Some intriguing theories describing the biological mechanisms leading to IFALD have emerged in the last 15 years. The observation that inflammation in the bowel rapidly leads to migration of inflammatory cells into the liver has led to the recognition that endothelial cells express molecules that encourage adhesion of the migrating leukocytes released by an inflamed bowel. The precipitating inflammatory event may be ischemia (as in volvulus or infarction), sepsis and small intestinal bacterial overgrowth (as in necrotizing enterocolitis), or inflammatory bowel disease; all appear to cause an increase in hepatic endothelial cell activation mediated via vascular adhesion molecule 1 (VAP-1), which in turn leads to the upregulation of other adhesion molecules such as E-selectin and intercellular adhesion molecule-1 and the secretion of the chemokine CXCL8 [51]. VAP-1 is strongly expressed by liver endothelial cells, which may explain why liver function is easily disturbed in patients on PN who are exposed to the additional stress of surgery and/or CRBSI. The relatively organ-specific nature of the interaction of the hepatic endothelium to VAP-1 provides a target for future therapies that block VAP-1 and may be useful in moderating the impact of inflammatory events on the liver [52].

Endosplasmic reticulum stress (ERS) has also been proposed as a biological mechanism that promotes IFALD. The signal for ERS glucose-regulated chaperone protein 94 (GRP94), which is a member of the heat shock protein 90 family contributing to protein folding in the endoplasmic reticulum, was measured in rabbits [53]. The animals were administered either standard soybean oil-containing PN or PN-containing ω3 fish oil. The investigators found that the GRP94 messenger RNA and protein levels in liver tissue were significantly higher (by a factor of 2) in the animals fed soybean oil PN, and these animals also had higher serum bilirubin and γ-glutamyl transpeptidase compared with rabbits receiving the fish oil PN and controls who were naturally fed rabbit milk. Another recently published study examined archived liver tissue from 20 adult patients with early and late IFALD and normal liver ($n = 3$). Much higher mean relative RNA levels of ERS markers (GRP78 and ERDj4) were found in those specimens with IFALD, especially those with more advanced IFALD [54].

Both mechanisms could be operating to cause IFALD in humans since they are linked with known risk factors such as sepsis, nutrient overload, and proinflammatory mediators. Emerging therapeutic options derived from these insights include vedolizumab, a humanized immunoglobulin G subclass 1 (IgG1) monoclonal antibody that interferes with leukocyte homing by blocking the 4b 7/mucosal vascular addressin cell adhesion molecule 1 (MAdCAM-1) interaction, which is currently in phase 2 human trials and numerous other antiadhesion agents in earlier stages of development [55]. Time will tell whether these agents will ultimately be useful in preventing and treating IFALD.

The bile salt sensor farsenoid X receptor (FXR) is a key regulator of hepatic lipid metabolism and may also play a role in the steatosis found in IFALD and that described in nonalcoholic fatty liver disease (NAFLD) [56]. FXR inhibits lipogenesis and bile salt synthesis by suppressing cholesterol 7 alpha hydroxylase when complexed with fibroblast growth factor 19 (FGF-19), which is secreted in the small intestine [57]. Reduced serum levels of FGF-19 are correlated with increased bile acid synthesis in patients with ileal dysfunction secondary to Crohn's disease. In children with NAFLD, serum FGF-19 levels inversely correlate with hepatic steatosis and fibrosis [58]. FXR has recently become a focus of interest for the pharmaceutical industry, where the possibility of using FXR agonists (e.g., obeticholic acid) to treat or prevent NAFLD has led to a number of phase 2 studies. FXR has not been well studied in SBS; however, since one of the target genes of FXR is intestinal FGF-19, patients with SBS are likely to produce less FGF-19 and the benefits of FGF-19 will be lost [59]. An abnormal feedback loop between FXR and bile acids and FGF-19 in SBS, especially where there is loss of the ileum [59], is another potential mechanism resulting in steatosis, hepatic fibrosis, and IFALD [60]. Further study in this area is clearly warranted.

TREATMENT AND MANAGEMENT STRATEGIES

There is a wide range of measures that are recommended for the avoidance of IFALD, but the best evidence for preventing IFALD is generally found in the neonatal practice and intensive care

Algorithm for managing IFALD in children (*see Table 26.5 for strength of evidence*)

Early/mild Type 1 IFALD
abnormal LFTs; bilirubin rising

- Screen for infection and primary liver disease
- Start antibiotics if infection likely
- Commence enteral nutrition unless concerns about NEC [1]
- Start ursodeoxycholic acid p.o. [61]
- Start cycling PN as soon as feasible [62]
- Use amino acid solutions which contain taurine supplements [39]
- Discuss PN prescription with NST

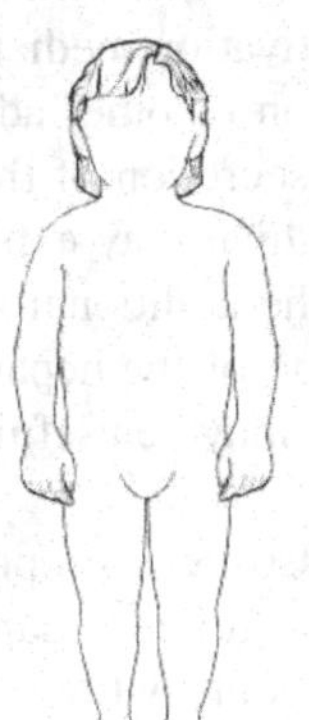

Worsening IFALD (Type 2/3)
abnormal LFTs; bilirubin >50 mmol/dL

- Screen for infection and treat as indicated, consider replacement of feeding catheter
- Review hygiene measures for feeding catheter
- Discuss with NST to reduce over exposure to PN calories [14,49]
- Consider second-line intravenous liquid with reduced ω6 linoleic acid
- Consider surgical strategies to enhance intestinal rehabilitation [18,66,67]
- Treat possible intestinal bacterial overgrowth with metronidazole p.o. or neomycin p.o. for 2–4 weeks [68]
- Stop intravenous lipid infusion for 1–2 weeks

Special circumstances
(a) High nasogastric losses in neonate or infant
Screen for and treat intestinal obstruction
Treat dysmotility with high-dose oral erythromycin 12.5 mg/kg/dose [7]
(b) Long-term intestinal failure (>3 months)
Discharge to home with NST supporting care of home PN [7,63]
Review prescription to reduce over exposure to PN calories [14,49]
Introduce lipid-free days/consider alternative type of PN lipid [64,65]

(c) IFALD worsens or does not resolve
Consult specialist center for advice reintestinal rehabilitation, nontransplant, bowel surgery and suitability of liver ± small bowel Tx [18,66]

FIGURE 26.2 Medical management algorithm for IFALD in children. See also Table 26.5 for details on strength of evidence. NST, nutrition support team; Tx, transplant.

settings because it is possible to recruit large numbers of subjects who tend to be less heterogeneous than patients who have been on PN for 3 months or more. Therefore, good clinical practice is often a matter of identifying high-risk groups (Tables 26.2 and 26.3) and extrapolating data from neonates and the intensive care practice. In particular, there is no doubt that care of these complex patients on long-term PN by experienced nutritional support teams makes a difference in the rate of CRBSI [69] and the likelihood of developing other serious complications. An algorithm for the management of IFALD is shown in Figure 26.2.

Apart from the use of oral erythromycin in patients with dysmotility [7] and ursodeoxycholic acid [61], the evidence base is insecure [10,14]. The suggested management approach typically represents a pragmatic approach to the problem guided mostly by expert opinion (Table 26.5). Ensuring that the patient is managed by a multidisciplinary team experienced in the management of SBS and intestinal failure is a top priority. Simple measures such as education and auditing of hygiene and the care of the central venous catheter when connecting and disconnecting from PN can be highly effective in reducing CRBSI by more than threefold [17,69]. The multidisciplinary team can

TABLE 26.5
Evidence-Based IFALD Treatment Options

Treatment of IFALD	Reference	Evidence Level (EL)
a. Drugs		
1. High-dose (12.5 mg/kg/dose) oral erythromycin for dysmotility in babies.	7	1+
2. Ursodeoxycholic acid (30 mg/kg/day) prevents IFALD Type 1 (bilirubin	61	1
<50 mmol/L) and improves established IFALD (Types 2 and 3).	70	2–
	71	2–
3. Cholecystokinin is not useful in preventing IFALD in neonates.	72	1
4. Metronidazole (25–50 mg/kg/day) prevents IFALD Type 1 and reduces	68	2–
Type 3 IFALD.	42	2–
b. Modifications to PN Solution		
1. Reduce soy-based IV lipid component of PN:		
a. Makes no difference to LFTs in infants on long-term PN	73	1–
b. Improves cholestasis in children >6 months	47	2–
c. Reduced to 1 g/kg/day to treat cholestasis in children	14	4
2. Use novel IV lipid emulsions enriched with fish oil:		
a. SMOF	64	1–
b. Omegaven	42	2–
c. Omegaven	48	2–
d. Omegaven	74	2–
e. SMOF lipid	65	2–
3. Limit lipids in PN:		
a. <3.5 g/kg/day in children	49	4
b. 9 g/kg per week in two divided doses (1.2 g/kg/day)	75	3
c. <1 g/kg/day in adults reduces development of fibrosis	4	2
4. Cycle PN—reduces risk of IFALD.	62	2–
5. Taurine prevents IFALD Type 1 and reduces Type 3 IFALD in patients with NEC.	39	2–
6. Choline (1–4 g/day) reduces steatosis.	40	2

Note: EL1, based on randomized controlled trials; EL2, cohort or observational studies; EL3, case series or case reports; EL4, expert opinion or consensus guidelines. Minus symbol signifies high risk of bias.

[a] See also Figure 26.2 treatment algorithm.

also be highly effective in reestablishing oral/enteral feeding through surgical and medical means [66], which reduces the risk of IFALD by stimulating the enterohepatic recirculation of bile acids, thereby providing a trophic stimulus to the intestinal mucosa and ultimately aiding weaning from PN altogether. The development of dedicated vascular access teams is another welcome development with good clinical outcomes in terms of reductions in the number of injuries to the cannulated vein (2.4%) and CRBSI, which was only 3.16 per 1000 line days in hospitalized children [76].

CONCLUSIONS AND PERSPECTIVES

Recognizing IFALD at an early stage and agreeing on the definition for early/Type 1, intermediate/Type 2 and advanced/Type 3 IFALD are important in determining the optimal treatment plan and facilitating multicenter clinical trials and registry studies. It also serves to highlight the treatable nature of IFALD. The use of multidisciplinary nutrition support teams offers great value to patients with intestinal failure at high risk of developing IFALD by minimizing exposure to excessive and/or deficient PN components, improving the standard of catheter care, thereby reducing CRBSI, enhancing intestinal rehabilitation medically and surgically, and, for patients with long-term intestinal failure, enabling discharge to the safer home environment. In the future, it may be possible to restore livers affected by IFALD to normality using treatments developed from molecular science such as antiadhesion molecules and chemical chaperones active in the endoplasmic reticulum or by manipulating the FXR. At present, the management of IFALD is more practically focused.

REFERENCES

1. Brown MR et al. Decreased cholestasis with enteral instead of intravenous protein in the very low-birth-weight infant. *J Pediatr Gastroenterol Nutr* 1989;9:21–27.
2. Sondheimer JM et al. Infection and cholestasis in neonates with intestinal resection and long-term parenteral nutrition. *J Pediatr Gastroenterol Nutr* 1998;27:131–137.
3. Kelly DA. Liver complications of pediatric parenteral nutrition-epidemiology. *Nutrition* 1998;14:153–157.
4. Cavicchi M et al. Prevalence of liver disease and contributing factors in patients receiving home parenteral nutrition for permanent intestinal failure. *Ann Intern Med* 2000;132:525–532.
5. Lumen W, Shaffer JL. Prevalence, outcome and associated factors of deranged liver function tests in patients on home parenteral nutrition. *Clin Nutr* 2002;21:337–343.
6. Nightingale JM. Hepatobiliary, renal and bone complications of intestinal failure. *Best Pract Res Clin Gastroenterol* 2003;17:907–929.
7. Ng PC et al. High-dose oral erythromycin decreased the incidence of parenteral nutrition-associated cholestasis in preterm infants. *Gastroenterology* 2007;132:1726–1739.
8. Beath S et al. Collaborative strategies to reduce mortality and morbidity in patients with chronic intestinal failure including those who are referred for small bowel transplantation. *Transplantation* 2008;85:1378–1384.
9. Hsieh MH et al. Parenteral nutrition-associated cholestasis in premature babies: Risk factors and predictors. *Pediatr Neonatol* 2009;50:202–207.
10. Barclay AR et al. Systematic review: Medical and nutritional interventions for the management of intestinal failure and its resultant complications in children. *Aliment Pharmacol Ther* 2011;33:175–184.
11. Lauriti G et al. Incidence, prevention, and treatment of parenteral nutrition-associated cholestasis and intestinal failure-associated liver disease in infants and children: A systematic review. *JPEN J Parenter Enteral Nutr* 2014;38:70–85.
12. Lacaille F et al. Intestinal failure-associated liver disease. A position paper by the ESPGHAN Working Group of Intestinal Failure and Intestinal Transplantation. *J Pediatr Gastroenterol Nutr* 2015;60:272–283.
13. Abu-Wasel B et al. Liver disease secondary to intestinal failure. *Biomed Res Int* 2014;2014:968357.
14. Wales PW et al. A.S.P.E.N. clinical guidelines: Support of pediatric patients with intestinal failure at risk of parenteral nutrition–associated liver disease. *JPEN J Parenter Enteral Nutr* 2014;38:538–557.
15. Khan KM et al. Developing trends in the intestinal transplant waitlist. *Am J Transplant* 2014;14:2830–2837.

16. Grant D et al. Intestinal Transplant Association. Intestinal transplant registry report: Global activity and trends. *Am J Transplant* 2015;15:210–219.
17. Puntis JWL et al. Staff training: A key factor in reducing intravascular catheter sepsis. *Arch Dis Child* 1991;66:335–337.
18. Torres C et al. Role of an intestinal rehabilitation program in the treatment of advanced intestinal failure. *J Pediatr Gastroenterol Nutr* 2007;45:204–212.
19. Bishay M et al. Intestinal failure-associated liver disease in surgical infants requiring long-term parenteral nutrition. *J Pediatr Surg* 2012;47:359–362.
20. Mercer DF et al. Hepatic fibrosis persists and progresses despite biochemical improvement in children treated with intravenous fish oil emulsion. *J Pediatr Gastroenterol Nutr* 2013;56:364–369.
21. Beath SV et al. Parenteral nutrition related cholestasis in post surgical neonates: Multivariate analysis of risk factors. *J Pediatr Surg* 1996;31:604–606.
22. Beath SV et al. Clinical features and prognosis of children assessed for isolated small bowel (ISBTx) or combined small bowel and liver transplantation (CSBLTx). *J Pediatr Surg* 1997;32:459–461.
23. Tulikoura I et al. Morphological fatty changes and function of the liver, serum free fatty acids and triglycerides during parenteral nutrition. *Scand J Gastroenterol* 1982;17:177–185.
24. Robinson DT et al. Parenteral nutrition-associated cholestasis in small for gestational age infants. *J Pediatr* 2008;152:59–62.
25. Fitzgibbons SC et al. Relationship between biopsy-proven parenteral nutrition-associated liver fibrosis and biochemical cholestasis in children with short bowel syndrome. *J Pediatr Surg.* 2010;45:95–99.
26. Duro D et al. Risk factors for parenteral nutrition-associated liver disease following surgical therapy for necrotizing enterocolitis. *J Pediatr Gastroenterol Nutr* 2011;52:595–600.
27. Andorsky DJ et al. Nutritional and other postoperative management of neonates with short bowel syndrome correlates with clinical outcomes. *J Pediatr* 2001;139:27–33.
28. Peyret B et al. Prevalence of liver complications in children receiving long-term parenteral nutrition. *Eur J Clin Nutr* 2011;65:743–749.
29. Wales PW et al. Neonatal short bowel syndrome: A cohort study. *J Pediatr Surg* 2005;40:755–762.
30. Dell-Olio D et al. Isolated liver transplant in infants with short bowel syndrome: Insights into outcomes and prognostic factors. *J Pediatr Gastroenterol Nutr* 2009;48:334–340.
31. Pierro A et al. Clinical impact of abnormal gut flora in infants receiving parenteral nutrition. *Ann Surg.* 1998;227:547–552.
32. Hermans D et al. Early central catheter infection may contribute to hepatic fibrosis in children receiving long-term parenteral nutrition. *J Pediatr Gastroenterol Nutr* 2007;44:459–463.
33. Fryer J et al. Mortality in candidates waiting for combined liver–intestine transplants exceeds that for other candidates waiting for liver transplants. *Liver Transplant* 2003;9:748–753.
34. Capron JP et al. Metronidazole in prevention of cholestasis associated with total parenteral nutrition. *Lancet* 1983;26:446–447.
35. Carlton G et al. The surgical management of patients with caute intestinal. Published by ASGBI 2010, asgbi.org.uk, accessed May 5, 2015.
36. Guglielmi FW et al. Catheter-related complications in long-term home parenteral nutrition patients with chronic intestinal failure. *J Vasc Access* 2012;13(4):490–497.
37. Gabe SM. Lipids and liver dysfunction in patients receiving parenteral nutrition. *Curr Opin Clin Nutr Metab Care* 2013;16:150–155.
38. Nightingale J et al. Guidelines for the management of patients with short bowel. *Gut* 2006;55(Suppl iv):1–12.
39. Spencer AU et al. Parenteral nutrition-associated cholestasis in neonates: Multivariate analysis of the potential protective effect of taurine. *JPEN J Parenter Enteral Nutr* 2005;29:337–343.
40. Buchman AL et al. Choline deficiency causes reversible hepatic abnormalities in patients receiving parenteral nutrition: Proof of a human choline requirement: A placebo-controlled trial. *JPEN J Parenter Enteral Nutr.* 2001;25(5):260–268.
41. Kosters A et al. The role of inflammation in cholestasis: Clinical and basic aspects. *Semin Liver Dis* 2010;30:186–194.
42. Sigalet D et al. Improved outcomes in paediatric intestinal failure with aggressive prevention of liver disease. *Eur J Pediatr Surg* 2009;19:348–353.
43. Cowles RA et al. Reversal of intestinal failure-associated liver disease in infants and children on parenteral nutrition: Experience with 93 patients at a referral center for intestinal rehabilitation. *J Pediatr Surg* 2010;45:84–87.
44. Clayton PT et al. Phytosterolemia in children with parenteral nutrition-associated cholestatic liver disease. *Gastroenterology* 1993;1105:1806–1813.

45. Wanten JA et al. Immune modulation by parenteral lipid emulsions. *Am J Clin Nutr* 2007;85:1171–1184.
46. Diamond IR et al. Novel lipid-based approaches to pediatric intestinal failure-associated liver disease. *Arch Pediatr Adolesc Med* 2012;166:473–478.
47. Rollins MD et al. Elimination of soybean lipid emulsion in parenteral nutrition and supplementation with enteral fish oil improve cholestasis in infants with short bowel syndrome. *Nutr Clin Pract* 2010;25:199–204.
48. Puder M et al. Parenteral fish oil improves outcomes in patients with parenteral nutrition-associated liver injury. *Ann Surg* 2009;250:395–402.
49. Koletzko B et al. Parenteral Nutrition Guidelines Working Group; European Society for Clinical Nutrition and Metabolism; European Society of Paediatric Gastroenterology, Hepatology and Nutrition (ESPGHAN); European Society of Paediatric Research (ESPR). ESPGHAN PN guidelines. *J Pediatr Gastroenterol Nutr* 2005;41(suppl 2):S1–S87.
50. Mutanen A et al. Serum plant sterols, cholestanol, and cholesterol precursors associate with histological liver injury in pediatric onset intestinal failure. *Am J Clin Nutr* 2014;100:1085–1094.
51. Lalor PF et al. Activation of vascular adhesion protein-1 on liver endothelium results in an NF-κB-dependent increase in lymphocyte adhesion. *Hepatology* 2007;45:465–474.
52. Welham ML. VAP-1: A new anti-inflammatory target? *Blood* 2004;103:3250–3251.
53. Zhu X et al. Parenteral nutrition–associated liver injury and increased GRP94 expression prevented by w-3 fish oil based lipid emulsion supplementation. *J Pediatr Gastroenterol Nutr* 2014;59:708–713.
54. Sharkey LM et al. Endoplasmic reticulum stress is implicated in intestinal failure-associated liver disease. *JPEN J Parenter Enteral Nutr* 2015 Feb 9. pii: 0148607115571014. Epub ahead of print.
55. Lobatón T et al. Review article: Anti-adhesion therapies for inflammatory bowel disease. *Aliment Pharmacol Ther* 2014;39:579–594.
56. Legry V et al. Yin Yang 1 and farsenoid X receptor: A balancing act in non-alcoholic fatty liver disease. *Gut* 2014;63:1–2.
57. Ali AH et al. Recent advances in the development of farnesoid X receptor agonists. *Ann Transl Med* 2015;3:5.
58. Lenicek M et al. Bile acid malabsorption in inflammatory bowel disease: Assessment by serum markers. *Inflamm Bowel Dis* 2011;17:1322–1327.
59. Mutanen A et al. Loss of ileum decreases serum fibroblast growth factor 19 in relation to liver inflammation and fibrosis in pediatric onset intestinal failure. *J Hepatol* 2015;62:1391–1397.
60. Fiorucci S et al. The nuclear receptor SHP mediates inhibition of hepatic stellate cells by FXR and protects against liver fibrosis. *Gastroenterology* 2004;127:1497–1512.
61. Arslanoglu S et al. Ursodeoxycholic acid treatment in preterm infants: A pilot study for the prevention of cholestasis associated with total parenteral nutrition. *J Pediatr Gastroenterol Nutr* 2008;46:228–231.
62. Jensen AR et al. The association of cyclic parenteral nutrition and decreased incidence of cholestatic liver disease in patients with gastroschisis. *J Pediatr Surg* 2009;44:183–189.
63. Hess RA et al. Survival outcomes of pediatric intestinal failure patients: Analysis of factors contributing to improved survival over the past two decades. *J Surg Res* 2011;170:27–31.
64. Antebi H et al. Liver function and plasma antioxidant status in intensive care unit patients requiring total parenteral nutrition: Comparison of 2 fat emulsions. *JPEN J Parenter Enteral Nutr* 2004;28:142–148.
65. Muhammed R et al. Resolution of parenteral nutrition-associated jaundice on changing from a soybean oil emulsion to a complex mixed-lipid emulsion. *J Pediatr Gastroenterol Nutr* 2012;54:797–802.
66. Sudan D et al. A multidisciplinary approach to the treatment of intestinal failure. *J Gastrointest Surg* 2005;9:165–176.
67. Cusick E et al. Small-bowel continuity: A crucial factor in determining survival in gastroschisis. *Pediatr Surg Int* 1997;12:34–37.
68. Kubota A et al. The effect of metronidazole on TPN-associated liver dysfunction in neonates. *J Pediatr Surg* 1990;25:618–621.
69. Stanger JD et al. The impact of multi-disciplinary intestinal rehabilitation programs on the outcome of pediatric patients with intestinal failure: A systematic review and meta-analysis. *J Pediatr Surg* 2013;48:983–992.
70. Chen CY et al. Ursodeoxycholic acid (UDCA) therapy in very-low-birth-weight infants with parenteral nutrition-associated cholestasis. *J Pediatr* 2004;145:317–321.
71. De Marco G et al. Early treatment with ursodeoxycholic acid for cholestasis in children on parenteral nutrition because of primary intestinal failure. *Aliment Pharmacol Ther.* 2006;24:387–394.
72. Teitelbaum DH et al. Use of cholecystokinin-octapeptide for the prevention of parenteral nutrition-associated cholestasis. *Pediatrics* 2005;115:1332–1340.

73. Goulet O et al. Long term efficacy and safety of new olive oil based intravenous fat emulsion in pediatric patients: A double-blind randomised study. *Am J Clin Nutr* 1999;170:338–345.
74. Gura KM et al. Safety and efficacy of a fish oil-based fat emulsion in the treatment of parenteral nutrition-associated liver disease. *Pediatrics* 2008;121;e678–e686.
75. Jakobsen MS et al. Low-fat, high-carbohydrate parenteral nutrition (PN) may potentially reverse liver disease in long-term PN-dependent infants. *Dig Dis Sci* 2015;60:252–259.
76. Arul GS et al. Ultrasound-guided percutaneous insertion of Hickman lines in children. Prospective study of 500 consecutive procedures. *J Pediatr Surg* 2009;44:1371–1376.

27 Central Venous Catheter Complications
Management and Prevention

Richard Gilroy, Jordan Voss, and Chaitanya Pant

CONTENTS

KEY POINTS

- Central venous access is necessary for the administration of parenteral nutrition and plays a central role in the management of short bowel syndrome with intestinal failure.
- Catheter-related complications continue to be a source of misery for patients with intestinal failure and include infection, malfunction, occlusion, and venous thrombosis.
- The relative frequency of catheter-related complications has declined, largely due to improved insertion techniques and refinement of line care practices.
- Reducing infection rates in long-term catheters focuses on catheter care, treating concurrent medical conditions that present risk for bacteremia or site infection, and addressing social and clinical support structures, thereby ensuring compliance.
- Ethanol and antimicrobial locks might be useful for preventing and/or treating catheter colonization, especially in individuals with a history of catheter-related bloodstream infection; however, insufficient data are currently available to recommend their routine use.

INTRODUCTION: BACKGROUND ON CENTRAL VENOUS CATHETER USE IN PARENTERAL NUTRITION

In 1968, Dudrick and associates [1] published their seminal experience with parenteral nutrition (PN) and provided a solution to the life-threatening consequences of intestinal failure. Since then, the indications and application of PN have increased exponentially, and home PN for those with long-term intestinal failure followed. It was, however, only 6 years later that John Ryan's article in the *New England Journal of Medicine* evaluating 200 consecutive patients receiving PN emphasized that this therapy was not without complications, some of which could be life threatening [2]. The most common nonprocedural complication identified was catheter-related bloodstream infection (CRBSI), which occurred in 7% of catheters. Over time, the relative frequency of CRBSI and other catheter-related complications has declined, largely due to improved insertion techniques and refinement of catheter care practices [3–5]. Nonetheless, catheter-related complications continue to be a source of misery for patients with intestinal failure. This chapter will outline an approach to the evaluation and management of the central line in the patient receiving PN, with particular attention to reducing the occurrence of complications.

INDICATIONS, LOCATIONS, AND TYPES OF CATHETERS AND PROCEDURE-RELATED COMPLICATIONS

Home PN is administered by a central venous catheter. The plastic or silicon catheter tip is optimally located between the lower third of the superior vena cava and the upper portion of the right atrium (i.e., near the cavo-atrial junction), as shown in Figure 27.1.

With the subclavian or internal jugular approach, the proximal extent of the catheter (either a subcutaneously implanted port or a tunneled catheter) is generally present at a subclavicular location. Tunneling in the subcutaneous fat allows placement of a protective cuff well away from the venous entry and cutaneous exit sites (Figure 27.1). The cuff is important as it reduces the risk of a CRBSI. An exit site in the neck might be used for short-term catheters but is not appropriate for long-term use in the home PN setting as the neck position both presents inconvenience and increases the risk for dislodgement of the catheter. Examples of tunneled catheters include the Hickman, Broviac, and Leonard catheters. As shown in Figure 27.2, the external portion of the catheter tube has a locking connection onto which a connection port from intravenous (IV) tubing can be connected. In some central venous access devices, the proximal end of the catheter connects to a subcutaneous reservoir, commonly known as a "port." This reservoir is then accessed by a needle (Figure 27.3). In some instances, because of loss of central venous access sites, alternate sites of central venous access paths are required. In these uncommon instances, the central venous system may be accessed through femoral or lumbar veins or, more rarely, via transhepatic access to the infrahepatic inferior vena cava [6–10]. Another very rare but occasionally necessary option is PN access through an arteriovenous fistula most often created for hemodialysis [11]. These locations should be avoided when subclavian or internal jugular veins are accessible.

Placement of the catheter tip more distally, i.e., within the right atrium, predisposes to greater risk for thrombosis, cardiac dysrhythmias, and catheter tip migration with hemopericardium and is not recommended [12]. During catheter insertion, transient atrial arrhythmias can be seen, and this generally indicates that the catheter tip is beyond the site of ideal insertion. Should the atrial

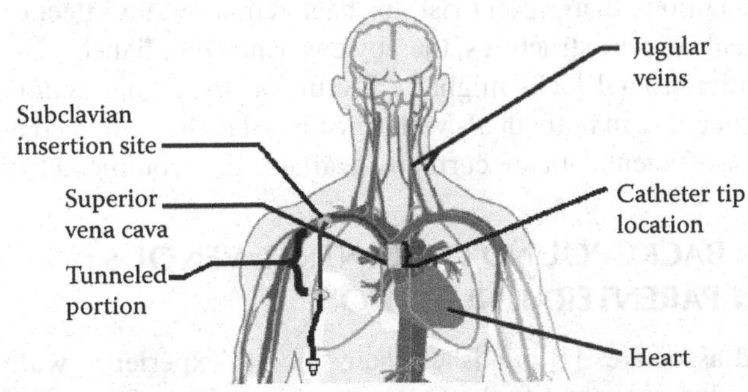

FIGURE 27.1 **(See color insert.)** The catheter tip should be between the lower third of the superior vena cava upper portion of the right atrium (yellow rectangle).

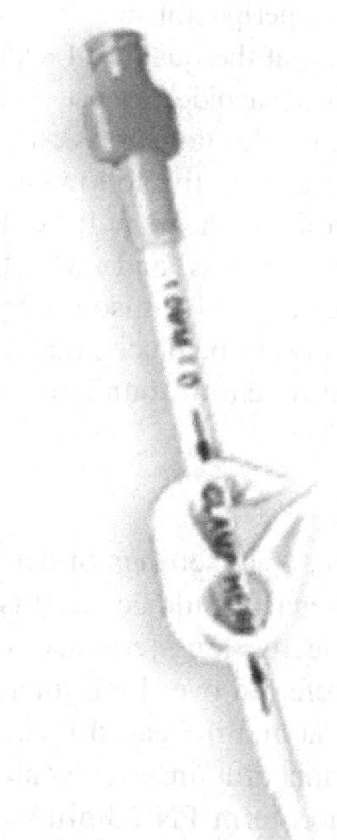

FIGURE 27.2 The external portion of a Hickman single-lumen catheter with a locking connection.

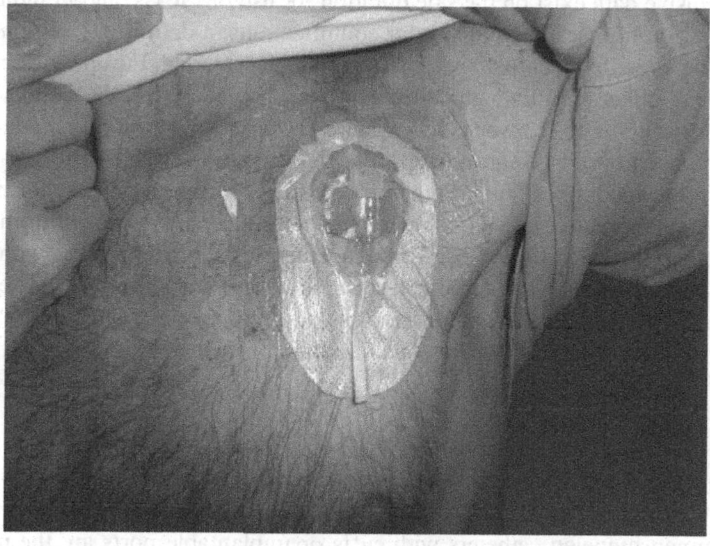

FIGURE 27.3 **(See color insert.)** A subcutaneous port is accessed via an external needle.

arrhythmias persist after removal of the insertion wire, this would theoretically signify risk for the previously mentioned complications. Other technical errors can lead to complications during the act of catheter insertion. For instance, loss of the guide wire, inadvertent arterial puncture and dilation with hemothorax, or pneumothorax during access have all been described. However, all of these have been significantly reduced with the common use of ultrasonic guidance during venous access.

The reasons for infusion of the PN solution into a large centrally located vein are to extend the venous access longevity (line-years) and because the hyperosmolar PN solutions being administered present a risk for phlebitis. Fluids with osmolarity greater than 900 mOsm/L are recommended for administration through a central venous catheter rather than a peripheral site, although more than one study has challenged this rationale, and it is acknowledged that the quality of supporting evidence is weak [13–16]. Short-length cannulas for peripheral PN should be avoided for use outside the hospital setting and should be very closely supervised in the inpatient setting due to their risk for dislodgement and phlebitis [17].

When determining which catheter type to use, the following should be considered: the indication for catheter placement, the duration the catheter will be used, the type used for any prior central venous access, complications of prior access, and the patient's preference. These circumstances influence not only the type of catheter used but also the location of the catheter placement. Importantly, all long-term catheters should always be placed under controlled, aseptic conditions by well-trained personnel preferably using real-time ultrasound guidance [18–23].

Short-Term Catheters

In the acute setting of new PN dependence, or in settings of active or presumed infection, placement of only short-term central venous catheters should occur. It is only after the resolution of acute management issues that planning of more elective long-term access should transpire. For short-term catheters, uncuffed subclavian lines are preferred over high internal jugular line insertion sites as the latter has a greater risk for dislodgement and increased inconvenience to the patient and staff managing the catheter. In recent years, peripherally inserted central venous catheters (PICCs) have largely supplanted subclavian lines for short-term PN administration in many centers. This has occurred as a result of their lower frequency of insertion- and infection-related complications in the acute care setting coupled with overall lower costs as hospital systems develop efficient practice service lines (often nurses) with concentrated expertise that place these on a frequent basis [24,25]. Although inconclusive data exist on the safe duration for use of PICCs, and in light of the relationship between duration of insertion and risk for complications, a definitive recommendation on the safe duration of their use in the outpatient setting cannot be provided. European Society for Clinical Nutrition and Metabolism (ESPEN) guidelines suggest, however, that PICCs may be used in the outpatient setting for up to 10–12 weeks [24]. There are case series but no randomized controlled data on PICC line use beyond 1 year; retrospective series show variable results for CRBSIs. Until additional data from randomized studies regarding the safety of these lines relative to cuffed catheters are available, this practice cannot be recommended [26,27]. When central lines are placed in the emergent setting, consideration of earlier replacement of short-term lines with catheters more appropriate for long-term use, when circumstances allow, appears warranted. When placing either short- or long-term catheters, no data support the use of prophylactic antibiotics at the time of insertion to diminish the rate of Gram-positive contamination of the catheter [28–30].

Long-Term Catheters

When considering the use of long-term central venous access devices, many of the same principles as for short-term catheters apply; however, there are also some unique elements that need consideration. Single-lumen tunneled catheters with cuffs or implantable ports are the most appropriate access devices when long-term catheters for PN are needed. There is evidence, although limited, that suggests that minimizing the number of lumens lowers the risk of infections. This is presumably due to the lower number of external connectors that serve as potential contamination sites as well as the decreased surface area for biofilm development in single-lumen compared with multilumen catheters [31]. Tunneled catheters with cuffs or implantable ports are associated with significant reductions in the risk of catheter-related infections derived from tracking of infections along the catheters length and also have a lower frequency of catheter dislodgement [32]. Lowering the risk of infection and reducing the risk of dislodgement of the catheter are seen to significantly benefit the patient at many levels. In the long-term setting, however, additional points also need to be considered when placing a catheter. Importantly, before placement of a long-term catheter, an awareness of the patency of the

TABLE 27.1
Catheter Insertion-Related Complications

	Frequency (%)			
Complication	**Internal Jugular**[a]	**Subclavian**[a]	**Femoral**[a]	**Overall**[b]
Arterial puncture	6.3–9.4	3.1–4.9	9.0–15.0	5
Hematoma	<0.1–2.2	1.2–2.1	3.8–4.4	1
Hemothorax	NA	0.4–0.6	Not applicable	1
Pneumothorax	<0.1–0.2	1.5–3.1	Not applicable	1
Failure to place	Not assessed	Not assessed	Not assessed	22
Malposition	Not assessed	Not assessed	Not assessed	4
Arrhythmia	Not assessed	Not assessed	Not assessed	Uncommon
Cardiac arrest	Not assessed	Not assessed	Not assessed	<1
Venous air embolism	Not assessed	Not assessed	Not assessed	<1
Total	6.3–11.8	6.2–10.7	12.8–19.4	

[a] McGee, D.C., Gould, M.K., *N. Engl. J. Med.*, 2348, 1123–1133, 2003.
[b] Safdar, N., Maki, D.G., *Intensive Care Med.*, 30, 62–67, 2004.

patient's central veins is needed, particularly in those with a history of prior central venous catheters. This can be established by Doppler ultrasound of the major neck vessels and upper torso vessels and, when needed, other large vessels being considered for access [33].

The specifics of the technique of inserting both PICC and other central venous access catheters are beyond the scope of this chapter. For the interested reader, the following references will provide more details [19–23,33]. Placement of catheters is not a benign event, and overall complication rates range from 15% to 33%. Table 27.1 lists central venous catheter insertion-related complications and additional mechanical complications associated with catheter insertion. Risk factors for procedure-related complications include not using ultrasound guidance for the puncture, placement in an emergent setting, use of less experienced personnel, and attempting access in locations of prior catheterization or partially occlusive thrombus [19–23,33,34]. In some instances, the relative frequency and type of complications are also related to the location and type of catheter being placed. In general, the frequency of all complications is reduced by greater operator experience.

When selecting the vessel through which the central venous access will be attained, a recipient's personal preference, dominant hand, history with catheters, and outcomes with these must be considered in the decision process. If a patient has a preference for a subcutaneous port versus tunneled catheter, this too must be considered in the planning for access. Although no randomized data in the PN literature exist to suggest greater safety of tunneled central venous access compared with ports, there are data in the oncology literature to suggest that ports and tunneled catheters have similar rates of complications [35]. As such, personal preference, local experience, and assistance at home are used to determine the preferred option [36].

EDUCATION AND CATHETER MANAGEMENT FOR THOSE WITH CENTRAL LINES

The Centers for Disease Control and Prevention (CDC) have outlined a series of recommendations for reducing the risk for catheter-related infections [37]. These include the following:

- Educate healthcare personnel regarding the indications for intravascular catheter use, proper procedures for the insertion and maintenance of intravascular catheters, and appropriate infection control measures to prevent intravascular catheter-related infections.

- Periodically assess knowledge of and adherence to guidelines for all personnel involved in the insertion and maintenance of intravascular catheters.
- Designate only trained personnel who demonstrate competence for the insertion and maintenance of peripheral and central intravascular catheters.

Beyond this, home PN patients, home health organizations associated with PN management, hospital centers managing PN patients, and care partners of home PN patients should be instructed on proper central line management. Specific recommendations might vary depending on the type and location of the catheter. When accessing the catheter either at home or in the healthcare setting, it is critical that the highest standard of catheter care is followed and a consistency to line care practice is maintained (i.e., the same steps should be followed each and every time). Figure 27.4 illustrates appropriate care for the exit site dressing. On average, this process takes between 5 and 7 minutes.

When handling the central line, patients, caregivers, and medical personnel should observe hand hygiene guidelines, including washing hands with soap and water and using sterile gloves prior to line access. Additionally, it has been suggested that access caps be scrubbed with 2% chlorhexidine gluconate in 70% isopropyl alcohol, which is allowed to rest for 40 seconds [13]. Accessing implanted ports requires the use of an aseptic technique, and supervised training is necessary. Centers placing ports are responsible for providing patients with education, training, and subsequent review of this important practice. Central venous catheters should be flushed with normal saline before and after use with a 10 mL syringe. For flushing, new syringes should be used only once, and a new syringe should be used for each lumen in the situation where more than one lumen is present and to be accessed.

LONG-TERM COMPLICATIONS OF CATHETERS: INFECTIONS

Catheter-related infections are the most common complication of long-term indwelling central venous catheters. Catheter-related infections are categorized by the principal site of infection, and management differs based upon the site. The infection categories are as follows:

- Exit site—cellulitis around the exit site without evidence of tenderness or erythema tracking along the tunneled catheter;
- Tunnel and cuff infection—tenderness, generally accompanied by inflammation, along the tunneled portion of the catheter; this may be associated with exit site inflammation;
- Catheter colonization—positive cultures from the central line in absence of clinical or laboratory evidence of infection; and
- CRBSI—bacteremia associated with clinical and laboratory evidence of infection.

CRBSIs are generally considered the most serious complication of PN and occur at a rate of 0.3 to 2.5 infections per catheter-year and account for 61% of all complications in PN [38,39]. Metastatic infections including septic thrombophlebitis and infective endocarditis may result from CRBSI. In all, the administration of PN is independently associated with an increased risk of bacteremia and sepsis as compared with those with intestinal resection who are enterally rather than parenterally fed. Risk factors identified for exit site, tunnel, and CRBSIs are listed in Table 27.2.

There are several points of importance for the prevention of catheter-related infections. The first of these is the insertion procedure and adhering to principles outlined previously. The reason for this is that insertion of a central venous catheter introduces a foreign object into a vessel, and around this object, a biofilm quickly develops. The formation of this biofilm begins as soon as the catheter is inserted and involves adhesion of plasma proteins, platelets, neutrophils, and fibrin to the catheter surface [40–42]. These patient-derived materials form a substrate that is conducive to bacterial attachment and subsequent growth while resistant to penetration by some commonly used antibiotics such as vancomycin. Once bacteria are fixed to the device, additional formation within

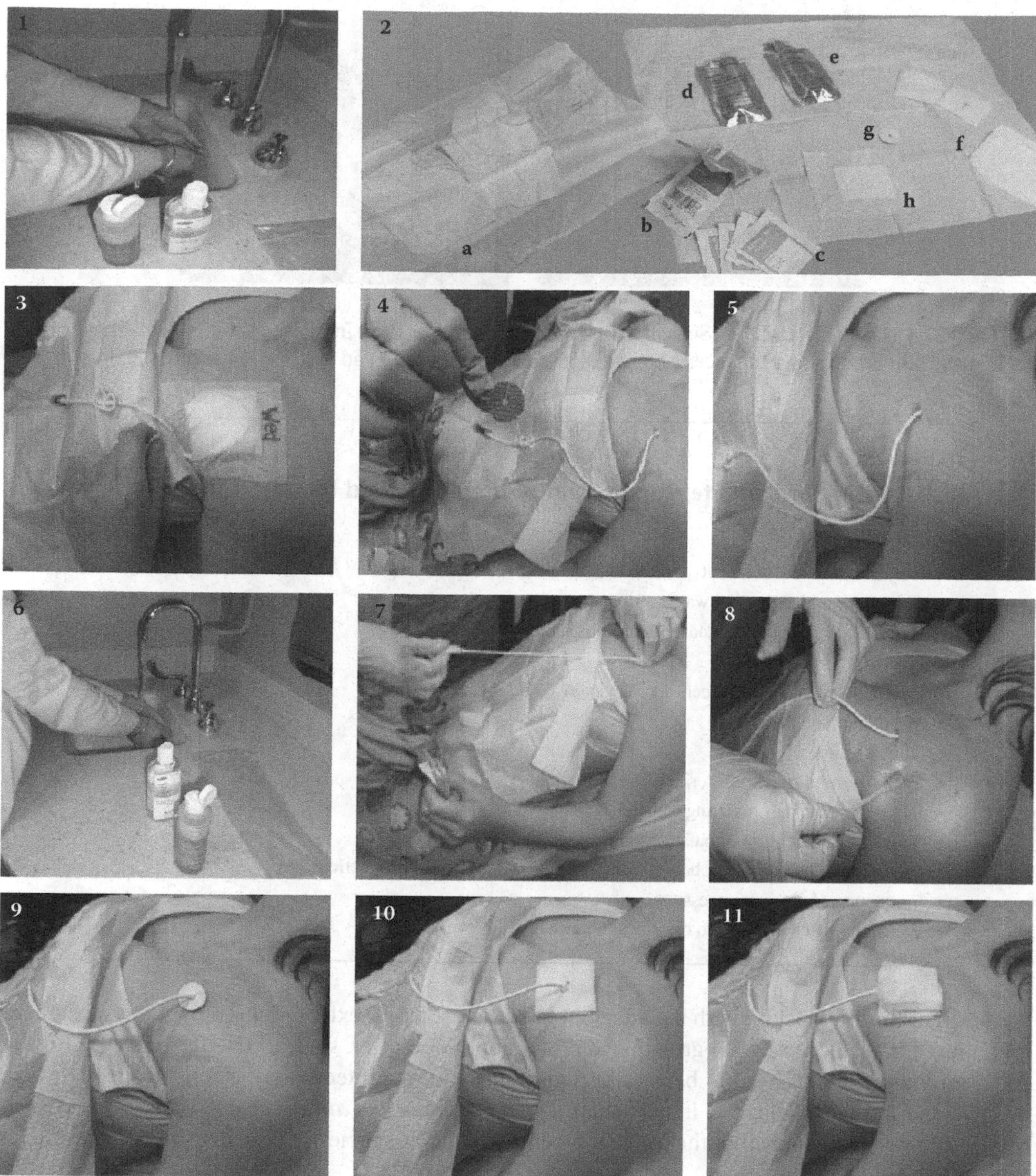

FIGURE 27.4 **(See color insert.)** Procedure for dressing change. 1. Hands should be thoroughly scrubbed for 40–60 seconds with soap after CDC hand hygiene guidelines. 2. The materials necessary for the dressing change are organized on a clean surface and sterile sheet: a. sterile gloves, b. skin barrier film, c. alcohol wipes, d. alcohol swab, e. chlorhexidine or povidone-iodine swabs, f. gauze pads, and g. chlorhexidine gluconate (CHG) impregnated disk. 3. Remove dressing. 4. Remove CHG-impregnated disk. 5. Inspect and palpate exit site and tunnel. 6. Repeat hand-washing procedure, then don sterile gloves. 7. Clean line with 70% alcohol wipe. 8. Prep area by first lightly scrubbing with the chlorhexidine (or povidone-iodine) swabs provided no allergy or hypersensitivity to these, and use all three swabs, working in circular motions, beginning at the exit site and radiating out to clean the area. Then, repeat with the 70% alcohol swabs, allowing the area to dry in between. Apply the skin barrier film using the same technique. Allow film to dry. 9. Apply the CHG disk around the catheter, noting which side of the disk should contact the skin. 10. Apply the gauze pad with a hole for the catheter. 11. A second gauze pad is placed on top. *(Continued)*

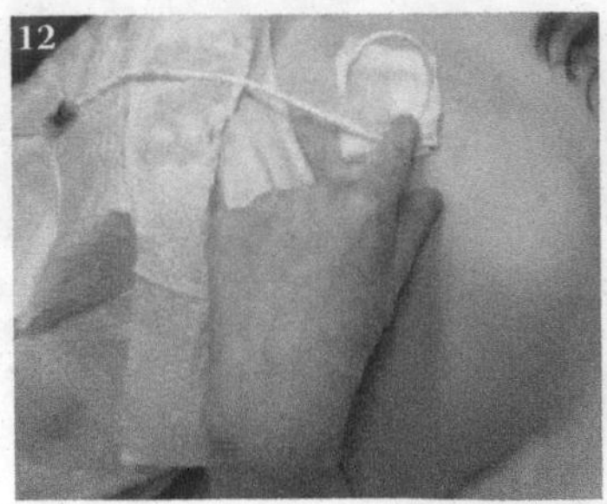

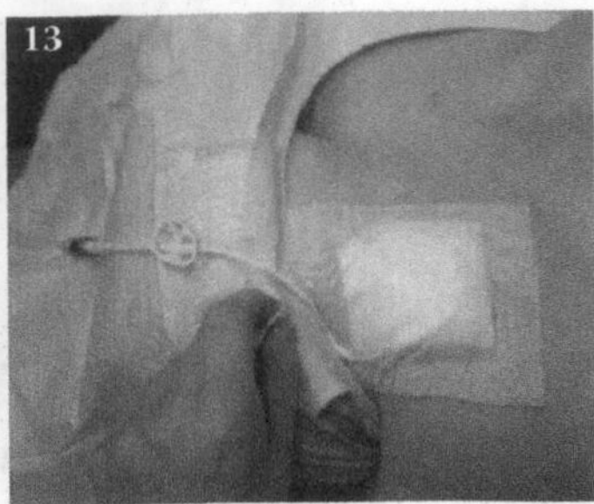

FIGURE 27.4 (CONTINUED) **(See color insert.)** Procedure for dressing change. 12. Patient's finger holds back of the second dressing in place. 13. A final outer adhesive gauze pad is placed to secure the dressing.

TABLE 27.2
Risk Factors for Exit Site, Tunnel, and Catheter-Related Bloodstream Infections

Risk Factors

- Duration of line placement
- Context in which the line was inserted
- Primary disease (e.g., fistulas, pseudo-obstruction)
- Line location (femoral)
- Prior history of access infection or thrombosis
- More than one lumen
- Uncuffed lines
- Lack of use of maximal sterile barrier technique
- Inexperienced staff inserting catheters
- Insufficient education of patient's family members or staff
- Improper technique as applied to catheter exit site care or PN connection
- Frequency of catheter access
- Proximity of central line to ostomy appliance

the original biofilm occurs, with the adherent bacteria excreting extracellular polymeric substances that allow for further bacterial growth and protection. Soon after, signs of CRBSI typically follow. As mentioned previously, this bacterially modified biofilm protects the bacteria from both host defense and antibiotic therapy, in particular the *Staphylococcus aureus* species, and is the reason for the compulsory removal of the catheter for this particular species of organism along with fungal species [40,42].

Infection Diagnosis

Clinical signs are the clue to identifying exit site and tunnel infections. Early diagnosis of these types of catheter infections is important as it presents an opportunity for line salvage and may prevent the more serious CRBSI. Patients, as part of their line care training, should be taught about these infections and to notify their care provider should these signs develop. To identify infections early, the exit site of the catheter should be visually inspected during dressing changes and the tunneled portion of the catheter palpated with any dressing change and with patient–physician clinical encounters. When an exit site infection is identified early, these rarely require line removal. In contrast, tunnel infections generally require removal. Unfortunately, CRBSIs often lack localizing clinical signs before the onset of symptoms and evidence of exit site and tunnel infections is not often present [41,43,44]. In all cases of new or worsening liver enzymes, in particular markers of cholestasis, in cases of unexplained pyrexia, chills, or malaise in the patient on PN, and when symptoms similar to a previous CRBSI occur in a patient on PN, a CRBSI must be suspected. Suspected exit site infections should be further assessed by culture of exit site drainage; however, given the potential for contamination by skin organisms, the organism cultured may not always reflect the culprit [44].

For proper diagnosis of CRBSI, simultaneous blood cultures from the catheter and a peripheral vein are helpful with time to a positive culture on the peripheral blood correlated with risk of line infection being present. For a defined CRBSI, either a greater than threefold increased colony count for the catheter sample or detection of growth 2 hours sooner for the catheter sample as compared with the peripheral sample is sufficient to establish the catheter as the source of the infection [45–47]. Caution must be exercised in attributing an infection to a catheter as the complicated nature of patients with PN-dependent intestinal failure reminds us that other sources of origin for bacteremia must always be considered, in particular in those with a history of multiple complicated abdominal surgeries and those in the early postoperative period. If the catheter is removed for a suspected CRBSI, a definitive diagnosis can be made by quantitative or semiquantitative culture of the catheter tip and the subcutaneous/tunneled portion of the catheter. It is critically important to note that almost one-third of patients presenting with a CRBSI do not present with a fever, and these infections are often heralded by laboratory abnormalities such as a fall in serum albumin from baseline or a rise in bilirubin above the previous baseline; less than a third have an elevated white blood cell count [44].

Infection Treatment

In instances of catheter infection, replacing the catheter with a new catheter over a guidewire is strongly discouraged [47,48]. In contrast, repairing the broken or malfunctioning catheter with a preprepared catheter repair kit is quite acceptable when there is no evidence of infection [47]. In instances where subsequent catheter tip cultures turn out to be positive in catheters that were exchanged, one should review the organism, identify if the organism is a suspected skin contaminant acquired during catheter removal by assessing the semiquantitative culture of the rolled tip, and consider a new catheter and insertion site in instances where a true infection is identified [49,50]. When performing a guidewire catheter exchange, the same maximum sterile barrier (see the "Prevention of Catheter-Related Infections" section) technique employed for an initial catheter insertion must be followed. A definitive treatment strategy for any catheter-related infection is removal of the catheter coupled to an empiric duration of IV antibiotics based upon the pathogen isolated and sensitivities identified. In all types of catheter-related infections, be it exit site or CRBSIs, oral antibiotics play no role in the management as the bioavailability of these in patients with intestinal failure precludes reliable systemic levels of antibiotics in these patients. If the infection is localized to the exit site only, initial management can be a topical antimicrobial therapy (e.g., mupirocin and clotrimazole), with the selection of an antibiotic guided by the sensitivities identified in the culture analysis of the swabbed exit site. When this approach is used, it is important that the patient remain under close clinical follow-up as risk for treatment failure leading to a more significant infection must not be ignored. In all other instances, IV antibiotics are generally sufficient to treat the infection and allow salvage of the existing catheter leaving line removal to refractory or recurrent infections. Of note, should the catheter be displaced or should the cuff become exposed, the central line should be removed. Finally, with CRBSIs, there can be the ability to salvage the catheter with IV antibiotics and without catheter removal in certain settings. Such cases are generally limited to the absence of overt sepsis, those where vascular patency is in no way compromised on ultrasound Doppler of the catheter, when the infection responds rapidly to IV antibiotics, and where the organism involved in the CRBSI is not recurrent and with sensitivities that support a reasonable probability for successful clearance. To assist in treating these infections, antibiotic locks may be considered (see below).

The type of catheter and site of infection also play a role in determining the most appropriate treatment. For nontunneled catheters, ESPEN guidelines [13] recommend catheter removal for cases where any of the following is present: erythema, pus at the exit site, clinical signs of septic shock, positive culture from a guidewire exchanged catheter, or positive paired blood cultures (i.e., positive cultures from both catheter-drawn and peripherally drawn blood). As with nontunneled catheters, tunneled and subcutaneous port catheters should be removed in cases of septic shock or metastatic infection. Additionally, these long-term catheters should be removed when paired blood cultures identify a fungal infection, *S. aureus* infection, or highly virulent bacteria such as a *Pseudomonas* species. In the absence of these aforementioned conditions and as outlined previously, an attempt may be made to salvage the catheter with or without use of an antimicrobial lock therapy in combination with systemic antibiotics [13]. It is to be noted that antibiotic lock therapy is complementary to systemic therapy and has been demonstrated to improve the likelihood of successfully eradicating CRBSI when used in combination with systemic antimicrobials. Antibiotic locks are not effective alone for clearing CRBSIs, and despite reports from single center case series, their role in preventing recurrent CRBSIs in long-term catheters is not established and cannot be recommended at this time [13]. High concentrations of antimicrobials for a dwell time of at least 12 hours and total duration of 14 days is a common approach employed for treating bacterial CRBSI [13]. If the salvage of an existing catheter is being considered, cultures should be repeated at 72 hours, at the end of treatment, and after completion of treatment. Ethanol locks have also been utilized in the setting of active infection, where 70% ethanol is left to dwell for 12–24 hours daily for 1–5 days. In one study, ethanol lock therapy led to 90% cure and 84% line salvage rates when used concurrently with systemic antibiotic therapy [51]. Close clinical follow-up is recommended.

The antibiotic to be used in the setting of a CRBSI should be guided by culture and prior organism sensitivity in those with a history of CRBSI, or the sensitivities on the current cultures when available. In the absence of cultures at the time of presentation, the antibiotic selection is best guided by prior positive cultures and a likely source of contamination, be it skin, site of a systemic source such as teeth, or gastrointestinal infection and prior antibiotic exposure. In instances of recurrent infections or in those with a history of significant resistance patterns, an infectious disease consultation should also be considered. Should a catheter removal occur in the setting of negative blood cultures and signs of ongoing infection, semiquantitative cultures should be obtained from the catheter tip at the time of removal to potentially assist in guiding therapy.

The duration of antimicrobial treatment should generally be longer for patients with persistent bacteremia >72 hours after catheter removal and longer in all cases where a conservative approach to CRBSIs is being followed and clinically the patient has failed to improve 48 hours after the offending line was removed. When catheter removal is required, temporary access should be obtained and, in this setting, a PICC is often used. In addition, when signs of infection persist beyond 48 hours, echocardiographic evaluation of the heart should also be considered; in instances of *S. aureus*, this is mandatory. It is recommended that for treatment of CRBSIs requiring line removal, a temporary source for PN administration be attained and a dual-lumen catheter placed for PN and antibiotic administration.

A final point to emphasize with long-term catheters relates to loss of vascular access. With any loss of a central vascular access site, a comprehensive review for cause is required and, following this, in instances where contributing factors are identified, a revision to clinical practices of the line or patient management implemented. The most common reason underlying access loss is infection, and catheter management practices in this setting must be reviewed. A less common cause of access loss is a hypercoagulable state, and a clue to this is a history of thrombotic events. These are usually identified in the patient's medical record. When identified, these disorders require hematology consultation, and the disorders present unique challenges and often limited therapeutic options in the patient with short bowel syndrome (SBS). In instances where more than two central venous access sites have been lost, referral to a center of excellence in PN care and intestinal transplantation is warranted. Finally, when placing catheters in the setting of procoagulant disorders, in particular where anticoagulation is in place prior to access being revised, anticoagulation management around the time of the procedure may be quite complex. In this setting, communication between the various groups managing the patient is important, and bridging of anticoagulation is generally recommended. It is also recommended in this setting that an expert is consulted for direction on periprocedure anticoagulation.

Prevention of Catheter-Related Infections

Attempts to prevent infections in central venous catheters in the setting of PN require that five main areas be addressed: catheter selection, catheter placement procedure, catheter maintenance, social issues, and other risk factors for bacteremia (Table 27.3).

Short-term, nontunneled catheters are susceptible to extraluminal colonization of the catheter by common skin microorganisms. It has been shown that proper antiseptic preparation of the insertion site using chlorhexidine gluconate solution reduces the risk of CRBSI and catheter colonization by 50% when compared with using povidone-iodine solution [52]. In addition to proper skin preparation, maximal sterile barrier (MSB) precautions are recommended. MSB precautions include use of cap, mask, sterile gown, sterile gloves, and a sterile full body drape. In a study comparing MSB precautions with use of sterile glove and a small drape, MSB resulted in lower rates of both catheter colonization and CRBSI.

Intraluminal colonization of the catheter has been shown to be the prominent cause of infections in catheters that have been in place for approximately 30 or more days [53]. Intraluminal colonization is believed to arise from bacteria that have entered through the catheter; thus, these infections may occur as a result of a contaminated infusate, contamination of connectors/hubs, excessive access to the hub, or inadvertent failure with catheter care leading to contamination.

Antimicrobial lock solutions have been shown to be effective at reducing catheter colonization and CRBSI, although the level of evidence is of low quality [42]. A lock solution contains a compound with antimicrobial activity, which is "locked" in the catheter for a time period rarely exceeding a day. The solution itself is held within the lumen of the catheter by the catheter's locking valve and resides between this point and the external hub that connects to the PN infusion cannulas. Various antimicrobials have been evaluated, with no single solution emerging as a best option and each antimicrobial solution having advantages and disadvantages, which vary based on catheter type and the suspected microorganism [54]. An important deficiency of all antimicrobial lock solutions is that the antimicrobial is within the tube and is therefore not active against biofilms that reside outside the catheter wall. A review of randomized controlled trials evaluating taurolidine lock solutions indicates that taurolidine results in lower rates of CRBSI and does not impact the rate of thrombosis [55]. The use of several antibiotics (including aminoglycosides, vancomycin, daptomycin, and tigecycline) in lock solutions has also been evaluated. These studies, including the taurolidine randomized trials, seem to be limited in number and sample size, but in general, the effectiveness of antibiotics in lock solutions seems to be species dependent. Larger prospective

TABLE 27.3
Prevention of Catheter-Related Infections

Areas to Be Addressed for Preventing Infections

- Ensure highest standard of clinical care during line insertion
- Appropriate care and maintenance of indwelling catheters
- Address any active issues in patients that present risk for bacteremia, such as:
  - Incompletely treated perirectal abscess in a patient with Crohn's disease
  - Acute allograft rejection in the pediatric patient with an intestinal transplant
  - Open or infected surgical wounds
- Appropriate catheter selection
- Social issues: insurance, illicit drug use, social support

in vivo studies are needed before definitive recommendations can be made. For more information on this subject, we recommend the 2015 review article by Vassallo et al. [54].

Ethanol as a lock solution has also been shown to be effective at preventing catheter infection, although the evidence to support this for routine prophylaxis is weak [37,41,56]. One advantage to ethanol locks is that they do not have specific microbial resistance issues and so provide a more pan-coverage. Although the ethanol lock appears to have some impact upon the biofilms, ethanol also may lead to damaging effects on polyurethane catheters; thus, ethanol locks should not be use with this type of central access (e.g., PICCs). Additionally, ethanol may result in a higher rate of catheter occlusion due to precipitation of plasma proteins, which occurs at concentrations of ≥28% ethanol [57]. In a review of studies from 2003 to 2013 by Tan et al. [51], ethanol locks were identified as effective for prophylaxis and treatment; however, in more recent reviews, evidence to recommend the routine use of ethanol locks remains insufficient [47,56,57]. Nevertheless, in pediatric patients experiencing recurrent line infections, the use of ethanol locks appears appropriate for secondary prevention [58,59]. In prevention studies, rates of infection were decreased by 53% to 91% using various ethanol lock regimens; use of 70% ethanol with a 2- to 4-hour dwell time daily was identified as the most effective approach [51].

Catheter Care

There are no data on the most effective dressing or optimal frequency of dressing change to reduce catheter-related infections. It is, however, important to keep the dressing adherent, clean, and dry and to change the dressing immediately should it become wet, disrupted, or dirtied. The use of topical antibiotics at catheter insertion sites is not recommended [41,43].

In addition to the gauze and tape dressing shown in Figure 27.4, polyurethane dressing has the advantages of requiring less frequent dressing changes (every 7 days compared with 2–3 days for gauze), and its transparency allows for visual inspection of the exit site without removing the dressing. Chlorhexidine-impregnated dressings or sponges (Biopatch) have been shown to reduce rates of catheter colonization and local infections. In managing the catheter hub during connection and disconnection of access to the catheter or port, the catheter hubs should be scrubbed using either 70% alcohol or 10% povidone iodine swabs before accessing. The skin overlying an implanted port should be scrubbed with chlorhexidine gluconate in alcohol prior to accessing. It is also recommended that catheter caps be changed every 5–7 days [42].

Catheter-Related Thrombosis

Central venous catheters disrupt blood flow and cause vascular trauma and inflammation and are therefore associated with a risk of thrombosis. Catheter-related thrombosis occurs at a rate 0.027 episodes per catheter per year. Larger and multilumen catheters are associated with an increased risk of thrombosis. To minimize risk in long-term PN users, single-lumen catheters are preferred. As stated previously, the catheter tip should be positioned between the lower third of the superior vena cava junction of the right atrium with the superior vena cava and the position confirmed by chest radiograph to further reduce the risk of thrombosis [13]. Catheter-related infections are the most common event leading to vascular thrombosis. In instances where thrombosis has occurred in the absence of a precipitant, we recommend evaluation for a hypercoagulable state. In instances where more than two access sites have been lost, this evaluation is critical. With axillary vein thrombosis, there is an 8–20% chance of pulmonary embolus and anticoagulation with a low-molecular-weight heparin is indicated with a recommended treatment duration of 3 months [60,61]. The limited data on the bioavailability of oral anticoagulants in SBS require cautious use in this setting. Catheter material also plays a role in thrombosis, with silicone and third generation polyurethane catheters associated with a lower risk of thrombosis than polyethylene or polyvinyl chloride (PVC) catheters [13]. Finally, in relation to catheter management in the setting of thrombosis, there are no specific recommendations, and the clinical context in which the thrombosis occurs must be considered. In situations where the catheter's function is compromised by the thrombosis or an active infection warrants removal of the catheter, removal should occur and an alternate site for temporary or permanent line placement is identified. In settings where partial thrombosis has occurred, a catheter might be removed and replaced at a different site or the catheter might remain in place and anticoagulation started. This most often occurs in settings where vascular access has become limited and the catheter remains functional.

Anticoagulants have been used prophylactically in an attempt to prevent thrombosis; however, their use is not supported by evidence from randomized trials. For instance, trials evaluating low-dose warfarin, unfractionated heparin, and low-molecular-weight heparin in cancer patients with central venous access indicate no consistent benefit [62–64]. There are, however, some data suggesting that both warfarin and low-molecular-weight heparin are equivalent in reducing thrombosis risk in individuals who are at an increased risk for thrombosis on long-term PN, although the data are quite limited [13].

Catheter Occlusion

Catheter occlusion is a broad term covering both partial and complete obstruction to the lumen of the central line. This occlusion limits or prevents the normal functioning of the catheter; 6.5% of PICCs and 1.8% of non-PICC central catheters will experience occlusion [64]. Catheter occlusion often occurs in the absence of vascular thrombosis, although occlusion is associated with an increased risk of CRBSI and catheter colonization. Signs of catheter occlusion include

- Inability to withdraw blood from the catheter or to flush the catheter;
- Increased resistance to flushing of the catheter and increasing frequency of alarms associated with PN or antibiotic infusions; and
- Slow infusion rate when the catheter is flushed.

If increased resistance to flushing or withdrawing blood is encountered, it is imperative that an attempt to overcome the resistance or clear the occlusion by excessively increasing the pressure on the syringe is avoided, the reason being that it is not of proven benefit and can result in damage or complete rupture to the catheter. The origin of catheter occlusions is divided into thrombotic and nonthrombotic types, with the thrombotic type accounting for approximately 60% of all occlusions [64,65]. The management of an occlusion is dependent on the occlusion type present and whether partial or complete. Figure 27.5 presents a flow diagram outlining an approach to the occluded catheter.

Blood reflux into the catheter lumen can lead to thrombus formation and occlusion. Appropriate flushing technique minimizes this risk. When flushing a catheter, both clamping under positive pressure and withdrawing the syringe while depressing the plunger and before the syringe is completely emptied lessen the probability of reflux into the catheter [64,66]. Most thrombotic occlusions can be cleared by administering alteplase [64]. Alteplase, a human tissue plasminogen activator, and urokinase are the best studied thrombolytics. Thrombolytics act by binding to fibrin within a thrombus and there convert the entrapped plasminogen to plasmin, which in turn degrades the fibrin matrix of the thrombus. Although the level of evidence generated from studies of thrombolytic therapies for catheter occlusions is limited by the quality of the studies [67], there is clearly a role for these agents in light of the fact that greater morbidity is derived from catheter replacement. Alteplase is typically administered in a dose of 2 mg/2 mL instilled as a 2-mL dose or to 110% of the catheter volume, if less than 2 mL, with a dwell time of 120 minutes. The thrombolytic is then aspirated and the catheter flushed [68].

Nonthrombotic sources of catheter occlusion include mechanical (kinking), drug/mineral precipitates, and lipid residue deposits [65,66]. In line with the origin of the mechanical problems previously

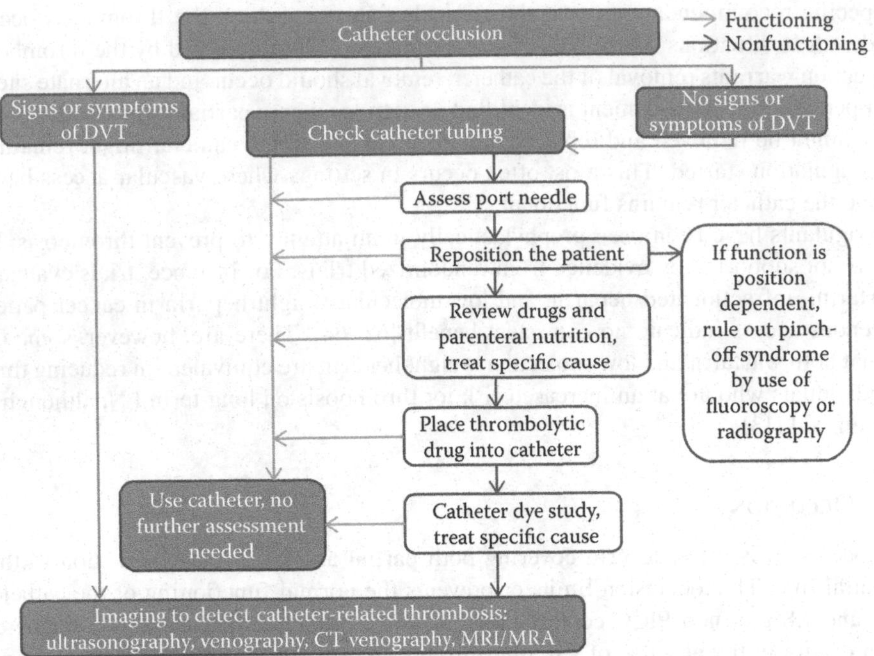

FIGURE 27.5 **(See color insert.)** Clinical algorithm approach to catheter occlusion.

described, prevention remains the most important management tool. Occlusion due to compression of the catheter between the clavicle and first rib is known as "catheter pinch-off syndrome" and should be suspected when a history of intermittent occlusion related to patient positioning is identified. To diagnose this syndrome, radiological contrast studies are needed and management usually consists of replacing the catheter through a different path of insertion. Drug and mineral occlusions are generally cleared by filling the catheter with solutions that generate chemical reactions designed to dissolve the precipitant that led to the occlusion. To clear mineral and some basic drug precipitates (i.e., those resulting from acidic drugs), including vancomycin precipitate and calcium phosphate (products in PN), 0.1 N hydrochloric acid is used [68–70]. Sodium bicarbonate is used to clear acidic precipitates of basic drugs, while lipid accumulations within catheters are best cleared with 70% ethanol [70]. It cannot be overemphasized that the optimal approach to occlusions is prevention, and fortunately, they have become quite uncommon in the modern PN era. The risk of catheter occlusion can be minimized by proper flushing techniques, avoiding administering solutions that appear cloudy, and use of a 1.2-μm filter when infusing three-in-one PN solutions.

CONCLUSION

The central venous catheter represents what could aptly be described as the "Achilles Heel" of parenteral support. Over the last 20 years, significant advances have been made in our knowledge of this vulnerability, and through this knowledge as outlined in this chapter, a variety of techniques are available to diminish line-related complications. Also described in this chapter are ways to approach the more common clinical aspects of the central venous access device, including line selection, insertion site selection, early identification of line-related complications, management of these complications, and, most importantly, prevention of these complications. Healthcare providers managing patients on PN should develop an intimate understanding of the principles outlined previously, as it is only through application of this knowledge that the associated morbidity and mortality associated with PN may be reduced or eliminated.

REFERENCES

1. Dudrick SJ et al. Long-term total parenteral nutrition with growth, development, and positive nitrogen balance. *Surgery* 1968;**64**:134–142.
2. Ryan JA et al. Catheter complications in total parenteral nutrition. *N Engl J Med* 1974;**290**:757–761.
3. Sutton CD et al. The introduction of a nutrition clinical nurse specialist results in a reduction in the rate of catheter sepsis. *Clin Nutr* 2005;**24**:220–223.
4. Bozetti F et al. Central venous catheter complications in 447 patients on home parenteral nutrition: An analysis of over 100,000 catheter days. *Clin Nutr* 2002;**21**:475–485.
5. Shirotani N et al. Complications of central venous catheters in patients on home parenteral nutrition: An analysis of 68 patients over 16 years. *Surg Today* 2006;**36**:420–424.
6. Grant JP. Anatomy and physiology of venous system vascular access: Implications. *JPEN J Parenter Enteral Nutr* 2006;**30**:S7–S12.
7. Rodrigues, AF et al. Management of end-stage central venous access in children referred for possible small bowel transplantation. *J Pediatr Gastroenterol Nutr* 2006;**42**:427–433.
8. Mortell A et al. Transhepatic central venous catheter for long-term access in paediatric patients. *J Pediatr Surg* 2008;**43**:344–347.
9. Detering SM et al. Direct right atrial insertion of a Hickman catheter in an 11-year-old girl. *Interact Cardiovasc Thorac Surg* 2011;**12**:321–322.
10. Yaacob Y et al. The vanishing veins: Difficult venous access in a patient requiring translumbar, transhepatic, and transcollateral central catheter insertion. *Malays J Med Sci MJMS* 2011;**18**:98–102.
11. Versleijen MWJ et al. Arteriovenous fistulae as an alternative to central venous catheters for delivery of long-term home parenteral nutrition. *Gastroenterology* 2009;**136**:1577–1584.
12. Fuchs S et al. Central venous catheter mechanical irritation of the right atrial free wall: A cause for thrombus formation. *Cardiology* 1999;**91**:169–172.
13. Pittiruti M et al. ESPEN guidelines on parenteral nutrition: Central venous catheters (access, care, diagnosis and therapy of complications). *Clin Nutr* 2009;**28**:365–377.
14. Kane KF et al. High osmolality feedings do not increase the incidence of thrombophlebitis during peripheral i.v. nutrition. *JPEN J Parenter Enteral Nutr* 1996;**20**:194–197.
15. Hoffmann E. A randomised study of central versus peripheral intravenous nutrition in the perioperative period. *Clin Nutr* 1989;**8**:179–180.
16. Boullat JI et al. A.S.P.E.N. clinical guidelines: Parenteral nutrition ordering, order review, compounding, labeling, and dispensing. *JPEN J Parenter Enteral Nutr* 2014;**38**:334–377.
17. Gura KM. Is there still a role for peripheral parenteral nutrition? *Nutr Clin Pract* 2009;**24**:709–717.
18. Calvert N et al. Ultrasound for central venous cannulation: Economic evaluation of cost-effectiveness. *Anaesthesia* 2004;**59**:1116–1120.
19. McGee DC, Gould MK. Preventing complications of central venous catheterization. *N Engl J Med* 2003;**348**:1123–1133.
20. NICE Technology Appraisal No 49: Guidance on the use of ultrasound locating devices for placing central venous catheters. 2002. Available at http://www.nice.org.uk/guidance/ta49/resources/guidance-guidance-on-the-use-of-ultrasound-locating-devices-for-placing-central-venous-catheters-pdf.
21. Bowen ME et al. Image-guided placement of long-term central venous catheters reduces complications and cost. *Am J Surg* 2014;**208**:937–941; discussion 941.
22. Bodenham AR. Can you justify not using ultrasound guidance for central venous access? *Crit Care Lond Engl* 2006;**10**:175.
23. Dariushnia SR et al. Quality improvement guidelines for central venous access. *J Vasc Interv Radiol* 2010;**21**:976–981.
24. Chopra V et al. The risk of bloodstream infection associated with peripherally inserted central catheters compared with central venous catheters in adults: A systematic review and meta-analysis. *Infect Control Hosp Epidemiol* 2013;**34**:908–918.
25. Seckold TL et al. A comparison of silicone and polyurethane PICC lines and postinsertion complication rates: A systematic review. *J Vasc Access* 2015;**16**(3):167–177.
26. Botella-Carretero JI et al. Role of peripherally inserted central catheters in home parenteral nutrition: A 5-year prospective study. *JPEN J Parenter Enteral Nutr* 2013;**37**:544–549.
27. Piper HG et al. Peripherally inserted central catheters for long-term parenteral nutrition in infants with intestinal failure. *J Pediatr Gastroenterol Nutr* 2013;**56**:578–581.
28. McKee R et al. Does antibiotic prophylaxis at the time of catheter insertion reduce the incidence of catheter-related sepsis in intravenous nutrition? *J Hosp Infect* 1985;**6**:419–425.

29. Ranson MR et al. Double-blind placebo controlled study of vancomycin prophylaxis for central venous catheter insertion in cancer patients. *J Hosp Infect* 1990;**15**:95–102.
30. Ljungman P et al. Peroperative teicoplanin for prevention of gram-positive infections in neutropenic patients with indwelling central venous catheters: A randomized, controlled study. *Support Care Cancer* 1997;**5**:485–488.
31. Saint S. Evidence Report/Technology Assessment Number 43. In *Making Healthcare Safer: A Critical Analysis of Patient Safety Practices.* Agency for Healthcare Research and Quality, AHRQ Publication 01-E058. Managing Editor Markowitz AJ. Rockville. MD. 2001, pp. 163–183.
32. Safdar N, Maki DG. The pathogenesis of catheter-related bloodstream infection with noncuffed short-term central venous catheters. *Intensive Care Med* 2004;**30**:62–67.
33. Ortega R et al. Ultrasound-guided internal jugular vein cannulation. *N Engl J Med* 2010;**362**:e57.
34. Eisen LA et al. Mechanical complications of central venous catheters. *J Intensive Care Med* 2006;**21**:40–46.
35. White AD et al. Implantable versus cuffed external central venous catheters for the management of children and adolescents with acute lymphoblastic leukaemia. *Pediatr Surg Int* 2012;**28**:1195–1199.
36. Van de Wetering MD et al. In *Cochrane Database of Systematic Reviews*. New York: John Wiley & Sons, 2013;**11**:1–37. Available at http://onlinelibrary.wiley.com/doi/10.1002/14651858.CD003295.pub3 /abstract.
37. O'Grady NP. Guidelines for the prevention of intravascular catheter-related infections. 2011. Available at http://www.cdc.gov/hicpac/pdf/guidelines/bsi-guidelines-2011.pdf.
38. Van Gossum A et al. Clinical, social and rehabilitation status of long-term home parenteral nutrition patients: Results of a European multicentre survey. *Clin Nutr* 2001;**20**:205–210.
39. Lloyd DAJ et al. Survival and dependence on home parenteral nutrition: Experience over a 25-year period in a UK referral centre. *Aliment Pharmacol Ther* 2006;**24**:1231–1240.
40. Tokars JI et al. Prospective evaluation of risk factors for bloodstream infection in patients receiving home infusion therapy. *Ann Intern Med* 1999;**131**:340–347.
41. Mermel L et al. Clinical practice guidelines for the diagnosis and management of intravascular catheter-related infection: 2009 update by the Infectious Diseases Society of America. *Clin Infect Dis* 2009;**49**:1–45.
42. Yousif A et al. Biofilm-based central line-associated bloodstream infections. *Adv Exp Med Biol* 2015; **830**:157–179.
43. Ryder M. Evidence-based practice in the management of vascular access devices for home parenteral nutrition therapy. *J Parenter Enter Nutr* 2006;**30**:S82–S93.
44 Clare A et al. What information should lead to a suspicion of catheter sepsis in HPN? *Clin Nutr Edinb Scotl* 2008;**27**:552–556.
45. Raad I et al. Differential time to positivity: A useful method for diagnosing catheter-related bloodstream infections. *Ann Intern Med* 2004;**140**:18–25.
46. Blot F et al. Diagnosis of catheter-related bacteraemia: A prospective comparison of the time to positivity of hub-blood versus peripheral-blood cultures. *The Lancet* 1999;**354**:1071–1077.
47. The Joint Commission. Preventing Central Line-Associated Bloodstream Infections: A Global Challenge, a Global Perspective. 2012. Available at http://www.PreventingCLABSIs.pdf.
48. Parbat N et al. The microbiological and clinical outcome of guide wire exchanged versus newly inserted antimicrobial surface treated central venous catheters. *Crit Care* 2013;**17**:R184.
49. Bishop L et al. Guidelines on the insertion and management of central venous access devices in adults. *Int J Lab Hematol* 2007;**29**:261–278.
50. Schiavone PA et al. Management of catheter-related infection in patients receiving home parenteral nutrition. *Pract Gastroenterol* 2010;**34**:22–34.
51. Tan M et al. Ethanol locks in the prevention and treatment of catheter-related bloodstream infections. *Ann Pharmacother* 2014;**48**:607–615.
52. Chaiyakunapruk N et al. Chlorhexidine compared with povidone-iodine solution for vascular catheter-site care: A meta-analysis. *Ann Intern Med* 2002;**136**:792–801.
53. Mermel LA. What is the predominant source of intravascular catheter infections? *Clin Infect Dis* 2011;**52**:211–212.
54. Vassallo M et al. Antimicrobial lock therapy in central-line associated bloodstream infections: A systematic review. *Infection* 2015;**43**(4):389–398.
55. Liu Y et al. Taurolidine lock solutions for the prevention of catheter-related bloodstream infections: A systematic review and meta-analysis of randomized controlled trials. *PLoS ONE* 2013;**8**:e79417.

56. Wales PW et al. A.S.P.E.N. clinical guidelines support of pediatric patients with intestinal failure at risk of parenteral nutrition-associated liver disease. *JPEN J Parenter Enter Nutr* 2014;**38**:538–557.
57. Mermel LA, Alang N. Adverse effects associated with ethanol catheter lock solutions: A systematic review. *J Antimicrob Chemother* 2014;**69**:2611–2619.
58. Pieroni KP et al. Evaluation of ethanol lock therapy in pediatric patients on long-term parenteral nutrition. *Nutr Clin Pract* 2013;**28**:226–231.
59. Oliveira C et al. Ethanol locks to prevent catheter-related bloodstream infections in parenteral nutrition: A meta-analysis. *Pediatrics* 2012;**129**:318–329.
60. Prandoni P et al. The long term clinical course of acute deep vein thrombosis of the arm: Prospective cohort study. *BMJ* 2004;**329**:484–485.
61. Guyatt GH et al. Executive summary: Antithrombotic therapy and prevention of thrombosis, 9th ed: American College of Chest Physicians evidence-based clinical practice guidelines. *Chest* 2012;**141**:7S–47S.
62. Schiffer CA et al. Central venous catheter care for the patient with cancer: American Society of Clinical Oncology clinical practice guideline. *J Clin Oncol* 2013;**31**:1357–1370.
63. Brandão LR et al. Low molecular weight heparin for prevention of central venous catheterization-related thrombosis in children. *Cochrane Database Syst Rev* 2014;**10**:3.
64. Gorski LA. Central venous access device occlusions: Part 1: Thrombotic causes and treatment. *Home Healthc Nurse* 2003;**21**:115–121; quiz 122.
65. Gorski LA. Central venous access device occlusions: Part 2: Nonthrombotic causes and treatment. *Home Healthc Nurse* 2003;**21**:168–171; quiz 172–173.
66. Hadaway LC. Major thrombotic and nonthrombotic complications. Loss of patency. *J Intraven Nurs Off Publ Intraven Nurses Soc* 1998;**21**:S143–S160.
67. Van Miert C et al. Interventions for restoring patency of occluded central venous catheter lumens. *Cochrane Database Syst Rev* 2012;**4**:CD007119.
68. Baskin JL et al. Management of occlusion and thrombosis associated with long-term indwelling central venous catheters. *Lancet* 2009;**374**:159–169.
69. Kerner JA et al. Treatment of catheter occlusion in pediatric patients. *JPEN J Parenter Enteral Nutr* 2006;**30**:S73–S81.
70. Werlin SL et al. Treatment of central venous catheter occlusions with ethanol and hydrochloric acid. *JPEN J Parenter Enteral Nutr* 1995;**19**:416–418.

28 Meeting the Unmet Needs of Home Parenteral and Enteral Nutrition Consumers

Education, Networking, and Support

Darlene G. Kelly, Joan Bishop, and Harlan Johnson

CONTENTS

KEY POINTS

- The need for home parenteral nutrition or enteral nutrition is a potential threat to normal longevity and quality of life.
- Support groups may be instrumental in helping patients adapt to new challenges that arise with various chronic disease states, including short bowel syndrome.
- This chapter provides information about reliable resources that might be helpful to those with short bowel syndrome.
- Similar not-for-profit home nutrition support organizations exist in other countries offering an opportunity to affiliate internationally, thus broadening resources, helping members to travel outside local areas, and facilitating the exchange of information.

INTRODUCTION

The events that lead up to the need for home parenteral nutrition (PN) or home enteral nutrition (EN) are frequently catastrophic for the patient and family, leaving them bewildered, helpless, and with a feeling of being alone. Very few individuals receiving these therapies know another person who requires home PN or home EN for survival, and often, the supporting clinical team does not either. Support groups may be instrumental in helping patients adapt to new challenges that arise with various chronic diseases, including short bowel syndrome (SBS). This chapter will highlight the experiences of one such support group with this patient population.

THE OLEY FOUNDATION

The Oley Foundation for Home Parenteral and Enteral Nutrition is a not-for-profit organization located at Albany Medical Center in New York that is celebrating 31 years of continuously serving consumers of home PN and home EN. It has more than 15,000 members (primarily from the

United States and Canada) consisting of persons receiving home PN and home EN, their caregivers, clinicians, and members from industry. The following are excerpts from a discussion among Oley's advisor for science and medicine (DK), the president (HJ), and the executive director (JB). Interspersed are comments received from home PN and home EN consumers, caregivers, and clinicians that are relevant to the text and are available on the Oley website [1]. The identifying names have been deleted.

DK: I asked the Oley president, Harlan Johnson, about the patient's and family's feelings early in the home PN experience.

HJ: My wife, Mary, had been on home PN for more than 35 years. She had not only been kept alive by the nutrition support but also she had a full life because of home PN. She had Crohn's disease with resulting short bowel syndrome (SBS) due to multiple intestinal resections. She described in a previously published article that with the benefit of home PN, the support of friends, excellent medical care, and a loving family, she was able to pursue a career, complete an advanced degree, work, buy a home, get married, and enjoy life [2]. In the article, she mentioned the importance of contact with others who had similar needs through the Oley Foundation. Oley introduced her "to a wealth of survivor stories—individuals who rise to meet challenges and face what could be debilitating circumstances with courage and style."

DK: Harlan mentioned that Mary's jejunostomy was her main challenge, and that it was always on her mind…she would have traded it "for anything." She never told anyone about her illness—not friends, not family, and she only told Harlan after 6 months of dating prior to their marriage. It was critical to her that she did not let her illness define her. Harlan described that because of the Oley Foundation, Mary felt free to share information with other attendees about her SBS, the jejunostomy, and the underlying Crohn's disease.

Harlan recalled that the first time he attended an Oley conference with his wife, he was surprised to hear her comfortably speak with others at a roundtable discussion about techniques she had learned over the years for dealing with her ostomy appliance and home PN. He indicated that from that day on, he began to learn not only about new techniques but also how Mary felt about her condition. Mary told him that Oley meetings were the only place where she could speak about diarrhea while eating lunch and not offend people; instead, the attendees were interested in what was being said! Mary and Harlan attended more than 20 annual Oley meetings and continued to learn at least one new thing at each meeting.

Mary was elected Oley president in 2010 and served in that capacity until her death in 2014 from an infection unrelated to her home PN. Mary was fully supportive of the Oley Foundation mission, which is to enrich "the lives of those requiring home intravenous and tube feeding through education, outreach and networking" [3].

Parents of a child wrote this to Oley: "When my son suffered a mid-gut volvulus at the age of five, the lives of my entire family changed in an instant. We were frightened in our darkest hour, and the Oley Foundation reached out to help us" [1].

Another couple told us: "Discharged from the hospital at 5 weeks old, our daughter was accompanied by an IV catheter, surgically implanted into her chest, and a stoma in her stomach with an exiting G-tube that emptied into a colostomy bag. She infused TPN for 20 hours a day just to stay alive. In spite of this new lifestyle, I consider us to be the lucky ones…a family fortunate enough to have been introduced to the Oley Foundation, the life preserver for people who require enteral and parenteral nutrition. I can't even imagine repeating her first year without them" [1].

DK: I visited with Dr. Lyn Howard, the founder of the Oley Foundation and one of the earliest United States (U.S.) clinicians to manage patients on nutritional support in the home setting, to discuss the history of Oley.

LH: The foundation dates back to the early 1980s, when I recognized the impact of home PN on the lives of my patients and how few of them had an in-depth understanding of the therapy that sustained them. It was also apparent that very few in the medical community were aware of the ability to move this hospital therapy into the home setting. A gentleman on home PN, Clarence "Oley" Oldenburg, and I discussed the need for an organization for "HPEN'ers" (those on home PN and/or EN) that would not only provide education to the patients and clinicians but also offer support with the psychological aspects and address their need for networking with others living with similar challenges.

These comments came from the parents of a young home PN consumer: "Through this invaluable organization, we learned what we needed most—how to improve our son's care and improve his outcome. Oley gave us support. Finally, here were families and experts who understood the challenges we faced… Over and over the experts available through Oley taught us the critical importance of sterile technique, how to carefully monitor his home PN, and countless details that have improved his life in ways we thought we could only dream of" [1].

DK: I have asked Joan Bishop, the executive director of Oley, to fill in more of the early story of the Foundation.

JB: From the beginning, the Board of Directors guiding Oley efforts consisted of a balance between patients, caregivers, clinicians from relevant disciplines, and leaders from the public. It is believed that this model has kept our focus targeted on the needs, issues and concerns of the true recipients of our efforts…the HPEN "consumers" and families.

DK: One of the first people I managed on home PN made it clear to me that when she is hospitalized, she is a "patient" but at home, she is a home PN "consumer." Indeed, this is the way she lives her life.

JB: The small, dedicated staff and a network of committed volunteers contribute greatly to the success and growth of Oley's efforts. Sixty-four Oley Ambassadors (home nutrition support consumers or caregivers themselves) are scattered throughout the U.S. and the world. These volunteers understand the challenges that those requiring HPEN face and recognize the value of Oley resources and connections. They freely share personal experiences, Oley information, and a positive outlook and provide a sense of community. Their contributions are integral to Oley efforts. The Foundation's medical director and advisor for science and medicine, both physicians with extensive experience in HPEN and chronic intestinal failure, provide insight and guidance to ensure that activity and efforts are appropriate. The staff enjoys close relationships with professional groups such as the American Society for Parenteral and Enteral Nutrition (A.S.P.E.N.), the American Vascular Association (AVA), the Intravenous Nurses Society (INS), as well as with the European Society for Clinical Nutrition and Metabolism (ESPEN), including the Home Artificial Nutrition and Chronic Intestinal Failure Work Group of ESPEN.

This comment came from a new home EN consumer: "I was really impressed with the knowledge, dedication, and professionalism of the Oley staff and the medical professionals who conducted the seminars/workshops. One thing that really impressed me was the chance to ask questions that related directly to my tube feeding in an open forum and also on a one-on-one basis with some of the nation's top medical personnel" [1] (Figure 28.1).

JB: Resources provided by the Oley Foundation include our website (http://www.oley.org), an equipment and product exchange program, a bimonthly newsletter (*LifelineLetter*), the volunteer network, connections to many home and healthcare providers, product manufacturers, and advocacy organizations and national and regional conferences. All of these position Oley to be an excellent and trusted source of information and support for the home PN and home EN community. Educational resources available through the Oley website include those for consumers of home PN and home EN, links to information for clinicians, complications charts for both types of feedings, information on enteral and

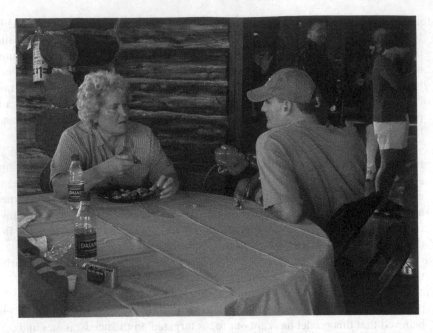

FIGURE 28.1 Dr. Lyn Howard, Oley medical director, discussing therapy with HPN parent/caregivers.

parenteral nutrition as well as on hydration, materials on traveling with these therapies, and materials on centers of experience with intestinal failure. Other professional and support groups have educational materials for clinicians, consumers, and caregivers (refer to the following list). Additionally, many of the infusion companies have educational materials for their consumers. There are published clinical guidelines on home PN from the Home Artificial Nutrition Work Group of ESPEN published in 2009 [4–6] and updated in 2015 [7] and from AuSPEN [8].

Professional and support groups with reliable educational materials available for clinicians and those with short bowel syndrome:

- Oley Foundation (http://www.oley.org)
- A.S.P.E.N. Clinical Guidelines (http://www.nutritioncare.org)
- ESPEN has updated Guidelines for Home Parenteral Nutrition and definition for Chronic Intestinal Failure forthcoming in 2015 (http://www.ESPEN.org)
- AuSPEN Clinical Guidelines (http://www.auspen.org.au)
- The National Institute of Diabetes and Digestive and Kidney Diseases (NIDDK) (http://www.niddk.nih.gov/health-information/health-topics/digestive-diseases/short-bowel-syndrome/Pages/facts.aspx)
- SBS Cure Project, which was developed to educate those with SBS and their families about treatments for short bowel syndrome (http://www.sbscure.org)
- Crohn's and Colitis Foundation for sample letters to appeal insurance issues (http://www.ccfa.org/science-and-professionals/programs-materials/appeal-letters/)
- Association for Vascular Access (materials available to members only)
- Intravenous Nurses Society (materials available to members only)
- Wound Ostomy & Continence Nurses Society (http://www.wocn.org)
- United Ostomy Associations of America (http://www.uoaa.org)
- Net of Care (http://www.netofcare.org)
- National Alliance for Caregiving (http://www.caregiving.org)

- National Family Caregivers Association (http://www.nfcacares.org)
- Family Caregiver Alliance (http://www.caregiver.org)

DK: A number of websites addressing a variety of health conditions are identified when one does a search for healthcare on the Internet. Care must be taken, however, when evaluating the veracity of these sites. When searching for websites, remember that for many search engines, the first few sites that are listed are typically paid advertisements. An article published in the Oley *LifelineLetter* gives pointers on how patient/consumers and others should critically read healthcare-related websites (http://oley.org/lifeline/Nutrition_and_You_Searching_the_Web.html) [9]. It is important to consider the source by observing the address: if it ends in .org, it is a not-for-profit organization, while .gov comes from the government, .edu is from an educational/academic institution, and .com is a commercial company. The .com locations generally have a primary role of selling a product or service, and usually, their educational material is dedicated to that role. The .org sites should be free of commercial influence, although this may not always be true. The educational materials in the .org sites should be carefully reviewed. The first questions about educational papers that should be considered are: Were the credentials of the author listed? Was educational material reviewed by qualified experts? Is there a medical or scientific advisor? The HONcode, sponsored by the Health on the Network Foundation, is an additional assurance that the not-for-profit websites have continual oversight to assure that they provide trustworthy medical information.

A parent of a consumer of HPEN said: "I LOVE, LOVE, LOVE getting the newsletter. It makes me feel connected, and not so alone" [1]!

Another consumer of Home PN noted that "The Oley newsletters are so interesting and helpful to me. From the intestinal centers to GLP-2 to what the blood tests mean—there is always something that I want to print up and save" [1].

Comments from the daughter of a consumer of home PN were as follows: "For the past number of years I have been receiving your *LifelineLetter*. When my mother was told that she would have to permanently feed through a Hickman line, she felt she could never cope. Here in Ireland I found it very hard to get any information and it was by going on the web I found out about your organization. It was like a lifeline for my family. Reading other peoples' stories and experiences, and seeing how well other people coped, gave my mother strength; she didn't feel like she was the only one having to live her life this way. Thank you for your newsletter. It helped a family greatly in their time of need" [1].

Several research studies have assessed the value of the Oley Foundation, demonstrating its importance for persons on home PN or home EN. Consumers of home PN and their families were the subject of a 1993 study by Smith [10], who interviewed 178 families and identified low quality of life, low self-esteem, poor family coping skills, and depression as prominent characteristics. Subsequently, the same researcher compared members of the Oley Foundation on home PN ($n = 49$) to individuals on home PN who were not members of a peer-support/education group ($n = 50$) matched for age, gender, duration of home PN, and diagnosis [11]. This case control study found that home PN patients affiliated with the Foundation had significantly fewer episodes of catheter infections, less depression, and better quality of life than the control group. In addition, a qualitative study of the value of the Oley Foundation that included 22 consumers of home PN or home EN identified Oley's programs, educational resources, and the competency, inspiration, normalcy, and advocacy gained from membership as factors that helped them adjust to life with HPEN dependency [12].

JB: The Oley national and regional conferences, held in varying locations in North America, are attended by HPEN'ers, their families, clinicians, board members, industry, as well as volunteers, many of whom attend annually. There are educational sessions, which are presented by well-known clinicians from the U.S., Canada, and on occasion from abroad. Breakout sessions give attendees an opportunity to ask questions and to learn more about specific topics (Figure 28.2). Exhibits introduce attendees to new technology that may be helpful to HPEN'ers. Importantly, there are opportunities for networking among those who are on these therapies. Friendships develop, and many become lifelong. Activities for adults, teens, and children allow mingling with consumers, clinicians, and staff (Figure 28.3). For the younger generation, child care and youth activities such as tours,

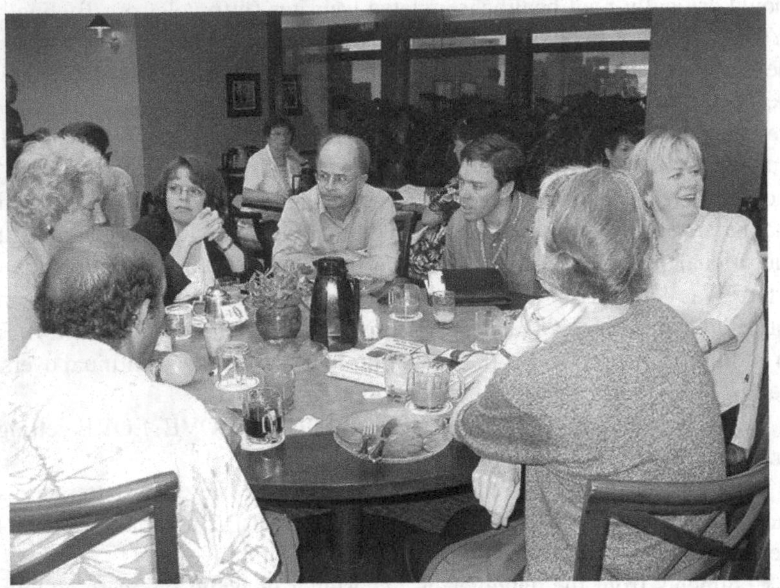

FIGURE 28.2 Round-table discussion at the Oley annual meeting.

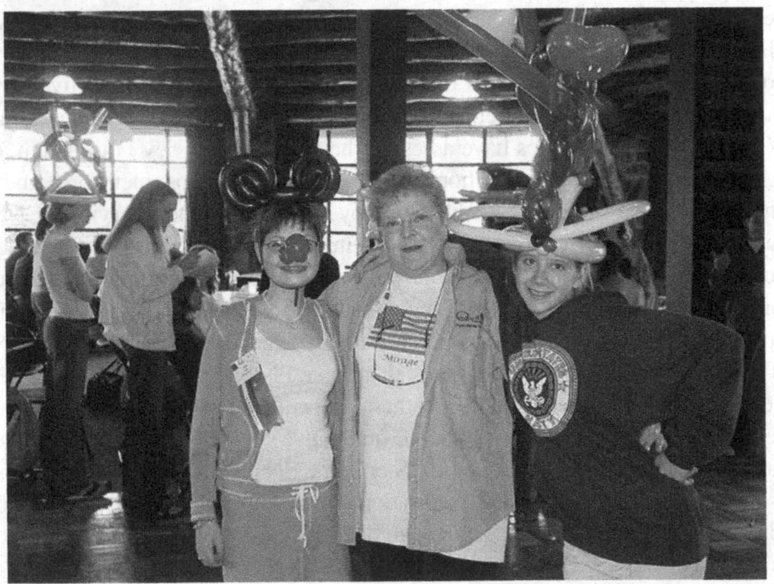

FIGURE 28.3 Oley youth participating in a balloon event with the Oley advisor for science and medicine (center).

crafts (Figure 28.4), a pajama party (Figure 28.5), and picnic (Figure 28.6) offer an opportunity to share, learn, and enjoy time together.

One first-time attendee's family commented: "Thank you so much for the wonderful conference. We made friends and got an education at the same time! It is good to know that we are not alone in this life we now live" [1].

A 9-year-old conference attendee said in response to an invitation to an Oley Foundation event: "Oley is my second family and we have to celebrate with one of our family members" [1].

JB: One physician who is very experienced in HPEN once told me: "I learn more from the Oley meetings, particularly from the consumers in attendance, than at many of the medical meetings I attend!"

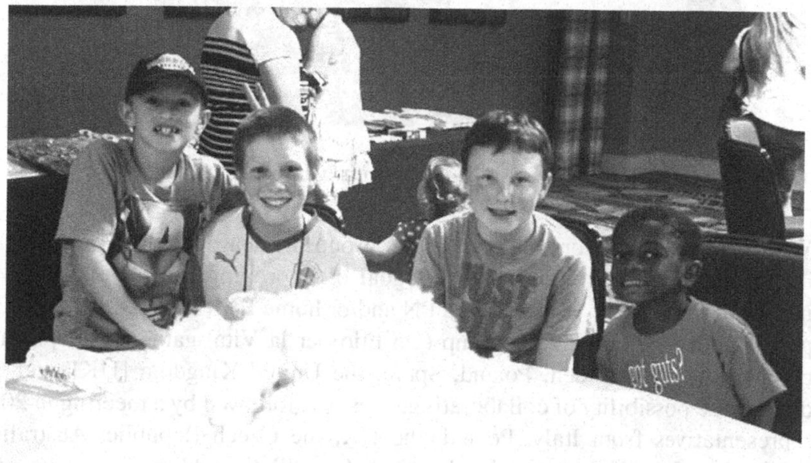

FIGURE 28.4 Oley kids gathering for the "build your bear" activity at the Oley meeting. Young Oley gentlemen preparing the bears' stuffing.

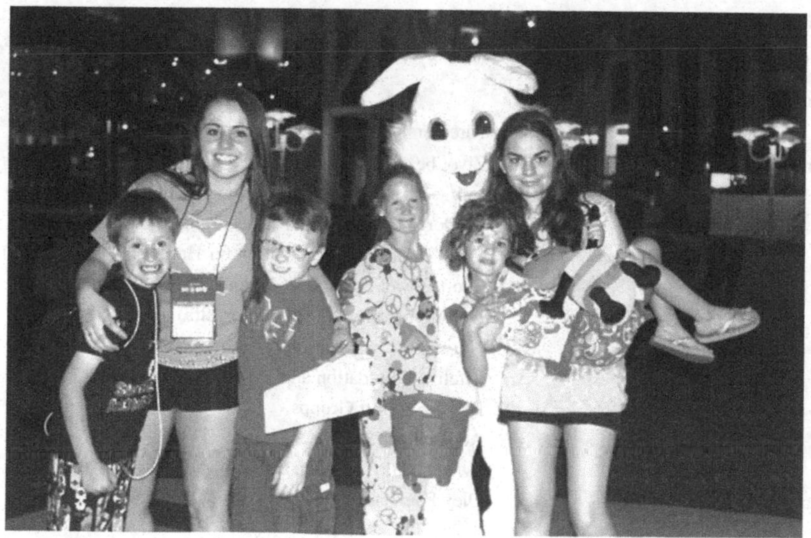

FIGURE 28.5 Oley volunteers coming together with the younger generation after the scavenger hunt.

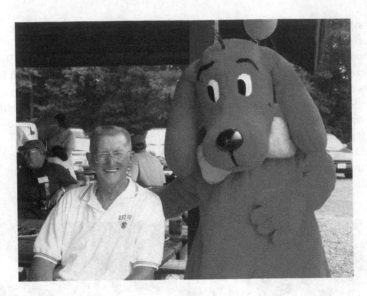

FIGURE 28.6 A long-term HPN'er discussing therapy with "Clipper" at the Oley picnic.

DK & JB: What is the next step for Oley and similar groups from around the world? There are many international patient groups with the goal of improving life for persons with chronic intestinal failure who rely on home PN and/or home EN (Table 28.1). In 2013, an Italian parent home PN caregiver's group (Un Filo per la Vita) gathered people from several countries (Italy, Sweden, Poland, Spain, the United Kingdom [UK], and the U.S.) to discuss the possibility of collaborating. This was followed by a meeting in 2014 in which representatives from Italy, Poland, the UK, the Czech Republic, Australia and New Zealand, and the U.S. met to develop plans for a "Patient Alliance for Chronic Intestinal Failure and Home Parenteral Nutrition," with the goal to unite efforts to establish communication and mutual projects and to educate each other, clinicians, and a segment of industry. Subsequent conference calls have taken place in the process of developing a

TABLE 28.1
Organizations for Consumers of Home Parenteral and Enteral Nutrition and Caregivers[a]

Country or Countries	Organization Name
Australia/New Zealand	Parenteral Nutrition Down Under (PNDU)
Czech Republic	Zivot bez střeva, z.s. (Life without gut Z.s.)
France	LaVie Par Un Fil (Organization for HomePEN Families)
Germany	Kinder and Schweiriger Ernaehrungssituation. V.-KISE
Great Britain	PINNT (British Organization for HomePEN Consumers)
Great Britain	Short Bowel Survivor & Friends (Great Britain)
Italy	Un Filo per la Vita (Thread for Life)
Norway	Norwegian Association for Home Parenteral Nutrition
Poland	Lifeline Foundation and Parenteral Nutrition in Poland
Poland	Polish Support Groups
Spain	Aepannupa (Spain)
Sweden	Swedish HPN-Association
United States and Canada	Oley Foundation

[a] This list may not be comprehensive due to the difficulty of obtaining information about some groups.

nonprofit structure. As the infrastructure is set up, other national groups will be invited to join the effort. Among the alliance's goals are to exhibit at future ESPEN meetings and to develop printed information regarding traveling with home PN and home EN that member groups can translate into their native languages.

CONCLUSION

The sudden need for home PN or home EN can be a frightening, life-changing experience for patients and their families that can have life-threatening consequences. Organizations such as the Oley Foundation that offer support to these persons can have a huge impact that leads to an improvement in quality of life and decreased complications while providing reliable education and educational resources.

One of the long-time Ambassadors summed up the Oley Foundation very well: "HPEN feeds my body; the Oley Foundation feeds my head, heart, and soul!" [1].

REFERENCES

1. The Oley Foundation. http://www.oley.org/about Oley/membertestimonials.
2. Patnode M. Flourishing in the face of chronic illness: A success story. *Dorland Health Case in Point Magazine*. 2013;33. http://www.dorlandhealth.com.
3. The Oley Foundation. http://c.ymcdn.com/sites/oley.org/resource/resmgr/Flyers/NewBrochure.pdf.
4. Staun M et al. ESPEN guidelines on parenteral nutrition: Home parenteral nutrition (HPN) in adult patients. *Clinical Nutrition* 2009;28:467–479.
5. Pittiruti M et al. ESPEN Guidelines on parenteral nutrition: Central venous catheter (access, care, diagnosis and therapy of complications). *Clinical Nutrition* 2009;28:365–377.
6. Van Gossum A et al. ESPEN guidelines on parenteral nutrition: Gastroenterology. *Clinical Nutrition* 2009;28:415–427.
7. Pironi L et al. ESPEN endorsed recommendations. Definition and classification of intestinal failure in adults. *Clinical Nutrition* 2015;34(2):171–180.
8. Gillanders L et al. AuSPEN clinical practice guideline for home parenteral nutrition patients in Australia and New Zealand. *Nutrition* 2008;24:998–1012.
9. Winkler M et al. Nutrition and you, Searching the web for reliable nutrition information. http://oley.org/lifeline/Nutrition_and_You_Searching_the_Web.html. Oley LifeLine Letter, Jan/Feb 2011.
10. Smith CE. Quality of life in long term TPN patients and their family caregivers. *JPEN Journal of Parenteral and Enteral Nutrition* 1993;17:501–506.
11. Smith CE et al. Home parenteral nutrition: Does affiliation with a national support and education organization improve patient outcome? *JPEN Journal of Parenteral and Enteral Nutrition* 2002;26:159–163.
12. Chopy K et al. A qualitative study of the perceived value of membership in the Oley Foundation by home parenteral and enteral nutrition consumers. *JPEN Journal of Parenteral and Enteral Nutrition* 2015;39:426–433.

29 Patient and Caregiver Perspectives

Learn and Live!

Lynn Ruse and Jim Ruse

CONTENTS

KEY POINTS

- Maintain a running log as an easy-to-refer-to file of important information.
- Learn how to use Internet searches to find current standard of care practices for specific conditions.
- Seek out experts specializing in short bowel syndrome.
- Change one treatment at a time and document cause and effects.
- Understand that everything you put in your mouth can either increase diarrhea or help diminish it.

HOW IT ALL BEGAN

Lynn, now 56, underwent a total colectomy at age 23 in 1983 due to atonic megacolon, resulting in a permanent ileostomy. More than 20 bowel resections, revisions, lysis of adhesions, and other failed surgical fixes later, she is now left with an estimated 180 cm of proximal small bowel ending in a terminal jejunostomy. Her last surgery was in 1999, 17 years ago.

Lynn was a flight attendant with USAir when she met and married her husband Jim, who is a research scientist. Jim has been her primary caregiver and patient advocate for the past 26 years. Although his degree is in microbiology, Jim has worked for more than 30 years as a biochemist in the biotechnology and biopharmaceutical industries. Sadly, Lynn had to retire from the airlines in 1991 after one of her major surgeries.

Due to the severity of Lynn's condition, it was difficult for Lynn to concentrate and remember everything doctors were telling her. Consequently, both Lynn and the physicians became increasingly dependent upon Jim to maintain and coordinate her care. Early in their relationship, several of Lynn's doctors and surgeons encouraged Jim to learn as much as he possibly could about Lynn's condition. They knew, as a scientist living with Lynn and focused on only one patient, through time and necessity, Jim was going to become an "expert in Lynn."

Because of a high-output end-jejunostomy, Lynn required intravenous (IV) support for many years, some of the time infusing IV nutrition (i.e., total parenteral nutrition [TPN]) and some of the time infusing IV hydration with added magnesium. From 2003 to 2006, a customized care plan was painstakingly developed and personalized for her needs. Over time, Lynn was able to wean completely from TPN, while still requiring IV hydration and magnesium replacement. Subsequently, by using an oral rehydration solution (ORS) and controlling fluid intake, Lynn was able to periodically wean from IV hydration for 6 to 18 months at a time.

Since 2006, Lynn has maintained a high-salt, high-calorie diet along with daily use of an ORS with added magnesium along with a histamine type 2 receptor antagonist (H2RA; e.g., ranitidine and famotidine) and chewable antacids as needed. She requires hospitalization due to dehydration and electrolyte imbalance about once or twice a year. In 2014, Lynn started using the recently approved glucagon-like peptide-2 (GLP-2) hormone replacement therapy (teduglutide or "Gattex"). In this chapter, we will discuss lessons we have learned that will hopefully provide practical suggestions for both patients and those who care for them.

TPN AND BLOODSTREAM INFECTIONS

Lynn had four very difficult surgeries from 1997 to 1999. After the first two surgeries, doctors did not think Lynn was going to live because of how much bowel they had removed and how many damaging cuts had been accidentally made in the remaining bowel. They were concerned because Lynn was receiving TPN and her heavily sutured bowel was exposing nutrient-rich blood to gut bacteria. Some doctors indicated that because of this, Lynn may have issues with "bacterial translocation," which could lead to a higher risk of infections, such as central venous catheter bloodstream infections, and TPN-related liver disease.

Lynn was given TPN from 1997 to 2003. In 1998, we had our first home TPN experience. Sadly, TPN was not a pleasant experience for us. Lynn had already experienced serious infections in the hospital…and now we were bringing this risk home.

At the time, home TPN services were not well coordinated. Pumps were bulky and always seemed to fail at the worst times—when no one was available to help (nights, weekends, and holidays). The home health nurse worked for a separate group from the TPN provider and came with her own supplies. The patient supplies were delivered by a different supplier and turned out to be different from what the nurse expected; the supplies that were provided were not always complete and it was difficult to maintain consistency. At the time, it was all very confusing and frustrating, verging on overwhelming. The majority of the responsibility for coordinating future supplies fell on the patient and caregiver, which was very difficult because we were confused and ill-prepared to deal with the complexities involved.

Once the home health nurse had connected Lynn to the TPN, she left and we were left to the confines of our home, but to Lynn, it did not feel like our home anymore—it felt like a hospital room, with hospital supplies and a refrigerator full of more hospital supplies. At one point, Lynn had a hospital IV pole and pump, which she had to wheel around her two-story home. Even when more portable pumps became available, it was very scary to leave home. There were constant fears of infection, someone would sneeze on you, or worse, they might pull the central line out. Lynn always had to have emergency supplies with her…just in case. She was always on guard and felt like a freak because everyone stared at the lady with the huge suitcase that had a tube full of white stuff going into her shirt.

From Lynn's reflection: "Most of your friends don't understand and you find yourself having to explain to everyone you see, over and over, again and again. It's difficult to have a normal conversation with people because your life is nothing like theirs and you have nothing in common to talk about. You just become the sick person that everyone whispers about and points at across the room. It becomes emotionally exhausting to leave your home, so you don't."

Yet Lynn still did her best to get out of the house, usually to see close friends or family who welcomed her into their home with their activities, where she felt safe and enjoyed a welcome change away from her "hospital home."

In 1998, because of Lynn's repeated blood infections, Jim went through additional medical training to be qualified to access Lynn's port. The hope was that with consistency and meticulous sterile technique, the risk of infection would be mitigated. But even after Jim took over the care of Lynn's central line, she continued to have one infection after another. Lynn and Jim (and her healthcare team) could not identify any pattern or failure in technique that could account for all of the episodes of bloodstream infection, which all cultured positive for gut bacteria (punctuated by the occasional opportunistic fungal infections, which occurred during IV antibiotic treatments).

From 1997 to 2005, every central line and port placed into Lynn's body became infected, necessitating weeks of IV antibiotic therapy and antifungal therapies with every infection. Lynn spent eight very difficult years living more than 60% of her days in the hospital, gravely ill. Over the years, having to replace multiple infected central lines took a toll on Lynn's veins. As her venous access sites diminished, there were serious mortality concerns. It became imperative to find some way to free Lynn from TPN and IV hydration. This became the driving force to get Lynn to the Intestinal Rehabilitation Center (IRC) at the University of Nebraska Medical Center in Omaha.

Consequently, in 2006, when Lynn was finally able to maintain hydration and electrolyte balance by mouth, Lynn and Jim, in agreement with her doctors at the time, decided to remove her portacath and Lynn has lived without a central venous catheter ever since. This has dramatically reduced her hospitalizations and greatly improved her quality of life. Once or twice a year, Lynn may have an acute exacerbation of diarrhea leading to dehydration and electrolyte imbalance, which necessitates IV hydration and magnesium replacement. As a consequence of this decision, when Lynn needs IV hydration, she has to be admitted to the hospital, for care and maintenance of a peripheral IV line, but usually for only a week or two at a time, as long as therapy is performed properly and secondary issues do not arise.

THE IMPORTANCE OF PROVIDING PATIENT EDUCATION

For many years, the only patient education we received were verbal conversations with Lynn's gastroenterologists and surgeons. Over time, we learned that it is extremely important to keep a detailed medical journal tracking information as we learned it. Otherwise, as the years went by, these conversations and long list of doctors all tended to meld together.

The lack of easily accessible information on short bowel syndrome (SBS) inhibited the discovery of others with problems similar to Lynn's. Prior to the advent of the Internet, most doctors had little to no exposure to short bowel patients like Lynn, and without comparable case histories, they could only rely on their own experiences. As such, and unbeknownst to us at the time, Lynn and I became medical pioneers, learning about her unique physiology through trial and error over years of discovery.

Lynn's doctors primarily treated her most acute and immediate symptoms, which were usually dehydration, due to her high ostomy output and muscle spasms. They did not seem to understand the causes of her diarrhea, and as a consequence, they were unable to control her diarrhea. Over the years, many different medications specifically for diarrhea and bowel motility were tried without success (see the "Medications" section).

As alluded to previously, Lynn and I spent time at the IRC in Omaha in both 2003 and 2005. The IRC was networked with other centers in the United States specializing in SBS patients like Lynn. They were able to provide current literature and scientific research, including comparison data from other SBS patients and their "typical" physiologic responses based on their remaining bowel anatomy. This type of information allowed us to quickly identify areas that were very similar to Lynn and other areas that did not apply at all. This gave everyone involved a more detailed understanding of Lynn's unique physiology.

The IRC staff spent time with both of us, helping us to understand not only what SBS patients needed but also why certain things were vitally important. The IRC was not just treating isolated symptoms, they also seemed genuinely concerned about improving Lynn's quality of life. They taught us how to make calculated adjustments in Lynn's care plan, one change at a time, and then monitor closely for cause and effect over time. It took a long time to learn what worked best for Lynn, but eventually, this led to the development of a customized care plan. Still today, we use these fundamental skills to continually improve Lynn's care plan as new information and treatments become available.

Finding a medical center with experience and expertise in SBS was vitally important for us to be prepared to properly address Lynn's condition. Importantly, it is not just about the information but *how* that information is delivered. It is noticeably different talking to knowledgeable professionals who genuinely understand the life of an SBS patient.

Imagine if you will from Lynn's perspective, a woman who has been chronically ill and has been hospitalized extensively to this point in her life. Lynn endured many years in numerous hospitals where the staff did not understand why she was "sick all the time." She was continually questioned because no one seemed to understand her condition and some even questioned her integrity. It became emotionally exhausting to have yet another time-consuming explanation with medical staff that had no understanding or willingness to learn about SBS. And then pause to imagine what it is like to walk into a facility like the IRC where the staff is very knowledgeable about SBS and they believe you rather than question your motivations. It made all the difference in the world to us.

MEDICATIONS—TOO MANY TO REMEMBER

Lynn has tried a number of the medications recommended to slow bowel motility and control diarrhea. Doctors prescribed medications with a specific dosage and regimen; however, it was then mostly left to us to determine if it was effective or not. Optimization of dose was attempted but not rigorously tracked by medical staff; the job of collecting and reporting data was left entirely to us. As expected, this caused numerous confrontations with medical personnel, who regularly questioned the validity of the data, and the integrity of both Lynn and me, because they could not believe the volume of Lynn's profuse diarrhea. That made optimization all the more difficult. Medications tried included the following:

H2RAs and proton pump inhibitors. Controlling the pH of Lynn's stool is important as it seems to prevent painful burning in her bowel, stoma, and skin surrounding stoma. The decision was made not to use proton pump inhibitors (e.g., omeprazole and pantoprazole) because, at the time, there were concerns about them worsening her existing hypomagnesemia and potentially causing small bowel bacterial overgrowth (SBBO). Instead, Lynn uses H2RAs (e.g., ranitidine and famotidine). On or off these medications, however, Lynn's volume of ostomy output appears to be about the same. These medications are now available over-the-counter and Lynn uses them as needed. Since starting teduglutide (see the "GLP-2 Hormone Replacement Therapy" section) in 2014, Lynn has not needed these medications, unless she has an exacerbation of high stool output, which has happened only once in the last 17 months, and was directly related to the ingestion of hyperosmotic contrast used for a radiology test.

Antibiotics for SBBO. Lynn was treated for SBBO from 1988 to 1991 due to chronic bothersome bloating and chronic pouchitis when she had a Koch pouch (continent ostomy) and again from 1997 to 2006 as she had dysmotile loops of bowel. Initially, she was on continuous treatment, then the IRC developed a plan of rotating a low dose of several different oral antibiotics for 14 days at the beginning of each month. The difficulty with this regimen over time, however, was an increase in diarrhea from the use of antibiotics, so it was decided to see if the treatment was worsening the diarrhea. In 2006, when Lynn was able to maintain her electrolytes and hydration by mouth using ORS, it was decided to end the rotation of oral antibiotics to reduce her output. Lynn has not been treated for SBBO since 2006.

Antidiarrheals. Lynn tried loperamide (Imodium) on multiple occasions since 1991 with the same result—regardless of the dose (Lynn has tried doses as high as 8–16 mg up to six times a day), it did not seem to significantly reduce the volume of her output. For Lynn, diphenoxylate with atropine (Lomotil) was more effective. This medication slowed her bowel almost to a stop without having to take a mouthful of pills. Unfortunately, the medication was too effective. Lynn could not find a dose of this medication that did not cause significant bowel problems: the output of stool would slow tremendously, then her abdomen would become distended, causing pain and nausea, and then she would "dump" a half liter or more of stool at a time. Therefore, we no longer use this medication.

Dicyclomine (Bentyl). For Lynn, this antispasm medication also slowed her bowel to a near stop, feeling like a bowel obstruction with nausea and vomiting. It was tried several times with similar results, so, once again, we no longer use this medication.

Morphine. Morphine consistently caused Lynn to have terrible vomiting and dry heaving, even in low doses. Because of this, the dose of morphine was never attempted to be optimized as an antidiarrheal medication for Lynn.

Codeine. By itself, this medication causes Lynn to be very nauseous. She can, however, use it in combination with an antinausea medication (e.g., promethazine and hydroxyzine). Lynn has used codeine for pain; however, codeine was never used in an attempt to lower her ostomy output.

Meperidine (Demerol). This was used for many years to slow the hyperactivity of Lynn's bowel. It worked very well to slow transit and the volume of output, but there was a constant concern of addiction. We found that taking a dose of meperidine followed by giving Lynn "real food" (e.g., potatoes, rice, white bread, oatmeal) would slow Lynn's ostomy output to a manageable 2.5 to 4 L per day. Fortunately, we eventually found other ways to control her stool output and Lynn has not used any opiate medication as an antidiarrheal since 2005.

Octreotide (Sandostatin). Octreotide is a medication administered by subcutaneous injection that slows gastrointestinal secretions and motility. In 1992–1993, Lynn endured daily injections of this medication. The formulation at that time burned very badly as the injection was delivered, leaving the injection site sore. Over the course of the 2 years of octreotide use, the stool output did not diminish substantially and it was discontinued.

Cholestyramine (Questran). Lynn was prescribed cholestyramine, a bile acid binder, by several doctors, multiple times over the years, with poor results each time. This medication is counterproductive for Lynn given her bowel anatomy, and our opinion is that this medication should not be used for anyone without a colon. When this medication was once again recommended for Lynn earlier this year (2015), as her patient advocate, I respectfully declined the medication and provided literature to support my reasoning. Unfortunately, it has been our experience that despite the fact that every facility makes you sign a form stating that you have "Patient Rights," when you actually exercise your rights, it does not usually go well. Medical staff and doctors may start treating you tersely, with indifference and disdain.

What well-informed patients and patient advocates want, crave, and desperately need are collaboration and respect from their medical team. We want medical treatments that will benefit the patient, but we are going to resist treatments that have proven to be ineffective or have proven to be harmful to the patient in the past. We want to be included in the decisions, and we would like to know that the information we bring to the discussion will be valued.

FUNDAMENTALS LEARNED

After the removal of Lynn's colon, followed by the removal of her end-terminal ileum in 1991, her bowel transit time from mouth to stoma was less than 30 minutes, with upward of 6–8 L of profuse, watery diarrhea every day. Her ostomy output was more than three times her urine output on a daily basis. Monitoring urine and ostomy output became a daily routine because no one could believe the volume of her ostomy output. Lynn was always hungry and had an unquenchable thirst. Lynn was able to maintain some nutrition by mouth, when she was allowed to eat, but hydration was nearly impossible to maintain orally, as the more fluid Lynn drank, the more ostomy output she had!

FINDING THE OPTIMAL DIET

Because of Lynn's profuse diarrhea, doctors continually debated the merits of giving her food. With only a 20- to 30-minute intestinal transit time, how much was she really able to absorb? For many years, doctors wanted to treat Lynn's diarrhea with "bowel rest." They would either immediately eliminate oral intake completely (i.e., nil per os/nothing by mouth [NPO]) or they would put her on a strict liquid diet, which usually included water (hypotonic), elemental nutrient drinks (hypertonic), and fruit juice (hypertonic). For nearly 20 years, this was the frontline treatment for Lynn. However, these protocols never worked and always made Lynn feel worse and more depleted. In reality, these care plans exacerbated Lynn's diarrhea and malabsorption. From repeated experience, it became clear that Lynn did better when she was given food; her stool would thicken and she would recover faster.

When Lynn went to the IRC in Omaha, we were pleased to find that the IRC doctors promoted eating. To this point, Lynn had been told by some doctors that she should not eat "real food." Once doctors encouraged Lynn to eat and drink the correct foods, she was eventually able to maintain her nutrition without needing TPN. Lynn still has issues with specific vitamin and mineral deficiencies, which require supplementation to be maintained in the normal range.

Prior to the IRC (starting back in 1991), Lynn had learned by trial and error many of the foods that worked well for her and she definitely knew what foods to avoid. She had a good but limited dietary plan. The IRC provided excellent information on ways to improve and provide variety to Lynn's diet specific to jejunostomy patients. Lynn was able to expand her diet and developed a relatively low residue diet, high in complex carbohydrates and proteins using white bread, rice, potatoes, oatmeal, quinoa, and grits as part of her meals to give her bowel some "substance," which could absorb part of the excess fluid and improve stool consistency.

All SBS patients have to design their own dietary plan based on their remaining bowel anatomy. A dietitian knowledgeable in SBS can be tremendously helpful to provide guidance in this regard; however, there will always be some element of trial and error when determining the optimal foods. As such, it is important to maintain a food log of cause and effect, to avoid repeating disasters. Also, keeping a 1-week food journal, periodically throughout your life, helps you to see what you are actually eating. Sometimes, looking at it on paper helps to correct issues you did not realize existed.

Thankfully, having documentation from the experts at the IRC provided much needed support for Lynn and Jim when confronted by other medical professionals who disagreed. It was no longer just Lynn and Jim begging doctors to "please give her food—she does better when she is allowed to eat!" The IRC also provided some basic "jejunostomy common sense" reminders about eating: (1) everything Lynn puts into her mouth can either cause more diarrhea or help diminish it, and (2) eat small meals, six to eight times a day, well cooked and well chewed.

FLUID BALANCE—HYPERTONIC, HYPOTONIC, AND ISOTONIC ORAL INTAKE

While at the IRC, both Lynn and I were educated about hypotonic, hypertonic, and isotonic fluids. Knowledge about the bowel's response to these different fluids enabled improved management of Lynn's hydration and control of her stool output.

Water, which had, in general, been encouraged for years, is hypotonic. However, for SBS patients like Lynn, without a colon, water depletes electrolytes in the blood by pulling them into the lumen of the bowel to create an osmotic equilibrium. With no place else to be reabsorbed back into the bloodstream, both water and electrolytes are expelled in the ostomy output. Because of this, and perhaps counterintuitive, water needed to be virtually eliminated from Lynn's diet. Instead, Lynn learned about and started using an isotonic ORS, a special blend of sugar and salt that is optimized to enhance the efficiency of fluid and electrolyte absorption in the upper small intestine. Lynn needed to drink 2–3 L of ORS every day, limiting hypotonic fluids to about 1 L per day and only with meals (Lynn likes Diet Coke). However, finding a palatable ORS was a challenge. Lynn tried many different commercially available ORS, most of which tasted like a mouthful of ocean water (or worse). An unpalatable ORS is not an acceptable option if this is needed as the primary source of hydration.

The World Health Organization recognizes a 50:50 mix of Gatorade and water plus a little added salt as an acceptable isotonic ORS (Powerade also works well and for Lynn seems to have a better mix of electrolytes). Additionally, some fruit juices can be diluted with water plus added salt to create an alternative ORS. Gatorade, Powerade, and fruit juices are all hypertonic drinks at full strength and would cause osmotic diarrhea, but using the right formulas to dilute them with water and add salt brings them into the isotonic range (see list below). Finding these modified ORS solutions palatable, Lynn was willing to drink 2–3 L of ORS a day.

Oral rehydration solutions Lynn found palatable:

Gatorade or Powerade mixture

- 2 cups Gatorade/Powerade
- 2 cups water
- 1/2 tsp salt

Grape juice and cranberry juice mixture

- 1/2 cup juice
- 3 1/2 cups water
- 1/2 tsp salt

Eliminating hypertonic drinks, limiting hypotonic drinks to meal time, and forcing 2–3 L of isotonic ORS freed Lynn from IV hydration for 6–18 months at a time (until she had an acute diarrhea event that knocked her system out of balance).

Slow Magnesium Replacement Therapy for Hypomagnesemia

Lynn has received IV magnesium replacement therapy literally hundreds of times and there is definitely a preferred method which has proven to be effective for Lynn. The goal is to prevent renal wasting of magnesium and limit the pain caused by magnesium replacement. We have learned some very important factors for Lynn.

Lynn tolerates IV magnesium best when delivered over longer periods of time; conversely, delivering IV magnesium in a high-concentration bolus over a short period of time causes her body to renally waste magnesium, exacerbating the issue.

For a very long time, our treatment for Lynn focused only on treating hypomagnesemia by giving IV magnesium replacement. Sometimes this worked and sometimes it did not. We thought that her low magnesium was "causing" her diarrhea, because when it was brought back into normal range with IV replacement, her diarrhea would stop. We did not fully understand the root cause. For years, we believed it was simply low-magnesium-related watery diarrhea, but that was just looking at the tip of the proverbial iceberg.

In 2012, Lynn was hospitalized due to an exacerbation of diarrhea with dehydration and hypomagnesemia. Despite aggressive IV fluids (IVF) and magnesium supplementation, her magnesium level remained low. In an attempt to assist with finding a way to help Lynn, I did extensive research online looking for root causes of hypomagnesemia in the setting of SBS and came across information relating to hyperaldosteronism, which is the natural result of the renin–angiotensin–aldosterone system (RAAS) response to dehydration and contributes to hypomagnesemia. Chronic dehydration and sodium depletion from large-volume stool losses and other insensible fluid loss (e.g., sweating) leads to a decrease in blood volume (hypovolemia). This causes the RAAS to respond to maintain blood pressure. Secondary hyperaldosteronism develops, causing the kidneys to retain sodium and lose magnesium (also known as tertiary hypomagnesemia).

Lynn's body seems to be hypersensitive to shifts in her blood sodium levels, which immediately affect her ostomy output. For Lynn, this means that management of sodium in her blood is of *immediate* and primary importance; it is not just about maintaining "fluid hydration." Just being outside for 10–15 minutes during the heat of the day starts a rapid downward spiral for Lynn. Sweating causes enough of a sodium deficiency in her blood to initiate the osmotic pull of water into her bowel and leads to watery diarrhea, which steadily increases by the minute unless she does something to stop it. Lynn typically has 30 minutes to an hour to correct the sodium imbalance (e.g., cool her body, stop sweating, eat a salty snack and/or table salt, and drink ORS) or else her high-volume output will lead quickly to hypovolemia, initiating the RAAS response yet again, and she will not be able to successfully rehydrate by mouth. If Lynn responds quickly to lower her body temperature and increase her serum sodium levels, her stool will become less watery and she can then rehydrate successfully with ORS alone.

We also learned that urine tests for random sodium, magnesium, and calcium were actually more beneficial to track electrolyte disturbances from secondary hyperaldosteronism, eliminating the need for daily blood tests. This was welcome news to Lynn who, after 30 years of IV hydration, is a "VERY hard stick." Daily blood tests (while in the hospital) are no fun for Lynn, and clinicians often forget just how many vials of blood they are requiring on a daily basis. In our experience, we have yet to find a facility that is capable or willing to track Lynn's progress using urine tests. All to date have remained resolute on tracking serum electrolytes, daily, because of insurance requirements.

Malabsorption of Nutrients and Pills

For Lynn, rapid intestinal transit results in minimal nutrient contact time. This, combined with her minimal intestinal surface area, means that at least 50% of her oral intake travels through her bowel without providing any nutritional benefit. Much has been documented about jejunostomy patients eating two to three times more than their pre-SBS diet to maintain their weight, simply because they are not absorbing nutrients. This is also true of oral medications and supplements, which need to be given in higher doses. Pills have also been a problem because they do not have time to dissolve, much less be absorbed. As such, liquid medications are preferred as long as they are not given in large volumes of hypertonic solutions such as sorbitol. Timed-release medications also need to be avoided as there is simply not enough transit time for them to release!

Since beginning the use of teduglutide in 2014, due to the associated increase in absorption, all of Lynn's nutrition and medications needed to be reevaluated and adjusted accordingly.

GLP-2 HORMONE REPLACEMENT THERAPY

The year 2013 was a difficult year for Lynn. It was unusually hot in southern California and Lynn was hospitalized several times for IV hydration and magnesium replacement. Over a few years, Lynn's stoma had atrophied and was, at that time, slightly inverted below the skin. Profuse, watery diarrhea caused daily appliance failures and, over time, created a recurring abscess in the skin below her stoma. This was underneath the appliance, where diarrhea would pool and eat away at her skin. This created severe discomfort for Lynn because her skin was badly blistered and infected around the stoma, where the appliance is supposed to "glue" to the skin. In Lynn's words, "it's like pouring rubbing alcohol on road rash, an awful stinging and burning feeling, all the time, with caustic stool spilling out on it and all around it, all the time." It was not a tenable situation. Doctors treated the infection with IV antibiotics (contributing to the diarrhea). Unfortunately, even with treatment, because of her stomal issues, Lynn's skin was not healing. Lynn's gastroenterologist and general surgeon agreed that Lynn needed a stomal revision to correct the root cause of the problem. Two colorectal surgeons were consulted, who both agreed she needed a revision; however, neither surgeon wanted to operate on Lynn and risk losing more bowel.

Again, searching online for a solution, I discovered that the Food and Drug Administration had recently approved a GLP-2 analog, teduglutide (a.k.a., Gattex), specifically for patients with SBS. This drug improves the ability of the intestine to absorb nutrients and fluid and had been shown in clinical studies to reduce IV fluid and TPN requirements in SBS patients. I dug further researching the clinical trial results and discovered that one of the "side effects" was stomal growth or enlargement. We presented this information to doctors and we were initially told that our insurance would never approve Lynn for this medication. In later discussions with a new gastroenterologist, although supportive, no immediate action was taken to pursue this.

Lynn was hospitalized in April 2014 with dehydration, failure to thrive, and several nutrient deficiencies (vitamin D was undetectable, vitamin B_{12} and vitamin E were quite low, and of course magnesium, an ongoing issue for Lynn, was also low). Lynn told me she felt like it was the end. In discussions with her doctors, we agreed to put Lynn on TPN to correct her deficiencies. After 3 days of TPN in the hospital, we were sent home once again on TPN.

I had contacted the manufacturer of teduglutide and we attended a meeting sponsored by the company (NPS Pharmaceuticals, Inc. [now Shire PLC]) to learn more about this medication. We discussed our plight with the representatives at the meeting and were put it touch with NPS Advantage. NPS Advantage coordinated the rest from that point. Representatives of the company contacted our gastroenterologist, providing information and training on this new product, and Lynn received approval for teduglutide in 2014. NPS Advantage then coordinated delivery of the medication and even applied for and received funding from the Patient Access Network Foundation to assist in paying for Lynn's portion of this very costly medication. Lynn received her first shipment of Gattex at the end of April 2014.

Remarkably, Lynn's physiology seemed to change with the first injection. Lynn was already a very well-managed SBS patient, and with this new medication, which she has tolerated very well, she was able to wean from TPN and has not needed TPN since. This started a brand new chapter—a new SBS physiology to learn and optimize. Here is a synopsis of some of the most dramatic changes:

Lynn's course since the 1991 removal of her terminal ileum and *prior* to use of teduglutide:

- Ostomy output *always* exceeded her urine output on a daily basis, sometimes 4–5 L per day.
- Transit time from mouth to stoma was 20–30 minutes maximum.
- Consistency of stool varied from a "light brown, oatmeal consistency" to extremely watery, high-volume diarrhea.
- Pills passed through without dissolving; even crushed, the pieces came through unaffected, floating in the ostomy pouch.
- Stoma was flat, flush with her abdomen or slightly inverted, and pink to slightly grey.
- Appliance adherence issues due to flat/inverted stoma, liquid stool, leaking under appliance.
  - Lynn had to use convex appliances with inserts to mitigate leakage and had to replace the appliance at least once a day due to leakage.

Lynn's course since 2014 *after* starting teduglutide:

- Urine output generally exceeds her ostomy output on a daily basis.
- Transit time (from mouth to ostomy pouch) increased to 3–5 hours.
- Stool became dark brown, thick, and pasty. The color, texture, and odor all changed.
- Pills no longer come out whole.

- After about a month of daily injections, Lynn's stoma began to enlarge, now protruding about 1.5 cm above her abdominal wall. The protruding stoma is convoluted, like a rose, and the stoma color changed to a darker, ruby red.
- Improved appliance adherence: protruding stoma + pasty stool = less leakage.

THE CAREGIVER PERSPECTIVE

Over the years, Lynn and I have learned two important things: (1) I will never be able to truly understand what it is like to have SBS and feel all of the things that she feels: physically, mentally, and emotionally; (2) conversely, Lynn will never truly understand what it is like to be her caregiver and patient advocate. Comedians often make light of their spouses who are always exhausted by the end of the day because they have a job and take care of the kids and the home, so that there is little to no time left for their spouse. Well, multiply that by about 100, and that is how both the SBS patient and their spouse feel. It has been my experience that SBS patients always feel run down and never feel energetic or "in the mood." You want to talk about someone who is *always* exhausted? Let me tell you… And the same is true for their spouse/caregiver, but for different reasons.

The caregiver is always on, and the only respite comes when the patient is in the hospital—which is a double-edged sword. As a caregiver, I found that I had two different modes, hospital mode and home mode—and each comes with its own set of responsibilities and problems.

Hospital mode is mental and is dominated by information. As the patient advocate, you try to stay informed about all of the tests and decisions that are happening, but in reality you are the outsider looking in. You may be a verbal participant in her care, but you have no authority to make changes and the medical staff can exclude you. If you hold a full-time job, you never get to talk to the doctor, because you are never at the hospital when they are. You feel powerless at times. And when you finally get home after visiting hours are over, you are all alone, and there is still everything left to do at home. You feel like you are running on a treadmill and going nowhere.

Home mode is both physical and mental. It is dominated by the overwhelming responsibilities of physically caring for a patient and maintaining a mountain of supplies that you absolutely cannot run out of. And if you have a full-time job, you have to make sure that everything is safe and cared for at home before you can leave. It is unbelievably stressful.

There are times you want to escape, run away, and hide and be done with all of the responsibilities. But no matter what you do, trying to momentarily escape, it never works. The responsibilities are still there. You still have to pay the bills. You still have to deal with insurance. And you still have to coordinate care.

This is where it is so important to have a network of family and friends who can help to shoulder some of the load. You cannot do it alone. Well, you can, but only for a while. I know from experience, this is not healthy and it will eventually break you, emotionally and physically. Help is necessary, and that requires that you swallow your pride, admit that you need help, and then accept the help when it is offered. This is where you will find your true friends…true friends do not wait for you to ask, they just come and help, and *you need to let them.*

Many people have told me, "if you need anything, please call." I know they meant it, but I rarely did (both because of pride and also because it was too difficult to have to explain what and why I needed help). I relied on only my closest and most trusted friends—others, I did not want to bother. What was truly humbling and greatly appreciated was when people saw what was needed and *they just did it*, without asking.

For example:

- My church brought two bags of groceries, more than once (stuff everybody uses and needs—tissues, toilet paper, bread, milk, butter, eggs, etc.).
- My neighbors mowed my lawn.

- My neighbors fed and walked my dog.
- Friends picked up our daughter after school and took care of her until I could get home.
- More than one of my friends took me away for the weekend, at their expense.
- An automotive service friend picked up and repaired my car for the cost of the parts.
- Friends planned visits to Lynn in the hospital so that I could take the night off.
- Friends coordinated and brought dinner several nights a week, so I did not have to cook.
- And one lovely lady from my church, whom I will never forget, came and told me that she had always wanted to do something to help for a very long time, but she never did. Lynn was coming home from the hospital after a long stay, and this lady told me that she was going to come to my house, while I was at work, and clean it from top to bottom, so that it would be clean for both of us when Lynn got home. It was something *she* could do, for *both* of us. She was an angel! What a true labor of love! I swallowed my pride, with tears in my eyes, I gave her my key, and I let her…

So please, if you are the friend, do not wait to be asked. The likelihood is that those in need will not ask. Listen to their plight and find something you can do—it does not have to be big, it just needs to lighten their load and show them you care.

My mother taught me that you should not be embarrassed or get angry over things you cannot control (easier said than done!). Well, living with SBS, there are going to be things that you cannot control. Ostomy appliances break (at the most inopportune times and in the most inopportune places) and then there is smelly diarrhea, everywhere. It can be humiliating, but the reality is it has to be cleaned up and dealt with. Why get angry about it? Lynn and I have learned to "roll with the punches," get the job done, and move on because "SBS happens," if you know what I mean!

Through it all, Lynn and I have endured a great deal, and we have also learned quite a bit, sometimes the hard way. We have developed tremendous compassion for others going through prolonged medical treatments, and we have had the opportunity to minister to, and encourage, other patients and caregivers we have met along the way. We have found that it is very important to "pay it forward" in this way. For years, we were the ones in need, but now, we have the opportunity to bless others. And I can tell you that you definitely receive your own blessing simply by helping someone else in need. Most people feel like no one else could possibly understand—well, let me tell you… we do!

QUALITY OF LIFE

Improvements in Lynn's condition and care always come with improvements in quality of life. Lynn has to live differently than others, but this is her "normal" life—it is not going to get "back to normal"—this is the new SBS normal, and any incremental changes help.

As someone with a high-output jejunostomy, Lynn had to live in a controlled climate; otherwise, simply sweating could put her back into the hospital. If the weather was warmer than 75°F outside, Lynn needed to live like a "pod person," moving quickly from air-conditioned home to air-conditioned car to air-conditioned building and back, never spending much time in the elements. Lynn had to plan every minute of her day because she typically only had two or three "good hours" each day. If Lynn chose to leave home to do anything, there were always preparations before hand, to make sure she could "put on her best face" and endure the time away from home. And after only a few hours away from home, Lynn was completely drained and needed to sleep, rehydrate, and recuperate. Lynn learned to prepare and recuperate, so that others would not see that she was sick and would treat her "normally." This was exhausting for Lynn. It is much better than living in a hospital, but her life at home was totally consumed by preparation and recuperation for a few good hours. Lynn also had to "empty" (i.e., her ostomy bag) every 30–40 minutes. This was particularly difficult at meal times when she would have to leave repeatedly to use the restroom, causing thoughtless people to accuse her of bulimia.

Since starting on teduglutide, Lynn has had more energy and is able to spend a little more time away from home. She can even spend a little time outside, in the elements. Unfortunately, feeling good can also lead to "overdoing it," which still causes Lynn to feel run down and sick for a few days—the benefit so far has been that she is able to recuperate and rehydrate at home (not in a hospital with IVF), and so far, environmental conditions have not knocked her system completely out of balance.

In addition, with teduglutide, Lynn's stoma grew! No need for surgical revision! And with a protruding stoma, Lynn's appliance now fits better and stays on for days, allowing the skin to heal. Thicker stool has also reduced the number of "accidents" caused by failing appliances and Lynn can empty at her leisure rather than panicking because her pouch is full and about to break. This means that Lynn does not have to run to the bathroom every 30–40 minutes. Now she can sit through an entire movie without leaving twice, to empty. We can drive for more than 90 minutes without stopping (huge difference—I used to have to know every freeway exit where there was a public restroom). And she can also sit through an entire meal without leaving the table.

Lynn still has some down times, but the increased energy and hydration levels have given Lynn a boost emotionally. Lynn has always "wanted to go out" (anything to get out of this house!), but now she actually has the energy to be able to go, rather than canceling because she just did not feel well enough. Lynn has always been a positive individual, but now I see more of Lynn the person and less of Lynn the SBS patient.

CAREGIVER + PATIENT = TEAM

I wish everyone could get to know my wife Lynn as a person, and not just an SBS patient. Lynn is the woman I love and she is one of the most humorous people I have ever met. She has a supremely positive, upbeat personality, which even comes out when she is deathly ill. She is welcoming, kind and considerate to everyone she meets even when she is hospitalized. She has an indomitable will to live. And she has the ability to make me laugh out loud, even in the intensive care unit just days after a major surgery. Marital experts have taught us that relationships are formed and strengthened through shared experiences—living with SBS, Lynn and I have had the advantage of sharing an abundance of experiences.

One of Lynn's favorite performers is Lucille Ball. Lynn has spent many days laughing during *I Love Lucy* reruns. Over the years, many people have commented that Lynn's expressive eyes, fun-loving humor, and the hilarious ways she handles unexpected circumstances remind them of Lucy. So, in a way, I have been able to enjoy a life where every week there are hilarious new episodes of *I Love Lynn*!

In the past, when Lynn lived in the hospital, our lives were totally consumed by Lynn's condition. And frequently, we were frustrated at our circumstances. In stressful and difficult circumstances, it was easy to act in ways that hurt each other's feelings. In 2004, we benefitted greatly from a wonderful counselor who spent 1 hour a week with each of us for about 6 months. She changed our lives and helped us immensely. She listened and allowed us to be brutally honest, and she compassionately helped us recognize that we were both hurting. In our own way, we were each grieving the loss of a relationship and a life that we had imagined together. The reality of our circumstances was nowhere near our expectations. We were fighting the same battle, not fighting each other, but we were both fighting for the opportunity to live life, together, to the fullest. Lynn and I have had a difficult path, but we have always enjoyed each other's company and we love to laugh. We have definitely found that a positive attitude and the ability to laugh despite our circumstances have helped us to enjoy our life together, wherever we are spending time (even in a hospital).

Early on, Lynn and I did not have the benefit of SBS support groups like the Oley Foundation. We were given literature from the Oley Foundation while we were at the IRC in 2003. However, at that time, we were told that the Oley Foundation was specifically for people on TPN, and since our focus was to get Lynn off of TPN, we did not pursue it further. Although we did not benefit from formal SBS support groups, we do have great friends, who have loved us and laughed with us throughout our lives. Trial by fire has a way of sifting through friendships. Some have burned out, while others have been refined and strengthened. Through 25 years of marriage, Lynn and I have dozens of wonderful friends across the United States with whom we still keep in touch and enjoy spending time whenever we can.

Through the process of writing this chapter, Lynn and I have both mentally "relived" some very difficult times—and that is not a bad thing—it is somewhat cathartic to talk about it. This is one of the wonderful things about having true friends. Whether patient or caregiver, you need to have loyal, trustworthy friends, and you need to go and talk with them. I believe that this is what a "support group" truly is—people who are understanding, with whom you can talk openly and honestly. What we have attempted to record here is information we wish we had known in 1991. What has been emotionally difficult about this process is the overwhelming realization that if we had known then what we know today, Lynn would not have lived 11 of the first 15 years of our marriage in a hospital, connected to an IV.

This information is second nature for us now, because we have lived it, together, every day, for 26 years. However, explaining it, in detail, for someone else to understand has always been difficult, and it takes time. Too often in our experience, Lynn and I have encountered medical professionals who simply do not have time. We now have an abundance of information available, and more coming out every year. In the last 15 years, medical science has learned a tremendous amount about the digestive system. Today, we know much more about SBS, but patients with SBS patients are still relatively rare, as are clinicians who truly understand how to care for them. We have listed below some tips and articles we found most beneficial over the years. Live and learn (and learn to live)!

What helped Lynn and me the most:

- *Clear explanation* of Lynn's jejunostomy physiology, what was happening and why, along with what to expect and look for in the future.
- *Find a medical center specializing in SBS* or at least clinicians who really understand SBS and how to treat it.
- *Build a medical team* who will collaborate with the patient and caregiver.
- The Internet—Learn to use search engines to find current best SBS practices and treatments.
- *Everything* you put in your mouth has the potential to increase or diminish diarrhea.
- *Medication tips*—Remind medical team to avoid timed/controlled/sustained release medications and medications delivered in highly osmotic solutions (sorbitol).
- Articles we found helpful are the following:
  - The Clinician's Guide to Short Bowel Syndrome
    - Parrish, C.R., *Pract. Gastroenterol.*, 29, 67–106, 2005
  - Guidelines for Management of Patients with a Short Bowel
    - Nightingale, J., Woodward, J.M., *Gut*, 55, 2006
  - Emerging Treatment Options for Short Bowel Syndrome: Potential Role of Teduglutide
    - Lee, C.T. et al., *Clin. Exp. Gastroenterol.*, 4, 189–196, 2011
  - Short Bowel Syndrome: Tailoring Nutritional and Medical Interventions to Improve Outcomes
    - Iyer, K.R., *Medscape Educ. Gastroenterol.*, 2013

Note: The following articles are all available at http://www.ginutrition.virginia.edu:

- Part 1: Short Bowel Syndrome in Adults—Physiological Alterations and Clinical Consequences
  - DiBaise, J., Parrish, C.R., *Pract. Gastroenterol.*, 38, 30, 2014.
- Part II: Nutrition Therapy for Short Bowel Syndrome in the Adult Patient
  - Parrish, C.R., DiBaise, J., *Pract. Gastroenterol.*, 38, 40, 2014.
- Part III: Hydrating the Adult Patient with Short Bowel Syndrome
  - Parrish, C.R., DiBaise, J., *Pract. Gastroenterol.*, 38, 10, 2015.

- Part IV-A: A Guide to Front Line Drugs Used in the Treatment of Short Bowel Syndrome
  - Chan, L.N., DiBaise, J., Parrish, C.R., *Pract. Gastroenterol.*, 39, 28, 2015.
- Part IV-B: A Guide to Front Line Drugs Used in the Treatment of Short Bowel Syndrome
  - Chan, L.N., DiBaise, J., Parrish, C.R. *Pract. Gastroenterol.*, 39, 24, 2015.
- Part V: Trophic Agents in the Treatment of Short Bowel Syndrome
  - DiBaise, J., Parrish, C.R. *Pract. Gastroenterol.*, 39, 56, 2015.

Index

Page numbers followed by f and t indicate figures and tables, respectively.

D

W

X

Z

Printed in the United States
by Baker & Taylor Publisher Services

Printed in the United States
by Baker & Taylor Publisher Services